Guide to
NURSING
MANAGEMENT
AND LEADERSHIP

Eighth Edition

Ann Marriner Tomey, PhD, RN, FAAN
Professor Emeritus
College of Nursing, Health and Human Services
Indiana State University
Terre Haute, Indiana

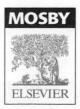

MOSBY

ELSEVIER

MOSBY
ELSEVIER

11830 Westline Industrial Drive
St. Louis, Missouri 63146

GUIDE TO NURSING MANAGEMENT AND LEADERSHIP, EIGHTH EDITION ISBN: 978-0-323-05238-2

Notice

Neither the Publisher nor the Author assume any responsibility for any loss or injury and/or damage to persons or property arising out of or related to any use of the material contained in this book. It is the responsibility of the treating practitioner, relying on independent expertise and knowledge of the patient, to determine the best treatment and method of application for the patient.

The Publisher

Previous editions copyrighted 2004, 2000, 1996, 1992, 1988, 1984, and 1980

Library of Congress Control Number: 2007942088

Acquisitions Editor: Yvonne Alexopoulos
Developmental Editor: Heather Bays
Publishing Services Manager: Jeff Patterson
Project Manager: Clay S. Broeker
Design Direction: Kim Denando

Printed in Canada

Last digit is the print number: 9 8 7 6 5 4 3 2 1

I want to thank my loving husband, H. Keith Tomey, for enriching my private life while supporting my professional activities and for helping me maintain balance. I'd also like to thank the students who stimulate my thinking.

REVIEWERS

Cathy Hoots Abell, MSN, RN
Assistant Professor
Department of Nursing
Western Kentucky University
Bowling Green, Kentucky

Martha Raile Alligood, BSL, BSN, MS, PhD, RN
Professor and Director
PhD Program in Nursing
School of Nursing at East Carolina University
Greenville, North Carolina

Kathleen Bobay, PhD, RN, BC
Assistant Professor
Marquette University
Milwaukee, Wisconsin

Judith Bonaduce, RN, MSN, BC
Assistant Professor
Center for Nursing Advocacy
Bryn Mawr, Pennsylvania

Valerie Brown-Krimsley, EdD
Director
Nursing Program
Brevard Community College
Cocoa, Florida

Ann Cook, RN, PhD
Professor
Columbia College of Nursing
Milwaukee, Wisconsin

Patricia Crane, PhD, RN, FAHA
Associate Professor
Adult Health Department
School of Nursing
University of North Carolina
Greensboro, North Carolina

Katherine Dimmock, JD, EdD, MSN, RN
Dean and Professor
Columbia College of Nursing
Milwaukee, Wisconsin

Susan Fox, PhD, RN, CNAA, BC
Senior Associate Dean for Community Partnership
   and Practice
College of Nursing
University of New Mexico
Rio Rancho, New Mexico

Mary Fuhrman, MSN, RN
Assistant Professor of Nursing
Clarke College
Dubuque, Iowa

Nancy Grove, RN, BSN, MEd, MSN, PhD
Director and Associate Professor
Nursing Program
University of Pittsburgh
Johnstown, Pennsylvania

Sharron Guillett, RN, PhD
Associate Professor and Chair
BSN Program
Marymount University
Arlington, Virginia

Ruth Hansten, RN, BSN, MBA, PhD, FACHE
Principal Consultant
Hansten Healthcare PLLC
Port Ludlow, Washington;
Adjunct Faculty
School of Nursing
University of Washington
Seattle, Washington

Patricia Horstman, RN, MSN, CNAA, BC
Director
Clinical Program Development
West Virginia University Hospital
Morgantown, West Virginia

Brenda Hosley, RN, PhD
Associate Professor
Department of Baccalaureate and Graduate
   Nursing
Eastern Kentucky University
Richmond, Kentucky

Suzy Lockwood, RN, MSN, PhD
Assistant Professor
Harris College of Nursing and
   Health Science
Texas Christian University
Fort Worth, Texas

DeAnne Parrott, RN, MEd, MS, CNE
Clinical Instructor
Kramer School of Nursing
Oklahoma City University
Oklahoma City, Oklahoma

Carol Reineck, PhD, CNAA-BC, COI
Associate Professor
Amy Shelton and V.H. McNutt Professorship
   in Nursing
University of Texas
San Antonio, Texas

Barbara Russo, MSN, RN
Clinical Faculty
School of Nursing
Indiana University
Bloomington, Indiana

Jean Ann Seago, PhD, RN
Associate Professor
University of California
San Francisco, California

Melissa Sherrod, RN, PhD
Assistant Professor
Harris College of Nursing
Texas Christian University
Fort Worth, Texas

Christina Leibold Sieloff, PhD, RN, CAN, BC
Associate Professor
College of Nursing
Montana State University
Bozeman, Montana

Joyce Simones, RN, EdD
Associate Professor
Department of Nursing Science
St. Cloud State University
St. Cloud, Minnesota

Janet K. Pringle Specht, PhD, RN, FAAN
Associate Professor and Practice Director
John A. Hartford Center for Geriatric Nursing
   Excellence
University of Iowa
Iowa City, Iowa

Jaynelle Stichler, DNSc, RNc
Associate Professor and Concentration Chair
Nursing Systems Administration
San Diego State University
San Diego, California

Dori Sullivan, PhD, RN, CAN, CPHQ
Department of Nursing Chair and Director
   of Interdisciplinary Studies
College of Education and Health Professions
Sacred Heart University
Fairfield, Connecticut

Marla Weston, PhD, RN
Weston Healthcare Consulting
Phoenix, Arizona

Elizabeth Woodard, RN, PhD
Research and Practice Consultant
New Hanover Regional Medical Center
Wilmington, North Carolina

PREFACE

Guide to Nursing Management and Leadership is designed to teach both undergraduate and graduate nursing students about the management process and leadership and to supply the practicing nurse with useful information about nursing administration. It can serve both as a textbook and as a reference and it presents theories as well as processes. The eighth edition of this text continues to provide a historical perspective to the evolution of leadership and management while also addressing the issues that influence this dynamic and evolving field.

BACKGROUND AND ORGANIZATION

The first edition was written during the 1970s, when nursing education emphasized clinical skills at the expense of managerial expertise and nurses who were interested in leadership and management had to turn to other disciplines. Now there are many books and journals about nursing leadership and management. The first edition, *Guide to Nursing Management,* was organized around the management process, which was then introduced to the nursing literature. The conceptual framework of the first edition was plan, organize, staff, direct, and control.

The rapid changes during the 1980s, with the increase in better-educated personnel and increased technology to handle management functions, brought about a focus on leadership, which was reflected with the fifth edition of *Guide to Nursing Management and Leadership* in 1996.

Continuous quality improvement, cost containment, free market competition, managed care, technology, increasing diversity, more focus on ethical issues, and the need for teams and transformational leadership were dominant during the 1990s, requiring a major transformation of the book for 2000. This sixth edition was divided into two major sections: leadership and management. The leadership section contained chapters about communications; stress management;

decision-making process and tools; motivation and morale; power, politics, and labor relations; conflict management and negotiations; and theories of leadership. The management section contained chapters about strategic and operational planning; financial management, cost containment, and marketing; organizational concepts and structures; organizational culture and change; selection and development of personnel, staffing and scheduling; evaluation and discipline of personnel; and continuous quality improvement, program evaluation and risk management. The content was refocused to differentiate leadership from management.

For the seventh edition in 2004, ethics, diversity, technology, and legal issues were integrated into several chapters. Protection from workplace violence, bioterrorism, sources and categories of law, continuum of multiorganizational arrangements, disease management, demand management, private management companies, cultural imposition and imperialism, generational differences, character development, the Health Insurance Portability and Accountability Act (HIPAA), employment-at-will, COBRA, and liability issues were added. Age, culture, and gender diversity; delegation; decision-making models; creativity techniques; ethics; emotional intelligence; politics; negotiation; mediation; arbitration; leadership; budgeting; variance reporting; recruitment and retention; staffing; and continuum of care were expanded. New features, such as Research Perspective boxes, were included to illustrate the findings of current research in the leadership and management field. The seventh edition also saw the addition of the Evolve website, providing course management software to teachers.

In this eighth edition, ethics, diversity, technology, and legal issue coverage has been updated and expanded and continues to be integrated into several chapters. Delegating, stress management, decision-making tools, research, evidence-based practice, and critical thinking coverage has also been expanded. Leadership and management roles are identified. There are also new introductions to the leadership and management sections and chapter summaries.

AUDIENCE

Both undergraduate and graduate students learning about leadership and management, as well as practicing leaders and managers, will benefit from this book. This book can serve as both a textbook and a reference for students and practicing leaders. Much of the content is useful for dealing with personal as well as professional issues.

FEATURES

- **A logical organization of 15 chapters,** separated into leadership and management parts, simulates the 15 weeks in a typical semester.
- A **brief overview** and **detailed listing of objectives** begins each chapter, communicating to students a clear purpose for each topic and offering guidelines for examination preparation.
- A **Major Concepts and Definitions** box outlines and summarizes the most significant ideas in that area of leadership or management and clarifies content-specific vocabulary.
- One or more **Research Perspective** boxes in each chapter summarize timely key studies, using a consistent format to outline the purpose, methods, and results and conclusions of each study and introduce the students to the expanding body of literature in nursing management.
- An online study guide contains **Practice Worksheets, Critical Thinking Activities,** and **Case Studies** that focus on realistic situations and application-oriented situations to help ensure content mastery.
- **Colorful quotations** interspersed throughout each chapter help place complex theories and issues into everyday contexts and provide food for further thought and analysis on various topics.

NEW TO THIS EDITION

- **Online instructor resources,** including a Test Bank, PowerPoint Presentations, and an Instructor's Manual with Chapter Overviews, Chapter Summaries, Chapter Objectives, Concepts and Definitions, and References, provide a wealth of information and tools for both the new and the experienced leadership and management instructor to enhance learning both inside and outside the classroom.
- **Expanded online student resources** include new self-assessment questions for quick study outside of the classroom and revised case studies and critical thinking activities to stimulate further discussion.
- **Updated two-color design** has been incorporated for increased visual appeal.
- **Tables, boxes, and illustrations** help synthesize and streamline complex issues and theories with easy-to-comprehend visual learning tools for students.
- **Information on succession planning** is provided, related to how the process can move beyond simply replacing positions to identifying and nurturing a pool of potential candidates for leadership positions to create a better future in the midst of a nursing shortage and a newly emerging multigenerational structure.
- **Emphasis on online resources and references** reflects modern-day teaching and learning styles, both of which rely heavily on the Internet for information and analysis.

ANCILLARIES

For the Teacher

- A test bank includes approximately 350 multiple-choice, NCLEX-style examination questions.
- PowerPoint lecture presentations feature approximately 25 slides per chapter to guide classroom lecture.
- Chapter Overviews, a Chapter Summary/Outline, Chapter Objectives, Concepts and Definitions, and References highlight the critical information found in the text.

For the Student

- Case Studies, Critical Thinking Activities, and Practice Worksheets provide students with an online study guide that focuses on critical analysis and application.
- Advanced organizers consisting of multiple-choice questions and discussion questions are used to sensitize the reader to important content and to guide study.
- Weblinks supply continuously-updated links to key sites for nursing management and leadership.

CONTENTS

PART
ONE

LEADERSHIP

Leadership is the inspiration for desired responses and getting work done through others. Leaders focus on purpose and doing the right thing. They are future oriented, challenged by change, and able to plan strategies and facilitate human potential. Leaders need good stress and time management to meet the challenges of leadership. They need to use good communication and decision-making skills. Leaders need to use their knowledge of power and politics to motivate people to act and to manage conflict. Knowledge of leadership theories helps leaders know how to adjust their leadership style to fit different situations. Leaders focus on doing the right things but may also be managers who help do things the right way.

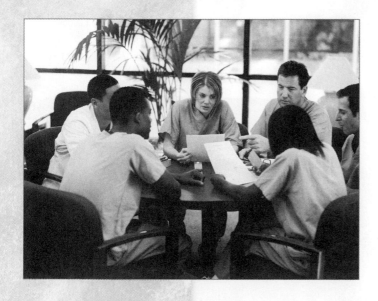

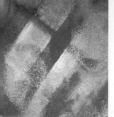

Communications

"He who influences the thought of his times influences the times that follow." —Elbert Hubbard

Chapter Overview

Chapter 1 describes the communication process, informational technology, communication systems, barriers to communications, gender differences, cultural differences, ways to improve communications, communicating with difficult people, assertiveness, transactional analysis, and life positions.

Chapter Objectives

- Describe the six steps in the communication process.
- Outline basic communication skills.
- Identify at least two issues related to the use of technology.
- Illustrate at least four communication systems.
- Summarize at least six barriers to communication.
- Formulate at least three ways to improve communication.
- Describe at least two ways to deal with hostile-aggressive people.
- Plan at least two strategies for dealing with a sniper.
- Describe at least two ways to handle complainers.
- Compare strategies for working with negative, unresponsive, and superagreeable people.
- Identify at least two barriers to assertiveness.
- Diagram complementary transactions.
- Analyze crossed transactions.
- Describe three games people play.
- Compare the four life positions.
- Differentiate how to use at least three assertive techniques.

Online Resources

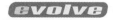

Critical thinking activities, worksheets, and case studies are available online at http://evolve.elsevier.com/Marriner/guide8e.

Major Concepts and Definitions

Communication *giving and receiving information via talk, gestures, writing, and so forth*
Ideation *decision to share an idea*
Encoding *putting meaning into symbols*
Transmission *sending the message*
Receiving *seeing and hearing a transmitted message*
Decoding *defining words and interpreting gestures*
Feedback *an evaluative response*
Grapevine *informal communication system*
Informal communications *casual, not according to prescribed ways*
Formal communications *according to prescribed rules*
Verbal *spoken*
Nonverbal *not spoken; space, appearance, body language, facial expressions, eye contact, posture, gestures, attentive silence, timing, pauses*
Assertiveness *the quality of being confident in stating one's opinions or needs*
Transactional analysis *a technique for analyzing discussions*
Life positions *an individual's assumptions about self in relation to others*
Passive *inactive, acted on*
Aggressive *active, bold, pushy*
Broken record *a technique involving repeating what one wants*
Fogging *agreeing with the truth*
Negative assertion *accepting negative aspects about oneself*
Negative inquiry *asking for more information about oneself*

COMMUNICATION PROCESS

All the leader's and manager's functions involve communications as both receivers and senders. The communication process involves six steps:

Ideation → Encoding → Transmission ⌐
⌐ Response ← Decoding ← Receiving ◄┘
└► Encoding → Transmission → Receiving ⌐
Response ← Decoding ◄┘

The first step, ideation, begins when the sender decides to share the content of a message with someone, senses a need to communicate, develops an idea, or selects information to share. The purpose of communication may be to inform, persuade, command, inquire, or entertain. Whatever the reason, the sender needs to have a goal and think clearly or the message may be garbled and meaningless.

Encoding, the second step, involves putting meaning into symbolic forms: speaking, writing, or nonverbal behavior. One's personal, cultural, and professional biases affect the goals and encoding process. Use of clearly understood symbols and communication of all the information that the receiver needs to know are important.

The third step, transmission of the message, must overcome interference such as garbled speech; unintelligible use of words; long, complex sentences; distortion from recording devices; noise; and illegible handwriting.

Receiving is next. The receiver's senses of seeing and hearing are activated as the transmitted message is received. People tend to have selective attention (hear the messages of interest to them but not others) and selective perception (hear the parts of the message that conform to what they want to hear), which cause incomplete and distorted interpretation of the communication.

Sometimes people tune out the message because they anticipate the content and think they know what is going to be said, or they are so busy formulating their response that they do not hear the message. The receiver may be preoccupied with other activities and consequently not be ready to listen. Poor listening is one of the biggest barriers in the communication process.

Decoding of the message by the receiver is the critical fifth step. The receiver defines words and interprets gestures during the transmission of speech. Written messages allow more time for decoding, thereby allowing receivers to assess the explicit meaning and implications of the message based on what the symbols mean to them. The symbols are subject to interpretation based on one's personal, cultural, and professional biases and may not have the same meaning to the receiver as to the sender. The communication process depends on the receiver's understanding of the information.

Response, or feedback, is the sixth and final step. It is important for the manager or sender to know that the message has been received and accurately interpreted (Rigolosi, 2005).

BASIC COMMUNICATION SKILLS

"The real art of communication is not only to say the right thing at the right place but to leave unsaid the wrong thing at the tempting moment." —Dorothy Nevill

One can *ensure understanding* by *assuming value, clarifying,* and *confirming,* and can then *enhance the value* by *identifying the merits, building* on the expressed ideas, and *balancing* the merits and concerns. One should *support* by expressing appreciation and being specific (Advanced Executive Leadership Skills, 1981). Both the sender and receiver should do this process, but the leader needs to be the role model (Box 1-1).

Ensuring understanding is facilitated by *assuming value, clarifying,* and *confirming. Assuming value* is an attitude that the person is worth listening to, which opens lines of communication so one can

---

> **BOX 1-1** Communication Skills
>
> **ENSURE UNDERSTANDING**
> Assume value
> Clarify
> Confirm
>
> **ENHANCE VALUE**
> Identify merits
> Build on ideas
> Balance merits and concerns
> Support

---

understand what the other person thinks and feels. It helps one understand what the other person is saying and why, and increases the chances that the other person will listen in return. *Clarification* is used when one is not sure what the other person is saying by asking a specific question such as "What do you mean when you say . . .," by making a statement such as "I don't understand what you mean," or by expressing open-ended interest by comments such as "and then?" *Confirmation* is used when one thinks there is understanding about what was said and why by checking for understanding and confirmation from the other person that one's understanding is accurate. Repeating what was said indicates one heard what was said but does not necessarily mean one understood. Saying "I understand what you said" indicates one thinks one understands what the other person said, but one's understanding may not be the same as the speaker's. Stating one's understanding of what the speaker said and why is a more accurate way of confirming.

Enhancing value differs from criticism by *identifying the merits, building,* and *balancing* instead of rejecting the other's ideas and actions. One often criticizes by telling others what one does not like about the other person's ideas, what is wrong, and what will not work. That leads to demoralization, defensiveness, and oppressed innovation. Refraining from criticizing may be more effective to enhance value.

To *enhance value, identify the merits* mentally and ask if the idea or action can be improved without mentioning concerns. If yes, *build* by specifying the merits verbally and adding value as a result of this building. A merit is anything one likes about what the other person said or did, or what one wants the person to keep doing despite the need for change. A merit may be a part of an idea, a good intention, an important issue that was addressed, or part of an action. If one has difficulty identifying merits, one can ensure understanding by asking people the value of their idea or act. Most people have good intentions. One can often enhance value by specifying the merits and suggesting slight refinements or changes to reach the goal without mentioning one's concerns. If a merit can be used as an example of what the leader wants, the change one suggests is an alternative to reaching the goal. If the person is not strongly committed to the previous idea or act, one can build by suggesting a minor change or refinement. Specify the merits verbally, add value by suggesting a refinement, and check back to confirm that the other person thinks that action is acceptable (e.g., "You wrote a good complete sentence here. Could you do that in other places where you have used phrases?").

However, if the person asks the leader for an evaluation or needs to know what is wrong to be able to make necessary changes, or if the situation requires a major change, one needs to *balance*. The leader should specify the merits and concerns, ask for suggestions or reactions, and check back. The leader then invites suggestions after identifying the merits and concerns to get the person involved in finding a solution, to get commitment to the leader's own ideas, and to get the other person's ideas instead of a confirmation of the leader's ideas. The leader does not invite suggestions unless those ideas will be considered for use or if the leader thinks the person needs to know one's ideas for the discussion. After the leader has invited and received suggestions, he or she gives reaction, confirms or clarifies, gives another itemized response, and asks for the other person's response.

Supporting promotes cooperation by giving timely and specific feedback about the positive aspects of another's ideas or efforts, and by acknowledging the value of the other's contributions. Most people need recognition for their efforts and accomplishments. There is a direct relationship between support given and cooperation. Less time is wasted if others know what is important to you. However, there are several reasons people are reluctant to support others. Some fear being perceived as weak or insecure, do not see a connection between giving and receiving, or fear generalization for a specific accomplishment to other situations. Giving support is appropriate when someone shows the first signs of improvement or meets minimum requirements not usually met, meets the basic requirements, or exceeds minimum requirements. Give support by expressing appreciation. Be specific in order to provide recognition, prevent others from misunderstanding one's intent, prevent others from thinking one likes everything, make the support believable, and let others know one pays attention to what others are doing. By mentioning personal qualities, one reinforces those qualities and earns goodwill and support. By mentioning how others' accomplishments are important, one helps others realize that their efforts make a difference and are valued, makes them feel more important, and increases their desire to continue contributing (Advanced Executive Leadership Skills, 1981).

COMMUNICATION PRINCIPLES

De Ann Gillies (1994, p. 187) identifies some communication principles. The effectiveness of various media differs with educational level, with less educated people relying more on aural and pictorial media and more educated people relying more on print. People with low self-esteem are more easily influenced by persuasive communications than are people with high self-esteem. People are more likely to hear messages that are compatible with their expectations and are more likely to listen to messages on topics about which they have read. The more trustworthy the speaker, the less manipulative the speaker is perceived to be. Majority opinion is more effective in changing attitudes than expert opinion.

METHODS OF COMMUNICATION

Whetten and Cameron (2004) present a "five s's" approach to effective oral and written presentations: *strategy, structure, support, style,* and *supplement.* The strategy develops the purpose for the specific audience and occasion. The structure translates the strategy into specific content. Examples and illustrations are used to support or reinforce ideas. Style, or the way ideas are presented, is as important as the ideas expressed. Supplement means to give informed responses to challenges and questions related to the presentation.

Strategy involves identifying the general and specific purposes of the presentation, understanding the needs and attitudes of the audience, and designing the message for the audience. Speech should be audience centered. More formal situations call for more formal presentations, whereas informal situations allow for slang. Both sides of issues should be presented if the audience is uncommitted or hostile.

Structure begins with a forecast of the main ideas to capture audience members' attention and give them a reason to listen or read. It gives the audience an outline of the message, making it easier for audience members to follow the presentation. Simple to complex, familiar to unfamiliar, and old to new are some ways to structure a presentation. Only a few main points should be made, transitions should be made among main points, and the presentation should end on a high note, calling for action or creating a good feeling.

Support from evidence and visual aids helps establish credibility. It is advisable to use a variety of supports and to keep visual aids simple and effective to aid comprehension and retention.

Style for oral communications involves preparing notes; practicing the presentation with the visual aids; and planning to engage the audience through use of eye contact, physical space, and body movement. Style for written communications involves mechanical and factual precision. Tone is related to word choice and should be adjusted to the formality of the situation. The proper format for the business letter, memo, proposal, or paper should be used.

Supplement the presentation by responding to challenges and questions by being prepared to answer questions in a specific format. First restate the objection, then state one's position. Offer support for one's position, and speak to the impact of adopting one's position.

INFORMATION TECHNOLOGY

Word processing is commonly used and allows electronic writing, revising, storing, and printing of documents. *Spreadsheet software* allows manipulation of information in columns and rows as in accounting, and allows writing, editing, graphing, storing, and printing of the data. *Database software* collects and catalogs information so that a large amount of well-organized data can be located and displayed. *Graphic software* allows use of clip art, icons, silhouettes, and line drawings to enhance written communications, whereas *presentation software* creates visual aids such as overheads and slides for oral presentations. *Electronic mail (e-mail)* allows users to send messages instantaneously using one-on-one interchanges, or it can connect staff throughout an organization at one or many sites. It can get information, including graphics and sound, to listservs and newsgroups. *Voice mail* answers the telephone automatically, plays a message, and accepts and stores voice messages. *Calendar and scheduling software* in conjunction with e-mail allows networked users to access each other's schedules. The software can identify common free time and allow one to immediately book a meeting. *Chat rooms* can be used for exchange of written messages in real time without having to find a physical location for a meeting. Much committee work can be done asynchronously through e-mail. The *World Wide Web* links computers around the world and is a major source of information (Roussel, Swansburg, & Swansburg, 2006). *Cell phones* can be used for text messaging. *Videoconferencing* can be used for live interaction. There is an initial start-up equipment cost and need to train staff, but videoconferencing can cut costs and travel time. *Web pages* are increasingly common and are used by organizations to communicate to not only the staff, patients, and their families, but also to health care providers and the public in general (Finkelman, 2006).

Handheld computers decentralize information to the point of care (Thompson, 2005). The use of standardized nursing languages becomes important for the use of electronic health care records to reduce differing terminology and increase understanding between separate data entries (Lunney, 2006). *Computerized order entry* can reduce medication errors (Jones & Moss, 2006). Participating nurses reported that online assignment sheets "saved time, energy, promoted teamwork throughout the hospital, and reduced the potential for errors" (Kalisch, Myer, Mackey, et al, 2006, p. 51).

Telehealth can be particularly helpful in home care and hospice care as it enables communication between the patients and the health care providers who are separated by geographic distances. Peck (2005, p. 339) reported that "Through telenursing a nurse can provide monitoring, education, follow-up, remote data collection, remote interventions, pain management, family support, and multidisciplinary care. . . ."

Ethics about how to use but not abuse the power of the aforementioned technology related to privacy, confidentiality, informed consent, and equity of access are important (Demiris, Oliver, & Courtney, 2006). Ethics involves making a value choice for doing the right thing. Curtain (2005, p. 350) identified what distinguishes an ethical choice from another choice: "Ethical choices share certain characteristics: (1) they always involve fundamental value conflicts; (2) because the choice involves fundamental values (matters of utmost importance) rather than facts (proven truth), scientific inquiry may influence the choice, but cannot provide answers; and (3) because these choices involve the placing of one value above another, and because by definition values are of the utmost importance, any decision reached will have profound, multiple, and often unanticipated impact on many areas of human concern."

Health care providers have a professional, legal, and ethical obligation to protect patient information. Confidentiality, by disseminating information only to authorized individuals or organizations that have a need to know, is a major issue. Most confidentiality violations involve fired workers or other insiders motivated by blackmail, curiosity, humiliation, or revenge. Breaches of confidentiality may also be unintentional disclosures, uncontrolled secondary usage such as for marketing, and unauthorized access such as use of another's password (Saba & McCormick, 2001). Telehealth also raises issues of confidentiality and

---

 RESEARCH Perspective 1-1

Data from Alexander JW, Kroposki M: Using a management perspective to define and measure changes in nursing technology, *Journal of Advanced Nursing* 35(5):776-783, 2005.

Purpose: The purpose of this study was to discuss the uses of the concept of technology from the management and medical science perspectives; to prepare a definition of nursing technology; and to present a study applying the use of the concept of nursing technology on nursing units.

Methods: A longitudinal study was done to measure the dimensions of nursing technology on nursing units 10 years apart. The 1980 and 1990 mean scores on the technology

dimensions for all the units were compared using t-tests. Of the 14 units used in both tests, four had significant changes in one or more of the technology dimensions. The four were a medical unit, two surgical units, and a labor and delivery unit.

Results/conclusions: The findings suggest that the dimensions of nursing technology change over time and support the need for nurse managers to assess nursing technology periodically before making changes on the unit.

reimbursement of health services across state lines and quality of care. Major challenges are keeping costs down while maintaining quality of care and privacy and confidentiality of data (Ball, Hannah, Newbold, et al, 2000).

COMMUNICATION SYSTEMS

Study of small-group process has revealed various communication networks (Box 1-2; Figure 1-1). The chain system is fast and accurate for simple problems. The middle person in the chain emerges as the leader, and the leadership position is stable. Unfortunately, morale is low, and so is the flexibility for problem solving.

In the Y, wheel, and circle communication systems, the leader emerges at the location of highest centrality, which is the fork of the Y, the

hub of the wheel, and the center of the chain; this provides fast, accurate problem solving. The coordinator, who is centrally located, is generally satisfied, but the peripheral members are less satisfied than members in less efficient systems. The wheel is an efficient, effective communication structure for simple problems.

The circular structure is slow and inaccurate. The structure does not influence the emergence of a leader. Because no one can communicate with everyone, there is no coordinator. However, morale is high, and there is considerable flexibility for problem solving (Borgatti, 1997).

Greater amounts of information must be processed as task uncertainty and complexity increase. Consequently, an adaptive structure such as the all-channel system is best for completing complicated and unpredictable tasks. When free to do so, groups tend to evolve to the all-channel network as problems become complex and shift back to a wheel structure as problems become simple. The right network is essentially the structure that facilitates the communication necessary to accomplish the task.

Downward Communication

The traditional line of communication is from the manager down through the levels of management (Figure 1-2). This downward communication is primarily directive and helps coordinate

---

BOX 1-2 Communication Systems

Chain
Y
Wheel
Circle
All-channel
Downward
Upward
Diagonal
Grapevine

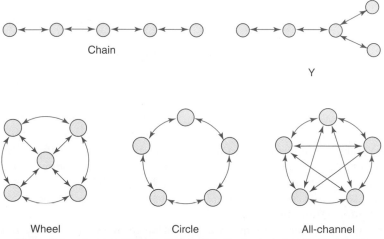

Chain

Y

Wheel   Circle   All-channel

Figure 1-1 • Communication systems: chain, Y, wheel, circle, and all-channel.

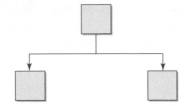

Figure 1-2 • Downward communication.

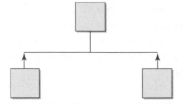

Figure 1-3 • Upward communication.

the activities of different levels of the hierarchy by telling staff associates what to do, and by providing the information needed by staff associates to relate their efforts to the organization's goals. It includes oral and written indoctrination, education, and other information to influence the attitudes and behaviors of staff associates. Common forms of downward communications are employee handbooks, operating manuals, job description sheets, performance appraisal interviews, employee counseling, loudspeaker systems, letters, memos, messages circulated with paychecks, posters, bulletin boards, information racks, company newspapers, annual reports, the chain of command, the grapevine, and unions. Downward communication contributes to greater staff member dissatisfaction than upward communication, regardless of the quality of the message (Sullivan & Decker, 2005; The Times 100, 2005).

Upward Communication

Newer management techniques encourage delegation of authority and more personal involvement in decision making, thus creating a need for accurate upward communication (Figure 1-3). Upward communication provides a means for motivating and satisfying personnel by allowing employee input. The manager summarizes information and passes it upward to the next level for use in decision making. That level then summarizes its action and transmits information to the next level. Because each level tends to bias the report by embellishing it with information that puts that level in the best light, there is a natural filtering process as information moves upward. By the time it reaches top management, it is highly refined.

In spite of this bias, staffs are often in a position to assess the situation more accurately than are their managers. An employee may have a better solution to a problem than the first-line manager, who may know more about a situation than a middle manager, and so on. Therefore, accurate upward communication is important for effective problem solving. Staff associates must feel free to communicate both solicited and unsolicited information upwardly and must have opportunity to do so, or management will lack needed information and both managers and staff will become frustrated. Upward communications are appropriate for work-related problems, and for expressing feelings, ideas, aspirations, attitudes, suggestions, and grievances. Common means for upward communication include face-to-face discussions; open-door policies; staff meetings; task forces; written reports; performance appraisals; grievance procedures; exit interviews; attitude surveys; suggestion boxes; counseling; the chain of command; ombudsmen; informers; the grapevine; unions; and participative, consultative, and democratic management in general (Quible, 2004; Sullivan & Decker, 2005).

Lateral Communication

Lateral, or horizontal, communication is between departments or personnel on the same level of the hierarchy and is most frequently used to coordinate activities (Figure 1-4). It is also used for face-to-face conversations, small-group meetings, problem solving, socialization, and electronic communications. The need for lateral communication increases as interdependence increases. For instance, it becomes more important when one worker starts a job and someone else finishes it.

It is also used by staff to transmit technical information to line authorities, and it may contain subjective and emotional aspects. Committees, conferences, and meetings are often used to facilitate horizontal communication (Kalisch, Myer, Mackey, et al, 2006; Sullivan & Decker, 2005).

Diagonal Communication

Diagonal communication occurs between individuals or departments that are not on the same level of the hierarchy (Figure 1-5). Informal in nature and frequently used between staff groups and line functions, and in project types of organizations, it is another facet of multidirectional communication that is common when communications flow in all directions at the same time. Diagonal communications allow individuals with diverse information to participate in problem solving with people from other levels in the organization. That informal communication system allows leaders and managers to monitor employee communications and to communicate with associates quickly, without going through a cumbersome, official communication system (Kotelnikov, 2007; Sullivan & Decker, 2005).

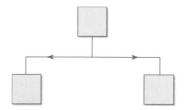

Figure 1-4 • Lateral communication.

The Grapevine: Informal Communication

Informal methods of communication coexist with formal channels and are referred to as the grapevine. Informal communications can move in all directions: within and outside of chains of command; between leaders, managers, and associates; and possibly within and outside of the organization. Informal communication is often rapid and subject to considerable distortion. The grapevine transmits information much faster than formal channels because it uses cluster chain pathways involving three or four individuals at a time, instead of going from one person to another, as in manager–staff member relationships. Information passes at an increasing rate as individuals from clusters inform other small groups of people who work nearby or with whom they have contact. Information spreads most quickly through the grapevine when it is recent, affects personnel's work (e.g., pay increases or changes in policies), and involves people they know. People who work near each other or come in contact with each other are likely to be on the same grapevine. In addition to clusters, rumors can be passed as a single strand from one person to another and from that person to another, and so on, or as gossip when one person tells many people.

Information becomes distorted for a number of reasons. Grapevine information is often fragmentary and incomplete. Because of this, there is a tendency to try to supply the missing pieces. Some people seize this opportunity to express

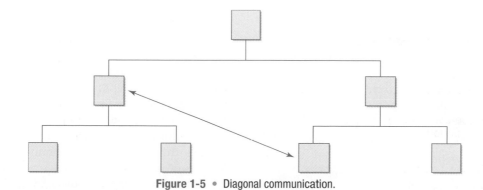

Figure 1-5 • Diagonal communication.

feelings of self-importance, thus compensating for feelings of insecurity but also distorting the message. Because the grapevine is informal, with no formal lines of accountability, individuals do not have to answer to their manager for misinforming others. Managers can learn much by listening to the grapevine and can remedy distortions by using the informal channels to pass on correct information (Borkowski, 2005).

BARRIERS TO COMMUNICATION

"No man has a good enough memory to be a successful liar."
—*Abraham Lincoln*

Thomas Gilovich (1991) indicates that misperception and misinterpretation of random data, misinterpretation of incomplete and unrepresentative data, biased evaluation of ambiguous and inconsistent data, seeing what we want to see, believing what we are told, and imagined agreement of others are *How We Know What Isn't So* (Box 1-3).

Common physical barriers to good communications are deafness, noisy environments, speech difficulties, poor eyesight, and poor cognitive abilities. Emotional barriers are aggression, fear perceptions, prejudices, and threats. Faulty reasoning and poorly expressed messages are major barriers to communication. Lack of clarity and precision resulting from inadequate vocabulary, poorly chosen words, platitudes, jargon, awkward sentence structures, poor organization of ideas, and

---

BOX 1-3 Barriers to Communication

Misperceptions
Misinterpretations
Faulty reasoning
Selective perception
False assumptions
Status
Gender differences
Cultural differences

---

lack of coherence are common. Talking too quickly or too slowly, slurring words, and not emphasizing important points lead to the faulty transmission of ideas. Arguing, blaming, interrupting, name calling, and threatening create psychological barriers and such things as beliefs, values, prejudices, jealousies, and fears can create personal barriers. Memos that are poorly organized, ramble, and lack summaries also complicate the communication process. Words mean different things to different people. Communication is complicated when the sender uses words with which the receiver is not familiar, does not communicate on the receiver's level, or makes the message long and complicated (McConnell, 2006).

If senders lack information or omit known information, they will pass on a distorted or filtered message. Filtering, whether intentional or unintentional, involves a biased choice of what is communicated. For instance, distortion is more likely when subordinates desire promotion, since they may pass on information about their merits and suppress less successful aspects of their work. Fear of the consequences of full disclosure contributes to such omissions. At other times individuals may not communicate some information because they do not believe it is important enough to do so. The receiver becomes confused when nonverbal cues such as facial expressions and posture conflict with the verbal communication, or when the sender does not admit to the intent of, or to the emotions underlying, the message.

People unconsciously use selective perception to hear what they want to hear in terms of their biases. Values, attitudes, and assumptions affect one's perception of the message. Making a value judgment about the worth of a message based on one's opinion of the sender or the expected meaning of the message allows the receiver to hear what one wants to hear. An attitude is a feeling toward someone or something that is based on experience or the lack thereof, and it is a common barrier to communication because of its screening effect (Maguire, 2002).

Uncommunicated assumptions are common and can make a considerable difference between the message sent and the one received. For instance, when program evaluation is mandated, personnel may fear that the results will be used to terminate workers, whereas management's actual intention is to use the results for recruiting purposes. Trust or distrust of the sender also influences how the message is received.

The sender is judged along with the message because the receiver has difficulty separating what one hears from how one feels about the sender. In fact, nonexistent motives can be attributed to the sender. Messages from higher echelons are often considered authoritative, even when they are not intended to be. The higher in the hierarchy a message originates, the greater are its chances of being accepted because of the status of the sender. If the sender has status with the listener, the message is usually considered credible. If the sender does not, the message may be discounted.

Staffs tend to pay attention to communications from managers, thus facilitating downward communication. Unfortunately, managers may give verbal and nonverbal cues about how busy and unapproachable they are. They may value communications from higher-level managers more than those from staff and may not reward staff for communications. In fact, staff is sometimes punished for communicating. Therefore, staff will be reluctant to report problems or potential problems when they believe these will be viewed as a weakness in their performance appraisal. Similarly, middle managers may not report problems that would reflect unfavorably on their managerial skills.

Status symbols indicate social and economic prestige and represent power. Such status symbols as titles; belonging to elite groups like management; name recognition; and a personal office magnify role and status barriers by increasing the psychological distance and the perceived organizational distance. Time pressures also become barriers that prevent communication. Managers do not have

time to see all their staff members as much as desired, and staff associates may not take the time to report to the manager. Time pressures are also used as an excuse for not listening. Premature evaluation of what is going to be said, preoccupation with oneself, lack of readiness to hear, lack of receptivity to new ideas, and resistance to change interfere with listening. Physical distance, organizational complexity, temperature, noise, physical facilities (such as offices, meeting rooms, and an informal coffee shop), and technical facilities (such as telephones, loudspeakers, and duplicating equipment) also affect communications (Marquis & Huston, 2006).

Gender Differences

Tannen (2001) indicates that women talk about their problems at length, whereas men want to find a solution or laugh the problems off. Women do rapport-talk, whereas men do report-talk. Women tend to be more talkative than men, initiate turn taking, make more frequent interruptions of others' comments, ask most of the questions, keep the conversations going, and use a larger vocabulary.

Gray (1992) indicated that men want to reason, whereas women want to be heard and validated. When stressed, men tend to become focused and withdrawn, whereas women tend to become emotionally involved and overwhelmed. Women have difficulty supporting a man who is not talking, whereas men have difficulty listening to women without giving advice.

Four stylistic modes of verbal communication between genders have been identified as follows (DeYoung, 2003):

1. Direct versus indirect style with males characterized as relatively direct, open, straightforward, and honest, and females characterized as relatively indirect, ambiguous, tactful, and face saving
2. Succinct versus elaborative style with males characterized as succinct and using elliptical sentences ("great movie"), whereas females are more elaborative and use metaphors, similes, and flowery expressions

3. Personal versus contextual style with males using the role-centered contextual style, and females using the personal style stressing equality
4. Instrumental or technical versus affective style with males using instrumental style with reference to quality, and females using affective style focusing on people's emotions

Cultural Differences

"There are hundreds of languages in the world, but a smile speaks all of them." —*Anonymous*

Culture is a learned pattern of beliefs, customs, language, norms, and values that is shared by a group of people. How that learned pattern of behavior is expressed distinguishes cultures from each other. Cross-cultural communication involves having respect for, tolerance of, and nonjudgmental attitudes toward people with different attitudes, behaviors, and values; obtaining knowledge of other cultures; and being sensitive to cultural differences. One should assume differences until similarity is found, emphasize description rather than evaluation and interpretations, and treat interpretations as working hypotheses to be tested.

Cross-cultural communication occurs when someone from one culture correctly understands a message sent by someone from another culture. Cross-cultural miscommunication occurs when someone from the second culture misinterprets the sender's message. No two people have exactly the same cultural background, so every communication is somewhat intercultural. The greater the cultural differences, the greater the communication challenges and probability that the message sent will not be the message received. As attitudes, behaviors, and values are shared, people change and the cultural process continues (LeBaron, 2003).

Americans of white European origin may speak English or any number of national languages. They tend to view eye contact as indicating trustworthiness. Silence can be interpreted to indicate respect or disrespect depending on the situation.

Hispanic Americans often speak Spanish or Portuguese. They may use dramatic body language using facial expressions and gestures to express emotions. Yet confrontation is believed to be disrespectful and expressing negative feelings is considered impolite. Eye contact with people in authority is considered disrespectful.

African Americans may speak English or Black Vernacular English, which has variation in grammar, pronunciation, and vocabulary. Direct eye contact may be viewed as rude or aggressive. Nonverbal communication is significant.

Asian Americans may speak Chinese, Korean, Japanese, Vietnamese, and/or English (as well as one of several other languages). Eye contact and saying no are considered disrespectful. Criticism or disagreement is not usually expressed verbally, and nodding yes does not necessarily mean agreement. Silence is valued.

Native Americans may speak English or tribal languages, and usually speak in soft voices with the expectation of attentiveness. Eye contact may be considered disrespectful. Body language is important. Silence is respectful to the speaker (Silvestri, 2005).

Our voices reveal our place of birth, geographic background, gender, age, level of education, emotional state, and relationship to others. Spoken language includes not only words but vocal paralanguage as well, including the regional accent, tone, pitch, emotion, hesitations, and so on. The way we view others is influenced by what we hear in their voices.

Slang terms can mean different things in different cultures, even when using what sound like the same words. For example, someone from Ireland might say, "Where is the crack?" when asking about where the party or fun is; this does not mean they are asking for drugs. Furthermore, "I was pissed" means "drunk," not "angry." "Dizzy" to someone from Britain has the same meaning as "scatterbrained" to someone from America. We interpret the speaker's voice by the pronunciation, accent, charisma, honesty, sarcasm, emotions, uniqueness, lifestyle, and geographic location (Denning, 2002).

Gestures may be friendly, angry, warning, or obscene, and may vary among cultures. When Japanese people put an index finger up above each side of the head, they are likely meaning they are angry while an American of white European descent may just be having fun playing a "devil." When the French put an index finger on their cheek, they likely mean they do not believe you, while in the United States that might mean "I am thinking." The thumbs up gesture Americans use to mean good luck or good job is an obscene Iranian gesture comparable to waving the middle finger in the United States (University of California, Nonverbal Communication Series, 2007).

The face is considered the organ of emotion. It communicates nonverbal communication. The emotions of anger, disgust, fear, sadness, and surprise are expressed in similar ways across cultures. Faces also give clues to heritage, region, age, and humor as well as emotions. While one needs to be sensitive to both verbal and nonverbal communications, one needs to also be wary about misinterpreting them (LeBaron, 2003; University of California, Nonverbal Communication Series, 2007).

Stereotypes form expectations regarding how strangers will act, and influence the way one processes information. Stereotypes may be positive or negative. One tends to remember more favorable information about in-groups (groups the individual belongs to, such as race, religion and family) and less favorable information about out-groups (groups to which the individual does not belong). Then the processing of information is biased in the direction of maintaining one's preexisting belief systems. That produces cognitive confirmation of one's stereotypes. One's stereotypes are automatically activated when one contacts strangers, and one unconsciously tries to confirm expectations when one communicates with others. Rigidly held inaccurate or negative stereotypes can lead to misunderstandings and inaccurate predictors of others' behaviors. Although one's stereotypes of in-groups

can be more accurate than one's stereotypes of out-groups, one tends to assume that people in a group are more alike than they really are. Consequently, even valid stereotypes can cause misinterpretations of the behaviors of atypical group members. One's stereotypes of others can influence one's own view of himself or herself. The more traits included in one's stereotype of a group that group members have of themselves, the more accurate one's predictions of that behavior (Gudykunst, 1998).

To form supportive environments in order to work better with others, one should be descriptive rather than judgmental, define mutual problems and express a willingness to find a solution collaboratively, be spontaneous instead of strategic, express empathy to show concern for others' welfare, treat others as equals, be open to different viewpoints, and be willing to experiment with other behaviors (Gudykunst, 1998). Through conversations, one can celebrate a togetherness by building something that is "ours" (Casmir, 1997).

IMPROVING COMMUNICATION

There are many ways one can improve communications (Box 1-4). Ideas should be clear before one attempts communication of the idea. What is the purpose of the message? Is it to seek information, inform, persuade, or initiate action? To formulate a message, one must gather the information needed and seek consultation from others as appropriate. Considering the goals and attitudes of the receivers helps the sender convey something of help or value to the

---

BOX 1-4 Improve Communications

Written
Oral
Gestures
Actions
Active listening
Build trust
Dictation etiquette
Telephone etiquette

receivers. One must also determine the mode of communication—by written or oral messages or through gestures. Face-to-face contact involves nonverbal behavior that further clarifies intent and allows for feedback to validate understanding of the message. Feedback through mutual exchange decreases the chance for misunderstanding. A climate that allows people to say what they think facilitates feedback.

One must also consider the setting in which one communicates and time one's messages for maximal impact. Should the communication be made in public or private? What is the social climate, and what effect will that have on the tone of the communication? What are the customs and practices of the audience, and how does one's message conform to audience expectations? It is helpful for the message to refer to something the receiver has experienced and for it to be timed for immediate use by the receiver. For example, a building evacuation plan will be better received during fire prevention week, when personnel are expecting a fire drill, than at most other times.

Communications should be well organized and expressed in simple words, a clear style, and the shortest sentences possible. Redundancy— the repetition of the message verbatim or its presentation in several different ways—ensures that the message is understood. The amount of redundancy depends on the content of the message and the experience and background of the receiver. Redundancy is especially important when the information is important and the directions are complicated. However, redundancy can become a barrier to communication if the message is simple and personnel are familiar with it. Employees are likely to stop listening because they know what is going to be said.

Because actions speak louder than words, the message is more forceful if the sender acts congruously. Communications should be followed up to make sure they were understood, and one should seek to understand as well as to be understood.

Listening, an active process that requires conscious attention, is critical to good communication. Trust is a prerequisite because people will not share feelings with those they do not trust.

The speaker must be convinced that disclosures will be kept confidential, that feelings will be respected and not judged, and that the information will be used appropriately and not used against the speaker.

Once trust is established, empathetic listening is needed. People think faster than they talk. As a result, when listening to another person talk, one has time left over for thinking, time that is frequently misused. Instead, if one concentrates on what is being said, one has less time for irrelevant thoughts. One can think ahead of the speaker, try to guess the points that will be made next, consider what the conclusion will be, listen between the lines, try to understand the speaker's point of reference, review, and summarize the points made.

Active listening involves refraining from talking while trying to understand the speaker's attitude and feelings. One should listen to the whole story, talking as little as possible and avoiding leading questions, arguing, or giving advice. Silent pauses encourage the speaker to continue. Attentiveness is indicated by comments such as "yes," "uh huh," and "go on"; restatement (repeating what was said); paraphrasing (saying what was said in different words); clarifying (asking the speaker what was meant); reflecting (responding to the feelings communicated); and summarizing (reviewing the major points made). By saying little, receivers can concentrate on listening instead of on what they are going to say in return (Ellis & Hartley, 2004).

Written communications usually have the advantage of being more carefully formulated than oral communications. They also may save time and money and can be retained as legal records and reference sources. Before writing, one must first consider the purpose of the communication. For a planned and organized message, the writer develops thoughts logically, gives evidence to back up statements, and carefully selects words. Writers must ask themselves whether the communication answers who, what, when, where, and why questions and should appraise the tone of the document. Because writing is not easy, one should expect to edit original drafts.

Dictation is a valuable communication skill. Dictating may require more effort at first, but it can soon become easier than writing in longhand. In dictation one must again consider the purpose of the communication, and plan and organize one's remarks. One starts dictation by indicating who is dictating what (letter or memo), the subject, type of paper needed (letterhead stationery, memo pad), and the number of copies needed. One should state the format (headings, double space, tabular outline, new paragraph), punctuation (capitalization, hyphen, period, commas, question marks, italics), and spell out unusual or unfamiliar words. Conversational instructions are given as one dictates. For example, "Mary, list the following statements and precede each with a dash." One should not smoke, eat, or chew gum while dictating. Background noises should be reduced as much as possible. Closing the office door during dictation can eliminate interference. Dictation should be given at a normal talking speed, with the words pronounced clearly and correctly. The sender can conclude dictation by saying "end of memo." If one cannot complete the dictation, instructions for the incomplete correspondence should be dictated. The dictator may want to keep a list of what is dictated and mark the items off as they are processed.

Telephone etiquette takes into account the needs of the sender and the receiver. One should answer the telephone promptly and cheerfully while smiling, and speak clearly and distinctly to identify the agency, unit, and self. One should listen politely, establish the purpose of the telephone call, determine the appropriate respondent, and ask questions to verify the message. One should answer questions with discretion, describe options appropriately, and identify actions for follow-up in a polite manner. Then the message is documented. To send a telephone message, one should gather the information needed and anticipate questions, call the number, identify the sender and receiver of the message, state the purpose of the call, exchange information, identify the follow-up, and document the call (Wywialowski, 2004).

Communications are critical for the functioning of an organization. Nurses need to be familiar with the communication process, communication systems, and directions communications can take. There are numerous barriers to communication. Leaders and managers need to know them and ways to overcome them.

 RESEARCH Perspective 1-2

Data from Chan MF: A cluster analysis to investigating nurses' knowledge, attitudes, and skills regarding the clinical management system, *CIN: Computers Informatics Nursing* 25(1):45-54, 2007.

Purpose: To explore nurses' knowledge, attitudes, and skills regarding the clinical management system by identifying profiles of nurses working in Hong Kong.

Methods: A total of 282 nurses from four hospitals completed a self-reported questionnaire between December 2004 and May 2005. A two-step cluster analysis revealed two clusters. The first cluster (n = 159, 54.4%) was labeled the "negative attitudes, less skill, and average knowledge" group. The second cluster (n = 123, 43.6%) was labeled the "positive attitudes, good knowledge, but less skillful" group.

Results/conclusions: There was a positive correlation in cluster 1 for nurses' knowledge and attitudes (re = 0.28) and in cluster 2 for nurses' skills and attitudes (re = 0.25) toward computerization. The study revealed that senior and more highly educated nurses generally held more positive attitudes toward computerization. The attitudes among younger and less well-educated nurses were generally more negative. Such findings can be used to formulate strategies to encourage nurses to resolve actual problems following computer training, to increase the depth and breadth of nurses' computer knowledge and skills, and to improve their attitudes toward computerization.

Johari Window

The process of giving and receiving feedback is illustrated by the Johari Window, named for its inventors, Joseph Luft and Harry Ingham (Figure 1-6). Two columns represent the self, and two rows represent the group. The left column represents things one knows about oneself. The right column represents things one does not know about oneself. As one solicits more feedback from the group, the pane moves to the right, enlarging the arena area, where what one knows about oneself and others also know is represented. The pane varies as the level of mutual trust and feedback in the group changes. The arena is characterized by free and open exchange of information between self and others.

The second pane, the blind spot, contains information one does not know about oneself but members of the group may know. One communicates to group members in verbal and nonverbal ways of which one may not be aware. The person with the large blind spot interacts primarily by giving feedback but solicits very little. The person may be a poor listener or may be insensitive to the feedback, or he or she may respond to feedback with undesirable responses, such as anger, crying, or leaving, which makes others reluctant to give feedback. Soliciting feedback can decrease this pane.

In the third pane, the façade, one knows something that the group does not know. The person with the large façade asks questions of the group but does not give information or feedback. The information may be hidden from the group because of fear of rejection, attack, or other hurtful behavior. When one perceives supportive elements in the group and does self-disclosure, the pane can decrease. One needs to disclose some information to test one's assumptions about the supportiveness of the group. Keeping information to oneself may be used to control and manipulate others.

In the fourth pane, unknown, neither the person nor the group knows. The person neither solicits nor gives feedback. As the arena gets larger through feedback and self-disclosure, the other panes get smaller. However, there will probably always be some unknown information, such as intrapersonal dynamics, early childhood memories, and latent potentialities that are unconscious. A receptive attitude to feedback and self-disclosure increases the arena and reduces the blind spot, the façade, and the unknown. The goal is to solicit self-disclosure and feedback to move information from the façade and the blind spot into the arena, making the information available to everyone (Yen, 1999).

COMMUNICATING WITH DIFFICULT PEOPLE

"It is easier to swallow angry words than to have to eat them."   —Anonymous

Hostile Aggressive

Bramson (1997) and Solomon (2002) have described working with difficult people (Box 1-5). One requires special communication skills to deal with some personalities, including hostile-aggressive, complaining, negative, unresponsive, and overly nice. Some hostile-aggressive types seem to attack in an abrupt, abusive, intimidating manner

	Self	
	→ Solicits feedback	
Group Self-disclosure ← or ← Gives feedback	Things I know	Things I do not know
	Arena	Blind spot
	Façade	Unknown

Figure 1-6 • Johari Window. (From Jones JE, Pfeiffer JW [editors]: *The 1973 annual handbook for group facilitators,* La Jolla, CA, 1973, University Associates.)

BOX 1-5 Difficult People

Hostile aggressive
  Exploders
  Snipers
Complaintive
Negative
Unresponsive
Superagreeable

that pushes others to acquiesce against their better judgment. These people tend to know what others should do, need to prove themselves right, and lack trust and caring. One must stand up to a hostile-aggressive person or one will feel overrun and frustrated. It is important to do this without fighting, or the conflict will escalate. It can be advantageous to give the hostile-aggressive person time to run down for a while and then interrupt to stand up for oneself. There may be no opportunity to speak between sentences, thus making it necessary to interrupt before the other person has finished speaking. It is also likely that the other person may interrupt. Then one must state firmly, "You interrupted me," and start again, preferably with a smile. One needs to get the other person's attention to do problem solving. Calling the person by name may help get the person's attention. Deliberately dropping a book is a more dramatic way to get attention. By standing up, one may also get attention. In addition, the other person may be less aggressive when sitting down. Then one needs to state ideas forcefully in a friendly manner that does not belittle the other person. It is important to avoid fighting with the hostile-aggressive person because such a battle will likely be lost. Even if the battle is won, the hostile-aggressive person's anger will likely increase, and the war may be lost. When one stands up to a bully, one may become a friend. When dealing with hostile-aggressive people, it is important to stand up for oneself without fighting.

Exploders

Exploders are a type of hostile-aggressive personality. Adult tantrums are the grown-up version of childhood tantrums that are a defense mechanism to cope with fear, helplessness, and frustration. Adult tantrums are sudden, almost automatic responses to feeling threatened. The exploder typically feels angry first and then blaming or suspicious. People act on their perceptions, but people are likely to perceive the same situation differently. Consequently, the other person may be unaware that the exploder has been threatened and be surprised by the outburst. The exploder should be given time to finish the tantrum and regain self-control. If the exploder does not finish, a neutral statement such as "stop" may interrupt the tantrum. Then one can show that the person is taken seriously by a comment such as "I can see this is important to you. I want to discuss this with you but not like this." Possibly one should change the pace by getting a cup of coffee and seeking a private place for a problem-solving session.

Snipers

Snipers use put-down remarks that are aggressive responses to an unresolved problem. It causes distress rather than positive actions. Unfortunately, the unsolved problems become worse, and the resulting stress causes more difficult behavior such as innuendoes, not-too-subtle remarks, and nonplayful teasing.

First of all, it is important to expose the attack by comments such as "That sounded like a put-down; did you mean it that way?" Usually snipers will deny any attack. Sniping is not possible without a camouflage that works. Standing up to the attack without escalating it will help one proceed with problem solving. It gives the sniper an alternative to a direct contest. It is appropriate to get other points of view that confirm or deny the sniper's criticism and then try to solve any problems that have surfaced. Sniping can be prevented by establishing regular problem-solving meetings.

Complainers

Complainers may dump on one directly or may complain about other "awful" people. Complaining helps people appear blameless and innocent, at least to themselves. One should listen attentively to the complaints, paraphrase an acknowledgment of what was heard, and confirm one's perception of how the complainer feels. One should not agree with or apologize for the allegations and should avoid the accusation-defense-reaccusation pattern. It is preferable to simply state and acknowledge the facts without comment and then proceed with problem solving.

Negative Thinkers

Negatively thinking people believe any task that is out of their hands will fail and that others do not care and are self-serving. One should beware of being dragged down by their despair. One can make optimistic but realistic comments about past successes in similar situations but should not try to argue negativists out of their 0pessimism. It is better not to offer solutions or alternatives until the problem has been thoroughly discussed or to ask people to act before they feel ready. During the problem-solving session, the negative events that could occur if the option is implemented should be explored. One should be ready to take independent action if the group refuses to do so and announce these plans without equivocation.

Unresponsive

Unresponsive people cannot or will not speak when input is needed from them. It is difficult to know what their silence means. The most important strategy is to get the silent person to speak by asking open-ended questions, waiting calmly for a response, and not talking to fill the silence. If an open-ended question gets no response, one should comment on what is happening, for example, "I'm not getting any feedback from you," and end the observation with another open-ended question such as "What are you thinking?" Attention should be given when the person does speak. If the person never speaks, one should terminate the meeting by stating what will be done because no discussion occurred.

Superagreeable

Superagreeable people are equally difficult because they lead one to believe that they are in agreement but let one down when it comes to taking action. They have a strong need to be liked and accepted, and to help others feel approved to get approval themselves. They run into trouble when their need for approval conflicts with negative aspects of reality. They commit themselves to actions that they do not complete. Once again, problem solving is important. One must try to learn what prevents people from taking action and let them know that they are

valued by telling them so, and by asking questions about their interests, hobbies, and family to get to know them better. One should ask them what is not as good as they would like it to be and what could interfere with good relationships. Listening to their humor for hidden messages in teasing remarks and being prepared to do problem solving are also important (Bramson, 1997; Solomon, 2002).

ASSERTIVENESS

Barriers to Assertiveness

Communication styles are passive (accommodating, avoiding, suppressing), aggressive (abusive, dominating, forcing), or assertive (collaborating, integrating) (Box 1-6). Assertiveness is the best style for nurse managers and the one they should foster in their personnel. However, there are barriers that nurses must overcome to become assertive (Box 1-7). The most pervasive barrier is female gender role socialization. Whereas men are often characterized as aggressive, competitive, independent, objective, analytical, task oriented, confident, self-disciplined, and emotionally controlled, women may be expected to be passive, dependent, subjective, intuitive, empathetic, sensitive, interpersonally oriented, weak, inconsistent, and emotionally unstable (Aphrodite Women's Health, 2005; Seventh District's Distance Learning Center of Excellence, 2007).

BOX 1-6 Communication Styles

Passive
Aggressive
Assertive

BOX 1-7 Barriers to Assertiveness

Gender roles
Nursing socialization process
Male-female role competition
Queen bees
Trashing

The nursing socialization process and the nature of nursing are additional barriers. Both nursing schools and health care agencies are likely to have had organizational hierarchies with authority and power concentrated at the top. This arrangement usually promotes compliance and conformity. Nurses have been taught to value sacrifice, humility, and service to others. They have been taught not to state their thoughts or feelings. Although they give intimate physical nurturing, they are taught not to become emotionally involved with patients. Nurses have been socialized into a subservient role. They are expected to follow physicians' orders and to be professional but not to anticipate equal financial reimbursement for their education and responsibilities. Nurses have been expected to be a part of the health care team but may not be allowed to make decisions or policies. They tend to keep so busy that they ignore their own rights.

In addition to these male-female role competition problems, nurses face female-female relationship problems. Men are more competitive with women than with other men, and women are more competitive with women than with men. Consequently, attempts to develop support systems for nurses are not usually successful. Instead, the queen bee and the trashing syndromes are likely to emerge.

The queen bee identifies with men, enjoys being told that one is different from most women, and feels superior to other women. The queen bee usually has to work very hard to become a success in a male-dominated society. One is likely to need to be cooperative and nonthreatening to achieve and maintain her successful position. The queen bee probably feels little animosity toward the system and the men who allowed her to become successful. Thus, she is likely to identify with her male colleagues instead of with other women. However, protective of her own position and aware of the high price she paid for it, she makes it no easier for other women to succeed (Wiseman, 2003).

Trashing is a form of character assassination that divides women against one another. It is self-destructive and leads to impotent rage.

Rather than exposing disagreements to resolve differences, trashing is done to destroy. It can be done to one's face or behind one's back, in public or in private. It questions one's motives, stresses one's worthlessness, and breaches one's integrity. The victim may be ignored, or anything the victim says or does may be interpreted in the most negative manner. Others' unrealistic expectations about another ensure failure. The trasher may give misinformation to others about what the victim does and thinks, or tell lies about what others think of the victim. Whatever method is used, it is manipulative, dishonest, and destructive. Women in general and nurses specifically need to become aware of what they are doing to each other, commit themselves to supportive instead of destructive behavior, learn to analyze interpersonal communication, and learn assertive behavior.

Transactional Analysis

Transactional analysis is a technique that can be used by nurses for analyzing and understanding behavior. It was developed by Eric Berne (1964, 1996) and popularized by Thomas Harris (1969) and Muriel James and Dorothy Jongeward (1996). Transactional analysis is an outgrowth of the Freudian concepts of id, ego, and superego—elements of the psyche that stimulate, monitor, and control behavior. Berne calls these ego states parent, child, and adult (Davidson & Mountain, 2007).

Ego States

The *parent* ego state controls and is the source of values, opinions, rules, regulations, and social conscience. The two major types of parent ego states are nurturing parent and critical parent. The nurturing parent guides, teaches, advises, and supplies "how to" information. The critical parent prohibits and supplies "should" and "should not" information. The parent ego state is a result of cultural traditions, social programming, and responsibilities. Parental judgments are drawn heavily from natural parents, older siblings, teachers, and other parent figures (Box 1-8).

BOX 1-8 Ego States

Parent
Child
Adult

BOX 1-9 Transactional Analysis

COMPLIMENTARY
Parent to parent
Child to child
Adult to adult

CROSSED
Parent to child

The *child* ego state is dominated by emotions and is the feeling state. It is the id ego state in which strong feelings are triggered by immediate experiences. People are in the child state when they are experiencing childlike natural impulses, such as joy, delight, and gaiety, or anger, hostility, and rage. The child ego state may be happy or destructive. The natural child is spontaneous, trusting, joyful, living, creative, and adventurous. The adapted child is suppressed and may express anger, rebellion, fear, or conformity.

The *adult* is the ego state that monitors one's behavior. It is the unemotional, thinking, problem-solving state. The adult ego state collects information, sets goals, compares alternatives, makes decisions and plans, and tests reality. The adult ego state is an unemotional state in which rational decision making takes place.

Every individual exhibits behavior from the three ego states at different times. A healthy individual maintains a balance among them. Unfortunately, some people are dominated by one or two of the ego states and are likely to create problems for leaders and managers. Parent-dominated individuals may not participate in problem solving because they think they already have the answer and know what is right and wrong. Child-dominated individuals may not engage in rational problem solving either. Screaming and being emotional have helped them get what they wanted before. It is likely to be difficult to reason with someone dominated by the child ego state. Working with adult-dominated individuals may be boring because they work so hard. A balance among the three ego states produces the healthiest worker (Chapman, 2007).

Transactions

When people interact, they participate as parent, child, or adult. A transaction or an observation unit is an exchange between people that consists of at least one stimulus and one response (Box 1-9). Transactional analysis is done to identify the participant's ego state and consists of complementary or crossed types (Figure 1-7). The basic principle of the complementary type is that the response to the stimulus is predictable and expected.

Adult-to-adult transactions are the manner in which much business is conducted (Figure 1-8). For instance, a supervisor says, "Would you please give Mr. Jones his prn medication before you give Mrs. Smith her 8 AM medications?" A staff nurse replies, "Yes, I understand that Mr. Jones is complaining of surgical pain."

Parent-to-parent interaction is often a short-term sharing of opinions (Figure 1-9). One staff nurse says to another, "Those new graduate nurses certainly don't know how to function." The other nurse replies, "That's for sure."

Child-to-child interactions usually involve an emotional exchange (Figure 1-10). As long as both parties are in a child ego state, they are unable to think rationally and solve problems. The first staff nurse says, "I just gave Mrs. Smith her 8 AM medications, and when I went to chart them, you had signed for giving them. Why don't you sign right after you give medications so they won't be repeated?" The second nurse answers, "Why don't you give me a chance to sign before you go and give them again?"

In *parent-to-child* interactions, one person takes a psychologically superior position over the other (Figure 1-11). A manager says, "I want to see you in my office." A staff nurse answers, "Yes, ma'am."

Crossed transactions result in closing communications at least temporarily (Figure 1-12). The response may be inappropriate or unexpected

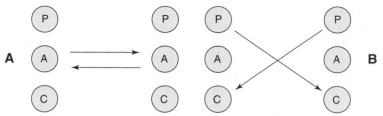

Figure 1-7 • Transactions. **A,** Complementary. **B,** Crossed.

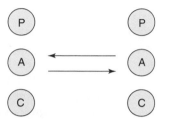

Figure 1-8 • Adult-to-adult complementary transaction.

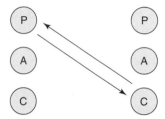

Figure 1-11 • Parent-to-child complementary transaction.

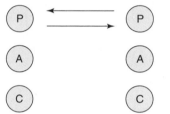

Figure 1-9 • Parent-to-parent complementary transaction.

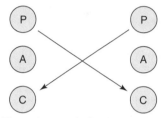

Figure 1-12 • Crossed transaction.

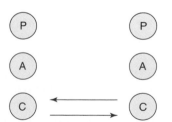

Figure 1-10 • Child-to-child complementary transaction.

and may confuse or threaten the sender of the stimulus. A supervisor says, "Miss Jones, could I see you about this in my office right away?" Miss Jones replies, "No! Can't you see I'm busy? You'll have to wait."

Transactions usually proceed in a programmed series, with rituals and procedures being the simplest kinds. Rituals are a series of simple, complementary transactions that provide mutual stroking with no real commitment. Most rituals have been used so often that the form has become more important than the content, but they provide structure for greeting people and expressing religious beliefs. Greeting rituals such as "Hi," "How are you?" and "I am fine" are not intended to supply information. The person who goes from office to office participating in rituals may get promoted because he or she is "a good guy." Rituals work for the person who can still get the job done. People who work hard to develop themselves may become apathetic when they realize socializing is more effective for obtaining promotions than hard work. Rituals may have started as a series of complementary adult transactions intended to manipulate reality, but they have lost their procedural validity over time (Davidson & Mountain, 2007).

Pastimes are pleasant ways to pass time with others to learn if you have enough in common to warrant further interaction. Common small talk includes topics such as cooking, fashions, costs, sports, recreation, and mutual acquaintances. There is no goal or emotional closeness involved. People who spend too much time participating in pastimes may sense that their lives are happy but empty, whereas the person who spends too little time making small talk may not have much fun and may feel harassed. Pastimes become a problem for the organization when they are an alternative to work (Chapman, 2007).

Game Playing

Berne (1996) stated: "A game is an ongoing series of complementary ulterior transactions progressing to a well-defined, predictable outcome." Games have a high stroke or recognition potential, but the payoff is usually negative. Games have hidden agendas that prevent both people and organizations from becoming winners (Box 1-10). While playing games, people dwell on their own sorrows and inadequacies, make

mistakes, catch others making mistakes, pass the buck, and fail to meet their obligations. People receive negative strokes and get hurt while real problems go unsolved. Productivity is limited because people use their energies to play games instead of completing the job. Attention is given to past events rather than to the present. While realities of the current situation go unperceived, problems go unsolved.

People need strokes, and negative strokes are better than no strokes. Consequently, in work environments that do not provide positive strokes, people have a need to play games. People who are bored with their jobs are also likely to play games. Games discourage openness, honesty, and intimacy. They take many forms. Games that blame others include "If it weren't for you" and "See what you made me do." Games that attack others include "Blemish," "Now I've got you, you SOB," "Bear trapper," "Corner," "Rapo," "Uproar," and "Let's you and him fight." Self-pity is reinforced by games such as "Poor me," "Kick me," "Stupid," "Wooden leg," "Harried," and "Lunch bag" (Berne, 1964).

Blame Others

"*If it weren't for you*" is a blaming game in which people who feel inadequate blame others for their inability to achieve. People who blame their inability to be innovative on rigid policies may fear their own creative abilities. "If it weren't for…" is a clue that the game is being played. When managers hear an employee say this, they should suspect that the complainer would not function better under different circumstances but would likely become frustrated and request a transfer or quit. Changes may be made on a trial basis to test suspicions.

"*See what you made me do*" and "*You got me into this*" are closely related blaming games. The player avoids responsibility by being vindictive. It is common for workers to blame managers for problems and for managers to blame workers for mistakes or poor decisions. The manager decides whether or not to use the input from the workers, and he or she needs to accept that responsibility.

BOX 1-10 Communication Games

BLAME OTHERS
If it weren't for you
See what you made me do
You got me into this

ATTACK
Blemish
Now I've got you
Bear trapper
Corner
Rapo
Uproar
Let's you and him fight

SELF-PITY
Poor me
Kick me
Stupid
Wooden leg
Harried
Lunch bag

Attack

Many games attack others. The *"Blemish"* player looks for inconsequential, unimportant flaws. Instead of looking at purposes, the player concentrates on minutiae and zeroes in on trivial mistakes. Any positive stroke is discounted with a blemish. Blemish players also play *"I was only trying to help you."*

The victims become resentful and may become the persecutor by playing *"Now I've got you, you SOB."* In this game the persecutor waits for the victim to make a mistake or sets the victim up for failure. The manager may be indulging in this game by setting standards too high to achieve, assigning people to work for which they are not qualified, creating impossible working conditions, or giving incomplete or unclear instructions. The worker may use grievance procedures or lawsuits against managers playing this game.

The *"Bear trapper"* often baits someone with false promises and then lets the trap fall. Organizations play this game in hiring practices when glamorous job descriptions are presented. This tends to result in high turnover. Workers learn the shortcomings of the job and become disillusioned. Presenting both the advantages and disadvantages of jobs is a more realistic approach.

The *"Corner"* player's victim is in a lose-lose situation. No matter what the victim does, it is wrong. A woman manager is damned if she is aggressive because that is not considered feminine and damned if she is not because aggressiveness is a desired managerial quality. A manager can corner someone into not completing work on time by not accepting the work that is done.

"Corner" can lead to *"Uproar."* Uproar often starts with a critical remark and results in an attack-defense dialogue that is often loud.

"Rapo" is a sexual game. A woman may wear revealing clothing and move in provocative ways. When a man responds, she rejects him. This game is problematic when men and women work together. Organizations require concentrating on equality and using human resources regardless of gender.

In *"Let's you and him fight,"* one person gets a second and a third person into a fight. When one person tells a second person the "bad" things a third person said about the second, the first person is fostering a fight.

Self-Pity

There are several versions of self-pity games. *"Kick me"* players provoke put-downs and make comments such as "I could kick myself for that." *"Stupid"* players collect put-downs about one's intelligence. Leaders and managers need to give immediate feedback and take corrective actions to prevent the "Stupid" game. The *"Wooden leg"* player uses a physical or social handicap to avoid work. A deprived background may be used as an excuse to underachieve. The manager needs to set and maintain standards to minimize this game.

Leaders and managers play *"Poor me"* games also. *"Harried"* executives work hard to maintain the sense of being OK. Harried executives are likely to work nights and weekends to appear competent and confident. "I'm not OK" feelings are hidden by appearing super OK.

The harried executive may also participate in the *"Lunch bag game."* Leaders and managers may carry leftovers in a used paper bag and eat at their desk instead of going to lunch with peers. This technique can be used to make other people feel guilty.

Games always involve putting someone down. To decrease games in organizations, one must stop putting oneself and others down. One should not play the complementary role but should give and receive positive strokes and invest time in activities and intimacy. Managers should integrate the goals of the workers and the organization and decrease boredom through job enrichment and personnel development. With good organization and management, positive strokes can become an intrinsic part of the job. Managers should foster an "I'm OK, you're OK" atmosphere.

Activities such as working and learning are goal directed and have a high stroke potential. They are a highly rewarding way to spend time. Workers must be careful not to take on so many activities that they neglect rituals and pastimes, and managers should not overload themselves with activities and leave the workers with idle time.

Intimacy is an open sharing of experience with others, usually by people with close relationships but sometimes by strangers. It is the most rewarding way to spend time. It is also the most risky. Although intimacy is without ulterior motives or exploitation, one needs high self-esteem to risk the openness of intimacy. It requires and fosters the "I'm OK, you're OK" atmosphere (Berne, 1996).

Life Positions

Harris (1969) identified life positions (Box 1-11). Life positions are more permanent than ego states. As individuals mature, they make assumptions about themselves and others. They consider themselves as OK or not OK and see others as OK or not OK. Four positions result: *"I'm OK, you're OK," "I'm OK, you're not OK," "I'm not OK, you're OK," and "I'm not OK, you're not OK."* OK feelings are associated with a sense of power, personal worth, well-being, capability, and lovableness. Not-OK feelings result from a sense of inability, weakness, helplessness, worthlessness, anxiety, and a feeling of being insignificant and unlovable. Most people develop a basic life position early in childhood that tends to be reinforced by the person's selective perceptions and reactions to experiences.

In the I'm OK, you're OK position, individuals feel interdependent with others and the environment. They are happy, active people with a positive outlook on life who like reinforcement for being OK but are not dependent on it. They use the happy child and nurturing parent ego states. Because they feel OK about themselves, they have little difficulty feeling that others are OK.

People in the I'm OK, you're not OK position do not believe they can rely on anyone but themselves. They think people are worthless and are likely to be enemies and consequently tend to blame others. The critical parent ego state is dominant. A manager in this position possesses a Theory X philosophy, implements a Likert type I system, and supervises people closely because they cannot be trusted.

People in the I'm not OK, you're OK position are burdened with self-defeating attitudes and a lack of confidence. They take a psychologically inferior stand to others and assume that they are less competent and less influential than others.

Individuals in the I'm not OK, you're not OK position are maladjusted. They think they are worthless and so are others. Lacking confidence in themselves and trust in others, they are suspicious and anxious, disconnected from others, alienated from the environment, and miserable, and they tend to give up.

During infancy, individuals have a mixture of OK and not-OK feelings, with the not-OK feelings predominating. The infant feels OK when physical needs are met and positive strokes are received. Most of an infant's experiences provide negative strokes and not-OK feelings. Because adults can satisfy the infant's needs, they are viewed as OK. For most people the I'm not OK, you're OK position is established early and continues into adulthood. Socialization of women and nurses particularly reinforces the position that they are not OK. Therefore they need a lot of positive reinforcement to move to an I'm OK, you're OK position. Assertiveness can help one achieve and maintain that position. Once it is learned, there will be less passive-aggressive behavior (Harris, 1969; Underwood, 2003).

Assertiveness Techniques

"If one tells the truth, one is sure sooner or later to be found out." —Oscar Wilde

Communication styles are commonly passive, aggressive, or assertive. Passive persons are often self-denying and inhibited and allow others to choose for them. Consequently, goals are not

---

BOX 1-11 Life Positions

I'm OK, you're OK.
I'm OK, you're not OK.
I'm not OK, you're OK.
I'm not OK, you're not OK.

achieved and feelings are hurt, anxious, and frustrated. Aggressive persons are self-enhancing at others' expense. Aggressors are expressive, choose for others, deprecate others, and achieve own goals by using others. Aggressive behavior generates hatred and sometimes revenge. Assertive persons are self-enhancing. Assertive people are expressive, choose for themselves, and can achieve their goals, and therefore are likely to feel good about themselves (Box 1-12).

Passive persons tend to be at a loss for words, do not say what is really meant, use many apologetic words, and hope people will understand what is wanted without telling others. Passive people tend to have a weak, hesitant voice; downcast eyes; and fidgety hands and nod frequently.

The aggressive person is loud; uses loaded, subjective words; makes accusations; and sends "you" messages that blame others. A flippant, sarcastic style with an air of superiority and rudeness is common. The person is likely to stand with hands on hips, feet apart, and narrowed eyes; pointing a finger; and talking in a superior, demanding, authoritarian manner.

Assertive persons initiate a discussion in a private environment; engage in an assertive dialog that separates facts from feelings; and clarify the central issues and differing viewpoints. Assertive people listen and seek a collaborative solution that balances power and satisfies both parties by using direct statements that say what they want or need. They use objective words, send "I" messages, and make honest statements about their feelings. They are attentive listeners who give the impression of caring. They use eye contact and spontaneous verbal expressions with appropriate gestures and facial expressions while speaking in a well-modulated voice (Huber, 2006).

BOX 1-12 Assertiveness Techniques

Broken record
Fogging
Negative assertions
Negative inquiry

The style used governs how situations will be handled. Suppose, for instance, that a leader or manager has noted that a staff nurse has been arriving at work late for the past 3 days. The passive leader or manager may not mention the problem at all. The aggressive leader or manager might say, "How about getting here on time or looking for a new job? What do you think we pay you for anyway?" The assertive leader or manager would be likely to speak to the staff nurse in private and might say, "I've noticed you have been late the past 3 days. Why haven't you been getting to work on time?" The last approach gives an impression of caring and facilitates problem solving.

Broken Record

Assertiveness is the most desirable style for a nurse manager. To achieve assertiveness, one must substitute verbal persistence for silent passivity or verbal abuse. Broken record is a technique managers can use to reach a compromise by indicating what they want and by keeping other people from talking them into what the others want to do. With the broken-record technique, managers keep repeating what they want:

Manager: I expect you to get to work on time.

Staff nurse: But I'm a night person. I stay up late, and it's difficult to get up so early to come to work. I'm so tired that I shut off my alarm and go back to sleep. Then when I do get up, I stumble around in the dark to find my clothes so I won't wake my husband.

Manager: You are scheduled to work the day shift this rotation, and I expect you to be at work on time. If you are a night person, would you like to be assigned to the night shift permanently?

Staff nurse: No. I wouldn't be able to see my husband then. He works 9 AM to 9 PM and gets home about 9:30 PM. I would have to come to work at 10:30, and I could see him for only about an hour. I would get home just in time for him to go to work.

Manager: You are scheduled to work the day shift this rotation, and I expect you to get to work on time. However, we could assign you to the evening shift permanently. Would you want that?

Staff nurse: Working the evening shift would allow me to see my husband after work and to sleep in. Yes, I would prefer the evening shift.

Manager: I will see how quickly we can get your schedule changed to permanent evenings. I do expect you to be here by 7 AM until we get your schedule changed (Straker, 2005).

Fogging, negative assertion, and negative inquiry are techniques for dealing with criticism, whether it is self-directed or from another source, real or imagined. They help minimize the negative emotional response of anxiety to criticism that manipulates one into defending what one wants to do instead of doing it. Accordingly, one feels less at conflict with oneself and more comfortable with both the negative and positive aspects of one's personality.

Fogging

Fogging is agreeing with the truth, agreeing in principle, or agreeing with the odds rather than denying the criticism, getting defensive, or counterattacking with criticism. It helps desensitize one to criticism and leads to a reduction in the frequency of criticism from others. It sets up psychological distance, is a passive skill, and does not encourage the other person to be assertive. It also encourages a person to listen to what the critic says, to respond only to what the critic says rather than to what is implied, and to consider probabilities. For example:

Staff nurse: You scheduled me to double back from evenings to days twice in a 2-week time schedule.

Manager: I see that I scheduled you to double back the first Wednesday and the second Friday (agreeing with the truth).

Staff nurse: When I double back, I have less than 7 hours of sleep. I get tired, have trouble functioning, and fear making mistakes.

Manager: I understand that you get tired when you double back and fear making mistakes. It seems logical that one would make more mistakes when tired than when alert (agreeing with the odds).

Staff nurse: We need a policy to prevent having just one shift off between shifts.

Manager: I agree. We do need staffing policies that would provide for adequate rest periods between shifts (agreeing in principle) (Louisiana State University Student Health Center, 2006).

Negative Assertion

With negative assertion people assertively accept negative aspects about themselves. This reduces the need to seek forgiveness for one's mistakes or the need to counterattack with criticism.

Staff nurse: Your new uniform really reveals how fat you are.

Manager: I'm overweight because I eat too much. I eat just about everything in sight except the kitchen sink. I've even seen the cat get worried (negative assertion).

Staff nurse: Well, that new uniform sure makes you look like a blimp.

Manager: These new styles don't complement my figure (negative assertion).

Negative assertion is not appropriate for physical or legal conflicts or for relating to people on a close interpersonal basis. The persistence of the critic will determine if one needs to use other assertive techniques (Louisiana State University Student Health Center, 2006).

Negative Inquiry

Negative inquiry fosters assertiveness in the critic. In an unemotional manner, the criticized person asks for more information that may be negative. This provides a basis for problem solving and consequently reduces repetitive criticism.

Staff nurse: You don't look good today.

Manager: Is it me or what I'm wearing?

Staff nurse: It's your face. You look so tired.

Manager: I don't feel tired. What about my face makes me look tired?

Staff nurse: Your eyes look so tired. They're so dark. There are bags under them.

Manager: What can I do to make them look less tired?

Staff nurse: If the problem isn't fatigue, I guess you could use a creme cosmetic over the bags and use light instead of dark-colored eye shadow.

RESEARCH Perspective 1-3

Data from Sa TL, Cohen J, Marculescu G: Nurse practitioners' attitudes and knowledge toward current procedural terminology (CPT) coding, *Nursing Economic$* 19(3):100-106, 2001.

Purpose: The purpose of this study was to describe nurse practitioners' attitudes and knowledge about current procedural terminology.

Methods: This research was an exploratory, descriptive, nonexperimental study. Data were collected using a mailed survey that was sent to nurse practitioners in California who were members of a state nurse practitioner organization. The instrument used was a self-administered questionnaire developed by the researchers.

All items in the attitudinal survey were placed on a continuum from positive to negative responses. Descriptive statistics using frequencies, percentages, and means were used.

Results/conclusions: Nurse practitioners lacked the required knowledge about coding and did not perceive the significance of this reimbursement strategy. Nurse practitioners need to be taught the coding and the importance of using it to get reimbursement.

Assertive behavior is more than demanding one's rights from others and keeping others from manipulating. In a social sense, assertiveness is the ability to communicate with others about who one is, how one lives, what one does, and what one wants and the ability to make others feel comfortable talking about themselves. Free information—information offered without being asked for—gives one something to talk about and reduces awkward silences. Self-disclosure reveals how one thinks, feels, and reacts to others' free information. This social conversation allows one to discover mutually rewarding relationships or to identify people with whom one has few common interests.

CHAPTER SUMMARY

Communication is important at all leadership levels. For this reason, it is important for nurse leaders to understand the communication process, to be able to identify barriers to communications, and to implement ways to improve communications. It is helpful to understand life positions, transactional analysis, and how to engage in an assertive dialog that separates facts from feelings, clarifies the central issues, and identifies differing viewpoints. There is a need to listen and seek a collaborative solution that balances power and satisfies both parties.

CRITICAL THINKING ACTIVITY

Reflective Journal: Make observations in a clinical setting, or reflect on past experiences. What communication system is in place? Describe it. Interview a staff nurse or manager about problematic barriers to communication. Ask staff nurses or managers what they think could be done to improve communications. What types of difficult people are involved? How are people dealing with them? How might they better deal with them? What do you think are the barriers to communication, and what could be done to improve communications? Do transactional analysis on some interactions you have observed. What games have you observed during a certain time at a specific place?

CASE STUDY

A staff nurse who works with you is frequently late to work. How will you assertively solve the situation with the nurse?

ONLINE RESOURCES

evolve Additional critical thinking activities, worksheets, and case studies are available online at http://evolve.elsevier.com/Marriner/guide8e.

REFERENCES

Advanced executive leadership skills, Stamford, CT, 1981, Xerox Learning Systems.

Alexander JW, Kroposki M: Using a management perspective to define and measure changes in nursing technology, *Journal of Advanced Nursing* 35(5):776-783, 2005.

Aphrodite Women's Health: *Male, female stereotypes created by media,* 2005 (website): www.aphroditewomenshealth.com/news/20050818234122_health_news.shtml. Accessed January 21, 2007.

Ball MJ, Hannah KJ, Newbold SK, et al: *Nursing informatics: Where caring and technology meet,* New York, 2000, Springer.

Berne E: *Games people play,* New York, 1964, Grove Press.

Berne E: *Games people play,* New York, 1996, Ballantine.

Borgatti S: Communication structure and its effects on task performance, 1997 (website): www.analytictech.com/networks/commstruc.htm. Accessed January 20, 2007.

Borkowski N: *Organizational behavior in health care,* Boston, 2005, Jones and Bartlett.

Bramson RM: *Coping with difficult people,* New York, 1997, Doubleday.

Casmir FL: *Ethics in intercultural and international communication,* Mahway, NJ, 1997, Lawrence Erlbaum Associates, Publishers.

Chan MF: A cluster analysis to investigating nurses' knowledge, attitudes, and skills regarding the clinical management system, *CIN: Computers Informatics Nursing* 25(1):45-54, 2007.

Chapman A: Transactional analysis: Eric Berne's transactional analysis—Early TA history and theory, 2007 (website): www.businessballs.com/transact.htm. Accessed January 21, 2007.

Curtain LL: Ethics in informatics: The intersection of nursing, ethics, and technology, *Nursing Administration Quarterly* 29(4):349-352, Oct/Dec 2005.

Davidson C, Mountain M: Eric Berne's transactional analysis—TA theory development explanation, 2007 (website): httpwww.businessballs.com/transactionalanalysis.htm. Accessed January 21, 2007.

Demiris G, Oliver DP, Courtney KL: Ethical considerations for the utilization of telehealth technologies in home and hospice care by the nursing profession, *Nursing Administration Quarterly* 30(1):56-66, Jan/Feb 2006.

Denning C: Polari, 2002 (website): http://www.chris-d.net/polari/. Accessed January 20, 2007.

DeYoung S: *Teaching strategies for nurse educator,* Upper Saddle River, NJ, 2003, Prentice Hall.

Ellis JR, Hartley CL: *Managing and coordinating nursing care,* ed 4, Philadelphia, 2004, Lippincott.

Finkelman AW: *Leadership and management in nursing,* Upper Saddle River, NJ, 2006, Pearson/Prentice Hall.

Gillies DA: *Nursing management: A systems approach,* Philadelphia, 1994, WB Saunders.

Gilovich T: *How we know what isn't so,* New York, 1991, Free Press.

Gray J: *Men are from Mars, women are from Venus,* New York, 1992, HarperCollins.

Gudykunst WB: *Bridging differences: Effective intergroup communication,* ed 3, Thousand Oaks, CA, 1998, Sage.

Harris TA: *I'm OK—you're OK: A practical guide to transactional analysis,* New York, 1969, Harper & Row.

Huber DL: *Leadership and nursing care management,* ed 3, Philadelphia, 2006, Saunders/Elsevier.

James M, Jongeward D: *Born to win,* Oxford, 1996, Perseus Press.

In Jones JE, Pfeiffer JW, editors: *The 1973 annual handbook for group facilitators,* La Jolla, CA, 1973, University Associates.

Jones S, Moss J: Computerized provider order entry: Strategies for successful implementation, *JONA* 36(3):136-139, March 2006.

Kalisch B, Myer KA, Mackey DM, et al: Online patient assignments enhance horizontal communication, *Nursing Management* 37(6):51, June 2006.

Kotelnikov V: Motivating and communicating, 2007 (website): www.1000ventures.com/business_guide/mgmt_motivating_comg.html. Accessed January 20, 2007.

LeBaron M: Cross-cultural communication, 2003 (website): www.beyondintractability.org/essay/cross-cultural_communication/?nid=1188. Accessed January 20, 2007.

Louisiana State University Student Health Center: Assertiveness, nonassertiveness, and assertive techniques, 2006 (website): http://healthyplace.com/Communities/Depression/suicide/asserting_ourselves_2.asp. Accessed December 19, 2006.

Lunney M: Helping nurses use NANDA, NOC, and NIC: Novice to expert, *JONA* 36(3):118-125, March 2006.

Maguire: Barriers to communication—How things go wrong, *The Pharmaceutical Journal* 268(23):246-247 (serial online): www.pjonline.com/pdf/cpd/pj_20020223_communication1.pdf2002. Accessed January 20, 2007.

Marquis BL, Huston CJ: *Leadership roles and management functions in nursing: Theory and application,* ed 5, Boston, 2006, Lippincott Williams & Wilkins.

McConnell CR: *Umiker's management skills for the health care supervisor,* Boston, 2006, Jones & Bartlett.

Peck A: Changing the face of standard nursing practice through telehealth and telenursing, *Nursing Administration Quarterly* 29(4):339-343, Oct/Dec 2005.

Quible Z: *The flow of communication.* In Gibson-Odgers P: *Administrative office management,* ed 8, Upper Saddle River, NJ, 2004, Prentice Hall.

Rigolosi ELM: *Management and leadership in nursing and health care,* ed 2, New York, 2005, Springer.

Roussel L, Swansburg RC, Swansburg RJ: *Management and leadership in nursing and health care,* ed 4, Boston, 2006, Jones & Bartlett.

Sa TL, Cohen J, Marculescu G: Nurse practitioners' attitudes and knowledge toward current procedural terminology (CPT) coding, *Nursing Economic$* 19(3):100-106, 2001.

Saba VK, McCormick KA: *Essentials of computers for nurses: Informatics for the new millennium*, New York, 2001, McGraw-Hill.

Seventh District's Distance Learning Center of Excellence, Director of Auxiliary West: Team Coordination Training, Assertiveness, 2007 (website): www.dirauxwest.org/TCTF/TCT8assertiveness.htm. Accessed January 21, 2007.

Silvestri LA: *Saunders comprehensive review for the NCLEX-RN examination*, St. Louis, 2005, Elsevier/Saunders.

Solomon M: *Working with difficult people*, Upper Saddle River, NJ, 2002, Prentice Hall Press.

Straker, D: Broken record, 2005 (website): http://changingminds.org/techniques/resisting/broken_record.htm. Accessed January 21, 2007.

Sullivan EJ, Decker PJ: *Effective leadership and management in nursing,* ed 6, Upper Saddle River, NJ, 2005, Prentice Hall.

Tannen D: *You just don't understand: Women and men in conversation*, New York, 2001, Quill.

Thompson B: Will technology change our practice?, *Nursing Administration Quarterly* 29(4):308-414, 2005.

Times 100: Communication, 2005 (website): www.thetimes100.co.uk/theory/theory.php?tID=173. Accessed January 20, 2007.

Underwood M: Life positions, 2003 (website): http://www.cultsock.ndirect.co.uk/MUHome/cshtml/ta/ta_life.html. Accessed January 21, 2007.

University of California, Nonverbal Communication Series: A world of gestures: Culture and nonverbal communications, 2007 (website): http://zzyx.ucsc.edu/~archer/vid3.html. Accessed January 20, 2007.

University of California, Nonverbal Communication Series: The human face, 2007 (website): http://zzyx.ucsc.edu/~archer/vid1.html. Accessed January 20, 2007.

Whetten DA, Cameron KS: *Developing management skills,* ed 6, Upper Saddle River, NJ, 2004, Prentice Hall.

Wiseman R: *Queen bees and wannabees*, London, 2003, Piatkus Books.

Wywialowski EF: *Managing client care,* ed 3, St. Louis, 2004, Mosby.

Yen D: Johari Window, 1999 (website): www.noogenesis.com/game_theory/johari/johari_window.html. Accessed July 21, 2007.

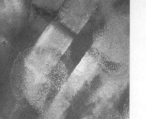

Stress Management

"There is little difference in people, but that little difference makes a big difference. The little difference is attitude. The big difference is whether it is positive or negative." —W. Clement Stone

Chapter Overview

Chapter 2 presents sources of stress, stress response, symptoms of stress, stress control, relaxation, time management, delegation, procrastination, and ways to maximize organization time.

Chapter Objectives

- Identify at least six sources of stress.
- Predict at least 12 symptoms of stress.
- Describe at least 12 stress management techniques.
- Evaluate how planning relates to time management effects.
- Delineate at least five ways to streamline paperwork.
- Formulate at least five ways to make telephone communication efficient.
- Select at least five ways managers can help meetings be effective and efficient.
- Assess responsibility, authority, and accountability as they relate to delegation.
- Explain the five rights of delegation.
- Explain reasons for procrastination.

Online Resources

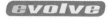 Critical thinking activities, worksheets, and case studies are available online at http://evolve.elsevier.com/Marriner/guide8e.

Major Concepts and Definitions

Stress *the body's nonspecific response to any demand*
Eustress *a positive form of stress that adds excitement and challenge*
Distress *a negative form of stress that threatens effectiveness*
Delegation *to entrust a task to another person who serves as one's representative*
Responsibility *obligation; what must be done to complete the task*
Authority *power to make final decisions and give commands*
Accountability *liability for satisfactory completion of work*
Planning *preparing a scheme for doing something*
Time *management controlling use of time for maximum productivity*

STRESS MANAGEMENT

Sources of Stress

Adjustment to change is stressful. Many events in life produce individual stress reactions. The death of a spouse or close family member, divorce, marital separation, marriage or remarriage, and personal injury or illness are highly stressful events. A change in the health of a family member, pregnancy, gain of a new family member, marital reconciliation, increased arguing with spouse, sexual difficulties, changes in financial state, mortgages, trouble with in-laws, a son or daughter leaving home, and the death of a close friend are stressful. Changes in living conditions and personal habits, such as changes in work, residence, school, recreation, church activities, social activities, sleeping habits, and eating habits, cause stress. Even personal achievements, vacations, and holidays are stressful. These personal stressors can affect one's job performance (Psychology Key Studies, 2007).

In addition to personal stressors, there are many sources of stress at work. Dismissal and retirement are highly stressful. Business readjustments such as changing jobs or responsibilities, changes in working hours or conditions, and problems with the boss are stressful. Even outstanding achievement is stressful. Poor physical working conditions; physical danger; work overload; time pressures; responsibility for people; role ambiguity and conflict; conflicts with superiors, peers, and subordinates; restrictions; little

participation in decision making; overpromotion or underpromotion; and lack of job security are stressors common to jobs.

Nurses face stress with life-and-death situations; heavy workloads involving physical and mental strain; knowledge of how to use numerous pieces of equipment and the consequences of equipment failure; reporting to numerous bosses; communication problems among staff members, physicians, families, and other departments; and awareness of the serious consequences of mistakes. A hospital is one of the most stressful work environments.

People often needlessly increase their own stress. The difference between the demands people place on themselves or perceive from others and the resources they perceive as available to meet the demands is a threat or stress. Individuals are typed by the demands they place on themselves. Type A people set high standards; are competitive; put themselves under constant time pressure; and are very demanding of themselves even in leisure and recreational activities. Type B people are more easygoing; relaxed; are less competitive; and are more likely to accept situations than fight them (Neill, 2005).

The classic *Holmes and Rahe's Social Readjustment Rating Scale* was developed by doctors by asking patients who were recovering from an illness if they had experienced any life events preceding the illness and by having the patients rate the events with a score. The doctors found a small correlation between life events and illness.

RESEARCH Perspective 2-1

Data from Aiken LH, Clarke SP, Sloane DM, et al: Hospital nurse staffing and patient mortality, nurse burnout, and job dissatisfaction, *JAMA* 288:1987-1993, 2002.

Purpose: The objective of this research was to determine the association between the patient-to-nurse ratio and patient mortality, failure-to-rescue among surgical patients, and factors related to nurse retention.

Methods: A cross-sectional analysis of linked data from staff nurses surveyed; general, orthopedic, and vascular surgery patients discharged between April 1, 1998 and November 30, 1999; and administrative data from nonfederal adult general hospitals in Pennsylvania. Risk-adjusted patient mortality and failure-to-rescue within 30 days of admission, and nurse-reported job

dissatisfaction and job-related burnout were measured.

Results/conclusions: After adjusting for patient and hospital characteristics, each additional patient per nurse associated with a 7% increase in the likelihood of dying within 30 days of admission and a 7% increase in the odds of failure-to-rescue. After adjusting for nurse and hospital characteristics, each additional patient per nurse was associated with a 23% increase in the odds of burnout and failure and a 15% increase in the odds of job dissatisfaction.

Even though the study was retrospective and relatively unreliable, the doctors concluded that major life events use up energy, leaving less energy to resist illness. This classic scale helps assess one's stressors and suggests that people with scores of over 300 life change units have a 90% chance of illness; those with 150-299 have a 50% chance of illness; and those with less than 150 have a 30% chance of developing a stress-related illness within 2 years (Doty, 2007; Holmes & Rahe, 1967; Psychology Key Studies, 2007).

Stress Response

Stress is impossible to avoid. It is a nonspecific response of the body to any demand. There are two types of stress: (1) eustress, a positive force that adds excitement and challenge to life and provides a sense of well-being, and (2) distress, a negative force caused by unrelieved tension that threatens effectiveness. Whether one will experience eustress or distress largely depends on the person's perceptions, physical activity or inactivity, mental activity or inactivity, nutrition, and relationships.

A stressor is anything an individual perceives as a threat. Stressors produce a state of stress by disrupting homeostasis. There are three stages in the stress response (Box 2-1). First, the alarm reaction is the mobilization of resources to confront

BOX 2-1 Three Stages in Stress Response

Alarm reaction: Mobilization of resources to confront threat
Resistance stage: Increase in energy consumption
Exhaustion: Depletion of the body's energy reserves

the threat. Second, in the resistance stage, there is a large increase in energy consumption. Once the reserve energy has been used, the body needs time to recover and to replenish the supply. When stress continues for long periods of time, the energy is used but not replaced, and the third stage, exhaustion, results because our body cannot maintain homeostasis and long-term resistance to combat prolonged stress.

Consequently, unrelieved stress interferes with one's physical and mental well-being. After the stress event the body returns to a state of equilibrium. Stable periods for bodies to restore adaptive energy allow one to meet new stressful situations (Seyle, 1965, 1976).

Symptoms of Stress

Numerous symptoms indicate that stress is becoming distress. These include but are not limited to those shown in Box 2-2. High stress

RESEARCH Perspective 2-2

Data from Murji A, Gomez M, Knighton J, Fish JS: Emotional implications of working in a burn unit, *J Burn Care Res* 27(1):8-13, 2006.

Purpose: The purpose was to determine the prevalence of burnout in health care professionals involved in primary burn care, and to gain an understanding of the stressors and pleasures they experience.

Methods: A cross-sectional survey was administered between February and March of 2004 to health care professionals working in a burn unit and a critical care unit. A demographic data sheet, the Maslach Burnout Inventory (MBI), and a questionnaire evaluating sources of stress, pleasure of work, and coping mechanisms used by staff were administered to 75 professionals.

Results/conclusions: There were no significant differences between units regarding emotional exhaustion and personal accomplishment subscales on the MBI. There were no significant differences in the perceived sources of workplace stressors, but differences existed in the coping mechanisms. The burn unit professionals exercised less, talked less with their families, ate less, and watched less television compared with the critical care professionals. The two units had comparable rates of emotional exhaustion and depersonalization but significantly different mechanisms for coping with workplace stress.

levels accumulated over several months are likely to result in physical and psychological reactions. The amount of stress necessary before one manifests symptoms varies, and depends on factors such as heredity, habits, personality, past illnesses, and previous crises and coping mechanisms. Well-educated, intelligent, creative people in management are at high risk for burnout. They may become workaholics but get little accomplished; experience chronic fatigue; feel they do not want to go to work; take increasing amounts of sick time; become negative; blame and criticize others; engage in backbiting; and talk behind others' backs (Jaffe-Gill et al, 2007).

Stress Control

"The secret of happiness is to count your blessings while others are adding up their troubles." —*Anonymous*

Nurse managers can prevent and control burnout by setting personal and professional goals, establishing priorities, practicing good health habits and relaxation techniques, improving the self-esteem by obtaining the skills they need, and using support systems (Box 2-3).

Values Clarification

Values clarification is a useful activity. Values should be chosen from alternatives with thoughtful consideration to the consequences of each alternative. They should be cherished and shared with others. The value should be integrated into one's lifestyle, and actions should be consistent with the values. To help clarify one's values, one may assign priorities to a list of values such as the following:

Affection	Pleasure
Duty	Power
Expertise	Prestige
Family	Security
Health	Self-realization
Independence	Service
Leadership	Spirituality
Parenthood	Wealth

One can also list in order of priority characteristics such as the following:

Ambitiousness	Honesty
Broadmindedness	Imagination
Cheerfulness	Independence
Cleanliness	Logic
Courage	Lovingness
Forgiveness	Responsibility
Helpfulness	

BOX 2-2 Symptoms of Stress
Fatigue Depression Tearfulness Restlessness Nervousness Withdrawal or sudden gregariousness Irritability Anger Feeling of being unloved Insecurity Feeling of vague anxiety Pessimism Self-criticism Frequent frustration Loss of interest in going out Loss of interest in people and things Decrease in self-care Disorganization Inability to relax or rest Accidents Arthritis Asthma Colds Colitis attacks Nightmares Early morning waking Feeling of not being able to get anything done Feeling that everything is too much Forgetfulness Lack of concentration Tendency to be demanding Loss of appetite or overeating Indigestion Constipation or diarrhea Nausea Headaches High blood pressure Rapid pulse Heart palpitation Perspiration Aching neck and shoulder muscles Low back pain Allergy problems Dermatitis Influenza Hives Menstrual distress Ulcers

BOX 2-3 Stress Control Measures
Values clarification Goal setting Time blocking Time management Assertiveness Feeling pauses Inner shouting Anchoring Sorting Thought stopping Compartmentalization Environmental changes Humor Centering Nutrition Exercise Sleep

Goal Setting

Goals should be consistent with one's values, and one should consider goal alternatives. To do this, one considers why a goal is desired. One may want a promotion for recognition or for economic reasons. If the promotion is not forthcoming, one may receive recognition through community service. Money might be generated through wise investments or fees for community services. The achievement of desired outcomes through different approaches increases flexibility and decreases stress caused by unmet goals.

Stress Avoidance and Regulation

When reappraising situations, one should avoid troublesome transactions. The frequency of stress-inducing situations should be minimized. Every change takes energy. Therefore during periods of high stress, routines and habits should be maintained as much as possible. One should be cautious about moving and starting a new job at the same time one is getting a divorce. That also would be a particularly poor time to try to stop smoking or lose weight. Unnecessary changes should be prevented during periods of high stress. Deliberately postponing some changes helps one deal with unavoidable change constructively and reduces the need for multiple adjustments at one time. However, increasing positive sources of tension that foster growth, such as learning a sport, can help offset the deleterious effect of negative tension.

Time Blocking

Time blocking is the setting aside of specific time for adaptation to a stressor. To reduce the stress from having been promoted to a management position, one can set aside time for reading about leadership and management or for observing a leader or manager. This helps ensure that concerns are addressed and tasks accomplished. It decreases anxiety, time urgency, and feelings of frustration. Define off-limit times, and set aside time when one will not be interrupted by phone calls or individuals except for emergencies. Schedule free time and exercise time, and put social events on the calendar like you would a business appointment.

Time Management

Time management helps control stress. Much time can be conserved when one knows one's value system and acts consistently with it, sets goals, and plans strategies for accomplishment of those goals. One can also use organizers such as to-do lists and calendars to plan good use of one's time.

Assertiveness

When one asserts oneself, one increases self-esteem and reduces anxiety, thus reducing stress. As with time management, assertiveness involves thinking through goals and acting consistently with one's values through the use of effective work habits, and by setting limits on others' attempts to block one's goals. It involves stating what one wants and how one feels, making requests, taking compliments, handling put-downs, and setting limits. An assertive person makes eye contact with others; stands straight; sits in an open, listening posture; and speaks in a clear voice. Assertive people choose for themselves and achieve desired goals through self-enhancing behavior that reduces stress.

Feeling Pauses

Feeling pauses are useful. One should take time to identify a feeling, label it, distinguish between thinking and feeling, and accept the feeling for what it is rather than talking oneself into what it should be. One should be aware of both positive and negative feelings and if one is feeling the following positive feelings:

Amusement	Hope
Calmness	Joy
Care	Love
Compassion	Passion
Elation	Relaxation
Excitement	Satisfaction
Forgiveness	Thrill
Happiness	

One should also acknowledge negative feelings, such as the following:

Anger	Fear
Anxiousness	Frustration
Confusion	Hurt
Depression	Jealousy
Embarrassment	Restlessness
Envy	Terror

Then one should determine whether the feeling is appropriate for the situation and decide how to express the feeling in a safe and appropriate way. Feelings can be expressed in "I feel" messages rather than "you" messages that blame or attack others. Feelings can be talked about with an uninvolved person. One can fantasize about how one would like to handle the situation better the next time. Negative feelings may be acted out symbolically by punching a pillow, drawing a picture, or writing a poem. One may set aside negative feelings by getting involved in something pleasant, such as exercise, hobbies, music, television, or talking to a friend. Feelings can also be experienced vicariously by getting involved in another's experience through reading a book, watching a movie, or listening to someone. Pausing to consider feelings can help create new beginnings (Kingsley, 2006).

Inner Shouting

Inner shouting is the process of shouting "I feel . . ." inside one's head or outloud privately. When the person blurts the feeling out spontaneously and publicly rather than saying it quietly inside one's head, adversary confrontation can occur. Anger should be viewed as a symptom. Pains should be focused on helping one take responsibility for feelings of hurt and humiliation; a person can try to humiliate you, but you do not have to feel humiliated. Assertive communication and problem solving can help resolve uncomfortable feelings. When you do…, I feel…. Could you do…? I will do…. One can change oneself but may not be able to change others. Then anchoring can be used to help establish the desired feeling.

Anchoring

Anchors are associated feelings that are initiated either by an event or by the memory of that event. Anchors may be sounds, sights, smells, tastes, or touches that stimulate positive or negative feelings. Birds chirping may remind one of happy, lazy mornings with the family. One may recall an awful accident at the sight of blood. A taste may revive memories of Grandma's home cooking. Our lives are filled with anchors that cause associations. We can use anchoring in a useful way to experience desired feelings. Because touch can be inconspicuous and easy to replicate, one can associate a positive feeling with a familiar touch to the body. This may be as simple as clasping one's hands and being reminded of soft music, beautiful colored glass, and the peaceful sanctuary of church. Pressures at different spots on the body can be conditioned to bring about different feelings. Exact pressure at a very specific spot makes the anchor work most accurately and should be done when one desires to bring back a pleasurable feeling. For example, when one wants to feel peaceful one might condition themselves to hold the palms of their hands together as in prayer. To establish a sense of patience, one might condition themselves to put the right hand over the left hand.

Anchoring is neurolinguistic programming. The anchor is a stimulus that triggers an emotion, and anchoring can create a new response to that stimulus by programming the subconscious to associate the desired feeling with specific words and gestures, which would then trigger the desired feeling. To create an anchor, identify the desired emotional state; think of oneself in that situation as if it were happening at this moment; feel the state build and then decline; repeat that process, but at the peak of the feeling make a unique gesture with the fingers of one hand and say a word or phrase to evoke the feeling before it declines; repeat that gesture and word or phrase at least five times; and then reinforce the gesture and word or phrase periodically to keep the intensity from fading over time (Murphy, 2007).

Sorting

Sorting is choosing the interpretation of an event. One can have an optimistic or pessimistic interpretation of events. Is the glass half full or half empty? We become what we think and therefore can make ourselves happy or miserable. To be happier and more fun loving, one should focus on the positive aspects of situations.

Thought Stopping

Thought stopping helps get rid of negative thinking. Excessive rehearsals in our minds of negative past events are unhelpful thoughts that waste time, reduce self-esteem, and encourage maladaptive behavior patterns. To prepare for thought stopping, one should think of beautiful, pleasant experiences: a sunrise, a waterfall, a flower, a pet, favorite music, baking bread, holding hands. One should also identify not-so-helpful thoughts: I'm stupid; I'm fat; nobody likes me. One should identify the negative thoughts that are most bothersome. In private one can think about a negative thought momentarily and suddenly yell, "Stop!" while clasping one's hands or hitting one's knee or thigh. This is startling, and the thought escapes. Immediately one should replace it with a pleasant thought. If the negative thought returns, the procedure can be repeated. It is reinforced when the negative thoughts are stopped. One can yell, "Stop" out loud, then try whispering, progress to just thinking, and then continue to use whichever works best. Thoughts lead to feelings that can lead to behaviors, so by changing the way one thinks, one can change the way one behaves. Thought stopping should not be used, however, when physical or emotional safety and grieving are involved (Messina & Messina, 2007).

Compartmentalization

Compartmentalization of thought is the deliberate decision to think negative thoughts at specified times of the day. During the allotted time one thinks about worry, guilt, or jealousy. One does not allow oneself to think these thoughts at other times of the day.

Environmental Changes

Environmental changes can be designed to reduce stress. This may be as extreme as changing jobs or residence, or as minor as painting a room a favorite color or adding a picture, candle, or basket. The short time inconvenience of remodeling may be worth the long-term stress reduction. Temporary changes in jobs can add variety and stimulation.

Humor

Humor related to an attitude toward life is most likely to reduce stress. There is a cluster of qualities that characterize this frame of mind, including flexibility, spontaneity, unconventionality, shrewdness, playfulness, humility, and irony. These are qualities that can be developed. Flexibility is the ability to examine all sides of an issue. One should try to look at a situation from several different viewpoints: the boss's, the subordinate's, the client's. Spontaneity is an uninhibited ability to swing from one mood to another. One might practice the body language of several emotions, including fear, anger, sadness, and love. One can free oneself from current values, places, and occupations through unconventionality and imagine living a day as a favorite animal, a famous historical person, an Eskimo, a Native American, or an astronaut. Shrewdness is being clever and artful. A shrewd person may refuse to believe that people or things are what they appear to be. One can think of a list of people and things and give an example of how each is not what it seems to be. Playfulness is the ability to see life as an amusing game. One

can visualize life as a game and give the game a name. One should identify times of various emotions—fun, enjoyment, fear, anger, sadness—and chart wins and losses. Humility is a willingness to question the importance of one's values, ideas, achievements, and existence. One must consider the meaning of one's life and consider how difficult situations have brought happiness, and how happy relationships have included suffering. Irony is the use of words to convey the opposite of their literal meaning and is an incongruity between what might be expected and what actually occurs. For example, when a friend appears in old clothes, one might say, "I see you wore your best clothes."

Centering

Centering helps reduce stress by bringing the mind and body back into balance. With left-sided dominance, intuitive, aesthetic, and creative functions are reduced under stress. To center oneself, one puts one's tongue on the "centering button," which is about one quarter of an inch behind the upper front teeth. This spot apparently stimulates the thymus gland, weakens the effect of stress, and balances the cerebral hemispheres. Other activities that seem to balance the two hemispheres of the brain include reading a poem in a rhythmic fashion; listening to a person with a soothing voice; listening to classical music; listening to natural sounds such as cats purring, birds chirping, or brooks or waterfalls babbling; looking at pictures of pleasant landscapes or smiling people making caring gestures; swinging one's arms during a vigorous walk; and taking a shower. Good posture and deep, slow breathing are also beneficial (Malloy, 2006).

Nutrition

Good nutrition helps maintain the body for full functioning. Eating a balanced diet, taking vitamin supplements, and drinking plenty of water are important. In general, people in the United States need to reduce fat and cholesterol, sugar, salt, and food additive consumption. Diets that contain high levels of fat and cholesterol are abundant in red meats, eggs, cheese, and prepared foods. Excessive consumption of fat is associated with cardiovascular diseases. People are obtaining an increasing proportion of their calories from sugar, which is associated with obesity, tooth decay, diabetes, and heart disease. There is a growing concern that additives and pollutants are related to cancer. Food additives include preservatives, coloring, flavoring, and stabilizers that extend shelf life and make processed food taste better. In addition, pesticides and other chemical pollutants are health hazards.

The increasing consumption of saturated fats and sugar, coupled with a decrease in activity levels, contributes to a widespread occurrence of obesity. In general, people in the United States need to increase exercise while decreasing caloric intake, particularly from fats and sugars. At the same time, the percentage of calories from foods containing fiber, such as fresh fruits, vegetables, and whole grains, should be increased. Canned and frozen prepared foods are usually devoid of their original fiber content and often have sugar and salt added. The grains we eat have often been refined to white flour and rice, thereby losing much of the roughage. Although improving eating habits may not prevent stress, it is one way to maintain the level of fitness needed to fight stress.

Exercise

Regular, vigorous exercise can also help one withstand chronic stress. Aerobic exercise elevates the heart rate during and for a period after the exercise. The range of elevation necessary to produce an aerobic effect is from 60% to 80% of the maximal heart rate the person can achieve, which is calculated at 220 beats per minute minus the person's age in years. Jogging, cycling, and swimming are particularly good aerobic exercises. Dance allows one to stretch and strengthen muscles and to reduce tension.

Regular exercise develops greater capacities in several areas of function. It increases the strength of cardiac contractions, the size of the coronary arteries, the blood supply to the heart,

the size of the heart muscle, and the blood volume per heartbeat. It decreases the heart rate at rest and with exertion and reduces vulnerability to cardiac dysrhythmias. It increases the blood oxygen content, blood volume, and efficiency of peripheral blood distribution and return. Exercise increases the blood supply to the lungs and the functional capacity during exercise. It increases lean muscle mass and functional capacity during exercise. Exercise also reduces strain and nervous tension resulting from psychological stress and reduces the tendency for depression.

Sleep

Sleep is also important for dealing with stress. Sleep needs decrease with age, and people may awaken several times during the night as they grow older. This should not be confused with insomnia, which is a prolonged inability to sleep. There are three types of insomnia: (1) initial, when it takes more than 15 minutes to fall asleep; (2) intermittent, with awakening during the night and difficulty returning to sleep; and (3) terminal, with early morning awakening and inability to go back to sleep.

Physical, emotional, and nutritional factors may contribute to insomnia. A lack of physical exercise, digestive problems, heart trouble, and high blood pressure interfere with sleep. Disturbing emotional states such as anger, fear, guilt, depression, and anxiety create tension that interferes with sleep. An unbalanced diet, alcohol, caffeine consumption, and a large meal shortly before bedtime can interfere with sleep.

To foster a good night's sleep, the day's activities should be tapered off before getting ready for bed. Regular exercise promotes deep sleep but should not be done for several hours before bedtime. Likewise, biofeedback and meditation have stress-reducing properties that foster sleep but should not be done before bedtime because they can boost energy and alertness. Chocolate, cola, coffee, tea, and other foods and beverages containing caffeine should be restricted, particularly in the evening. Overeating, particularly heavy foods, should also be avoided at night.

The bed should be associated with sleep, and the room should be dark and quiet (Scott, 2007).

Relaxation
Abdominal Breathing

Numerous techniques can be used to foster relaxation. Deep breathing is a quick method. When stressed, people tend to breathe in short, shallow breaths. Thus, the lungs do not fill up completely. The remaining air is stale, and oxidation of tissues is incomplete. Muscle tension results. Without being conspicuous, one can take a few abdominal breaths almost anywhere at any time. It is best to do abdominal breathing for 5 to 10 minutes once or twice daily while sitting upright. It may be done during normally quiet times or to reverse the stress response when it has been triggered. To do abdominal breathing, one should inhale slowly through the nose while keeping the back straight. First the abdomen expands, then the chest, and possibly the shoulders. Then one should exhale slowly and hold the breath for 1 or 2 seconds before starting another inhalation (Box 2-4).

Massage

Massage can relieve tension, provide a passive form of exercise, and foster tactile communication. It stimulates relaxation and flexibility. Self-massage can be done from a chair. It can be done as a full-body massage or to a part of the body that is particularly tense. To do a full-body massage, one may start by placing both hands on the top of the head and moving them in slow circular motions down the back of the head, neck, and shoulder area. The neck and shoulder are common sites for tension. They may be most easily massaged by crossing hands over so that the right hand massages the left shoulder and the left hand massages the right shoulder. Then the hands are returned to the top of the head and moved forward in circular motions over the forehead, face, neck, and chest. To relax the right arm, one grasps the fingertips of the right hand with the left hand and moves up the hand and arm to the shoulder in circular motions with the fingers on top and the thumb on the underside. Then one massages down the right side of the chest. The procedure is repeated up the left arm and down the left side. Then hands are placed on the lower abdomen with fingertips touching. Circular motions are used up to the chest.

The lower back is another area that is commonly tense, particularly from sedentary work. One places the hands on the lower back with fingertips touching at the coccyx. The fingertips then massage up as high as one can reach. A foot should be massaged with the massage continuing up the foot, over the ankle, and up the calf and thigh. Then the massage should be repeated on the other foot and leg. This full-body massage can be done after a warm bath at bedtime to foster sleep (Otis, 2002).

Progressive Relaxation

Progressive relaxation may also be used to foster sleep. It is the conscious contraction and relaxation of muscles. By deliberately tensing muscles, one can learn to identify what muscles are tight and learn to relax them. It can be used before, during, or after an anxious situation. If done routinely once or twice daily, it can help keep one's anxiety level down.

Progressive relaxation can be done in a standing, sitting, or lying position. There is greater likelihood of falling asleep in a lying position. In a sitting position, one should keep the head squarely on the shoulders, back against the chair, feet on the floor, legs uncrossed, and hands on the lap in a relaxed position. During progressive relaxation, one tenses specific muscles to a maximal degree and notes how tight the muscles feel for about

---

BOX 2-4 Relaxation Techniques

Abdominal breathing
Massage
Progressive relaxation
Biofeedback
Autogenic training, self-hypnosis
Meditation
Visualization and mental imagery
Poetry
Music
Baths

5 seconds. Then the muscle is relaxed, and the pleasant feeling of relaxation is enjoyed for about 10 seconds. For a head-to-toe progression, one starts by wrinkling up the forehead and noting where it feels particularly tense. Then one relaxes that part slowly, identifies the muscles that are relaxing, notes the difference between tension and relaxation, and enjoys the relaxed feeling (Box 2-5).

With experience in progressive relaxation, one can also learn to relax without tension. One first concentrates on relaxing each body part and then on generalized relaxation with deep breathing. One takes a deep breath, holds it, and then exhales slowly while relaxing the entire body from head to toe, saying "relax" so that the "x" is said as the focus reaches the toes (Center on Aging Studies, The University of Maryland Medical System Corporation, 2001a).

Biofeedback

Biofeedback uses mechanical devices to gain self-regulation to control autonomic responses. The galvanic skin response uses electrodes attached to the fingertips to measure skin resistance, which is moisture of the skin that indicates nervousness. Arteries contract under stress and dilate with relaxation. A thermistor on the finger detects changes in peripheral skin temperature that are associated with activity of the smooth muscles in peripheral arteries. This skin temperature is particularly useful for control of migraine headaches. The electroencephalograph uses electrodes attached to the scalp to detect electrical activity on the brain's cortex. Different brain wave patterns are associated with different states of mind. The electromyograph uses electrodes attached to the forehead or forearm to measure muscle tension from electrical impulses generated by muscles. People with migraine and tension headaches, hypertension, and gastrointestinal problems have responded well to biofeedback. Because the instruments convert skin resistance, skin temperature, brain waves, and muscle tension into readily observable signs, people can tell if they are controlling their body responses or not. They can also learn to read and interpret body signals without the use of instruments to modify their autonomic responses.

Autogenic Training: Self-Hypnosis

Autogenic training produces deep relaxation through self-hypnosis. These regular but brief sessions of passive concentration on physiologically adapted stimuli reduce other extraneous stimuli, and they have helped people with asthma, arthritis, constipation, hypertension, migraine headaches, and sleep disturbances.

To do self-hypnosis, one should lie down with eyes closed in a quiet room and take a few deep breaths. Each autogenic training session should last 2 to 20 minutes, preferably 20 minutes two or three times daily. There are six phrases; when learning autogenic training; only one phrase should be added at a time, one per week, until all six are being used each session.

The first phrase focuses on heaviness, the second on warmth, the third on heartbeat, the fourth on breath, the fifth on solar plexus, and the sixth on the forehead. Supporting phrases such as "I am relaxing" or "I am at peace" are

---

BOX 2-5 Progressive Muscle Relaxation in Sitting Position

Close eyes tightly.
Wrinkle nose.
Place teeth together, and press lips into a forced smile.
Press tongue hard against the roof of the mouth.
Clench teeth.
Pucker lips.
Pull chin toward chest.
Put head back as far as it will go.
Press head to right shoulder.
Press head to left shoulder.
Hold arm out straight, make a fist, and tighten the whole arm or pull elbow tightly into side.
Repeat with the other arm.
Push shoulder blades toward each other.
Pull chest in.
Pull stomach in.
Tighten muscles in lower abdomen, buttocks, and thighs and raise self in the chair.
Push foot against the floor; then point toes toward the head and repeat with the other leg and foot.

interspersed between induction phrases. For the heaviness induction, one systematically concentrates on thinking that each part of the body feels heavy: "My face is heavy. I am relaxing. My neck is heavy. I am at peace. My shoulders are heavy. I am resting. My chest is heavy. I am quiet." For the warmth induction phrase, one substitutes "warm" for "heavy" in the previous phrases. The heart induction phrase is, "My heartbeat is calm and regular." Then one concentrates on "My breathing is relaxed and comfortable." Next one puts one's hands on one's abdomen to create warmth and repeats, "My solar plexus is warm." Finally, one thinks, "My forehead is cool." To return to an alert state, one takes a few deep breaths and thinks, "I will arise refreshed and alert," then moves one's arms and legs, opens one's eyes, and slowly gets up (Manktelow, 2003a; Richmond, 2007).

Meditation

Meditation focuses attention on an experience, helps one become aware of one's response, and facilitates the integration of the physical, mental, emotional, and spiritual aspects of one's life. There are many methods for meditating. One may focus on an object such as a candle or chant, listen to music, or meditate on one's own breath. To meditate on one's breath, one can count while breathing: one on inhalation, two on exhalation, three on inhalation, and four on exhalation. That process can be repeated until the allotted time for meditation is over. Usually people experience an inner calm and sense of well-being from meditation (Calder, 1998).

Visualization and Mental Imagery

Visualization and mental imagery can be used to relax. One starts in a relaxed position and visualizes pleasant thoughts. One can meditate on a visualized colored object such as a blue sky, white cloud, green tree, red apple, or pink flower. One can imagine being in a favorite place such as on a sandy beach, in the mountains, or in front of a fireplace in a favorite room listening to music. One can concentrate on the sights, sounds, smells, tastes, and feelings of the pleasant thoughts (Gawain, 2003; The University of Maryland Medical Corporation, 2001b).

Poetry

Poetry reading or writing is useful for reducing tension, particularly if one is depressed and movement and verbalizing have not worked sufficiently. Poems are chosen for their rhythm, their mood, and the feelings expressed. Poems can be read in a one-to-one or group meeting. Discussions about the meaning can help verbalize feelings.

Music

Soft classical music can help release feelings and emotions and bring about relaxation.

Baths

Water is a relaxant. One should fill the bathtub with water that is body temperature and immerse oneself up to one's neck for about 15 minutes. Hot tubs and swimming pools can also be used for water therapy.

Enhancing Self-Esteem

"You yourself, as much as anybody in the entire universe, deserve your love and affection."
—Buddha

Positive affirmations can be used to enhance one's self-esteem. One can become more comfortable with positive thoughts about oneself and decrease the amount of self-devaluation. Several methods can be used. One might imagine positive scenes and see oneself as one wants to be. One can repeat positive affirmations such as "I am happy," "I am healthy," or "I am beautiful." One can also write positive affirmations on cards, put them in conspicuous places, and read them often. People may take turns making positive comments about each other (Box 2-6).

Support Groups

Support systems are synergistic. Some can accomplish more through support groups than by themselves. Support groups provide a feeling of being accepted, valued, loved, and esteemed, as well as a sense of belonging. In addition to providing emotional support, support systems help provide a social identity and are a source of information, services, and material aid.

Wheatley (2002) says that many people feel isolated or invisible and want to talk about concerns and struggles. Telling our stories creates a relationship and helps us move closer to one another. It's difficult to hate someone whose story we know. Wheatley (2002) encourages the following principles: (1) acknowledging each other as equals, (2) staying curious about each other, (3) recognizing that we need each other's help to become better listeners, (4) slowing down to think and reflect, (5) understanding that conversations are a way to think together, and (6) expecting messiness.

There are several types of support systems. The family is usually the natural support system that constitutes the primary support group. Peer support groups are also important. They are composed of people who have had similar experiences, have adjusted, and want to share their insight. A manager may receive support from other managers or a jogger may receive support from other joggers. Religious organizations provide a congregation that sets guidelines for living, shared values, and provides traditions. Voluntary service groups and self-help groups provide support for specific purposes such as to lose weight, to stop drinking alcohol, to quit smoking, or to adjust to a mastectomy or a stoma. Family, friends, and peers are usually sought out before professional support systems, but the helping professions are available when support from others is inadequate.

It is extremely important that managers take excellent care of their own well-being. They can function at their best if they are healthy. They need considerable energy to be supportive of others and will not have strength to share if they are hurting. Likewise, staff nurses need a sense of health and well-being to provide the best nursing care. Managers are responsible for providing care to the caregivers.

The manager should help protect personnel from undue work-related stress. Personnel may be taught identification of stress symptoms and stress management. Annual physical examinations and vacations could be encouraged or required and possibly provided. Counseling and referral services can be provided as support systems. Nutrition, educational, and health promotional programs can be presented, and nutritious food can be served in the cafeteria. Exercise programs can be provided and encouraged. Leaders and managers should monitor stress levels by asking staff about their stressors periodically and allowing staff to discuss their stressors. Then the leader or manager can explain what support systems are in place, refer staff to appropriate help, and encourage the development of support systems. For example, staff might appreciate the opportunity to buy food at the cafeteria to take home and feed their family to alleviate the stress of having to prepare a meal. Leaders and managers could encourage this if the staff would like that benefit and could alert kitchen personnel to prepare amounts of food accordingly.

Protection from Workplace Violence

Dysfunctional families, anger about illness and dying, disgruntled workers, and subsequently workplace violence are too common. People may express their stress through violence. Sheehan (2000, p. 24) suggests asking the following questions to assess the risk of violence: "Does the patient have a history of aggressive behavior? Does the patient exhibit anger, irritation, or illogical thought processes? Does the patient exhibit confusion and agitation? Does the patient lack emotion or have a dull demeanor?" These questions can also be asked about a patient's family members, visitors, and staff. Then Sheehan recommends the following strategies to reduce the risk (Sheehan, 2000, p. 25):

Establish a zero-tolerance policy for violent behavior. Identify patients with a history of aggressive or violent behavior, and communicate this behavior to staff while maintaining confidentiality. Transfer violent patients to units with higher staffing ratios or with staff trained to deal with violent behavior. Enforce visiting hours and visitor passes. Don't let employees work alone in isolated units or units with walk-in patients. Don't allow employees to be alone with patients during intimate physical examinations. Don't let employees enter seclusion rooms alone.

TIME MANAGEMENT

If productivity were a function of time only, one would expect all to produce equally. And yet, although everyone has the same number of hours in a day and the same number of days per week, some people accomplish more than others. Granted, some people work longer and harder than others to accomplish more, but some just make better use of their time. Because nurses work long hours, they should work smarter—not harder—to get more done in less time.

PERSONAL TIME MANAGEMENT

Covey (1989) said one needs to start by being proactive and accepting responsibility for one's actions and attitudes. The more one exercises freedom to choose responses, the more proactive one becomes. Then opportunities are fed and problems are starved.

Second, one should begin with the end in mind. One should begin with a clear understanding of the desired direction and destination. Things are created mentally before they are created physically. Quality is designed and built in. Ineffective people use old habits and environmental conditions. One may climb the ladder to success only to find once one got to the top that the ladder was against the wrong wall.

Third, put first things first. Personal management is organizing and managing according to personal priorities to get where one wants to go.

It is important to give less time to things that are urgent but not important, such as pressing matters and nonproductive meetings, because they do not have long-term benefits and to spend more time on things that are important but not urgent, such as relationships, prevention, planning, preparation, taking opportunities, and recreation.

Fourth, think win-win. Effectiveness is often accomplished by cooperative efforts of two or more people. A win-win attitude explores options until a mutually satisfactory solution is reached. Desired results, guidelines, accountability, resources, and consequences are made explicit. It is an abundance mentality that builds on synergy rather than a scarcity mentality that leads to win-lose strategies.

Fifth, seek first to understand, then to be understood. Communications are important to building win-win relationships. Our perceptions come from our experiences. Credibility problems usually involve differences. Empathetic listening is therapeutic. Once people feel they are understood, they lower their defenses. Once one understands the other person's point of view, it is easier to arrive at a win-win solution by problem solving.

Sixth, synergize. Synergy comes from teamwork or creative cooperation. Diversity can produce a synergy, where the whole is greater than the sum of its parts. Synergy results from bringing different perspectives together in a spirit of mutual respect to seek the best solution.

Seventh, sharpen the saw. The longer one saws, the duller the saw gets and the harder one works to get less and less accomplished. People need physical, spiritual, mental, social, and emotional self-renewal. One needs to give priority to a balanced program for self-renewal.

Habits involve knowledge, attitudes, and skills. Effective habits can be learned, and ineffective habits can be unlearned. As one practices *The 7 Habits of Highly Effective People*, one is changed from the inside out (Box 2-7).

Covey (1994) taught the six steps to empowerment by putting first things first. Start by connecting to the mission. Write a personal mission

---

BOX 2-7 Personal Time Management

Be proactive
Begin with the end in mind
Put first things first
Think win-win
Seek to understand first
Synergize
Sharpen the saw

From Covey SR: *The 7 habits of highly effective people: Power lessons in personal change*, New York, 1989, Simon & Schuster.

BOX 2-8 Managerial Time Management

Inventory activities
Set goals
Plan strategies
Plan schedules
Say no
Use transition times
Accelerate learning
Improve reading
Do critical thinking
Streamline paperwork
Use computers
Use telephone calls
Schedule office visits
Control visit time
Use meetings effectively
Delegate
Stop procrastinating

---

statement. Identify up to seven roles. Second, review one's roles. Third, identify one's goals related to each role. Concentrate on relationships, prevention, preparation, planning, seizing opportunities, and recreation. Fourth, organize one's week by prioritizing activities to reach one's goals for each role. Schedule one's priorities on the calendar. Fifth, exercise integrity toward the first things in one's life. Start each day by previewing the day, prioritizing, and being sensitive to important commitments. Watch for opportunities to live one's mission. Sixth, evaluate, learn, and live.

Meyer (1993) discussed how to align purpose, strategy, and structure for speed and for working smarter rather than just working faster. He indicated that analyzing strategy and core processes enables management to detect and correct problems earlier and leverage knowledge toward improved innovations and increased value.

MAXIMIZE MANAGERIAL TIME

"From what we get, we make a living; what we give, however, makes a life." —Arthur Ashe

Inventory Activities

Nurse managers may start a plan for maximizing use of their time by conducting an inventory of their activities. After recording what they did every 15 minutes for a typical week, they assess how they spent their time. How much time was spent in which activities? Was the way

the time was spent determined by conscious decisions, habit, work demands, default, or spontaneity? What do they like to do? What activities do they want to increase? What do they want to decrease? How can they reduce the time wasters (Box 2-8)?

Set Goals

Next, nurses determine their short-, medium-, and long-range goals. What does one want to accomplish? What does one want to do soon? Which goals must be completed before others? Which will take the longest to achieve? Setting priorities helps resolve goal conflicts and directs how one will spend time.

Plan Strategies

Once one has determined and ranked the goals, one plans strategies for how to accomplish them. What activities must one do? What are low-priority activities that can be eliminated? Next, the nurse leader or manager schedules activities. A tickler box with divider cards for months and weeks can be used by filing task cards behind the appropriate month and week card. As they look at their major responsibilities for a whole year, nurses may have some flexibility in determining when certain jobs are done and can use the cards to help balance the workload around tasks that have to be done at certain times, such as preparing the budget. Various calendar systems can also be used: one may do major project planning on a year-at-a-glance calendar; desk ink blotters that depict a month at a time can help regulate that month's work; a week-at-a-glance or a day-at-a-glance calendar is convenient for carrying in one's bag or pack. Daily worksheets depicting what work should be done during which hour may also be useful. Commercial planning systems such as Filofax, Franklin Day Planner, Day Runner, and Day Timer are available. Computer software packages are also available for desktop or hand-held computers. Calendars can be on computer systems so that meetings can be scheduled when the most people are available. Computer files of correspondence, reports, or other documents can be stored on the computer in readily retrievable ways (Grohar-Murray & DiCroce, 2003; Marquis & Huston, 2006; Sullivan & Decker, 2005).

Plan Schedule

Nurse leaders and managers need to assess their peak and low times to plan a detailed schedule more effectively. Is one most alert and creative in the early morning or late at night? Is one a slow starter in the morning? Does one reach a low energy point in the middle of the afternoon? The nurse's prime internal time—the most creative time for working alone—is a good time to schedule work that is difficult or should not be interrupted. When is the prime external time, the best time to work with others? If one reaches a low point in the afternoon, that may be a good time to schedule office visits. One may offer guests a cup of coffee or tea, which tends to facilitate communication, sip on one's own drink, and listen.

Time should be set aside for certain activities each day. Scheduled activities are recorded. Scheduled and unscheduled times are noted, and contact and thinking times are identified. The secretary may be given available hours for scheduling office visits.

A few minutes at the beginning of each day should be allowed for planning. A running list of what the nurse manager needs to do in order of importance can be made each morning to plan what will be done that day. Desk-organizing files—which are merely folders with such labels as urgent, return calls, dictate, read, file, and low priority—can help determine what to do each day. Scheduled free time can be used to deal with these activities. A few minutes at the end of the day are used to evaluate what happened.

Say No

Learning how to say no graciously, especially regarding low-priority work, saves time. It is advisable for nurse leaders and managers to acknowledge the request, state and explain their position, check back for understanding with the other person, and avoid defensiveness. For example, when asked to speak at a meeting, one might respond, "I would love to discuss our institutional goals with your committee. However, I have another commitment at that time. Barbara Jones and Sue Smith are both very familiar with the institutional goals. Perhaps you could ask one of them to speak. Does that sound agreeable to you?"

Use Transition Times

Managers can accomplish much during transition times. Incoming mail may be read while one is on hold when returning phone calls. Reports can be read while commuting to and from work, or audiotapes can be listened to while driving. Isometric exercises can be done at almost any time. Lunch and coffee breaks may be used for personal business. Because many people are watching their weight, lunch breaks may include exercise such as walking and jogging, or time for meditation in concert with eating lunch.

Accelerate Learning

Leaders and managers need to be familiar with relevant information. An accelerated learning program includes *clear, realistic learning goals* that can be achieved in days. It is often better to quickly learn and act on the available information in a few days or weeks rather than to wait to retrieve all the information and wait for months or years to act. *Collect the information in one place.* Discard irrelevant and redundant materials, and rapidly skim the rest. Organize the materials into a logical sequence, and use speed-reading techniques to reread it. *Group the material into small study units.* Abstract the study unit information into a short paragraph. *Format the material* into a style you will study repeatedly. *Review the material,* preferably at least twice daily, to quickly comprehend and memorize it. Accelerated learning can help leaders learn a large volume of information without anxiety and overload (Tracy, Rose, 1997).

Improve Reading

Common reading problems include reading one word at a time, rereading, subvocalization of words as one reads, and difficulty concentrating. People usually read a block of words and can increase their speed by increasing the number of words read in each block. One may be able to expand the number of words read in each block by holding the reading material further from the eyes. Pushing oneself to reduce the fixation time to read each block will help one acquire information more quickly. Running a finger, pen, or pencil along the line one is reading can decrease skipping back. The speed of moving the pointer influences the speed of reading. So reading more words in each block, reducing the time to read each block, and using a pointer to smooth the way the eyes move over the reading reduce skipback and help increase reading speed and concentration (Manktelow, 2003b).

It helps to know what one needs to know to select the appropriate reading material. The table of contents, indexes, and glossaries can help locate desired information. Then one needs to consider how deeply to study the content. Skimming material is appropriate for shallow knowledge; scanning can be used for moderate knowledge; and studying for detailed knowledge. To read in detail, it helps to skim the reading first to get an overview and an understanding of the structure. It is appropriate to highlight or underline important information to review it later

and to keep one's mind focused on the material. Photocopying may be considered if the text is borrowed or should not be marked up.

Different types of documents have different depths and breadths of information in different places. News articles generally have the most important information first and then fleshes it out in more detail later. Opinion articles present the author's point of view first, support the argument in the middle, and repeat the most important information in the summary. Usually the most important information in feature articles is in the body of the text.

One can create a table of contents for what one is reading if it is not already provided. Mind mapping is another useful way to take notes to consolidate and summarize information and think through complex information. To develop a mind map, write the title of the subject in the center of a page and draw a circle around it, then draw lines out from the circle and label subheadings. Link another level of information to lines of the appropriate subheadings. For individual ideas or facts, draw lines out from the appropriate topic. One can use single words, simple phrases, symbols, and images, and can color code different ideas. A line can be drawn to connect information in one part of the mind map that is related to other information to show the association. Mind maps can help people make associations; people therefore may remember the picture better than they can remember conventional notes (Centre for Independent Language Learning, 2007; Manktelow, 2003c).

Improve Memory

Listening and memory techniques also save time. When listening for understanding, one should assume value in what the speaker is saying by being attentive, delaying judgment, maintaining eye contact if culturally appropriate, and using attentive body language. One then needs to assess the content of the information by focusing on central ideas, looking for relationships between ideas, and selecting an organizing structure such as main and supporting ideas, advantages and disadvantages, or putting information into chronological order. One should analyze the information by listening to what is being said, identifying how it is being said by inferring emotions from body language and tone of voice, and considering the speaker's motivation for saying it. Distractions may have to be reduced so the listener can concentrate.

Verbal, physical, and mental techniques can be used to stimulate memory (Box 2-9). Repeating, clarifying, and summarizing are effective verbal techniques. Physical techniques for stimulating memory are note taking, filing, and follow-up memos. Focusing, linking, imaging, locating, and chunking are mental techniques. Mnemonics are devices such as formulas or rhymes that assist memory.

Focusing by putting attention on one thing at a time helps block out distractions. Forming acronyms by using the first letter of the words to be remembered to form a new word can be helpful.

Linking is a common memory technique that makes associations between things that make them easier to remember later. One codes information to be remembered into images and then links the images together. Associations may be cause and effect, parts of a whole, or things that are near each other, logically go together, contrast with each other, or happen concurrently. Creating an association that leads from point one to point two to point three and creating an image of those associations will help one remember a speech. One may remember the steps in a procedure by visualizing them. The image in the mind is easier to remember than a list of steps in a procedure manual.

BOX 2-9 Memory Techniques

VERBAL
Repeating
Clarifying
Summarizing follow-up memos

PHYSICAL
Note taking
Filing

MENTAL
Focusing
Linking
Imaging/locating
Chunking

Linking information to a sequence helps ensure that one does not forget part of the information. One may begin by linking rhymes to numbers like 1 for fun, 2 blue, 3 tree, 4 more, 5 hive, 6 sticks, 7 heaven, 8 late, 9 mine, and 10 hen. Then one links those images to the sequence to be remembered. For example, if one wants to recall the sequence 515, you would link together hive-fun-hive. One imagines playing with hives, having fun, and then getting hives from the hive, which helps one remember 515. The sillier and more nonsensical the image, the easier it is to remember. This is also known as a peg system, pegging, or linking ideas to a known sequence.

Shapes can also be pegged to numbers like 1 for stretcher, 2 curved neck, 3 heart, 4 sail, 5 big belly on body, 6 tennis racket, 7 edge of bed, 8 hour glass, 9 big head, 10 open mouth. One can also mix the rhymes and shapes. Images can also be pegged to the alphabet. It is best to choose the strongest image and use it rather than change the images.

Imaging creates a vivid mental image that helps one remember something by strengthening associations. For example, when introduced to Leona Dean, the nurse might picture her leaning on a dean of a specific school to help remember her name. Roman room is a technique used to store lists of unlinked information. One associates images that one wants to remember with images in a room. To recall the information, one just takes a tour around the room again in one's mind and visualizes the known objects with the associated information. Other rooms can be used to store other information.

Locating is a memory technique that uses a known structure, often one's home, to arrange and remember information by putting it in specific locations. One might progress through an orientation program by visualizing the hallway in the office and thinking of who is in each office as one walks through the hall and what service that person provides for new staff. The journey method combines the narrative of the link method with the structure of peg systems.

Chunking helps one remember by dividing large amounts of information into smaller, more manageable pieces. One could chunk information needed into separate sections of a report, or the nurse could locate what items are needed in specific, separate offices. One can find information about memory techniques by looking up mnemonics or memletics on the Internet. There are many additional techniques (Manktelow, 2003d).

Critical Thinking

Critical thinking is needed to excel in the information age. It is a reflective problem-solving style of thinking. One should *focus on the right questions,* define terms, and list critical issues. *Analyze arguments* by identifying and examining assumptions, positions, reasons, and conclusions. *Question, challenge,* and *clarify* by asking who, what, when, where, and why questions. Distinguish between facts and inferences, relevant from irrelevant, and similarities from differences. Because one understands that feelings influence thoughts and thoughts influence feelings, it is important to consider what those feelings and thoughts are. Request more information as needed. *Judge the credibility of the sources.* Consider the reputation, expertise, and possible conflicts of interest of the source. *Use logic,* including inductive and deductive reasoning. Evaluate the related research. *Use high-level thinking strategies,* such as analyzing, clarifying, comparing, inferring, and problem solving.

Avoid faulty thinking such as overgeneralization, use of selected cases instead of a wide-based foundation of facts, and use of inadequate sources. Emotion-laden words that elicit strong emotions can camouflage weaknesses. Highly ambiguous language and poorly defined terms can lead to multiple interpretations. Unrelated and irrelevant points can cause distractions from the key points of an argument. Repetition in a variety of places by a number of people becomes more believable regardless of its truthfulness. Acceptable statements make unacceptable conclusions more believable. Expert opinion is not necessarily the truth. Denigration of opponents is sometimes used to discredit another's arguments, so conclusions should be separated from the person presenting the issues (Paul et al, 1990).

Streamline Paperwork

Much time can be saved by streamlining paperwork. Scheduling a block of time to answer mail prevents interruptions. If the situation warrants, a standard reply can be used. Some responses can be made on the query memo if no file copy is needed, or in a query e-mail that can be saved in a computer file as necessary. Keeping as little as possible and only what is needed saves time. Color coding is useful, and recording the destruction dates on files reduces the need to review the materials later. Dictation usually takes less time than writing by hand, and calls can be used when a record is not necessary. Computerization and e-mail also save time. Invisible information (spoken word) can be recorded on a steno pad kept by the phone with each page dated sequentially. Unfortunately that information is difficult to move to priority areas. A spiral-bound message pad with no carbon required can be used to tear off the top sheet and send wherever needed while still keeping a chronological record. The disadvantage is that there is little space for writing on the form. Recycled paper by each phone can be used when a permanent record is not needed. Some calendar systems have forms for recording conversations and can be treated like phone message sheets. Selective reading by scanning the table of contents in documents and reading summaries at the end of long responses and reports saves time. Managers should not concentrate on details unless necessary, because they are quickly forgotten. Scanning for major points is often adequate.

Use Computers for Time Management

Computers can replace a hodgepodge of record-keeping procedures with a uniform system. With the use of a computer, printer, and accounting or accounts payable software, information can be entered one time into a database and sent electronically anywhere that the technology is available. A graphic interface program can merge a computerized mailing list of names and addresses into letters, address envelopes and mailing labels, do mathematical calculations on the screen while the letter is being composed, spell check the entire document, identify more interesting words using the on-screen thesaurus, print out multiple copies, make global changes in all documents if the letter is revised, and preview the letter on the screen before printing it. It can also check a calendar for a date or schedule an appointment; set an alarm for the appointment; dial a phone number; send and receive faxes; calculate figures; address envelopes; create a macro of often-used addresses or phrases; create, save, and delete files; and locate a file and insert it into another document. Computer software can be used to organize projects and keep and track the progress relative to performance objectives. Files should be saved frequently and backed up on a hard drive, compact disc, thumb drive (also flash drive), or tape. Computer files can duplicate the paper files. Clutter should be removed from both computer and paper files. Portable printers and fax machines or a phone jack and a fax-modem board inside a portable computer allow receiving and sending data anywhere the technology is available, as do wireless connections.

Use Telephone Calls

Telephone calls instead of office visits or correspondence save time. Secretaries can screen calls so that other activities are not interrupted and, in fact, may be able to handle much of the business. A call-back system can be used to complete the business the secretary cannot handle. If late morning and late afternoon are chosen for returning calls, calls are likely to be kept short, because people are eager to eat lunch or to go home.

Paging and beeping systems, call forwarding, call back, call waiting, speed dialing, three-way calling, voice mail, and conference calls make telephoning more efficient. A cell or portable phone allows one to move around and work while using the telephone. Mobile phones can be used at the patient's bedside or while walking between patients.

Forms for telephone messages are less likely to get lost than scraps of paper. It is helpful for phone messages to be collected in one place. A secured pen or pencil by the phone is convenient. One should keep a list of commonly called phone numbers handy. If major topics for conversation are outlined before making a call, it is less likely that one will forget something and need to call back. One can set the tone of the call. A business-like call started by "What can I do for you?" will accomplish more in less time than a friendly call started with "How are you?" Conference calls also save time by focusing more on business than socializing. The purpose for the conversation helps determine whether a meeting or a conference call is necessary.

Schedule Office Visits

Secretaries may also screen office visits. Again, the secretaries may be able to handle much of the business themselves. When leaders or managers schedule reception hours, secretaries can schedule appointments for the appropriate length of time and inform leaders and managers of the purpose of the meeting so that they can be adequately prepared. One may need to close the office door to complete a task without interruptions. Sitting with one's back to the door may decrease interruptions because people will note that the manager is busy.

Control Visit Time

The length of a meeting can be better controlled if it is not in the manager's office. Managers may go to the staff's work area or meet visitors in a reception area, where they are free to leave whenever they think it is appropriate. By standing up when someone drops into the manager's office, managers prevent the visitor from sitting down, thus controlling the situation. They can assess the priority, make an appointment for another time, keep the visit short, or invite the visitor to sit down for a longer discussion. Many drop-in visits can be prevented by scheduling lunch with staff members on a regular basis. This allows the manager an opportunity to keep informed, discuss matters of common interest, and eat lunch at the same time. Staff can be informed through memos and routing slips.

Use Meetings Effectively

Managers spend considerable time in meetings, much of which is wasted. Meetings are used for participative problem solving, decision making, coordination, information sharing, and morale building. Managers should first consider the purpose of the meeting; if it is not necessary, they should not conduct it. Key participants are identified, and if they cannot attend, the meeting should be cancelled. People who do not need to attend should not be invited. Managers should consider alternatives to a meeting, such as a memo, telephone call, or conference. Staff associates can represent the manager at some meetings both to save managerial time and to develop the staff associates. Managers may limit their time in meetings by attending only that segment when they are to make a contribution. Scheduling meetings before lunch and quitting time facilitates ending meetings on time. A centrally located meeting place saves travel time. The purpose of the meeting should be clearly defined, and an agenda should be circulated before the meeting.

The agenda is the order of business and should have a title for the meeting. It should state the date, time, and place of the meeting. Organizations and businesses may prescribe the topics or format to be used to set agendas, such as a call to order, approval of minutes from the last meeting, officer and standing committee reports, special committee reports, unfinished business, new business, and adjournment. The chairperson can develop an agenda that identifies the person responsible for each topic. For example, committees may be listed under committee reports, and the chairperson of a committee may be identified as the person who is to give that committee's report. That way people know in advance that they are responsible and can come to the meeting prepared to present and with the appropriate materials. The chairperson can also identify timelines as guidelines. The time allowed for the report can be recorded to the right of the presenter's name. That helps keep the meeting on time. A specific time may be identified for when a topic will be discussed, so interested parties will know which portion of the meeting to attend (Huber, 2006; Robert et al, 2000).

Meetings may be primarily for information giving or for discussion, brainstorming, and problem solving. For the first type an agenda with the topic, presenter, and time frame works well. A less structured agenda is needed for discussion and problem solving as people need to be encouraged to express their thoughts and feelings freely. Covey (2004) stresses the importance of finding one's voice to express one's thoughts and feelings and helping others find theirs. One first finds one's own voice and unique significance and appreciates others' potential. Then one helps others find their voices and creates an environment of engagement by developing trust and a shared vision. That facilitates the evolution from "my voice" and "your voice" to "our voice."

Meetings should start on time, because time is expensive. Starting a meeting 15 minutes late for 20 people who earn $30 an hour costs $150 in downtime. Stating the purpose of the meeting and following the agenda are the manager's responsibilities. The leader or manager should start with high-priority items so that only low-priority items will be left over. The leader or manager should control interruptions, restate conclusions, make assignments and deadlines clear, and end the meeting on time. If the business is completed early, the leader or manager dismisses the meeting. Minutes are circulated preferably within 1 day after the meeting; this allows people to be informed without having to attend the meeting unless their input is specifically needed. Minutes also remind participants of their assigned tasks (Ellis & Hartley, 2004).

Delegation

The leader or manager decides what task should be done when, where, and by whom. Responsibility and authority should be assigned. The leader or manager needs to evaluate the risk involved in delegating by assessing the criticality of the expected results and the confidence in resources. The planning strategy ascertains specifications, including the expected results, rationale, requirements, and constraints. The delegated authority should be specified, and support needed should be anticipated. When communicating the delegated assignment, the leader or manager should ensure understanding, give and receive feedback, and address concerns. To monitor the delegated assignment, the leader or manager should set up a milestone-tracking system, review scheduled status reports, and give feedback on the interim reports. Support is provided by responding to the delegatee's needs, acknowledging the status reports, and being available for guidance and problem solving. The leader or manager should intervene only when the action seems warranted and, even then, by avoiding interference and explaining one's actions. Reverse delegation should be avoided by clarifying specifications, transferring authority, and expressing confidence in the delegatee. The results should be evaluated by examining the specifications, evaluating the monitoring results, and giving feedback on the final results.

Establishing routines improves learning curves, success, and productivity. Routines can reduce tension, errors, and wasted time. The leader or manager decides what to delegate, selects the appropriate person, communicates the responsibilities to that person, grants authority with the responsibility, provides support, monitors the situation, and evaluates the results (Sullivan & Decker, 2005).

Reasons for Delegating

Delegation saves time and can help develop others. Delegation maximizes the use of the talents of staff associates. It can build trust and increase self-esteem, pride, and job satisfaction. It uses latent abilities in personnel that contribute to their growth and development. Staff members learn by doing. Their involvement tends to increase their management skills, motivation, and commitment to accomplish goals while increasing group cohesion. It helps identify future leaders and managers and frees the manager to manage. This also reduces managerial costs (Box 2-10).

Five Rights of Delegation

The five rights of delegation are (1) task, (2) circumstance, (3) person, (4) direction/communication, and (5) feedback/supervision. The right

---

BOX 2-10 Reasons for Delegating

Saves time
Helps develop others
Builds trust
Increases self-esteem
Increases pride
Increases job satisfaction
Uses latent talent
Develops skills
Increases managerial skills
Helps identify future leaders
Increases motivation
Increases commitment to goals
Increases group cohesion
Frees manager's time
Reduces managerial costs

---

task should be within the scope of the person's practice and consistent with the job description. In addition, organizational structure, policies, procedures, and standards should be considered. Staff should not be assigned an activity outside their defined role or something they have not been taught. To achieve the right circumstance, the health status and complexity of the care needed should be matched to the skill of the staff member assigned the delegation (National Council of State Boards of Nursing, 1995).

The right person should have the appropriate license or certificate, an appropriate job description, and a demonstrated skill that is to be checked off on the skill checklist before the skill is delegated to that person. Registered nurses can delegate activities of daily living such as positioning, bathing, grooming, dressing, ambulating, toileting, and feeding to unlicensed assistive personnel. The unlicensed assistive personnel can also do bedmaking, take vital signs, measure intake and output, and do some specimen collection. A registered nurse can delegate updating the RN assessment of a patient; teaching from the care plan; administering medications; initiating and maintaining intravenous lines, blood transfusions, and in some states IV push and IV piggyback medications; removing stitches; and inserting feeding tubes to licensed practical/technical nurses (Handel, 2007).

The right direction/communication should be clear, concise, complete, and correct. It should specify the activities to be performed, the expected results, timelines, and follow-up communications. The right feedback should ask for input, get the person's recommended solution to the problem, and recognize the person's efforts. The registered nurse may give direct or indirect supervision when that responsibility is delegated to another licensed nurse. The manager should monitor the performance, give and receive feedback, intervene if necessary, and confirm clear documentation (Box 2-11).

Delegation Decision-Making Process

A National Council of State Boards of Nursing (1995) position paper described the assessment, planning, implementation, and evaluation of delegation. First, the Nurse Practice Act should permit the delegation, authorize the task or tasks to be delegated, and authorize the nurse to decide delegation. The delegator needs the appropriate education, skills, and experience; the appropriate scope of authority; and demonstrated and documented evidence of current competency.

The delegator needs to assess the needs of the patient, the circumstances, and availability of adequate resources. Then the delegator needs to plan for the task or tasks to be delegated by specifying the knowledge and skills required to do each task, by requiring documented or demonstrated current competency to do each delegated task, and by determining the implications for the patient and others. To ensure appropriate accountability, the delegator accepts accountability for the performance of the delegated task or tasks and verifies

that the delegatee accepts the delegation and accountability for the delegated task or tasks. Then the delegator supervises performance of the task by providing directions and clear expectations about how the task or tasks are to be performed; monitoring the performance to ensure compliance to established standards of practice, policies, and procedures; intervening as necessary; and ensuring documentation of the task or tasks. Finally, the delegator evaluates the delegation process, evaluates the patient and the performance of the task or tasks, and receives and gives feedback. The delegator adjusts the plan as necessary (Hansten, 2004; Sullivan & Decker, 2005).

Conditions That Facilitate Delegation

Several conditions facilitate delegation. First, leaders and managers need to understand the concept of delegation and have a generally positive attitude toward people. They need to overcome feelings of loss of prestige through delegation and develop a positive atmosphere for their staff. They should help achieve results through effective communication instead of by doing the job themselves. Thus they concentrate on the accomplishment of overall goals and objectives rather than the day-to-day details.

Top leaders clarify policies, goals, and objectives, and these are further developed by each succeeding lower level. For example, top management sets the overall budget, but each department then works with its own budget. Specifying goals and objectives directs personnel and determines priorities and the use of resources. Management by objectives promotes this.

Job descriptions provide a definition of the responsibility and authority involved with each position. Everything that must be done for the organization to meet its goals is part of someone's job. Thus, job descriptions are based on the functional needs of the agency and clarify the responsibility of the individual's position and the objectives of the work.

Before writing job descriptions, management decides which assignments to delegate. To do

---

BOX 2-11 Five Rights of Delegation

Task
Circumstance
Person
Direction
Feedback

so, leaders and managers should be aware of the capabilities and characteristics of their staff associates. Testing employees to ascertain what can and cannot be done and providing the necessary training help overcome many personnel failures. Staff members are often not qualified to do nor interested to do certain tasks. People tend to put off tasks they find unpleasant and then do the tasks poorly. It is not necessary to delegate equally. By knowing individual capabilities, the leader or manager can delegate according to the member's interests and abilities.

Job descriptions are not always advantageous in small or rapidly changing organizations because those staffs often assume different roles at different times. Generalization is more common than the specialization required in larger, more stable organizations. Some employees outperform the requirements of their job descriptions, whereas others are not able to do some of the duties described. Job descriptions can be redefined according to the person's capability, individual profiles, and organizational needs. If employees are unable to handle the required duties, they may be transferred to another area, given further training, supplied with an assistant to supplement their weak areas, or fired.

Controls based on goals, rather than means, are important. The leader or manager checks on how well the delegated responsibilities are being performed, and the staff know whether or not they are meeting their responsibilities. Performance standards clarify how the leader or manager measures achievement. These standards cover the quantity and quality of work expected and the time allowed for its accomplishment. The standards should be broad enough to allow individuality. If the standards are perceived as reasonable and fair by both the leader or manager and staff, both will be happier with the jobs. Staff like their work to be noticed and appreciated. The leader or manager meets the need for recognition and appreciation by having a general knowledge of what is happening, using an open door policy, expressing willingness to give assistance and support, and taking a personal interest in the problems. A "snoopervisor," however, is not appreciated.

It is the leader's or manager's responsibility to assess the results of delegation. One of the most satisfactory ways of being aware of what is happening is by being among the staff members. Formal and informal meetings, systems of reporting, quality control, and statistical sampling are other means. Although inspection is perceived as unpleasant, most staff associates accept it as necessary. However, people do object to unnecessary inspections that disturb routines.

Even though one may receive satisfaction from knowing that one is doing a good job, having those efforts recognized by others is appreciated. A leader or manager errs if one does not give praise for work well done. People should also be rewarded for their continued contributions to the agency through raises and promotions. If a staff associate errs, the person should be corrected as soon as possible. But when staff associates participate in goal setting, when the emphasis is on the goal rather than individual personalities, and when training is a continuous process, corrections that otherwise would have been made by the leader or manager may be unnecessary. The system encourages self-correction.

Learning to live with differences may be difficult for leaders and managers, especially if the leader or manager once performed the staff's tasks and now finds that the tasks are being done differently. It is even more threatening when the staff does a better job than the manager once did. It has to be recognized that there will be differences in quantity and quality of work accomplished and methods used between the leader or manager and staff or between staff.

Responsibility, Authority, and Accountability

Assignment of responsibility, delegation of authority, and creation of accountability are the three concepts most often mentioned in relation to the delegation process (Box 2-12). Responsibility denotes obligation. It refers to what must be done to complete a task and the obligation created by the assignment. The leader or manager and the staff member must understand the activities for which the staff member is responsible, what results are

BOX 2-12 Aspects of Delegation

Responsibility
Authority
Accountability

expected, and how performance is to be evaluated. Leaders and managers need a clear idea of what is to be done before they can communicate to others. To clarify ideas for themselves, leaders and managers may put their ideas in writing. By so doing, the leaders and managers are less likely to give incomplete directions. The assignment of responsibility is not complete, however, until the staff decides to accept the obligation.

Authority is the power to make final decisions and give commands. People to whom responsibility has been assigned need the authority to direct the performance of delegated duties. People need authority of sufficient scope to include all related activities without frequent consultation with the leader or manager. The granting of too little authority is a common problem, because organizational policies and procedures are often limiting, and sometimes the person may have little control over the actions of others.

People with delegated authority perform for the leader or manager. Although authority is delegated so that the staff can fulfill their responsibilities, the leader or manager maintains control over the delegated authority and may recall it. Delegation of authority involves the staff's knowledge, abilities, skills, and potential contribution and the leader's or manager's guidance. During the initial phase of delegating authority, staff presents ideas and plans. The leader or manager raises questions, explores alternatives, and helps identify potential problems and ways to prevent them. Then mutual agreement is reached. The leader or manager offers continuing support by providing staff, resources, and information needed by the staff for the completion of the delegated responsibility. Good communications, sharing of information and feedback, are important.

Accountability refers to liability. Staff incurs an obligation to complete work satisfactorily and to use authority appropriately when they accept delegated responsibility. They are accountable to their leader or manager. Leaders and managers are accountable for the performance of the task, the selection of the person to complete it, and both the staff's and the leader's or manager's own performance. Managers are responsible for delegation to team leaders, who are accountable for delegation to team members. Each remains accountable for the work delegated (Marquis, Huston, 2006).

Cultural Considerations for Delegation

Communication is affected by culture. Context of speech, dialect, kinesics (stance, gestures, eye movement), use of touch, and volume have cultural variables and influence how one is perceived. Delegation given in a soft voice may not be considered as important as directions given in a louder tone. A quiet, passive worker may be perceived as unable to do the work. Asian Americans and Native Americans may be more quiet while Hispanic Americans may be more verbally expressive.

Interpersonal space varies among cultures and within cultures with French, African Americans, and Hispanics often being comfortable with closeness and middle class Caucasian Americans tending to want 2 to 3 feet of personal space. Asian Americans are likely to prefer formal space except for family and close friends. They usually do not touch during conversations and it is not acceptable to touch members of the opposite sex. Native Americans often want personal space and use a light touch of another's hand as a greeting while European Americans are likely to use a firm hand shake for a greeting. Hispanic Americans tend to value physical presence, are very tactile, and use embraces and handshakes.

Past, present, and future orientations vary among cultures and within cultures. European Americans tend to value the future, time, and tend to be on time. Asians, Hispanics, and Native Americans tend to value the past and the elderly but focus on the present. Depending on age and socio-economic situation, African Americans may be past, present, or future oriented. They may be late because they value relationships more than time. The same is true for the Hispanic culture. People with a past orientation may be particularly good for having elderly people reminisce, but a future-oriented person will be better adapted for strategic planning.

Social organization differs among cultures. Some are more individualistic, and others are more family oriented. African Americans tend to appreciate large extended family networks. Households are often headed by a single-parent woman. The elderly are usually respected. Church affiliation and religious beliefs are often a source of strength.

Asian Americans tend to be devoted to the traditional family unit hierarchical structure. Men often have the power and authority while women are expected to be obedient. Education is highly valued. Religions may include Taoism, Buddhism, Islam, and Christianity, among others. Social organizations are strong in Asian American communities.

Hispanic Americans tend to value the nuclear and extended family. The needs of the family tend to take precedence over the individual's needs. The older, less acculturated men are the decision makers and bread winners while the women are the homemakers and caretakers. Hispanics usually have strong church affiliations and strong social organizations within the Hispanic community.

Native Americans are often family oriented, have extended families, and the grandparents are sometimes considered the family leaders. Elders are honored and children are taught to respect traditions. Myths and legends give spiritual guidance and religion and healing practices are integrated into their culture. The father tends to work outside the home while the mother is responsible for the homemaking. Community social organizations are usually important to Native Americans.

Americans of white European origin value the nuclear and extended family. Traditionally the man is the dominate figure, but there are variations. Judeo-Christian beliefs are common and community social organizations are often considered important.

Some cultures are more individualistic, and others more family oriented. People also differ in internal and external control, with some thinking people can control the environment and others leaving that to fate, luck, or God's will. There are also biopsychosocial differences, putting some people at more risk for some conditions than others. It is important to be cognizant of cultural differences among individuals within a culture as well as among cultural groups because these differences can affect the relationship between the delegator and delegatee (Huber, 2006; Marquis, Huston, 2006; Silvestri, 2005). When problems arise, one should use these ideas on culture as guidelines to take the opportunity to learn more about another's culture and promote cultural competence. This tends to also increase self understanding.

Reasons for Underdelegating

There are numerous reasons for underdelegating. Leaders and managers may think they can do the job more quickly themselves, resent interruptions to answer questions, or not want to take the time to check what has been done. They may get cooperation from other departments more easily than from staff associates or be unwilling to take risks for fear of being blamed for others' mistakes.

Some leaders and managers do not have confidence in the staff associates and are afraid that the staff associates will not keep the leaders and managers adequately informed. Or the leader or manager may not trust the staff associates and complain about a lack of training and sufficient experience. Leaders and managers may argue that the staff associates have little understanding of the organizational objectives and are specialists without the general knowledge needed for problem solving. In some cases, someone may even be afraid that the staff associates will outperform the leader or manager.

Therefore some leaders and managers may like to do the work and think that will get the work done better. Some receive personal recognition for and satisfaction from the work and prefer to do the real things instead of just plan with others. Such people often expect perfection, consider themselves indispensable, and desire to dominate. Some are afraid of losing power and prestige and are aware that poor operating procedures and practices may be exposed.

Reasons for not Accepting Delegation

Staff has their reasons for not accepting delegation. Some depend on the leader or manager and find it easier to ask the boss. Others lack self-confidence and fear failure and criticism. This fear is often related to how mistakes have been handled. Emphasis on the mistake itself is more threatening than using the situation as a learning experience.

Lack of guidelines, standards, and control are additional problems. Duties are not always clearly defined, authority is not specified, or necessary information and resources are not readily available. Some staff is already overworked. The incentives are inadequate, and they do not want to perform work if the leader or manager receives the credit. Good delegation is not dumping, which is giving employees repetitive, mundane work that feels like being a "gofer" instead of doing something of value that helps develop the person (McConnell, 2006). Procrastinators may not do what was delegated.

PROCRASTINATION

"What we see depends mainly on what we look for." —Sir John Lubbock

Reasons for Procrastination

Reasons for procrastination may be divided into two basic categories: emotional reasons and non-emotional reasons (Box 2-13).

Emotional Reasons

There are several emotional causes of procrastination. People may fill present moments with trivia to escape an overwhelming task or choose a pleasant task to escape an unpleasant one. Procrastination can be used as an excuse for poor

---

BOX 2-13 Reasons for Procrastination

EMOTIONAL
To escape an overwhelming task
To escape an unpleasant deadline
To excuse poor work
To gain sympathy
To get someone else to do the job

NONEMOTIONAL
Lack of goals
Goals without time estimates
Unrealistic time estimates
Insufficient information
Inadequate follow-up
Overcommitment

---

work with comments such as "I just couldn't get to it until the last minute." Some play victims of circumstances to gain sympathy. Although it is preferable to delegate than to play "poor me," there are those who try to get someone else to do the job through procrastination.

Nonemotional Reasons

Lack of goals, goals without deadlines, and unrealistic time estimates are some reasons for procrastination. Some people have insufficient information to do a job, do inadequate follow-up, or have so many interruptions they cannot get a job done. Others are just so overcommitted that they do not have time to do everything they have agreed to do.

Techniques to Stop Procrastination

Dividing and conquering, or breaking a large job down into smaller, more manageable tasks, is a good way to overcome procrastination. Doing a start-up task to get in the mood and taking advantage of moods help. Starting with what one does not like to do and the highest priorities and giving oneself incentives are helpful. Considering the consequences of not doing the job can motivate some people into action.

Consider using the money one will earn by doing things one likes to do to hire someone to do what one does not like to do. Consider switching jobs with someone, or divide up the job so one can do what one likes to do, such as the review of the literature, while someone else does what that person likes to do, such as the statistical analysis of the data. Make a commitment to someone or a wager to help overcome procrastination (Yoder-Wise, 2007). It is appropriate to ask yourself, "What's the best use of my time now?" Then set goals, plan realistic time schedules, and gather the necessary information to do the job. Avoid over commitment and reward oneself for jobs well done (Box 2-14).

MAXIMIZE ORGANIZATION TIME

Plan

Much time can be saved through appropriate organizational planning. The purpose for the existence of the agency should be determined, and the goals and objectives should be defined and ranked in order of importance. Nurse leaders and managers determine who is responsible for coordinating activities, who makes what decisions, and who needs to be informed about certain decisions. Management also determines what decisions need to be made before others, what action needs to be taken first, and what deadlines must be set. The determining and ranking of goals focus activities and prevent people from spending time doing inappropriate or unimportant tasks.

BOX 2-14 Techniques to Stop Procrastination

Break a large job down into smaller tasks.
Do a start-up task.
Take advantage of your moods.
Consider the consequences of not doing the job.
Consider hiring someone to do the task.
Consider switching jobs with someone.
Divide up the job to do what one likes to do.
Make a commitment to someone or a wager with someone.
Set goals.
Set realistic time schedules.
Gather necessary information.
Avoid over-commitment.
Give yourself rewards.

People who are adequately informed of what is expected do not waste time wondering what needs to be done. Making time estimates and setting time limits help regulate work flow. Through appropriate planning, problems can be prevented. The decreased amount of time spent in crisis management increases the time available for creative work.

Organize

The leaders and managers structure the agency to accomplish the tasks necessary to meet the agency's goals. Organizational charts help clarify who is responsible to whom and for what. Job descriptions further clarify these matters. Multiple bosses, confusion over who is responsible and who has authority for what, and duplication of tasks can be prevented with planning. Autonomy and independence reduce the amount of time otherwise spent in conflict management. Policies and procedures help clarify expectations.

Staff

Selection of well-qualified staff is critical for time saving because they require less supervisory time for development and corrective action. Staff development further reduces time lost by better preparing staff to do their jobs. Appropriate use of personnel through assessment of work to be done, careful planning of the number and mix of personnel, and matching staff members' interests and abilities to the job further reduce waste. When nurses' interests are matched to the organizational goals and people feel appreciated, staff is likely to have increased job satisfaction. Consequently there is little absenteeism and fewer turnovers. Nurse leaders and managers should watch for chronic absenteeism, try to determine the reason, and correct it. Leaders and managers also expect punctuality, because tardiness is a loss of time and money. If nurse managers find that employees' personal problems are affecting the work, the leader or manager should refer personnel for appropriate assistance.

Direct

It is the nurse leader's and managers' responsibility to delegate what a less qualified, lower-paid person can handle. The leader or manager identifies the task to be delegated, determines the best person to do the job, and communicates the assignment clearly. The leader or manager allows the staff member to help determine how the task will be accomplished and keep authority commensurate with responsibility. The leaders and managers set controls, monitor results, and provide support as needed. It is essential that leaders and managers teach others how to do the work instead of doing it themselves. Considerable time can be saved by streamlining communication systems and by not holding any more meetings than necessary. Nurse leaders and managers should also facilitate open communications and assertive behavior and handle conflict immediately before it drains time and energy.

Control

Nurse leaders and managers set standards, monitor results, and give feedback. The leaders and managers adjust closeness of supervision to the needs of the employee, take disciplinary action as soon as it is justified, and fire personnel who are not meeting minimum standards. Good management conserves time and energy, lack of which leads to management by crisis.

CHAPTER SUMMARY

There are numerous sources of stress such as stress related to change, personal, professional, and self-imposed stresses. Stress can be positive or negative depending on a person's perceptions, physical stamina, mental health, nutritional status, and social support. Numerous physical and mental symptoms indicate that stress has become distress. Fortunately there are many techniques to control stress such as relaxation, time management, and delegation. There are ways to prevent procrastination, and ways to maximize organization time through the management processes of planning, organizing, staffing, directing, and controlling were identified.

CASE STUDY
A number of nurses on your staff are married, raising small children, taking classes toward a degree, and feeling stressed. They are starting to develop some negativism. How will you approach this problem?

CRITICAL THINKING ACTIVITY

Reflective Journal: Identify what time and stress management techniques you are using. Review others, and decide if there are others you should try. Plan your strategies for experimenting with additional time and stress management techniques. Write your personal mission statement. Identify up to seven roles. Identify up to four goals for each role. Schedule your priorities into your calendar.

ONLINE RESOURCES

evolve Additional critical thinking activities, worksheets, and case studies are available online at http://evolve.elsevier.com/Marriner/guide8e.

REFERENCES

Aiken H, Clarke SP, Sloane DM, et al: Hospital nurse staffing and patient mortality, nurse burnout, and job dissatisfaction, *JAMA* 288:1987-1993, 2002.

Calder C: *Meditation handbook*, 1998 (website): http://home.att.net/~meditation/MeditationHandbook.html. Accessed July 28, 2007.

Center on Aging Studies: Relaxation, no date (website): http://cas.umkc.edu/casww/relaxatn.htm. Accessed November 15, 2007.

Centre for Independent Language Learning: *Mind maps*, 2007 (website): http://elc.polyu.edu.hk/CiLL/mindmap.htm. Accessed July 28 2007.

Covey SR: *The 7 habits of highly effective people: Powerful lessons in personal change*, New York, 1989, Simon & Schuster.

Covey SR: *First things first*, New York, 1994, Simon & Schuster.

Covey SR: *The 8th habit: From effectiveness to greatness*, Tampa, FL, 2004, Free Press.

Doty R: *Scoring for the Holmes-Rahe Social Readjustment Scale*, 2007 (website): http://www.cop.ufl.edu/safezone/doty/dotyhome/wellness/HolRah.htm. Accessed July 28, 2007.

Ellis JR, Hartley CL: *Managing and coordinating nursing care*, Philadelphia, 2004, Lippincott.

Gawain S: *Creative visualization: Use the power of your imagination to create what you want in your life*, Novato, CA, 2003, New World Library.

Grohar-Murray ME, DiCroce HR: *Leadership and management nursing*, ed 3, Upper Saddle River, NJ, 2003, Prentice Hall.

Handel K: *RN assignment decision tree: Assignment to unlicensed assistive personnel (UAP)*, 2007 (website): http://www.sos.state.ga.us/plb/rn/decision_tree.htm. Accessed July 28, 2007.

Hansten RI: *Clinical delegation skills: A handbook for professional practice*, ed 3, Boston, 2004, Jones & Bartlett.

Holmes TH, Rahe RH: The social readjustment rating scale, *Journal of Psychosomatic Research* 11:213-218, 1967.

Huber DL: *Leadership and nursing care management*, ed 3, Philadelphia, 2006, Saunders/Elsevier.

Jaffe-Gill E et al: Stress: Signs and symptoms, cause and effects, 2006 (website): www.helpguide.org/mental/stress_signs.htm. Accessed January 10, 2007.

Kingsley N: The power of a pause, 2006 (website): www.noelkingsley.com/blog/archives/2006/07/post_47.html. Accessed January 10, 2007.

Malloy J: *Centering room*, 2006 (website): http://www.meditationcenter.com/center/index.html. Accessed July 28, 2007.

Manktelow J: *Self-hypnosis*, 2003a (website): http://www.mindtools.com/stress/RelaxationTechniques/SelfHypnosis.htm. Accessed July 28, 2007.

Manktelow J: *Speed reading*, 2003b (website): http://www.mindtools.com/speedrd.html. Accessed July 28, 2007.

Manktelow J: *Reading strategies*, 2003c (website): www.mindtools.com/rdstratg.html. Accessed July 28, 2007.

Manktelow J: *Memory improvement tools*, 2003d (website): http://www.mindtools.com/memory.html. Accessed July 28, 2007.

Marquis BL, Huston CJ: *Leadership roles and management functions in nursing*, ed 3, Philadelphia, 2006, Lippincott.

McConnell CR: *Umiker's management skills for the new health care supervisor*, ed 4, Boston, 2006, Jones & Bartlett.

Messina JJ, Messina CM: *Coping: Thought stopping in recovery*, 2007 (website): http://www.coping.org/selfesteem/lifestyle/stop.htm. Accessed July 28, 2007.

Meyer C: *Fast cycle time*, New York, 1993, Free Press.

Murji A, Gomez M, Knighton J, Fish JS: Emotional implications of working in a burn unit, *J Burn Care Res* 27(1):8-13, 2006.

Murphy P: Anchoring-neuro-linguistic-programing, 2007 (website): http://www.whitedovebooks.co.uk/nlp/anchoring.htm. Accessed July 28, 2007.

National Council of State Boards of Nursing: *Delegation concepts and decision-making process: National Council position paper*, 1995, (website): https://www.ncsbn.org/323.htm. Accessed July 28, 2007.

Neill J: *Personality types*, 2005 (website): http://www.wilderdom.com/personality/L6–1PersonalityTypes.html. Accessed July 28, 2007.

Otis D: *Self-massage techniques*, 2002 (website): http://www.coolnurse.com/massage.htm. Accessed July 28, 2007.

Paul R, et al: *Critical thinking handbook: A guide for remodeling lesson plans in language arts, social studies and science*, Rohnert Park, CA, 1990, Foundation for Critical Thinking.

Psychology Key Studies: *Holmes and Rahe's Study of Stress and Life Events*, 2007 (website): http://www.qeliz.ac.uk/psychology/holmes%20and%20rahe.htm. Accessed July 28 2007.

Richmond RL: Autogenics training. In Richmond RL: *A guide to psychology and its practice*, 2007 (website): http://www.guidetopsychology.com/autogen.htm. Accessed July 28, 2007.

Robert HM, et al: *Robert's rules of order*, ed 10, New York, NY, 2000, HarperCollins Publishers.

Scott E: *About stress management*, 2007. (website): http://stress.about.com. Accessed July 28, 2007.

Seyle H: *The stress of life*, Toronto, 1965, McGraw-Hill.

Seyle H: *Stress in health and disease*, Boston, 1976, Butterworth.

Sheehan JP: Protect your staff from workplace violence, *Nurs Manage* 31:24-25, March 2000.

Silvestri LA: *Saunders comprehensive review for the NCLEX-RN examination*, ed. 3, St. Louis, 2005, Elsevier.

Sullivan EJ, Decker PJ: *Effective leadership and management in nursing*, ed 6, Upper Saddle River, NJ, 2005, Prentice Hall.

Tracy B, Rose C: *Accelerated learning techniques*, Niles, IL, 1997, Nightingale Conant.

The University of Maryland Medical System Corporation: *Relaxation techniques: Guided imagery*, 2001a (website): http://www.umm.edu/sleep/relax_tech.html. Accessed July 28, 2007.

The University of Maryland Medical System Corporation: *Relaxation techniques: Progressive relaxation*, 2001b (website): http://www.umm.edu/sleep/relax_tech.html. Accessed July 28, 2007.

Wheatley MJ: *Turning to one another: Simple conversations to restore hope to the future*, San Francisco, 2002, Berrett-Koehler.

Yoder-Wise PS: *Leading and managing in nursing*, ed 3, St. Louis, 2007, Mosby.

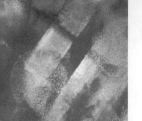

Decision-Making Process and Tools

3

"Indecision is the graveyard of good intentions." —Anonymous

Chapter Overview

Chapter 3 describes the decision-making process, critical thinking, creative decision making, consultation, ethics, moral reasoning, ethics committees, decision-making tools, computers, group factors in decision making, and committee aspects of decision making.

Chapter Objectives

- Identify the five steps in the decision-making process.
- Differentiate between committees, ad hoc committees, and task forces.
- Compare advantages and disadvantages of group participation in decision making.
- Describe at least six techniques to increase creativity.
- Compare and contrast at least two ethical positions that can be used to consider moral dilemmas.
- Describe at least five decision-making tools.
- Delineate at least three models that can be used to describe phenomena.
- Summarize how to use a Gantt chart.
- Identify how computers can be applied in nursing.

Online Resources

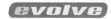 Critical thinking activities, worksheets, and case studies are available online at http://evolve.elsevier.com/Marriner/guide8e.

Major Concepts and Definitions

Ad hoc committee *a temporary committee to make recommendations*

Decision-making process *the process of selecting one course of action from alternatives*

Committee *a group of people chosen to deal with a particular topic or problem over time*

Critical thinking *the ability to question philosophically and exercise careful judgment when evaluating a situation*

Creativity *intellectual inventiveness*

Consultation *an interactive, helping relationship between two parties*

Ethics *a moral philosophy that examines how means are related to ends and how to control means to serve human ends*

Morality *a personal standard for what is right and wrong*

Values *beliefs and attitudes about the worth of something that may influence decision making*

Task force *a group of people with a time-limited assignment*

Tool *an instrument used to accomplish an end*

Model *an abstraction or representation of something more complex*

Probability *the likelihood of an event's occurrence*

Simulation *an imitation of an event or process*

Game theory *a simulation of system operations*

Gantt chart *a tool used to visualize multiple tasks that need to be done*

Decision tree *graphic tool to visualize alternatives available, chance events, and probable consequences*

PERT *program evaluation and review technique*

CPM *critical path method to calculate time estimate for activities*

Computer *an electronic machine that performs rapid calculations or compiles, correlates, and selects data by means of stored instructions and information*

Vroom and Yetton model *a tool used to identify autocratic, consultative, and group decision processes*

DECISION-MAKING PROCESS

Decision making, the process of selecting one course of action from alternatives, is a continuing responsibility of nurse leaders and managers who are confronted by a variety of situations. Hospital or agency policies provide guidelines for dealing with routine situations. Exceptional circumstances, however, can make decisions more difficult and may require a mature sense of judgment. Problem solving is a skill that can be learned, and because staff nurses can learn by observing their leaders, good decision making by the leader may do more than solve immediate problems; more important

for the long term, it can foster good decision making by staff nurses. Decision making relies on the scientific problem-solving process: identifying the problem, analyzing the situation, exploring alternatives and considering their consequences, choosing the most desirable alternative, implementing the decision, and evaluating the results (Finkelman, 2006; Huber, 2006; Roussel, Swansburg, & Swansburg, 2006; Sullivan & Decker, 2005) (Box 3-1).

The first step in the decision-making process is defining the problem. What is wrong? Where is improvement needed? Sometimes the problem seems obvious and can be dealt with routinely.

BOX 3-1 Decision-Making Process

Identify the problem, and analyze the situation.
Explore the alternatives.
Choose the most desirable alternative.
Implement the decision.
Evaluate the results.

If the employee repeatedly reports late to work or abuses the privilege of sick leave, the leader or manager can respond in accordance with agency policies. However, leaders and managers who are concerned only with the infraction may be dealing with the effect rather than the cause of the problem. Consequently, similar situations may continue. It is important to define the factors that are causing the problem. For instance, two staff nurses may each complain about the intrusion of one into the other's work. Initially the problem may appear to be a personality clash or a political power struggle. However, the cause may be the leader's or manager's failure to define the job responsibilities of each nurse. As long as the leader or manager concentrates on the symptom instead of the problem, the difficulties will arise. It is only when the real problem has been identified that effective decision making can be initiated.

Nurse leaders and managers can identify the problem by analyzing the situation. All too frequently decisions are made and implemented before all the facts have been gathered. To prevent this, the leader or manager should have a questioning attitude. What is the desirable situation? What are the presenting symptoms? What are the discrepancies? Who is involved? When? Where? How? With answers to these questions managers can develop tentative hypotheses and test them against what they know. Progressive elimination of hypotheses that fail to conform to the facts reduces the number of causes to be considered. Feasible hypotheses should be further tested for causal validity. When managers believe they have identified the cause or causes of the problem by analyzing available information, they should begin exploring possible solutions.

Explore the Alternatives

There are usually a number of ways to solve a problem. Some may be quick and economical but less effective than their alternatives. Others may be more effective but less economical. If various alternatives are not explored, the course of action is limited.

When solving a problem, managers should determine first whether the situation is covered by law, policy, or standards. If it is not, they must draw on their education and experience for facts and concepts that will help them determine alternatives. Using one's experience is probably the most common approach to solving problems, but it may be inadequate. The more experience the leader or manager has had, the more alternatives may be suggested to solve a variety of problems. However, health care changes rapidly, and solutions to yesterday's problems may not work today. As a result, leaders and managers should look beyond their own experiences and learn how others are solving similar problems. This can be done through continuing education, professional meetings, review of the literature, searching the Web, correspondence, and brainstorming with staff. Inductive and deductive reasoning are both appropriate.

Choose the Most Desirable Alternative

The number and quality of alternatives depend largely on the creativity and productivity of leaders or managers and their staff. Leadership that prevents immediate acceptance of an apparently obvious solution and facilitates group exploration of decision-making opportunities (such as problems to solve) usually increases the number of alternatives and the quality of problem solving.

Eagerness to reach a decision may lead to premature solutions; on the other hand, considering only a few alternatives in haste blocks good decisions. Avoidance of the real problem, lack of clear problem definition, insufficient data, early statement of attitude by a status figure, mixing of idea generation and idea evaluation, lack of staff

TABLE 3-1 Decision-Making and Problem-Solving Models and Nursing Process

Decision Making	Problem Solving	Nursing Process
1. Identify the problems, and analyze the solution.	1. Assess: define the problem.	1. Assess.
2. Explore the alternatives.	2. Plan: generate a list of alternatives and evaluate for cost, feasibility, and risk.	2. Select nursing diagnosis.
3. Choose the most desirable alternative.	3. Choose the best solution.	3. Plan care.
4. Implement the decision.	4. Implement the apparent best solution.	4. Implement the care plan.
5. Evaluate the results.	5. Evaluate the effectiveness.	5. Evaluate the outcomes.

commitment because the superior who makes the decision does not implement it, and decisions made by large groups also interfere with reaching effective solutions.

One alternative is not always clearly superior to all others. The leader should try to balance factors such as patient safety, staff acceptance, morale, public acceptance, cost, and risk of failure. Criteria for calculating the value of decisions are useful. The following questions may be asked: Will this decision accomplish the stated objectives? If it does not, it should not be enforced and another option should be used. Does it maximize effectiveness and efficiency? One should use available resources before seeking outside assistance. Finally, can the decision be implemented? If not, it obviously will not solve the problem.

Implement the Decision

After a decision has been made, it must be implemented. A decision that is not put into action is useless. The leader or manager will need to communicate the decision to appropriate staff in a manner that does not arouse antagonism. The decision and procedures for its implementation can be explained in an effort to win the cooperation of those responsible for its implementation. The leader or manager will need to select the staff to implement the decision and provide the direction to initiate action. Leaders or managers may need to control the environment so staff can function as planned. Once the decision has been implemented, it should be monitored and evaluated.

Evaluate the Results

The final step of decision making is evaluating the results of the implementation of the chosen alternative. Evaluative criteria may have to be developed. Audits, checklists, ratings, and rankings can be used to review and analyze the results. Because solutions to old problems sometimes create new problems, making and evaluating additional decisions may be required. The decision-making and problem-solving models and the nursing process are very similar (Table 3-1). They are all scientific problem solving.

ORGANIZATIONAL MODELS FOR DECISION MAKING

There are several organizational models for decision making including: (1) the rational model, which uses deliberate actions to select the best solutions; (2) the political model, where the goal is to win; (3) the collegial model, that facilitates decisions by a group of peers; (4) the bureaucratic model, which uses routines; and (5) the garbage can model, which is based on pure chance (Box 3-2).

Rational Model

The rational model is based on the premises of common goals, technical competence, and sequential process to achieve goals when individual values are consistent with organizational values. It is a deliberate action to select the best solution to achieve the desired outcome. Feedback increases the understanding of causal relations, which can then be used in future

BOX 3-2 Organizational Models
Rational
Political
Collegial
Bureaucratic
Garbage can

decision making. The advantage is that it helps unify associates with the goals of the agency. Disadvantages include unrealistic expectations of how people function, a large amount of time for processing, and narrow thought processes that can become counterproductive.

Political Model

The political model is built on the premises of a win-win situation, diversity of interests, even dispersion of power, and available forums for people with multiple, conflicting values that are protecting their own self-interests. A lobby majority makes the decisions. Changes are based on negotiations rather than causal links and are unpredictable. Statesmen with political skills provide information to associates who may not share the organizational values. Decisions may be limited to the statesmen's narrow views. This takes less time than consensus models. This model can promote creative solutions with majority support that can be implemented even if there are differences in viewpoints.

Collegial Model

The collegial model involves full participation of a community of peers for decision making. It is based on the premises of group consensus, mutual respect, and adequate time. It is common in an academic community. There are shared responsibilities for organizational goals based on the professional background and interests of the participants. Decisions tend to support general welfare. Feedback is usually informal and dependent on participants' observations and priorities. This shared governance approach with professionals who have diverse and specialized information takes considerable time because of numerous group meetings. When there is consensus, implementation tends to go smoother than when there is no consensus.

Bureaucratic Model

The bureaucratic model is common in health care. It is based on the premises of historical norms and operating routines. The value is for operational efficiency based on history and tradition. Implementation of change is through use of routines as determined by policies and procedures that lead to predictable outcomes and only slight adaptations to operations. The hierarchical bureaucracy dictates the key players. Information is from history, tradition, and norms. Time for implementation depends on the efficiency of the operations. This model does not recognize informal channels of communication and ignores political struggles for power. Alternative solutions generated may be limited and depend on the historical success of the agency and the corporate memory. A past inefficient operation may be perpetuated. If there is a history of efficiency, changes consistent with history and norms may be made with little resistance.

Garbage Can Model

The garbage can model is based on the premise of pure accident. Decisions are unplanned and coincidental based on multiple diffuse values. Implementation is incidental with no planning. The outcomes occur by chance and may repeat errors. Key players may be associates who perceive an opportunity and contribute to organization anarchy and adhocracy. Outcomes depend on key player creativity. Because there are no goals or criteria for evaluating outcomes, errors may be repeated. It is also possible to consider creative solutions to problems (Franz, 1998).

CRITICAL THINKING

Scriven and Paul (2004) have defined critical thinking for the National Council for Excellence in Critical Thinking Instruction as "Critical

---

BOX 3-3 Elements of Critical Thinking and Reasoning

Purpose or goal
Central problem or question at issue
Point of view or frame of reference
Empirical dimension
Conceptual dimension
Assumptions
Implications and consequences
Inferences and conclusions

Data from Paul R: *Critical thinking,* Santa Rosa, CA, 1993, Foundation of Critical Thinking.

---

thinking is the intellectually disciplined process of actively and skillfully conceptualizing, applying, analyzing, synthesizing, and/or evaluating information gathered from, or generated by, observation, experience, reflection, reasoning, or communication, as a guide to belief and action. In its exemplary form, it is based on universal intellectual values that transcend subject matter divisions: clarity, accuracy, precision, consistency, relevance, sound evidence, good reasons, depth, breadth, and fairness."

Elements of reasoning are essential dimensions that provide general logic to reason. They include the purpose or goal; central problem or question at issue; point of view or frame of reference; empirical dimension; conceptual dimension; assumptions, implications, and consequences; and inferences and conclusions (Box 3-3). Critical thinking contributes to quality decision making and problem solving.

Purpose or Goal

All reasoning has a purpose or goal and requires clarity, significance, achievability, and consistency of purpose.

Central Problem or Question at Issue

All reasoning is an attempt to prevent or solve a problem, figure something out, or answer a question. To answer a question or solve a problem one must understand what it requires. Clarity, significance, relevance, and answerability of the question are needed.

Point of View or Frame of Reference

All reasoning is done from a point of view. Reasoning is improved when multiple relevant points of view are sought and when those points of view are articulated clearly, emphasized logically and fairly, and applied consistently and dispassionately.

Empirical Dimension

Reasoning is only as sound as the evidence on which it is based. The evidence should be clear, relevant, accurate, adequate, fairly gathered and reported, and consistently applied.

Conceptual Dimension

Reasoning is only as relevant, clear, and deep as the concepts that form it. Concepts are general ideas and should be clear, deep, neutral, and relevant.

Assumptions

All reasoning is based on assumptions, which are suppositions or statements accepted without proof. Reasoning can only be as sound as the assumptions on which it is based. Assumptions should be clear, consistent, and justifiable.

Implications and Consequences

All reasoning has implications, consequences, and direction. Understanding the implications and consequences is important to reason through a decision or issue. One must consider the clarity, completeness, precision, reality, and significance of articulated implications.

Inferences and Conclusions

All reasoning has inferences by which one draws conclusions and gives meaning to the data. Reasoning is only as sound as the inferences it makes and the conclusions to which it comes. Inferences should be clear and justifiable. Conclusions should be consistent, profound, and reasonable (Paul, 1993; Paul & Elder, 2005).

Critical Thinking for the Nursing Process

Critical thinking skills used in the assessment phase of the nursing process include observing; distinguishing pertinent and important data from other data; and validating, organizing, and categorizing data. To make the diagnosis, one must find patterns and relationships, make inferences, and state the problem while suspending judgment. To plan the care, one generalizes by transferring knowledge from one situation to another, develops evaluative criteria, and hypothesizes. During implementation of the plan of care, one applies knowledge and tests the hypotheses. To evaluate outcomes, one makes criterion-based evaluations to decide if hypotheses were correct (Alfaro-Lefevre, 2003; Huber, 2006; Sullivan & Decker, 2005).

GROUP DECISION MAKING

Group Factors

Within an organization, it is unusual for an individual to complete the decision-making process alone. Even if one makes the decision, others will probably be involved in the implementation. Commitment to the decision is important to its implementation and may be increased by participation in the decision-making process. One should be aware that there are always disadvantages as well as advantages to group participation in decision making (Huber, 2006; McConnel, 2006; Roussel, Swansburg, & Swansburg, 2006; Sullivan & Decker, 2005) (Box 3-4).

Advantages

Because of their broader experience, groups have a wider range of knowledge to draw on than does the individual, can do more complete data collection, and can generate more possible solutions. Participation allows one to express one's views and attempt to persuade others, thereby increasing self-expression, innovation, and development. The discussion helps differentiate between the ideal and the real and makes consensus possible. People are

---

BOX 3-4 Group Decision Making

ADVANTAGES
Broader experiences
Wider range of knowledge
Possibility for more complete data collection
Increases the expression of one's views
Allows attempt to persuade others
Increases self-expression
Can increase innovation
Practice develops critical thinking
Discussion helps differentiate between the idea and the real
Consensus becomes possible
Increases commitment to implementation
Opportunity for high-quality results

DISADVANTAGES
Time consuming
Social pressures
Desire for group acceptance
Attempts to appease superior
Hierarchical pressures to acquiesce to manager's desires
Formal status can inhibit interaction
Matching abilities to degree of participation
Varying levels of competence
Varying levels of expertise
Minority may rule
Interest in winning
Acceptable solution may maintain status quo

---

more apt to be committed to implementation if they have had the opportunity to share in the decision-making process. Group decisions are time consuming and expensive. However, if group members have diverse backgrounds, it may be less time consuming for a group to make a decision than for an individual to talk to several people individually, gather information, and analyze it. In the long run, it may be no more expensive than having a higher paid manager make the decision or having to deal with resistance to change because of lack of input. Practice can help develop critical thinking skills by thinking out loud; thinking outside the box; questioning; raising ethical, financial, social, and political issues; seeking out others who have creative ideas; and through discussions that lead to high quality results.

Disadvantages

Group decisions are time consuming and may result from social pressures. The staff may be influenced by a desire for group acceptance or by an attempt to appease their manager. Hierarchical pressures can reduce the subordinate's participation to acquiescence to the manager's desires. Formal status is likely to inhibit interaction even when the supervisor has less expertise than the staff. A competent superior is more likely to possess self-confidence and allow interaction. It is not always easy to determine another's competence, nor can one always expect the level of expertise to match the degree of participation.

Group participants change and so do the problems. A minority may rule if an individual or a few people dominate the group. Members may become more interested in winning an argument than in determining the best alternative. Choosing the most acceptable solution may produce consensus, which is not necessarily the optimal alternative, and may simply serve to foster the status quo.

Committee/Task Force Aspects

Committees are one way to do group decision making. To be most effective, committees and task forces should have members who have the appropriate educational background and variety of work experience, interest in the task, as well as enough members to do the work. The purpose and goals should be clear. Responsibilities and tasks should be identified, and assignments should be clear, with deadlines. Effective chairpersons use agendas, and minutes are helpful.

A committee is a group of people chosen to deal with a particular topic or recurring problems over time. A task force has a time-limited assignment. The authority delegated to committees and task forces varies widely. A committee may have advisory, informational, coordinating, or decision-making responsibility. A staff committee serves merely in an advisory capacity. A line committee is an executive group responsible for making decisions affecting subordinates. Formal committees are part of the organizational structure and have specific duties and authority. Informal committees have not been delegated authority and are often primarily for discussion. Formal committees tend to be permanent; informal committees are more likely to be temporary. Committees are usually most useful when appointed for a specific purpose. A committee appointed to collect data, analyze it, and make recommendations is an ad hoc committee. Task forces are assigned a specific task and disband when that task is accomplished. There are advantages and disadvantages to decision making by committees (Huber, 2006; Marquis & Huston, 2006; Roussel, Swansburg, & Swansburg, 2006, Sullivan & Decker, 2005).

Advantages

Although the ultimate responsibility for a decision is the top administrator's, that burden can be shared through the use of committees and shared governance councils. Group deliberation and judgment can be advantageous for decision making. Complex problems may be more manageable when department heads, specialists, and staff participate. Sharing in the decision-making process increases the department heads' and others' understanding of the situation and commitment to the decision. Most decisions based on consensus after deliberations are widely satisfactory. The unanimity of committee decisions helps increase the support and confidence of subordinates. It is appropriate for committee members to use critical thinking, creative decision making, and related tools to come to moral and ethical decisions.

Disadvantages

Although committees can share the top administrator's burden for decision making, more leadership ability is required to conduct business in that manner. Committee members' decisions may make the manager appear to be a figurehead and decrease the person's prestige in the community. They may in fact control a weak administrator. The manager may use committees to avoid responsibilities or to delay decisions. A committee may have a fixed responsibility, but it is the group rather than the individual that is held accountable because it is difficult to identify who is responsible for a poor committee decision. A committee decision is a slow, ponderous process that is consequently expensive. Pressure for unanimity may discourage input from more aggressive and creative members. Consensus through compromise may decrease the quality of the decision. Indecisiveness can result in an adjournment without action taken and can contribute to a minority tyranny of the strongest members.

Committee Functioning

"The goal of committee functioning is not to think alike but to think together." —Ann Tomey

Despite the obvious disadvantages and misuses of committees, there is an increasing emphasis on group participation. Committee decisions are particularly useful for policy formulation and planning. Thus, the leader and manager should consider how to maximize the use of committees. To build consensus, the chair listens to all committee members, uses the ideas, and gets people onto the team by involving them in critical thinking, creative thinking, and realistic critiquing of ideas.

Defining the scope and authority of the committee helps members know what their responsibilities are. Members should know if they are to simply discuss an issue, provide the manager with ideas, make recommendations, or be responsible for the decision. Given the above, there is less chance that committee members will waste their time dealing with issues beyond the scope of their responsibility. Moreover, an awareness of the limits placed on them allows committee members to evaluate their work. It may be advisable to review committees periodically, dissolve those no longer needed, consolidate those duplicating responsibilities, and create new ones that are needed.

The size of the committee is important. It should be large enough to facilitate deliberation and have a membership with a breadth of knowledge and expertise. If it is too large, however, that

encourages indecision and inefficiency. Effective committee size may range from five to fifteen members. Five is considered an ideal size if the five members have adequate knowledge and skill. The larger the group, the more time it takes to allow each member to participate and for the group to reach consensus. Appropriate membership is critical for effective committee functioning. Members need the necessary knowledge and skills, should possess authority, must be suitably representative, and should be able to work well within a group.

Good chairpersonship can increase the effectiveness of a committee. The chairperson can facilitate committee work by preparing agendas, circulating reports before the meeting, making research results available to members, collecting necessary facts before the meeting, defining the proposal for action, and conducting the meeting efficiently. Agendas circulated to members well in advance of meetings allow committee members to know what to expect and to come to the meeting prepared to deal with the subject. There should be an opportunity for members to add to the agenda items at the beginning of a committee meeting. The circulation of reports and other information before the meeting helps prevent wasting meeting time while members review studies or think aloud. It reduces the chances of a decision being railroaded, a report being meekly accepted, or a decision being postponed until after members have had more opportunity to study the proposal.

The chairperson should keep the discussion on the subject and help integrate committee deliberation. Thus, rather than resorting to compromise, members may develop a point of view that differs from the preconceived notions they brought to the meeting. The chairperson should not force members to take a position until after the subject has been fully considered. Members who take a premature stand may feel the need to defend that position for the sake of winning an argument rather than for the quality of the decision. The chairperson can encourage each member to be a critical evaluator and to consider the consequences of the action. Outside experts may be invited in or task forces can be selected to study issues and report back to the committee. It may be useful to have a follow-up meeting after a consensus has been reached to allow for and to deal with any second thoughts.

Committees permit simultaneous participation, and yet people may still leave the meeting with varying interpretations of what happened. Consequently, it is advisable to have a secretary take minutes of the meeting and for the chairperson to circulate the draft for modification before having the minutes approved by the committee. There should be a procedure for keeping a copy of minutes and relevant papers for future reference. The chairperson should also follow up on the decisions made and report the findings to the committee. Was the recommendation implemented? If so, what were the results? If not, why not? (Swansburg & Swansburg, 2002; Young & Cooke, 2002).

Consensus Building Versus Groupthink

Consensus building is collaborative problem solving accomplished by bringing people together, identifying issues and alternatives, listening to each person's ideas, realistically considering the positive and negative aspects of each idea, using critical thinking, and resolving conflicts. Consensus is reached when everyone agrees each person can live with the decision even if it is not the first choice for everyone. It takes time to build consensus.

On the other hand, groupthink seeks fast solutions with little critical thinking or input from group members. The people may feel invulnerable, ignore negative feedback, stereotype differing views as misinformed, and use peer pressure to suppress doubters. Dissenting members who self-censor and remain silent are not represented by what becomes a unanimous decision. People conform rather than challenge ideas, and poor decisions can result.

There are ways to prevent groupthink. The leader or manager should not state their opinion; each committee member should be a critical evaluator; one person should be assigned the role of the devil's advocate; several small groups may work on the same problem at the same time and then share their recommendations; consultants can be invited in; and each committee member may discuss issues with trusted colleagues outside the committee. The committee should try to come to consensus through problem solving and creative thinking (McConnell, 2006; Roussel, Swansburg, & Swansburg, 2006; Swansburg & Swansburg, 2002).

CREATIVE DECISION MAKING

The Creative Process

The creative process has steps similar to those of the problem-solving process, but the emphasis is different (Box 3-5). Decision making stresses choice of a solution, whereas the creative process emphasizes the novelty and uniqueness of the solution. Creativity is a latent quality, activated when a person becomes motivated by the need for self-expression or by the stimulation of a problem. Thus the first phase of the creative process is a *felt need*. Similarly, when decision makers are confronted with a problem, they start seeking a solution.

The second phase of creative problem solving is a work stage known as *preparation*, from which creative ideas emerge. Innovation partially depends on the number of options considered. By exploring relationships among potential solutions, one may identify additional solutions. Many decisions are made after slight preparation and therefore result in commonplace solutions. Superficial analysis of obvious information does not facilitate creative answers. Extensive use of libraries for data collection is useful; the creative person may take notes on readings, develop them into files with other clippings and ideas, review these materials, and combine the most appropriate aspects of old solutions into new answers.

BOX 3-5 Creative Decision-Making Process

Felt need
Preparation
Incubation
Illumination
Verification

Incubation, the third phase, is a period for pondering the situation. Repetition of the same thoughts with no new ideas or interpretations is a sign of fatigue and indicates that it is a good time to start the incubation period. Switching one's attention provides a necessary respite, and yet the unconscious mind continues to deal with the problem. A time should be set to reexamine the situation and review the data collected during the preparation phase.

Illumination is the discovery of a solution and the fourth step. It may come to mind in the middle of the night or during the performance of another task. It is recommended that the idea be written down so the details can be preserved. Having paper and pencil readily available at all times (including in the bedside stand) is helpful.

It is rare for an illumination to be ready for adoption. *Verification,* the fifth and final phase of creative decision making, is the period of experimentation when the idea is improved through modification and refinement. The advantages and disadvantages of each alternative must be weighed; resources and constraints such as personnel, finances, facilities, and equipment have to be evaluated; and potential technical and human problems should be considered. Some decisions have failed at implementation because potential problems were not anticipated and dealt with. It would be unfortunate for an otherwise useful alternative to be rejected for a disadvantage that could be easily overcome. By comparing the advantages and disadvantages of the options, the leader, manager, and/or group can choose the most desirable alternative (Huber, 2006; McConnell, 2006; Roussel, Swansburg, & Swansburg, 2006; Sullivan & Decker, 2005).

Encouraging Creativity

The thinking mechanism of the human brain has been conceptualized as having two sides. The right side is intuitive and conceptual and is used for uninhibited creative thinking. The left side is analytical and sequential. If we use the analogy of driving a car, the right side of the brain is a green light that keeps us going until we have generated a multiplicity of ideas. The left side is a red light that says stop and questions whether this is worthwhile. The judicial left side of the brain analyzes and evaluates the creative ideas generated by the right side of the brain. We need to use both sides. We are usually socialized to use the left side more than the right side, but the right side can be stimulated. To encourage creativity we can consider how to adapt, combine, eliminate, rearrange, reverse, or substitute ideas or put something to other uses (Josephson, 2007) (Box 3-6).

BOX 3-6 Creative Thinking Techniques

DIVERGENT THINKING
Meditation
Brainstorming
Reverse brainstorming
Brain writing
Collective notebook technique
Stepladder technique
Stepladder of abstraction
Forced association
Visual trek/visual confirmation
Think tanks
The Delphi technique

CONVERGENT THINKING
Lists
Drawing
Sequencing
   Ranking
   Continuous scale
   Series of events chain
   Cycle
   Bridging snapshots
   Problem/solution outline
Compare/contrast
   Venn diagram
   Know, Want to know, Learned, How can we
     learn (KWLH)
Morphological matrix
Musts/wants
Highlighting
Short, medium, long term (SML)
Synetics
Visualization
Visually identifying relationships
Forecasting alternative future scenarios
Self-interrogation checklist
Modeling
Evaluation matrix
Advantages, limitations, unique qualities, overcome limitations (ALUo)
Pared comparison analysis

Divergent Thinking

"The mind is like a parachute. It functions only when open." —Anonymous

Divergent thinking is a spontaneous, free-flowing generation of random, unorganized thinking. The goal is to generate many different ideas quickly. It breaks a topic down into components to gain insights. One's view of the problem is expanded because the problem is considered in different ways (Treffinger, Isaksen, & Stead-dorval, 2006).

Six Thinking Hats

The six thinking hats technique facilitates looking at decisions from a number of perspectives and forces people out of their habitual thinking styles to get a 360-degree view of the situation. "Many successful people think from a very rational, positive viewpoint. This is part of the reason they are successful. Often, though, they may fail to look at a problem from an emotional, intuitive, creative, or negative viewpoint. This can mean that they underestimate resistance to plans, fail to make creative leaps, and do not make essential contingency plans. Similarly, pessimists may be excessively defensive, and more emotional people may fail to look at decisions calmly and rationally" (Labelle, 2005).

The six hats are white, red, black, yellow, green, and blue. The white hat is for analyzing past trends, looking for available information and considering what can be learned from it, looking for the gaps and closing them or noting them, and trying to extrapolate from the historical data. The red hat is for using intuition, gut reactions, and emotions to think about how other people who do not know your reasoning might react emotionally. The black hat is for using pessimism, judging, looking for the bad points, and being cautious and defensive. It facilitates finding the faults, which allows people to eliminate them, alter them, or to prepare contingency plans. The yellow hat is for positive, optimistic thinking that identifies the benefits and values of the decision and motivates people to keep going

when the going gets tough. The green hat is for a freewheeling way of creative thinking that can generate a number of creative alternatives. The blue hat is used by the meeting facilitator for process control and to direct people back to different hats for continual processing.

Meditation

The optimal state for peak performance of athletes is relaxed concentration, or "playing loose." Meditation can generate a more focused state of relaxed attention. It is often identified as a component of Eastern religions and is a practice of focusing the mind. It involves contemplation. Different physical positions are recommended for meditation. The most famous are the cross-legged postures. The ritual involves freeing the mind of all thoughts, focusing the mind on a single object, opening the mind up, and doing a reasoned analysis of the new thoughts. It focuses on developing oneself. The goals of meditation can range from spiritual enlightenment, through transformation of attitudes, to better health. It helps integrate the mind, body, and spirit. Meditation is a method of stress reduction that contributes to mindfulness and creates a more flexible attention span, increased awareness of the situation, and objectivity in emotional and morally difficult situations. It can ready one for divergent and convergent thinking.

Brainstorming

Brainstorming creates a list of ideas in an unstructured way. A description of the task may be sent to participants before the brainstorming session so that participants could be brainstorming ideas. It is appropriate to start the brainstorming session by clarifying the task verbally and by writing it so the participants can easily view it. Guidelines for generating options should be clarified. Participants should defer judgment; generate as many ideas as possible and then try to identify a few more ideas; look at how to combine, separate, rearrange, and so on; and focus on quality of decisions. Ideas could be recorded on a chalkboard, flip chart, or Post-its. Using Post-its can speed up the process by having participants write their own ideas on Post-its, and having someone collect them and post them rather than having one person record all the ideas. The ideas are easier to move around and to converge, diverge, and rearrange.

Under favorable circumstances a group working together can identify more ideas than an individual or that group of individuals working separately. Brainstorming is a technique leaders can use to create a free flow of ideas. They should encourage the members to contribute a large number of freewheeling ideas without fear of criticism or ridicule. This can improve the quality of ideas offered and result in new combinations through rearrangement, reversal, substitution, and other modifications.

Brainstorming seems to work best for simple and specific problems. Complex problems can be divided into parts that are handled separately. If the problem is too complex, the discussion may lack focus and be very time consuming. Brainstorming may be most useful when group members understand at least part of the problem. Although the session may not produce a viable solution, its stimulation may continue beyond the meeting and cause employees to take another look at their routine activities.

Creativity is probably fostered best in a permissive atmosphere in which mutual respect prevails and people are encouraged to express their views and ideas even if they are at variance with current policies and practices. A free interchange of ideas with considerable borrowing and adaptation fosters the production of creative ideas. This is a divergent way of thinking that apparently generates the largest number of creative ideas when people look for what can be used from "wild" ideas, rather than criticizing them because they will not work. Piggybacking uses one idea to stimulate other ideas and is a key to good brainstorming (Treffinger, Isaksen, & Stead-dorval, 2006).

Reverse Brainstorming

Reverse brainstorming or negative brainstorming can turn negativism into creative problem solving. Start by identifying a problem. Then reverse the problem or challenge by asking what causes the problem instead of how to prevent it by saying something like "What causes low staff morale?" instead of "What can we do to improve staff morale?" Once that list has been generated, reverse those ideas into solutions for solving the original problem by more brainstorming. After that list is generated, evaluate the suggestions.

Brain Writing

Brain writing encourages free association and recording of ideas without verbal interaction. A problem is identified. Participants are given a blank piece of paper and told to write at least four ideas, suggestions, solutions, and so forth. The paper is then passed to someone else. The paper can be systematically passed to the right or left or can be put in the center of the table for selection. Reading others' ideas is intended to stimulate more ideas, which are then written on the page. The process continues until the pages are full, the time period has elapsed, or no one can think of anything else to write. There are variations where people can write on Post-it notes or small cards and put them in a central location like a table, bulletin board, or poster board (Treffinger, Isaksen, & Stead-dorval, 2006).

Collective Notebook Technique

People can keep an ideas diary or an ideas notebook that is small and portable. A poster notebook of drawings and lists of ideas can be put in a central location for people to view, allowing participants to come up with alternative ideas and to become open to discussion. In a group, a problem is identified, and participants are instructed to record thoughts and ideas about the problem for a specified period. Participants give their notebook to another person, who reads it, looks for patterns, and synthesizes the content. The participants then meet, analyze the results, and make recommendations to solve the problem (Mycoted, 2006).

Stepladder Technique

The stepladder technique structures the entry of group members into the group to ensure that each member contributes to the decision-making process. Initially two group members try to solve a problem. Then a third member joins the core group and presents a preliminary solution to the problem. The entering person's presentation is discussed by all three persons. The process is repeated as group members are added.

Each member is given the group's task and time to think about it before presenting to the group. The entering person presents preliminary solutions before the group comes to a final decision. There is a discussion after each entering person presents. The final decision is delayed until all members of the group have presented and are available to participate in the final decision (Treffinger, Isaksen, & Stead-dorval, 2006).

Ladder of Abstraction

A ladder of abstraction helps participants explore the task in broader or narrower ways or at varying levels of abstraction. It encourages making abstract options more concrete, focused, and specific and making specific narrow options broader and more abstract. Discussing concepts, then the definition of the concepts, followed by concrete examples of the concepts is going from abstract to concrete. For example, a broad discussion of staff participation narrows to a discussion of committees and more specifically to a discussion of the personnel committee. That is going from abstract to more concrete. Then the appropriate level of abstraction can be considered. "Why" questions help broaden an idea, whereas "how" questions help it to become more specific. Post-its can be used to speed the generation of ideas. If not many ideas are generated, the facilitator may ask, "What is preventing you from accomplishing this task?"(Treffinger, Isaksen, & Stead-dorval, 2006).

Forced Association or Fitting

The situation requiring improvement is identified. Participants use free association to generate a list of words associated with the situation, and then a list of associated words is generated and recorded. The participants look for relationships between the original list and the associated list. The lists are critically analyzed to choose words useful for addressing the situation requiring

improvement. People can be requested to force a relationship between a random item and the task at hand (Straker, 2007).

Visual Trek/Visual Confrontation

Visual trekking is good for stretching to generate original and unusual options. The participants make new connections by making a mental journey away from a task and then connecting back to the original task. A word is chosen to create an image and then to stimulate fuzzy connections back to the task, or participants may do a physical journey to find something tangible to stimulate images. Participants may draw pictures rather than use written words. For example, the beach may stimulate people to think about the sun, blue sky, warmth, and good feelings. Fuzzy connections, such as thinking about a sunny, warm work environment with good feelings, could be made. Then more concrete connections are made to find novel options (Treffinger, Isaksen, & Stead-dorval, 2006).

Think Tanks

In think tanks, five to eight people are gathered together in an exotic or different place to stimulate innovation. A relaxed atmosphere is encouraged to stimulate divergent and unusual ideas. The problem or goal is clearly stated. This is particularly useful for future projections (Wenger, 2004).

Delphi Technique

The Delphi technique allows members who are dispersed over a geographical area to participate in decision making without meeting face to face. A problem is identified, and members are asked to suggest potential solutions through the use of a questionnaire. Members anonymously return the first questionnaire, and the results are centrally compiled. Each member is sent a copy of the results; after viewing them, members are asked for their suggestions again. Review of the results of the first questionnaire typically triggers new solutions or stimulates changes in original positions. This process continues until consensus is reached. Little change usually occurs after the second round.

The Delphi technique insulates group members from one another's influence and does not require physical presence, so it is particularly appropriate for scattered groups. Unfortunately, it is time consuming and may not develop as many alternatives as the other techniques (Polit & Beck, 2007).

Convergent Thinking

After using divergent thinking to generate many ideas, the ideas need to be organized and structured using convergent thinking to select the best solution. The problem is divided into smaller and smaller pieces to find a more manageable perspective. The group considers what is most important, what is the essence, and if there are strands, clusters, groupings, or patterns (Treffinger, Isaksen, & Stead-dorval, 2006).

Lists

The checklist method is used to assemble criteria on a checklist, sort it, prioritize it, eliminate items, and add others. An attribute list records characteristics. They are then rearranged in possible combinations of ideas. The SCAMPER technique lists verbs that are idea generating. SCAMPER is an acronym for substitute, combine, adapt, modify-magnify-minify, put to other uses, eliminate, and rearrange or reverse (Infinite Innovations Ltd, 2006).

Drawings can be used to evoke and record creative insight. Intuitive consciousness communicates more readily in symbols and impressions than in words.

Ranking is a sequential graphic organizer. Items may be ranked by order of hierarchy, gradation, rank, seriality, succession, etc (Figure 3-1, *A*).

A continuum scale can be used when items have a relative position. It can be from more to less importance, younger to older age, less to more achievement, or by chronological historical events (Figure 3-1, *B*).

Sequencing in a series of events can show the steps in a linear procedure or the stages of something (Figure 3-1, *C*).

A cycle shows how a series repeats itself again and again. One needs to identify the key events and consider how they relate to each other and how they reinforce each other (Figure 3-1, *D*).

Sequencing in bridging snapshots shows changes over time. It reveals the sequence of methods, can illustrate complex processes, and may indicate cause and effect (Figure 3-1, *E*).

Sequencing in the problem/solution outline illustrates the who, what, where, when, why and how of the problem-solving process and projects solutions and results (WriteDesign, 2007a) (Figure 3-1, *F*).

Comparing and contrasting can be done with a Venn diagram, which is two overlapping circles. Characteristics of two things such as ideas, people, places, etc., are put in the right or left circle with common characteristics in the overlapping section (Figure 3-1, *G*). It can also be done with a compare/contrast matrix. The two names of the things being compared and contrasted are put at the top of the columns, and the rows are labeled with attributes. Then one considers how the attributes are similar and different in the two columns (WriteDesign, 2007b) (Figure 3-1, *H*).

A KWLH grid can also be used to identify what we know about the situation, what we want to learn, what we have learned, and how we can learn more. KWLH can label the columns, and the information can be written into the rows (WriteDesign, 2007c) (Figure 3-1, *I*).

Morphological Matrix

The morphological matrix helps combine elements from various attributes by creating a framework for new options. Each parameter is listed as a column heading in the matrix. For a patient's diet, appetizer, salad, soup, entrée, vegetable, fruit, dessert, drink, and bread could be listed as parameters. Then specific examples are listed below each parameter. Patients' meals are then individualized by mixing one item from each column (Treffinger, Isaksen, & Stead-dorval, 2006).

Musts and Wants

Musts and wants is a way to narrow down a large number of alternatives quickly. Make two columns, and label one "musts" and the other "wants." Items that are essential, indispensable,

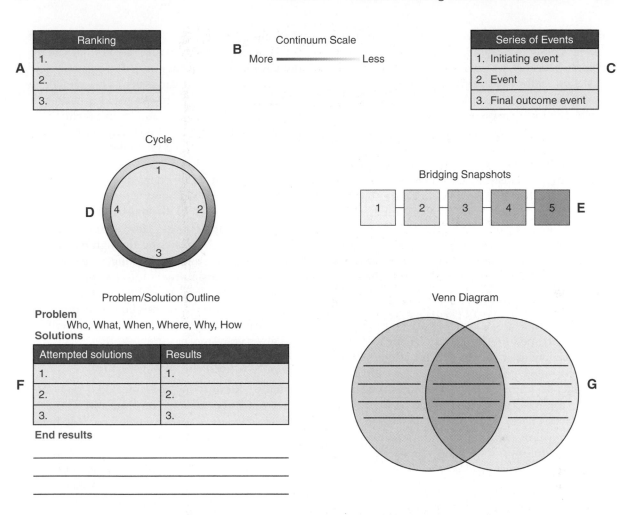

Figure 3-1 • Covergent thinking for creative decision making.

and vital are listed under musts. Desirable and preferable items are listed under wants. Musts are what have to be considered. Failing to consider a must jeopardizes the desired outcome. Wants are nice to consider for polishing or strengthening actions that are not critical to the outcomes. Post-its are a useful tool for categorizing options (Treffinger, Isaksen, & Stead-dorval, 2006).

Highlighting

Highlighting is a focusing tool that condenses a variety of options into themes, thus compressing a large number of options into a more manageable number of categories. First the best options are identified and called "hits." Screening options from a long list or selecting options for further consideration can do this. Participants can be given bright-colored sticker dots with different colors representing different priorities, colored markers, or gold stars for frequency of selection, or they can draw symbols by the listed items. When more people are doing the hitting, fewer hits per person are recommended. When there are a larger number of options under consideration or more themes, more hits per person are recommended. Then those that are related to each other are clustered into themes called "hot spots." Numbers can be used to cluster options related to each other into hot spots initially. The theme is used to name the category. Each hot spot should have only one theme. Not all hits need to be placed in hot spots. Post-its are an efficient way to put hits into hot spots (Treffinger, Isaksen, & Stead-dorval, 2006).

SML

SML (short, medium, long) is a focusing tool used to determine the order in which options should be deliberated, to compare alternatives in relationship to timing, and to sequence alternatives within time frames. Options could be sequenced into first, second, and third order for consideration; morning, noon, and nighttime sequencing; short-, medium-, and long-term time frames, and so on. Alternatives can also be sequenced in each time frame. Post-its can facilitate the sequencing process. Some options may span time frames (Treffinger, Isaksen, & Stead-dorval, 2006).

Synetics

Synetics is the joining together of apparently irrelevant elements. A problem is identified, and a brief analysis is given. The problem is then simplified to clarify it and reinterpreted as an analogy or metaphor. The group then plays with the analogy. The analogy or metaphor chosen to represent the problem is considered in depth. The problem is thus redefined in a new light.

Visualization

Free association can be used to create a big dream approach. First, desired outcomes are visualized and then visually run backward to identify a new approach. Imagine what you would like: a phone that tells you who is calling before you answer it; that shows who is talking to you; that you do not have to touch to answer; that rings wherever you are (office, home, car, beach). Once you have imagined what you want, you can begin dreaming about how to make your dream a reality. This technique allows you to pretend that you already have what you want and facilitates concentration on the outcomes.

Visualization helps one think in pictures, develop imagination, and dream. Meditation allows one to listen to the heart and the creative self. Focus helps one get clear about intention. Visual research by browsing through magazines and pictures stimulates thinking visually. Collage making puts a dream into a tangible form. Poetic wordplay stimulates the right brain, intuitive powers, and creative thinking. Creative journaling can include drawing as well as writing and gives voice to vision.

Visually Identifying Relationships

Visually identifying relationships provides quiet reflective time to generate options. It is particularly good for visual learners. It helps to start with a relaxation exercise and to then show participants a few pictures sequentially. The participants record their observations and reactions to each picture on a worksheet. The group then connects their observations back to the task in an effort to generate original ideas. Stepping away helps participants find a new perspective for the task (Treffinger, Isaksen, & Stead-dorval, 2006).

Forecasting Alternative Future Scenarios

The future is often more a matter of choice than of chance. The choice is enhanced by forecasting potential scenarios—status quo, least preferred, most preferred, and not likely—and selecting the most desired. The process includes assessing the present situation, identifying its strengths and weaknesses, recognizing the driving forces in the environment, constructing possible alternative future scenarios, identifying the preferred future, developing a plan of action, implementing the plan, and evaluating the implementation.

Self-Interrogation Checklist

Questions are used to stimulate new perspectives about a situation. Questions help define and refine situations. They help obtain information, assess options, generate new ideas, and make decisions. Questions could include the following: Is it practical? Is it cost effective? Is it efficient? Is it effective? Can we do more? Can we streamline? Can we improve the situation?

Modeling

Look at how others are doing what one wishes to do. However, be cautious: what works for someone else, somewhere else, may not work for one here and now. Similarly, what worked for one somewhere else or at some other time may not work now. Seek out what can be used or adapted, given the current situation and the preferred future.

Evaluation Matrix

The evaluation matrix structures a way to evaluate several options against specific criteria. The criteria (such as cost, time, legality, ethics, feasibility, risk) label columns across the top of the matrix. Alternatives label rows down the left side of the matrix. A rating scale such as 0 for low and 5 for high is used to specify how well each alternative meets the criteria. Happy or sad faces, colors, or shapes could also be used for evaluating each alternative against the criteria. It is preferable to go down each column rather than across each row for better comparisons when scoring the options. Each group member can complete a matrix. Scores can be averaged or consensus determined before the alternative is evaluated and scored on the primary grid. Then ideas can be generated for ways to strengthen options, so that the best option or options can be selected, implemented, and evaluated again (Treffinger, Isaksen, & Stead-dorval, 2006).

Advantages, Limitations, Unique Qualities, Overcome Limitations (ALUo)

This focusing tool helps evaluate options by identifying strengths, weaknesses, and unusual qualities. It is particularly useful when choices have been narrowed down to two or three that need further development. Instead of just listing strengths and weaknesses, ask questions such as "How can we overcome the weakness?" By identifying and planning how to overcome weaknesses, novel solutions are generated and supported instead of discounted. The unique qualities are to be preserved (Treffinger, Isaksen, & Stead-dorval, 2006).

Paired Comparison Analysis

The paired comparison analysis is a focusing tool that systematically compares or ranks several options against each other a pair at a time to prioritize them. This helps assess the importance of options. Columns are labeled with options across the top of the matrix. Rows are labeled with the same options down the left side of the matrix. Two decisions are made for each comparison. First, which one is more important? Then, how much more important is one option over the other when total scores are calculated? Total scores help understand the priorities. Let's say a is compared with b and c and outranks both. The letter a is written in the box where a, b, and c converge. One sums the number of a's in the row and gets 2. Then one compares b with c. Let's say b outranks c. One has one b in that row. If one now ranks a, b, and c, a is first with a score of 2, b is second with a score of 1, and c is third with a score of zero. Each group member can do his or her own paired analysis. Then options can label columns across the top of a grid, and group member names can label rows down the left side of the grid. Their score for each option can be put in the box where the option and their name converge. Total the scores for each option at the bottom of each column to determine the group consensus. Circle or highlight the highest and lowest scores for each option. Have the people giving the highest and lowest scores for each option discuss their reasons for their ranking and how they respond to the other person's rationale. Summarize the outcomes of the conversation, and confirm the group's understanding of the priorities. High scores usually have a higher priority (Treffinger, Isaksen, & Stead-dorval, 2006).

RESEARCH Perspective 3-1

Data from Kramer M, Maguire P, Schmalenberg C, et al: Excellence through evidence: Structures enabling clinical autonomy, *JONA* 37(1):41-52, 2007.

Purpose: This research was to identify the structures, practices, elements in environment, and interventions that nurses, nurse managers, and physicians identify as promoters of staff nurse clinical autonomy to enable clinical decision making.

Methods: Three sources of evidence were explored: (1) published literature, (2) operational and evaluation data provided by co-investigators at each research site, and (3) consensus of experts.

Results/conclusions: Both clinical autonomy and RN-MD collaboration are partnerships that value recognition and acceptance and combined spheres of accountability, activity, and responsi-

bility that need to be articulated and recognized. Formal and informal RN-MD or interdisciplinary meetings to define boundaries and domains of responsibility can be helpful; documents such as career ladder criteria, scope or practice, and performance appraisal forms are as well. Hiring nurses who are intelligent, well educated, and want to be held accountable; providing guidance to the newcomer to develop self-confidence; and providing continuing education, continuing research activities, and evidence-based practice are important. Job autonomy with support of autonomous decision making by peers in a nurturing culture seems to foster autonomous nursing decision making.

Developing Creative Thinking Attitudes

Creative thinking can develop novel solutions. People need to be open minded about new ideas and the ideas of others. Inquiring minds are never satisfied. Creative people are not unduly concerned about the opinions of others, because many great ideas are first ridiculed and later accepted. People need to put aside critical, analytical, and judicial thinking while working creatively and move beyond their personal habits and attitudes. After numerous ideas have been generated, they can be judged and the best selected. Trust, acceptance, and good humor help create an environment conducive to creative problem solving. Creative people have an inner motivation, mental ability, objectivity, tolerance for complexity, enjoyment of risk taking, and ability to find problems.

Blocks to Creativity

There are numerous blocks to creativity. Negative attitudes, self-censorship, inflexibility, lack of confidence, misconceptions, lack of effort, habits, conformity, and reliance on authority all block creativity (Harris, 2002).

CONSULTATION

"Information is not, of course, an end in itself, it is the basic input to decision-making." —Henry Mintzberg

Consultation is a helping relationship. It is a process of interaction between the consultant, who has the specialized knowledge and skills, and the consultee, who asks for assistance with problem solving. It has a beginning and an end and is a temporary, voluntary, educational relationship. The consultee identifies a problem and seeks help from an expert. Because the consultant is usually not a part of the hierarchical structure of the organization, the consultant is an outsider who advises. Implementation of the recommendations depends on the consultee, thus giving the process a take-it-or-leave-it quality. The consultative process usually involves problem solving, but the consultant may play several roles: helping identify problems, educating staff about related issues, identifying obstacles to problem solving, offering advice about how to solve problems, acting as a change agent, developing interpersonal relationships, mediating conflicts, or performing tasks that organizational members do not have the skill to perform. The consultant typically collects and analyzes data, recommends or intervenes, and then terminates the relationship.

Consultants become known by doing something and telling others about it, volunteering to present workshops and speeches, publishing books and articles, being active in professional organizations, circulating flyers and announcements, and being included in lists of consultants.

An internal consultant knows the system, history, political realities, norms, and language better than an outside consultant and will probably devote more time to the problem. Internal consultants are viewed as less costly because they are usually not compensated extra for consultative services. Unfortunately, there are disadvantages to hiring internal consultants. They may be part of the problem; lack perspective to see the whole; have no independence of movement; have no adequate power base; encounter resistance because of their relationship with the hierarchy, vested interest, or organizational politics; or have a limited background.

An external consultant has a more diverse background, brings new ideas and a different perspective to the situation, is independent of the power structure, and is consequently high powered. Unfortunately, the external consultant does not know the history and politics of the institution and may not care about them.

Once it has been determined that there is a need for consultation, what the purpose is, and who the consultant should be, a contractual agreement is necessary. The agreement may be verbal or written, but it should determine the fee, hours of the consultant's time, expected outcome, and criteria for termination. The fee may be negotiated as a flat fee, a fee based on hours spent at the agency that includes travel and preparation time, or an hourly rate for all the time the consultant spends on the project, including research and report writing. The hours are largely controlled by the compensation structure. The consultant may have a regular schedule or be "on call." In most cases the outcome is accepted whether it is judged acceptable or not. A common outcome is a written analysis with recommendations, decisions reached, systems devised or revised, and projects completed. Usually the termination occurs at a natural closure point, such as the resolution of the problem or completion of the project. However, contingency plans should be made in case there are personality conflicts or the project takes too long and exceeds the budget (Huber, 2006).

ETHICAL ASPECTS OF DECISION MAKING

"Justice is always violent to the party offending, for every man is innocent in his own eyes." —Daniel Defoe

Ethics is a moral philosophy, a science of judging the relationship of means to ends, and the art of controlling means so they will serve human ends. It involves conflict, choice, and conscience. When there is a conflict, there is a choice between conflicting alternatives. The choice is influenced by values. Values are learned first from important adults in one's life and are modified by association with people of different values. Value modification and reinforcement are lifelong processes. A value is consciously prized and cherished, freely chosen from alternatives, and acted on in a variety of ways. Ethical choices must also consider wants, needs, and rights: people may want what they do not need. Someone may want a dessert but not need it; in fact, it may be harmful. People often need what others also need. One who needs food to keep from starving may have a right to receive food from people who have plenty but not from someone who would starve without it. That would infringe on the other person's rights, and duty and rights are correlated: it is one's duty to protect rights. A legal obligation is legislated, but it may not be ethical. A moral dilemma occurs when a decision has equally unsatisfactory alternatives.

Ethical Theories

Deontological (from the Greek "deon" or duty) theories focus on the intent of the action and are duty and rights based. Emphasis is on individual rights, duties, and obligations and the dignity of human beings. The intention of the action rather than the end of the action is considered. The intent is considered moral if it follows an impartial and objective principle (Kay, 1997a). *Teleological* (from the Greek "telos" or end) theories derive the rules and norms for conduct from utilitarian consequences of actions. They favor the common good. Right has good consequences, and wrong has bad consequences. The greatest amount of good and the largest amount of happiness are good. *Principlism* is a deontological theory that includes ethical principles. The ethical principles control ethical decision making more than the ethical theories. The principles are moral norms, including autonomy, beneficence, fidelity, justice, nonmaleficence, paternalism, respect for others, utility, and veracity. Each principle can be used individually, but they are often used in concert.

Utilitarianism is a consequentialist theory that considers a good act as one that causes the least harm and brings the most good to the most people (Kay, 1997b). *Egoism* is based on self-interest and self-centeredness. Decisions are made for personal comfort. It is based on the principle that the right decision is the one that brings pleasure to the decision maker (Kay, 1997c). *Relationships* is a caring-based theory that emphasizes generosity and promoting common good for the welfare of the group rather than individual rights. *Obligationism* is a theory that tries to balance distributive justice (dividing equally among all citizens regardless of age, gender, race, religion, or socioeconomic status) and beneficence (doing good and not harm). One should do what is good and prevent harm and evil. It is useful for determining public policy. Social contract theory is based on a concept of original position and considers the least advantaged persons in society as the norm. The determination of what is right or wrong is from the perspective of the least advantaged people, such as children or handicapped people. It is based on distributive justice and supports giving the most to the least advantaged (Friend, 2006). Natural law is called the virtue of ethics. Actions are considered right when in accord with human nature. People should do good, avoid evil, and

BOX 3-7 Ethical Theories
Deontological
Teleological
Principlism
Utilitarianism
Relationships
Egoism
Obligationism
Social contract
Natural law

have opportunities to reach their potential. Happiness occurs when people think rationally and make conscious choices rather than responding to instincts (Simms, Price, & Ervin, 2000) (Box 3-7).

Ethical Principles

Autonomy involves personal freedom, freedom of choice, and responsibility for one's choices. Informed consent and progressive discipline recognize autonomy.

Beneficence indicates that the actions one takes should be in an effort to promote good. This principle can support providing extensive, painful treatments to increase quantity and quality of life or allowing a person to die peacefully without life support. It can be used to promote employees' positive attributes instead of their shortcomings. The act benefits others.

Confidentiality is securing the person's privacy through silence.

Fidelity is keeping one's commitments and promises. One should not make a promise to a patient or worker that cannot be kept.

Justice means treating people equally and fairly. Equals should be treated equally, and unequals should be treated according to their differences. It is useful to apply when making decisions about competition for scarce resources or benefits. Pay raises should reflect performance as well as time of service. Holidays, vacation time, and attendance at conferences should reflect performance as well as who is next on the list.

Distributive justice implies that benefits and burdens should be distributed equally regardless of gender, race, religion, or socioeconomic

BOX 3-8 Ethical Principles
Autonomy
Beneficence
Confidentiality
Fidelity
Justice
Distributive justice
Nonmaleficence
Paternalism
Respect
Utility
Veracity

BOX 3-9 Ethical Positions
Utilitarianism
Egoism
Formalism
Rule ethics
Fairness

status. This raises the issue of conflict between cost containment and equal distribution of scarce resources regardless of ability to pay.

Nonmaleficence means if you cannot do good, at least do no harm. Nurses may need to remember that even pain and suffering can bring about good for the patient when they are performing painful procedures for the patient's benefit. Performance appraisals should emphasize the employee's good qualities and give positive direction for improved performance instead of destroying self-esteem.

Paternalism allows one to make decisions for another, limits freedom of choice, and is seen as an undesirable principle. Most see it as justified only to keep another person from harm. It is not appropriate for a paternalistic manager to set the personal goals for employees.

Respect for others is considered the highest principle that incorporates all the other principles. Respect for others acknowledges the rights of people to make their own decisions and to live by their decisions. It transcends cultural, gender, and racial issues.

Utility indicates that what is best for the common good outweighs what is best for the individual. It could justify paternalism. One using utility needs to be careful not to become less humanistic.

Veracity indicates that people should be honest and tell the truth. It applies to telling patients and staff the truth so they can make well-informed decisions (Marquis & Huston, 2006; Sullivan & Decker, 2005; Wywialowski, 2004; Yoder-Wise & Kowalski, 2006) (Box 3-8).

Ethical Positions

An ethical dilemma occurs when there is no correct decision, there is a conflict between two or more ethical principles, or a decision needs to be made between two equally unsatisfactory choices. There are several ethical positions that do not solve dilemmas. However, they do provide ways to structure and clarify them.

Utilitarianism is a community-oriented position that focuses on the consequences and prefers the greatest amount of good and happiness for the most people, or the least amount of harm.

In contrast, *egoism* seeks solutions that are best for oneself without regard for others. One's own pleasure is the concern.

Formalism considers the nature of the act and the related principles without thought to personal position or consequences of the actions: be honest; remember the golden rule.

Rule ethics expects obedience to laws, rules, professional codes, and authority.

Fairness considers distribution of benefits and liabilities from the viewpoint of the least advantaged population. Benefit to the least advantaged group is the norm in this type of decision making (Box 3-9).

Ethical Relationships and Decisions

There are also models for ethical relationships. In the *priestly model* the manager is paternalistic and makes decisions without considering others' values or seeking others' input. Although nurses may have expertise that qualifies them to make some decisions, they have no right to make moral decisions affecting other people. Autocratic leadership may use the priestly model. The *engineering model* suggests that one person presents facts to another and sets aside his or her own code of ethics to do what the other wants; staff working for line authority may provide an example of this model. The *contractual model* provides a contract that identifies general obligations and benefits for two or more people. It deals with the morals of both parties and is appropriate for superior-subordinate relationships. In the *collegial model* individuals share mutual goals and reach decisions through discussion and consensus. When there are shared values, this model helps build teams and minimize conflict (Velch, 1980).

To make an ethical decision, one must first consider what is intended to be a means and an end and then determine what good or evil is found in the means and the end. If a major evil is intended either as a means or an end, it is an unethical decision.

If the ramifications of the decision are probable but not willed as a means or an end, there are several factors to consider. The good or evil of each alternative should be evaluated: a necessary good outweighs a useful good; paying workers' wages outweighs paying for profit sharing. Urgency increases the necessity; therefore physical needs must be met before self-actualizing needs. An agency should provide adequate wages for food and shelter before providing continuing education. The probability of an outcome should be considered: a possible negative outcome is outweighed by a probable good; one will work to earn a living even though there is a slight risk of back strain. The intensity of one's influence is considered because one's impact on someone else may have undesirable consequences; for instance, if an employee is fired for incompetence, it may cause a hardship for the employee's family. If the manager did not tell the employee what was expected or how to do the job, the manager would have been a considerable factor in that employee's poor job performance. Firing the employee would seem evil. If, however, the staff member is frequently tardy or absent through no fault of the manager, the consequences of firing the worker seem justified. If there is no proportionate reason for permitting an evil, the act is unethical. If there is an alternative that provides more good and less risk of evil, it should be chosen; if there is not, there is proportionate reason for risking an evil (Aroskar, 1980) (Box 3-10).

BOX 3-10 Ethical Relationship Model

Priestly
Engineering
Contractual
Collegial

BOX 3-11 Levels of Moral Development

Premoral
Conventional
Autonomous

MORAL REASONING

Levels of moral development have been identified by Lawrence Kohlberg as (1) premoral or preconventional when behavior is motivated by social or biological impulses with no sense of obligation to rules; (2) conventional when the person accepts standards of the group with little critical reflection, uses literal obedience to the rules, and feels obligation; and (3) autonomous when the person thinks and judges for himself or herself, considers the purpose and consequences of the rules, and does not accept the group standards without reflection (Anders, 2007).

Moral choice involves selecting one of two or more values that conflict. Ten universal moral values are distributive justice, law, liberty, life, property, punishment, roles and concerns of affection, roles and concerns of authority, gender, and truth.

The level of moral development determines what one finds valuable, how one defines the value, and why one finds it valuable. First, a person considers the power of the person involved. Second, one looks at satisfying one's own needs. Third, the individual considers relationships with others and then sees life as inherently worthwhile aside from other considerations. Moral judgment is necessary but not sufficient for mature moral action. People may do wrong even when they know better (Box 3-11).

MORAL AND ETHICAL LEADERSHIP

Values are the worth, merit, or importance one places on something. Morals are deliberate choices made that are consistent with one's perceptions of moral values and ethical norms. When one deliberately chooses to do what that person believes is wrong, the person is immoral. Ethics is related to an analysis of what is right or wrong. One must consider what is important to one's self and to others. Accordingly, human interdependence is an important issue for ethical behavior.

Staff nurses use individual justice to care for individual patients, but staff nurses and nursing leaders need to use distributive justice to address the professional responsibility for the collective practice of nursing on the unit, in the facility, and throughout the profession and all of health care. Nursing management in health care involves many ethical components as managers deal with complex interactions among themselves, the organization, the community, and the society. The primary ethical dilemma for nurse managers is balancing high quality care with fiscal responsibilities. Nurse managers need to act as client advocates while helping staff create a climate of ethical behavior. The managers need to be able to ask the right ethical questions, make the right ethical decisions, and do the right thing by applying ethical principles.

Typical approaches to distributive justice include rendering the same thing or treatment to everyone. It requires that all people are treated the same way without considering distinguishing particulars. This is not very practical in a health care setting. Rendering justice to each according to his or her works requires consideration of professional and social utility. It does not consider need or merit. It is appropriate in an emergency. Rendering justice according to merits is based on personal excellence and can include awards, merit raises, and promotions. Rendering justice according to rank does not require equality and is questionable. Recognizing education, experience, and competence can be appropriate. Justice may also be rendered according to legal entitlement, but legal and ethical are not necessarily the same. Rendering justice according

to need is appropriate for caring for clients in a health care setting but may not be appropriate in other situations. Distributive justice is important to staff nurses and especially important to nursing leaders who have the moral obligation to provide competent caregivers and services (Curtin, 2005).

UNIVERSAL PRINCIPLES OF ETHICS IN A MULTICULTURAL WORLD

Laws tell us what to do, and ethics tell us why. Ethical principles involve both human rights and responsibilities. Personal ethics or morality reflects the general expectations of a person in society. These are instilled in children through culture, education, and religion and are expected of one another. They include values and concerns for the well-being of others, respect for others' autonomy, trustworthiness, honesty, compliance with the law, justice, fairness, benevolence, altruism, aesthetics, equality, dignity, respect for human rights, and preventing harm. Professional ethics have additional responsibilities such as impartiality, objectivity, openness, confidentiality, diligence, fidelity, and avoiding conflict of interest. The principles of global ethics are controversial but may include global justice through international laws, social responsibility, environmental stewardship, interdependence, responsibility for the whole, and reverence for place. The principles only provide guidance and should be considered in the context of universality. There are selective violations of the principles that may be considered acceptable by society. Murder is illegal but may be considered acceptable in war. Lying is wrong but may be considered acceptable to save someone from harm. Most cultures seem to value trustworthiness but have different beliefs about truth telling. Eastern cultures value harmony whereas Western cultures prefer forthrightness. Hence, misunderstandings can occur because underlying principles are embodied in diverse ways that reflect differences in cultural values. Morality is a matter of opinion, and opinions do vary from culture to culture. However, these principles of ethics, which are recurring patterns of ethically responsible behavior, can serve as land-marks for our consciences (Sheikk, 2003).

ETHICS COMMITTEES

Complex ethical issues regarding patient care and policy making must be addressed. Institutional ethics committees deal with ethical questions that often require painful choices for patients, particularly for infants and those older adults who are unable to make their own decisions.

The following issues must be addressed within the institution's philosophy, both when forming an institutional ethics committee and through ongoing study and evaluation of the existing committee: responsibility; accountability; eco-nomic costs; efficacy; role of the committee in patient care decisions; privacy for the patients and families; and committee composition, structure, meetings, and access. In addition to ethical deci-sion making, the committee may do case reviews, consult, make policies, provide education, and enact Health Insurance Portability and Account-ability Act (HIPAA) policies. An ombudsman, or a community leader such as a minister, may be appointed. Nursing should be represented on the multidisciplinary committee. Ethics committees are likely to deal with ethical issues in nursing practice such as do-not-resuscitate orders, pa-tients' rights, professional practice issues, death and dying, and allocation of resources. Common ethical issues in health care include but are not limited to abortion, breaches of client confiden-tiality, cost containment, enactment of HIPAA policies, end-of-life decisions, end-of-life pain management, informed consent, organ transplan-tation, and rationing of care (Yoder-Wise, 2007).

NURSING CODE OF ETHICS AND STANDARDS OF PRACTICE

American Nurses Association's Code of Ethics for Nurses

The American Nurses Association (ANA) House of Delegates approved the new *Code of Ethics for Nurses* at its June 30, 2001 meeting in Washington,

DC. In July 2001, the Congress of Nursing Prac-tice and Economics voted to accept the new lan-guage of the interpretive statements. The revised *Code of Ethics for Nurses with Interpretive State-ments* has the following nine provisions:

1. The nurse, in all professional relationships, practices with compassion and respect for the inherent dignity, worth, and uniqueness of every individual, unrestricted by considerations of social or economic status, personal attributes, or the nature of health problems.
2. The nurse's primary commitment is to the patient, whether an individual, family, group, or community.
3. The nurse promotes, advocates for, and strives to protect the health, safety, and rights of the patient.
4. The nurse is responsible and accountable for individual nursing practice and determines the appropriate delegation of tasks consistent with the nurse's obligation to provide optimum patient care.
5. The nurse owes the same duties to self as to others, including the responsibility to preserve integrity and safety, to maintain competence, and to continue personal and professional growth.
6. The nurse participates in establishing, maintain-ing, and improving health care environments and conditions of employment conducive to the provision of quality health care and consistent with the values of the profession through indi-vidual and collective action.
7. The nurse participates in the advancement of the profession through contributions to practice, education, administration, and knowledge development.
8. The nurse collaborates with other health professionals and the public in promoting com-munity, national, and international efforts to meet health needs.
9. The profession of nursing, as represented by associations and their members, is responsible for articulating nursing values, for maintaining the integrity of the profession (American Nurses Association, 2003).

International Council of Nurses' International Code of Ethics for Nurses

The International Council of Nurses (ICN) first adopted an international code of ethics for nurs-es in 1953. It has been revised and reaffirmed several times since then. It identifies that the need for nursing is universal and that nurses have four fundamental responsibilities: to promote health, prevent illness, restore health, and alleviate suffering. It reaffirms that nurses give services to the individual, family, and community and coordinate services with related groups unrestricted by age, color, creed, culture, disability or illness, gender, nationality, politics, race, or social status. The 2006 *ICN Code of Ethics for Nurses* has four principal elements that outline the standards of ethical conduct: nurses and people, nurses and practice, nurses and the profession, and nurses and co-workers. They are as follows:

1. Nurses and people
   The nurse's primary professional responsibility is to people requiring nursing care.
   In providing care, the nurse promotes an environment in which the human rights, values, customs and spiritual beliefs of the individual, family, and community are respected.
   The nurse ensures that the individual receives sufficient information on which to base consent for care and related treatment.
   The nurse holds in confidence personal information and uses judgment in sharing this information.
   The nurse shares with society the responsibility for initiating and supporting action to meet the health and social needs of the public, in particular those of vulnerable populations.
   The nurse also shares responsibility to sustain and protect the natural environment from depletion, pollution, degradation, and destruction.
2. Nurses and practice
   The nurse carries personal responsibility and accountability for nursing practice, and for maintaining competence by continual learning.
   The nurse maintains a standard of personal health such that the ability to provide care is not compromised.
   The nurse uses judgment regarding individual competence when accepting and delegating responsibility.
   The nurse at all times maintains standards of personal conduct which reflect well on the profession and enhance public confidence.
   The nurse, in providing care, ensures that uses of technology and scientific advances are compatible with the safety, dignity, and rights of people.
3. Nurses and the profession
   The nurse assumes the major role in determining and implementing acceptable standards of clinical nursing practice, management, research, and education.
   The nurse is active in developing a core of research-based professional knowledge.
   The nurse, acting through the professional organization, participates in creating and maintaining safe, equitable social and economic working conditions in nursing.
4. Nurses and co-workers
   The nurse sustains a cooperative relationship with co-workers in nursing and other fields.
   The nurse takes appropriate action to safeguard individuals, families, and communities when their care is endangered by a co-worker or any other person. (International Council of Nurses, 2006)

DECISION-MAKING TOOLS

"Choices are the spice of life." —Anonymous

Most decisions involve varying degrees of uncertainty. Decision-making tools help visualize options to facilitate evaluation of the options. Leaders and managers use research of various kinds to minimize the uncertainty of their decisions. Probability theory, which is applied to risk and uncertainty, queuing theory, which deals with waiting lines or intermittent servicing problems, and linear programming, which implements matrix algebra or linear mathematical equations are beyond the discussion of this chapter.

Simulation, Models, and Games

Simulation is a way of using models and games to simplify problems by identifying the basic components and using trial and error to determine a solution. Through simulation the manager may compare alternatives and their consequences. The computer may be used to help solve simulations. These methods may be used to study organizational changes, scheduling, assembly line management, and time sequences.

A model represents something else, most commonly objects, events, processes, or systems. It is a technique of abstraction and simplification for studying something under varying conditions.

Manipulation is used to test the impact of proposed changes on the system without disturbing the subject of the model. Almost all quantitative methods used to guide decision making are models. They are particularly useful because of their convenience and low cost compared with manipulating real occurrences. Although models vary considerably in the accuracy with which they represent real situations, they increase predictive capabilities over such methods as guesswork and intuition.

Models are developed to describe, explain, and predict phenomena. The critical element of model building is conceptualization. Consequently, models can provide abstractions that facilitate communication. Models vary in the degree of abstraction used: a life-size mannequin is a realistic model that nursing students use to learn how to make occupied beds; a model of a building or a piece of equipment built to scale is quite concrete, whereas blueprints or photographs, organizational charts, and mathematical models are abstract.

The more variables added to the model, the more realistic but cumbersome it becomes. The objective of modeling is to provide a simplified, abstract version of reality. Managers must strive for the appropriate level of abstractness. They may base their decision on an oversimplified model if they do not attempt to expand their knowledge of the situation. Simplified models may be useful for quantitative analysis and prediction, but one must be cautious, because a person with the least knowledge of a situation may be the most certain about how to solve the problem. If description and understanding are important, more comprehensive models should be developed. Continuing to research a problem may contribute to a more realistic model, but it may also delay the decision too long. The cost of gathering additional information may be prohibitive; therefore balancing the cost of model refinement against the benefits obtained is required.

Game theory is a simulation of system operations. The player tries to develop a strategy that will maximize gains and minimize losses, regardless of what the competitor does. War games are commonly used to train personnel and to test plans and equipment under field conditions. Management games are used primarily to train personnel rather than to solve competitive problems. They are particularly useful for training in decision making by simulating real-life operations in a laboratory setting. Some of these examples are computer simulation games.

Gantt Chart

"Luck is where preparation meets with opportunity." —Anonymous

Gantt charts, named for their developer, Henry Gantt, are highly developed schedules that allow one to visualize multiple tasks that have to be done. A Gantt chart (Figure 3-2) is a grid with rows for tasks or assigned responsibility and columns for the time frame, which may be minutes, hours, days, weeks, months, years, or decades, depending on the longevity of the project. A line is drawn through the time frame while a task is in progress. An X is put at the point where that task is completed. One typically works backward from due dates.

A person is told on Monday that a report is due Friday at 4 PM. The person needs to collect information, type the report on the computer, revise the report, and submit it. The person will use 3 days to collect the information and 1 day to type or word process it, incubate the ideas overnight, do any revision needed Friday morning, and submit the report Friday afternoon. Gantt charts can be created in Excel (Huber, 2006; McConnell, 2006).

Decision Trees

A decision tree (Figure 3-3) is a graphic method that can help managers visualize the available alternatives, outcomes, risks, and information needs for a specific problem over a period of time. It helps them to see the possible directions that actions may take from each decision point and to evaluate the consequences of a series of

Task	Responsible	Mon	Tue	Wed	Th	Fr
Collect information	ME	– – – – – – – – ·				
Type report	ME				X	
Revise report	ME					X
Submit report	ME					X

Figure 3-2 • Gantt chart.

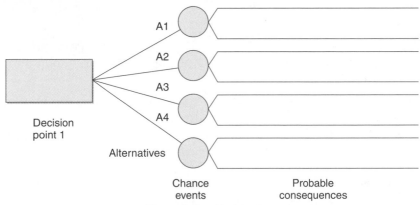

Decision point 1

Alternatives

Chance events

Probable consequences

Figure 3-3 • Decision tree.

decisions. The process begins with a primary decision having at least two alternatives. Then the predicted outcome for each decision is considered, and the need for further decisions is contemplated. The matrix resembles a tree as the decision points are diagrammed.

The results diagrammed on the tree are founded on the manager's experience and judgment but may be supported by computational data. For complex problems, probability statistics may be used to explore further factors that favor or oppose expected events. Although the decision tree does not depict an obviously correct decision, it allows managers to base their decision on a consideration of various alternatives and probable consequences. It helps them realize that subsequent decisions may depend on future events. Decision trees are useful for short- and

medium-range planning, as well as for decision making. Unfortunately, decision trees for longer than 2 or 3 years become cumbersome and speculative.

In Figure 3-4 the nursing staff decides to have a ward picnic for the psychiatric patients. The alternatives are to hold the picnic indoors or outdoors, and the chance events are rain or no rain. If the picnic is scheduled indoors and it rains, the patients may be crowded but dry; there will be no bugs; and the staff will be proud of their decision. If the picnic is scheduled indoors and it does not rain, the patients may feel crowded; the room may seem stuffy; the party will lack a picnic atmosphere; and the staff may regret not scheduling it outside. On the other hand, if the picnic is scheduled outdoors and it rains, the participants will get wet; the food will be ruined;

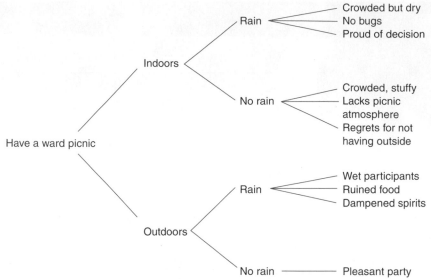

Figure 3-4 • Decision tree for psychiatric ward picnic.

and spirits will be dampened. If the picnic is scheduled outdoors and it does not rain, it will be a pleasant experience (Marquis & Huston, 2006). The American Nurses Association and the National Council of State Boards of Nursing have developed a decision tree for delegation to nursing assistive personnel (American Nurses Association, 2006).

Program Evaluation and Review Technique

Program evaluation and review technique (PERT) is a network system model for planning and control under uncertain conditions. It involves identifying the key activities in a project, sequencing the activities in a flow diagram, and assigning the duration of each phase of the work. It is particularly appropriate for one-of-a-kind projects that involve extensive research and development.

PERT recognizes that certain tasks must be completed before the total project can be completed and, further, that subtasks must be completed before others can be started. The key events are identified, numbered, labeled, or numbered and labeled on the flow chart. The activities that cause the progress from one event to another

are indicated by arrows, with the direction of the arrow showing the direction of the work flow.

PERT also deals with the problem of uncertainty with respect to time by estimating the time variances associated with the expected time of completion of the subtasks. Three projected times are determined: (1) the optimistic time (t_o), which estimates the completion time without complications; (2) the most likely time (t_m), which estimates the completion time with normal problems; and (3) the pessimistic time (t_p), which estimates the completion time given numerous problems. Thus the shortest, average, and longest times needed to complete an activity are calculated. The expected time (t_e) is calculated from these figures by the following formula:

$$t_e = \frac{t_o + 4(t_m) + t_p}{6}$$

If the optimistic time is 2 weeks, the most likely time 4 weeks, and the pessimistic time 6 weeks, the expected time is as follows:

$$t_e = \frac{2\,weeks + 4(4\,weeks) + 6\,weeks}{6}$$

$$= \frac{24\,weeks}{6} = 4\,weeks$$

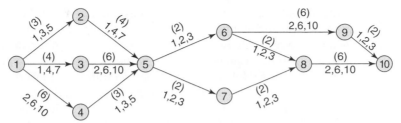

Figure 3-5 • Program evaluation and review technique (PERT) model. This PERT model indicates that subtask 1 must be completed before 2, 3, and 4 can be done; 2, 3, and 4 before 5; 5 before 6 and 7; 6 before 9; 6 and 7 before 8; and 8 and 9 before 10. A coding system can be used to determine what the numbers mean. For example, 1 = program planned, 2 = staff informed. Arrows show direction of work flow. Optimistic, most likely, pessimistic, and expected times are recorded for each activity. The expected time is in parentheses.

The PERT model helps the manager determine priorities (Figure 3-5). Use of resources can be considered when setting priorities. Assignments may be changed temporarily, overtime may be allowed, or temporary help may be hired to facilitate the activity flow and to manipulate the time required to move from one event to another.

PERT is a good tool for construction projects. Foundations need to be laid before walls can be put up. The plumbing and electrical wiring need to be done before the drywall is put up. Then the drywall can be painted and cabinets installed, etc. PERT helps determine when to hire subcontractors. It can also be used to plan a move, to renovate, or to do a new service or project. There would need to be a decision to do the new service. A facility might need to be built or renovated. A manger would need to be appointed, policies created, staff hired and trained, etc. A manager might be able to develop policies and interview staff while the building is being built or renovated (McConnell, 2006; Yoder-Wise, 2007).

Critical Path Method

Critical path method (CPM), closely related to PERT, calculates a single time estimate for each activity, the longest possible time. A cost estimate is figured for both normal and crash operating conditions. Normal means the least-cost method, and crash refers to conditions in less-than-normal time. Simple sequences can be worked out manually and more complex ones by computer. CPM is particularly useful where cost is a significant

factor and experience provides a basis for estimating time and cost. Managers can observe the critical path and compare the progress with the projected dates.

Critical paths have been used to indicate standard practices of care. They predetermined the course of progress for patients with specific diagnoses and treatments. They would indicate the length of stay and the interventions that should occur at specific times. For example, a patient would be admitted the day of the surgery a couple of hours before the surgery is scheduled. An EKG, and blood and urine tests would be run. An IV would be started. The patient would have a specific time in surgery and the recovery room and be discharged to home. If there were complications, the patient might be in surgery or recovery longer and more medications and supplies might be used, or the patient might be admitted to another health care facility. That would increase the costs. Critical pathways are more useful for conditions that require longer recovery times, like fractured hips or body part replacements. Critical pathways have been able to help reduce some cost by reducing radiology and laboratory tests and by reducing the length of stays. They allow both clinical and financial projections. Unfortunately, there are sometimes justifiable differentiations between unique patients that cause more paperwork and utilization reviews that add to administrative costs.

Network analysis techniques facilitate planning and result in objective plans by making it possible to identify the critical path and show interrelationships among parts, thus facilitating improvements in structure and communications. They are particularly useful for task force or project forms of organization and for projects (Huber, 2006; Marquis & Huston 2006).

Advantages and Limitations of Quantitative Tools for Decision Making

Quantitative tools lend themselves to a rational, systematic approach to problem solving for decisions that can be expressed mathematically. They encourage disciplined thinking. They are not limited to the six or seven variables the human mind can consider at one time, and they may evaluate thousands of interrelationships simultaneously. Decisions made with the use of quantitative tools are likely to be superior to those that rely heavily on judgment. Unfortunately, many managerial problems involve intangible, nonmeasurable factors that reduce the effectiveness of the tools. The mathematical expressions are based on assumptions; if those assumptions are not true for a given situation, the tool becomes useless.

COMPUTERS

Computers can facilitate complex decision making. Computers provide several advantages over paper-based record systems. Information can be stored in smaller areas, search and analytical tasks can be performed, and information can be obtained quickly and efficiently. Unfortunately, if used improperly, computers can magnify weaknesses in an organization.

Computers can be applied in nursing in three major categories: (1) clinical systems; (2) management information systems; and (3) educational systems. In clinical systems, computers help with patient histories, medical records, and patient monitoring. Computerized record systems can improve the usability of patient information because data from the chart can be rearranged to be useful to various health care professionals. Physicians can enter their diagnoses, protocols,

and notes directly into the computer, saving nurses transcribing time. The instructions can be printed out at the appropriate auxiliary department. Nurses can also record their notes directly into the computer and spend less time and energy accumulating and summarizing data to develop care plans. Standard screens with standard choices increase efficiency for recording observations and doing care plans. Nurses are made aware of changes that require their intervention quickly because information from ancillary departments can be sent automatically to the nursing station terminal. The computer can sort and analyze data and facilitate communication about the patients among health care providers.

An integrated clinical system allows patient data to be quickly available to health care providers. The system should be easy to use, have standardized data elements, have data repositories and archival systems for information that should be retained long term, and have stand-alone or departmental system accessibility to patient information.

Emergency department systems can triage patients based on assessment criteria. The system can calculate the level of severity based on the assessment and historical data entered by the triage person. The data can be readily available to all clinical personnel, such as those in the laboratory, pharmacy, and radiology departments. The marketing and planning departments can use the statistics to evaluate the market share information. The *laboratory system* allows ordering, collecting, analyzing, and storing of laboratory information, as well as reporting of results. *Pharmacy systems* can be used to order, check allergies, check dosage based on the patient's height and weight, check drug-to-drug interactions, check drug-to-food interactions, label medications, do inventory control, do drug utilization monitoring, and dispense medications. It allows medication cart fill, update, and check functions; printing of written orders; electronic recording of administration of medications; and an alert system for when medications are overdue. *Radiology systems* allow for ordering, scheduling, recording results, and tracking radiology exams. They can generate notices to send to patients and

RESEARCH Perspective 3-2

Data from Genrich SJ, Banks JC, Bufton K, Savage ME, Owens MU: Group involvement in decision-making: A pilot study. *The Journal of Continuing Education in Nursing,* 32(1):20-26, 2001.

Purpose: The purpose of this study was to determine if leadership could be taught regarding using the appropriate level of group involvement in decision making using the Vroom-Yetton-Jago Leadership Model.

Methods: A convenience sample of 27 health care leaders who attended a 90-minute class offered in one agency were eligible for inclusion in the pretest and posttest on similar case studies for this quasiexperimental study. A paired t-test resulted in statistically significant findings.

Results/conclusions: The results indicate that participating in a class on the use of the Vroom-Yetton-Jago Leadership Model may help leaders gain the skill needed to appropriately delegate decision making to groups.

schedule repeat exams. Transcription can be done electronically with an electronically attached signature. Some transcription systems allow for filling in the blanks to eliminate excessive typing. The systems can also track the location of various exam results and has the capability to store images directly on the radiology system, making digitized images readily available. *Cardiology systems* are similar to radiology systems and can be used for the collection, analysis, and reporting of cardiology exams. Transcription capabilities, ability to display and store digitized images, and telemedicine to transmit the report to physicians are desirable.

Dietary systems can assess nutritional status and facilitate ordering and preparing diets. They can create, maintain, and print menus; enter modifiers about restrictions or limitations to basic diets; place a diet on hold for a period of time; print a worksheet for the tray preparation area; and print out diet information for patient and family education.

Respiratory therapy systems can be used to order equipment and treatments, schedule procedures, document responses to treatments, and record interventions. The system can track routine cleaning and maintenance of equipment, and disposable and reusable equipment and supplies.

Computer systems can also be used in *operating rooms, ambulatory clinics, physician offices, and case management systems.* They are good for scheduling and materials management. Transcription and patient billing are useful functions. Systems can handle scheduling appointments with several different services with one phone call, which can also obtain basic data, such as insurance information, which can be verified later. They can track missed appointments.

Patient care documentation systems are the largest application of computer systems in health care. Point of care or bedside systems document patient assessments, treatments, medication administration, response to treatments and medications, and other progress notes. They can be used in home care as well as critical care. They allow for integration of care by several care providers.

Patient monitoring systems record patient responses and can alert nurses to changes. Computers can record the patient's progress on paper or on the monitor, sound an alarm, and often transmit information from the patient's bedside to monitors at the nursing station. In addition to monitoring patients continuously and detecting changes, computers can analyze and interpret the data. Through computer monitoring, nurses can respond quickly to changes in patients' conditions.

Computers have many applications in management information systems. They can be used for tracking patient acuity and calculating patient care requirements; for patient classification systems, inventory control, supplies and material management, staff scheduling, policy and procedure changes and announcements, patient charges, budget information and management, personnel records, statistical reports, administrative reports, memos; and record location and tracking.

In *educational systems,* computer-assisted instruction allows students to proceed at their own speed, provides immediate feedback, and allows dissemination of information to remote areas. When using computers as decision-making tools, nurses should take advantage of good commercial software that is available and should investigate the possibility of using existing systems. Securing the confidentiality of patient and personnel records by carefully locking up data storage (e.g., DVDs, CD-ROMs, diskettes) or by constructing a password system is very important (Kreider & Hasselton, 1997).

The Vroom and Jago model (1988) is a computer-friendly revision of the Vroom and Yetton model (1973) (Box 3-12). It provides an additional number of problem attributes, deletes the decision rules, changes dichotomous variables to continuous variables, and provides mathematical formulas to determine decisions (Ratzburg, 2007).

"The only exercise some minds get is jumping to conclusions!" —Pansy Torrance

---

BOX 3-12 Vroom and Yetton Normative Model

Vroom and Yetton address decision making as a social process and emphasize how managers do rather than should behave in their normative model. They identify the following alternative decision processes: A=autocratic, C=consultative, G=group, I=first variant, and II=second variant.

TYPES OF MANAGEMENT DECISION STYLES*

AI   You solve the problem or make the decision yourself, using information available to you at that time.

AII   You obtain the necessary information from your subordinate(s), then decide on the solution to the problem yourself. You may or may not tell your subordinates what the problem is in getting the information from them. The role played by your subordinates in making the decision is clearly one of providing the necessary information to you, rather than generating or evaluating alternative solutions.

CI   You share the problem with relevant subordinates individually, getting their ideas and suggestions without bringing them together as a group. Then you make the decision that may or may not reflect your subordinates' influence.

CII   You share the problem with your subordinates as a group, collectively obtaining their ideas and suggestions. Then you make the decision that may or may not reflect your subordinates' influence.

GII   You share a problem with your subordinates as a group. Together you generate and evaluate alternatives and attempt to reach agreement (consensus) on a solution. Your role is much like that of chairperson. You do not try to influence the group to adopt "your" solution, and you are willing to accept and implement any solution that has the support of the entire group.

(GI is omitted because it applies only to more comprehensive models outside the scope of the article.)

DECISION RULES

Vroom identifies seven rules that do most of the work of the model. Three rules protect decision quality, and four protect acceptance.*

1. The information rule
   If the quality of the decision is important and if the leader does not possess enough information or expertise to solve the problem alone, AI is eliminated from the feasible set. (Its use risks a low-quality decision.)

2. The goal congruence rule
   If the quality of the decision is important and if the subordinates do not share the organizational goals to be obtained in solving the problem, GII is eliminated from the feasible set. (Alternatives that eliminate the leader's final control over the decision reached may jeopardize the quality of the decision.)

BOX 3-12 Vroom and Yetton Normative Model—cont'd

3. The unstructured problem rule

   In decisions in which the quality of the decision is important, if the leader lacks the necessary information or expertise to solve the problem alone, and if the problem is unstructured (that is, the leader does not know exactly what information is needed and where it is located), the method used must allow the leader not only to collect the information but also to do so in an efficient and effective manner. Methods that involve interaction among all subordinates with full knowledge of the problem are likely to be both more efficient and more likely to generate a high-quality solution to the problem. Under these conditions AI, AII, and CI are eliminated from the feasible set. (AI does not provide for him or her to collect the necessary information, and AII and CI represent more cumbersome, less effective, and less efficient means of bringing the necessary information to bear on the solution of the problem than methods that do permit those with the necessary information to interact.)

4. The acceptance rule

   If the acceptance of the decision by subordinates is critical to effective implementation, and if it is not certain that an autocratic decision made by the leader would receive that acceptance, AI and AII are eliminated from the feasible set. (Neither provides an opportunity for subordinates to participate in the decision, and both risk losing the necessary acceptance.)

5. The conflict rule

   If the acceptance of the decision is critical, and an autocratic decision is not certain to be accepted, and subordinates are likely to be in conflict or disagreement over the appropriate solution, AI, AII, and CI are eliminated from the feasible set. (The method used in solving the problem should enable those in disagreement to resolve their differences with full knowledge of the problem. Accordingly, under these conditions, AI, AII, and CI, which involve either no interaction or only one-on-one relationships and therefore provide no opportunity for those in control to resolve their differences, are eliminated from the feasible set. Their use runs the risk of leaving some of the subordinates with less than the necessary commitment to the final decision.)

6. The fairness rule

   If the quality of the decision is unimportant and if acceptance is critical and not certain to result from an autocratic decision, AI, AII, CI, and CII are eliminated from the feasible set. (The method used should maximize the probability of acceptance because this is the only relevant consideration in determining the effectiveness of the decision. Under these circumstances, AI, AII, CI, and CII, which create less acceptance or commitment than GII, are eliminated from the feasible set. To use them is to run the risk of getting less than the needed acceptance of the decision.

7. The acceptance priority rule

   If acceptance is critical and not ensured by an autocratic decision, and if subordinates can be trusted, AI, AII, CI, and CII are eliminated from the feasible set. (Methods that provide equal partnership in the decision-making process can provide greater acceptance without risking decision quality. Use of any method other than GII results in an unnecessary risk that the decision will not be fully accepted or receive the necessary commitment on the part of subordinates.)

   As one asks the diagnostic questions and applies the rules to specific situations, one may eliminate all but one decision style from the feasibility set. However, it is more likely that several decision styles could be used and still protect both the decision quality and acceptance requirements. Then the time factor is used to determine which of the feasible options will require the least time.

   Vroom and Yetton focus on three classes of outcomes that influence the ultimate effectiveness of decisions: (1) the quality of the decision, (2) acceptance of the decision by the subordinates, and (3) available time needed to make the decision. The authors found that managers can diagnose a situation quickly and accurately by answering the following seven questions*:

Continued

BOX 3-12 Vroom and Yetton Normative Model—cont'd

PROBLEM ATTRIBUTES	DIAGNOSTIC QUESTIONS
A. The importance of the quality of the decision:	Is there a quality requirement such that one solution is likely to be more rational than another?
B. The extent to which the leader possesses sufficient information/expertise to make a high-qualtiy decision by herself:	Do you have sufficient information to make a high-quality decision?
C. The extent to which the problem is structured:	Is the problem structured?
D. The extent to which acceptance or commitment on the part of subordinates is critical to the effective implementation of the decision:	Do you need the acceptance and commitment of others to implement the decision?
E. The prior probability that the leader's autocratic decision will receive acceptance by subordinates:	If you were to make the decision by yourself, is it reasonably certain that it would be accepted by your subordinates?
F. The extent to which subordinates are motivated to attain the organizational goals as represented in the objectives explicit in the statement of the problem.	Do subordinates share the organizational goals to be obtained in solving this problem?
G. The extent to which subordinates are likely to be in conflict over preferred solutions:	Is conflict among subordinates likely in preferred solutions?

CHAPTER SUMMARY

The decision-making process can help prevent problems while the problem-solving process applies the decision-making process only after there is already a problem. The nursing process is decision making and problem solving applied to nursing. They are all scientific processes. There are several components to critical thinking to facilitate sound decision making. Divergent thinking generates ideas, while convergent thinking identifies the best solution. Creative thinking generates novel solutions. Not making a decision is also a decision. Consultation can be useful, and ethics committees can provide moral and ethical leadership. Group factors and committee aspects in decision making are similar. Computers can be used to facilitate complex decision making. Numerous decision-making tools are available, and leaders can use the objectives for the activity to determine which tool to use.

CASE STUDY

Your organization has limited funds for personnel raises. You represent your unit on the agency budget committee. Should you give everyone the same dollar amount raise, thus giving a lower percentage raise to personnel with larger salaries? Should you give the same percentage raise across the board, thus giving people with higher salaries more money? Should the raises be stratified, giving different categories of people different dollar or percentage raises? What are other options?

CRITICAL THINKING ACTIVITY

Reflective Journal: Make observations in a clinical setting, or reflect on past experiences. Answer the following questions: What creative-thinking techniques have you observed being used? What decision-making tools have you observed being used? How are ethical issues addressed in an agency with which you are familiar? What departments are represented? Is there a nurse member on an ethics committee? How does that committee function?

REFERENCES

Alfaro-Lefevre R: *Critical thinking in nursing: A practical approach,* Philadelphia, 2003, Saunders.

American Nurses Association: *Code of ethics for nurses with interpretive statements,* Washington, DC, 2003, American Nurses Association.

American Nurses Association, National Council of State Boards of Nursing: *Joint statement on delegation,* 2006 (website): http://www.ncsbn.org/Joint_statement.pdf. Accessed July 24, 2007.

Anders MD: Kohlberg's ideas of moral reasoning, 2007 (website): http://web.cortland.edu/andersmd/KOHL/kidmoral.HTML. Accessed July 24, 2007.

Aroskar MA: Ethics of nurse-patient relationships, *Nurse Educ* 5:18, 1980.

Curtin LL: A framework for analysis: Part I, *NAQ* 29(2):183–187, 2005.

Finkelman AW: *Leadership and management in nursing,* Upper Saddle River, NJ, 2006, Pearson/Prentice Hall.

Franz M: *Organizational models of decision making,* 1998 (website): http://www.viterbo.edu/perspgs/Staff/MFranz/chap4_fast/tsld017.htm. Accessed July 24, 2007.

Friend C: *Social contract theory,* 2006 (website): http://www.iep.utm.edu/s/soc-cont.htm, Accessed July 24, 2007.

Genrich SJ, Banks JC, Bufton K et al: Group involvement in decision-making: A pilot study, *The Journal of Continuing Education in Nursing* 32(1):20-26, 2001.

Harris RA: *Creative problem solving: A step-by-step approach,* Los Angeles, 2002, Pyrczak.

Huber DL: *Leadership and nurisng care management,* ed 3, Philadelphia, 2006, Saunders/Elsevier.

Infinite Innovations Ltd: *SCAMPER technique training for lateral thinking,* 2006 (website): http://www.brainstorming.co.uk/tutorials/scampertutorial.html. Accessed July 24, 2007.

International Council of Nursing (ICN): *The ICN code of ethics for nurses,* 2006 (website): www.icn.ch/icncode.pdf. Accessed July 24, 2007.

Josephson B: *Right brain vs. left brain,* 2007 (website): http://coe.sdsu.edu/eet/articles/dominance/start.htm. Accessed July 24, 2007.

Kay CD: *Notes of deontology,* 1997a (website): http://webs.wofford.edu/kaycd/ethics/deon.htm. Accessed July 24, 2007.

Kay CD: *Notes on utilitarianism,* 1997b (website): http://webs.wofford.edu/kaycd/ethics/util.htm. Accessed January 23, 2007.

Kay CD: *Varieties of egoism,* 1997c (website): http://webs.wofford.edu/kaycd/ethics/egoism.htm. Accessed July 24, 2007.

Kramer M, Maguire P, Schmalenberg C, et al: Excellence through evidence: Structures enabling clinical autonomy, *JONA* 37(1):41-52, 2007.

Kreider NA, Hasselton BJ: *The systems challenge,* Chicago, 1997, American Hospital Association.

Labelle S: *Six thinking hats,* 2005 (website): http://members.optusnet.com.au/~charles57/Creative/Techniques/sixhats.htm. Accessed July 24, 2007.

Marquis BL, Huston CJ: *Leadership roles and management functions in nursing: Theory and application,* ed 5, Philadelphia, 2006, Lippincott.

McConnell CR: *Umiker's management skills for the new health care supervisor,* ed 4, Boston, 2006, Jones & Bartlett.

Mycoted: *Notebook,* 2006 (website): http://www.mycoted.com/Notebook. Accessed July 24, 2007.

Paul R: *Critical thinking,* Santa Rosa, CA, 1993, Foundation of Critical Thinking.

Paul R, Elder L: *Critical thinking: Learn the tools the best thinkers use,* Upper Saddle River, NJ, 2005, Prentice Hall.

Polit DF, Beck CT: *Nursing research: Generating and assessing evidence for nursing practice,* Philadelphia, 2007, Lippincott.

Ratzburg W: *The Vroom and Yetton's leadership model,* 2007 (website): http://www.geocities.com/Athens/forum/1650/qvroom.html?200713. Accessed July 28, 2007.

Roussel L, Swansburg RC, Swansburg RJ: *Management and leadership for nurse administrators,* ed 4, Boston, 2006, Jones & Bartlett.

Scriven M, Paul R: *Defining critical thinking,* 2004 (website): http://www.criticalthinking.org/aboutCT/definingCT.shtml. Accessed July 24, 2007.

Sheikk A: *Universal ethics: Dealing with ethics in a multicultural world,* 2003 (website): http://www.studentbmj.com/back_issues/1200/editorials/438.html. Accessed July, 2007.

Simms LM, Price SA, Ervin NE: *Professional practice of nursing administration,* ed 3, Albany, NY, 2000, Delmar.

Straker D: *Bisociation: Forced association,* 2007 (website), http://creatingminds.org/principles/forced_association.htm. Accessed July 24, 2007.

Sullivan EJ, Decker PJ: *Effective leadership and management in nursing,* ed 5, Upper Saddle River, NJ, 2005, Prentice Hall.

Swansburg RC, Swansburg RJ: *Introduction to management and leadership for nurse managers,* ed 3, Boston, 2002, Jones & Bartlett.

Treffinger DJ, Isaksen SG, Stead-dorval KB: *Creative problem solving: An introduction*, ed 4, Waco, TX, 2006, Prufrock Press.

Velch R: Models for ethical medicine. In Aroskar MA: Ethics of nurse-patient relationships, *Nurse Educ* 5:18, 1980.

Vroom VH, Jago AG: *The new leadership: Managing participation in organizations*, Englewood Cliffs, NJ, 1988, Prentice Hall.

Vroom VH, Yetton PW: *Leadership and decision-making*, Pittsburgh, 1973, University of Pittsburgh.

Wenger W: *High thinktank,* 2004 (website): http://www. winwenger.com/htt.htm. Accessed July 24, 2007.

WriteDesign: *Sequence,* 2007a (website): http://www. writedesignonline.com/organizers/sequence.html. Accessed July 24, 2007.

WriteDesign: *Compare and contrast,* 2007b (website): http://writedesignonline.com/organizers/ comparecontrast.html. Accessed July 24, 2007.

WriteDesign: *Evaluate graphic organizers,* 2007c (website): http://www.writedesignonline.com/ organizers/evaluate.html. Accessed July 28, 2007.

Wywialowski EF: *Managing client care*, ed 3, St. Louis, 2004, Mosby.

Yoder-Wise PS: *Leading and managing in nursing*, ed 4, St. Louis, 2007, Mosby.

Yoder-Wise PS, Kowalski KE: *Beyond leading and managing in nursing*, St. Louis, 2006, Mosby.

Young AP, Cooke M: *Managing and implementing decisions in health care*, Edinburgh, 2002, Bailliere Tindall & Royal College of Nursing.

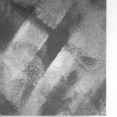

Motivation and Morale

4

Chapter Overview

Chapter 4 explains theories of motivation, including Taylor's monistic theory, Maslow's hierarchy of needs theory, Alderfer's modified need hierarchy, McClelland's basic needs theory, Herzberg's motivation hygiene (two-factor) theory, Argyris's psychological energy theory, Vroom's expectancy theory, Skinner's positive reinforcement theory, equity theory, intrinsic motivation, McGregor's Theory X and Theory Y, Likert's participative management theory, Theory Z, and the historical development of motivation theory. Emotional intelligence, genetic predisposition to personality, morale, workplace incivility and horizontal violence, workplace violence, burnout, and job satisfaction are discussed.

Chapter Objectives

- Locate Maslow's five needs in Alderfer's three categories of existence, relatedness, and growth needs.
- Identify at least five hygiene and five motivation factors in Herzberg's theory.
- Describe Vroom's expectancy theory.
- Explain how Skinner's positive reinforcement theory works.
- Describe ways people deal with perceived inequities.
- List at least three beliefs each for McGregor's Theory X and Theory Y.
- Describe emotional intelligence.
- Discuss the relationship between morale, burnout, and job satisfaction.

Online Resources

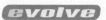 Critical thinking activities, worksheets, and case studies are available online at http://evolve.elsevier.com/Marriner/guide8e.

Major Concepts and Definitions

Burnout *a state of emotional exhaustion*
Climate *a general atmosphere or attitude*
Dissatisfaction *discontent*
Motivation *given impetus to incite, impel, or spur on*
Intrinsic *essential, inherent, not dependent on external circumstances*
Extrinsic *not inherent, not essential, external, extraneous*
Job satisfaction *contentment with one's work and job climate*

MOTIVATION

Why do people work? Why do some employees achieve high productivity whereas others are content with mediocrity or less? What can a manager do to stimulate intrinsic and extrinsic motivation? These questions are important to the leader and manager. They elicit complex and uncertain answers. Unfortunately, there are no simple rules that a leader and manager can follow to stimulate the staff.

Taylor's Monistic Theory

> *"He who has no money is poor, but he who has nothing but money is the poorest of all"* —Anonymous

Monistic theory is derived from the principles of scientific management. Frederick Taylor, a pioneer in this field, believed that if energetic people with high productivity learn that they earn no more than a lazy worker who does as little as possible, they will lose interest in giving optimal performance. Taylor argued that an incentive is needed to prevent this loss. It should be possible to earn more by producing more, so that pay would depend on productivity. Incentives such as merit increases, bonus systems, profit sharing, savings sharing, and piece rates are examples of monistic methods. With implementation of payment by piece rate, the employer must be certain that wage costs do not increase more rapidly than production supports. This system can place considerable pressure on the worker and create tensions that lead to undesirable behavior. Payment by piece rate almost certainly guarantees that some workers will be paid more than others. A larger paycheck may increase one's self-esteem and even serve as a status symbol as well as help meet physiological needs by being able to purchase food, clothing, and shelter (Taylor, 1903, 1911) (see Chapter 7).

Maslow's Hierarchy of Needs

In contrast to Taylor's belief that money is a primary motivator, Abraham Maslow maintained that people are motivated by a desire to satisfy a hierarchy of needs. Maslow hypothesized that satisfaction of the basic physiological needs triggers the emergence of more abstract needs and that a satisfied need is no longer a motivator. The five basic needs he identified are physiological, safety/security, social/belonging, esteem, and self-actualization. He later added the following needs: understand for the cognitive need of academic types, aesthetic beauty for the emotional need of artists, and transcendence that is beyond realizing one's own potential to helping others achieve their potential (Huber, 2006; Roussel, Swansburg, & Swansburg, 2006; Sullivan & Decker, 2005; Maslow, 1987) (see Chapter 7) (Figure 4-1).

Physiological Needs

The body needs water, food, oxygen, elimination, rest, exercise, sex, shelter, and protection from the elements. People have a strong drive

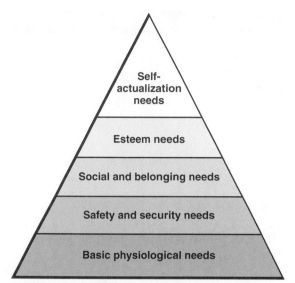

Figure 4-1 • Maslow's hierarchy of needs. (Modified from Maslow AH: *Motivation and personality.* Copyright 1954, 1970, 1987 by Abraham H. Maslow. Modified by permission of Prentice-Hall, Upper Saddle River, NJ.)

for self-preservation, and whenever their basic physiological needs are threatened, the needs become prepotent. These needs are relatively independent and must be met repeatedly to remain fulfilled. In an affluent society, physiological needs are probably not the most common motivators. However, the nurse manager should determine whether physiological needs are being met. Personnel should not be overworked. Meal breaks and rest breaks should be provided. Pay should be adequate for food, shelter, health care, and recreation.

Safety/Security Needs

People need physical, emotional, and financial safety. They need a stable environment in which they are protected against the threats of danger and deprivation. People do not want to worry about inadequate income because of loss of job, accident, or old age. Arbitrary management actions, favoritism toward or discrimination against employees, and unpredictable administration of policies are dangerous to safety needs and should be avoided.

Social/Belonging Needs

Social needs include a feeling of belonging, acceptance by one's peers, recognition as an accepted member of a group, being an integral part of the operation, giving and receiving friendship, and affectionate relations with others. A cohesive work group is likely to be more effective than an equal number of people working separately. Yet management, fearing hostility toward its objectives, may control situations to prevent esprit de corps. Thwarting of the social needs, however, may stimulate resistance and antagonism that further defeat management's objectives.

Esteem Needs

Achievement, competence, knowledge, independence, status, recognition, prestige, appreciation, reputation, and respect contribute to one's self-confidence and self-esteem. Management can help meet these needs by giving praise when it is deserved and through the use of constructive evaluations, pay raises, and titles. Unlike the lower physiological and safety needs, the esteem needs are not so easily satisfied.

Self-Actualization Needs

It is doubtful that one ever achieves all that of which one is capable. Feelings of accomplishment, responsibility, importance, challenge, advancement, and new experiences and opportunities for growth contribute to self-fulfillment.

Alderfer's Modified Need Hierarchy

Clayton Alderfer proposes a modified need hierarchy theory that collapses Maslow's five hierarchical levels into three (Box 4-1). His existence-relatedness-growth (ERG) theory suggests that in addition to a satisfaction-progression

TABLE 4-1 Comparison of Maslow's Hierarchy of Needs and Alderfer's Existence, Relatedness, and Growth

Maslow	Alderfer
Self-actualization needs	Growth needs
Esteem needs	Relatedness needs
Social/belonging needs	Existence needs
Safety/security needs	
Physiological needs	

BOX 4-2 McClelland's Basic Needs Theory

NEED FOR:
Achievement
Affiliation
Power

process, in which people are constantly frustrated in their attempts to satisfy one level of needs, they can redirect their energy toward a lower-level need. Alderfer's model is less rigid than Maslow's and suggests that more than one need may be operative (Huber, 2006; Roussel, Swansburg, & Swansburg, 2006; Sullivan & Decker, 2005) (Table 4-1).

McClelland's Basic Needs Theory

David McClelland has identified three basic needs that all people have in varying degrees: the need for achievement, power, and affiliation (Box 4-2). The need for achievement involves a desire to make a contribution, to excel, and to succeed. People with high achievement needs are eager for responsibility, take calculated risks, and desire feedback about their performance. People who have a high need for power want to be in control and desire influence over others. They are more interested in personal prestige and power than effective performance. For contrast, people with high affiliation needs desire working in human environments and seek out meaningful friendships. They want to be respected and avoid decisions or actions that oppose group norms. They are more interested in high morale than productivity. Leaders and managers should match personnel needs with assignments. If a project has well-defined objectives and specific tasks, a person with a high achievement need may be appropriate. If a project involves unpleasant tasks with personnel (such as retrenchment), a person with high power needs may do the job best. A person with high affiliation needs would not want to

make decisions that would alienate peers but would be good for fostering morale (Huber, 2006; Roussel, Swansburg, & Swansburg, 2006).

Herzberg's Motivation Hygiene (Two-Factor) Theory

"Let me give so much time to the improvement of myself that I shall not have time to criticize others." —Anonymous

Frederick Herzberg found that work motivators include achievement, growth, responsibility, advancement, recognition, and the job itself. According to Herzberg, if people are satisfied with their job, they are receiving positive feedback, developing skills, and improving their performance. Herzberg maintains that employees can be motivated by giving them challenging work in which they can assume responsibility (Figure 4-2 and Box 4-3).

Dissatisfaction results when people perceive that they are being treated unfairly in pay, benefits, status, job security, supervision, and interpersonal relationships. Herzberg classifies all of the above as hygiene factors and argues that they are not motivators because they do not cause any improvement in attitudes or performance. They can only prevent dissatisfaction and poor morale. Hygiene factors do not make a job more interesting. If people are highly motivated and find their job interesting and challenging, they can tolerate dissatisfaction with hygiene factors. When there is high hygiene and low motivation, workers are likely to view the job as a paycheck. According to Herzberg, when the motivating factors including achievement,

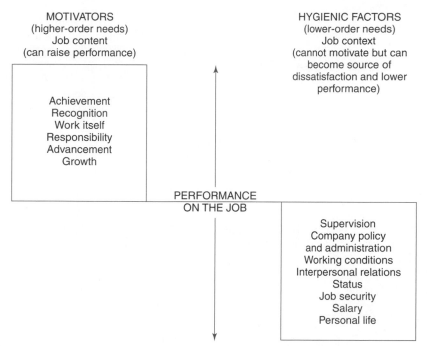

MOTIVATORS
(higher-order needs)
Job content
(can raise performance)

HYGIENIC FACTORS
(lower-order needs)
Job context
(cannot motivate but can
become source of
dissatisfaction and lower
performance)

Achievement
Recognition
Work itself
Responsibility
Advancement
Growth

PERFORMANCE
ON THE JOB

Supervision
Company policy
and administration
Working conditions
Interpersonal relations
Status
Job security
Salary
Personal life

Figure 4-2 • Herzberg's two-factor motivation hygiene theory of needs motivation. (From Claus KE, Bailey JT: *Power and influence in health care,* St Louis, 1977, Mosby.)

BOX 4-3 Herzberg's Motivation Hygiene Theory

MAINTENANCE FACTORS
Dissatisfiers
Hygiene factors
Job contest
Extrinsic factors

MOTIVATIONAL FACTORS
Satisfiers
Motivators
Job content
Intrinsic factors

recognition for achievement, responsibility, interesting job, growth, and advancement are high, and hygiene factors are high, workers are likely to be highly motivated with few complaints. High complaints and lack of motivation accompany low hygiene and low motivation factors (Herzberg, Mausner, & Snyderman, 1959; Herzberg, 1977; Huber,

2006; Roussel, Swansburg, & Swansburg, 2006; Sullivan & Decker, 2005) (see Chapter 7) (Figures 4-3 and 4-4).

Argyris's Psychological Energy Theory

"You must look into people, as well as at them." —Anonymous

Chris Argyris believes that people will exert more energy to meet their own needs than those of the organization. According to Argyris, the greater the disparity between the individual's and the organization's goals, the more likely it is that the employee will feel dissatisfaction, tension, conflict, apathy, or subversion. Argyris suggests that management match personnel and jobs by taking advantage of people's talents and interests, make jobs interesting and challenging, help personnel satisfy their needs for self-actualization, improve interpersonal relationships, and use a

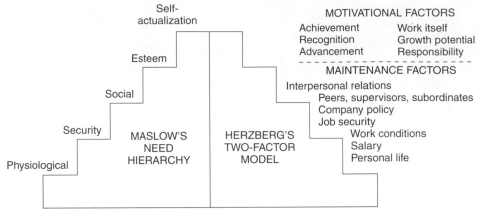

Figure 4-3 • Comparison of the Maslow and Herzberg models. (From Donnelly JH Jr, Gibson JL, Ivancevich JM: *Fundamentals of management: Functions, behavior, models,* ed 4, Dallas, 1990, Business Publications.)

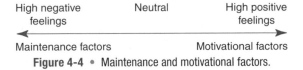

Figure 4-4 • Maintenance and motivational factors.

management style consistent with McGregor's Theory Y (which will be discussed later) (Argyris & Schon, 1974) (see Chapter 7).

Vroom's Expectancy Theory

"Argue for your limitations, and sure enough they're yours." —Richard Bach

Victor Vroom popularized the expectancy theory during the 1960s. It is based on Kurt Lewin's (1951) field theory and has been expanded by Lyman Porter and others (Porter, Bigley, & Steers, 2003; Porter & Lawyer, 1968). Expectancy theory states that motivation depends on how much people want something and their estimate of the probability of getting it (Figure 4-5).

Valence is the strength of a person's preference for something. It may be negative or positive from −1 to +1. If the person does not want something, there is a negative valence. If the person is indifferent, the valence is zero. A positive valence indicates a desire for something (Figure 4-6, *A*).

Expectancy is the probability of getting something through specific actions. If a person believes that an action will result in an outcome, expectancy has a value of 1. If no probability is perceived, the expectancy is zero. Expectancy varies from one situation to another (Figure 4-6, *B*).

If someone has a high valence and a high expectancy, the motivation will be high. If there is a low valence and a low expectancy, the motivation will be low. If one is high and the other low, moderate motivation will result.

The expectancy theory has been further developed to include the importance of the outcome factor. To be highly motivated, a person needs to find an outcome attractive, believe that certain actions will lead to the desired outcome, and assess that the result is worth the effort. To motivate personnel, managers should clarify connections between work and outcome and should reward desirable behavior (Huber, 2006; Sullivan & Decker, 2005; Vroom, 1960, 1964) (see Chapter 7) (Figure 4-7).

Skinner's Positive Reinforcement Theory

"To accomplish great things we must not only act, but also dream; not only plan, but also believe." —Anonymous

Operant conditioning and behavior modification are other names for B.F. Skinner's positive

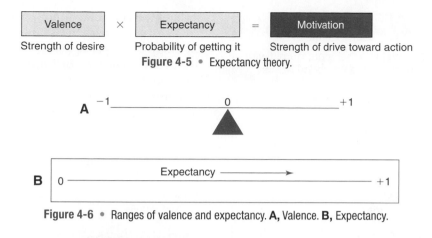

Figure 4-5 • Expectancy theory.

Figure 4-6 • Ranges of valence and expectancy. **A,** Valence. **B,** Expectancy.

M = Motivation
EP = Belief that effort will lead to desired performance
PO = Anticipation that performance will lead to a particular outcome
V = Value of reward

Figure 4-7 • Vroom's Expectancy Theory Regarding Motivation. (Adapted from Vroom VH: *Work and motivation*, New York, 1964, John Wiley & Sons.)

reinforcement theory. According to Skinner, behavior may be strengthened or weakened depending on what follows it. Positive reinforcement strengthens behavior. Withholding positive reinforcers weakens behavior, whereas intermittent reinforcement increases resistance to extinction. Punishment will help reduce behavior, but it cannot teach new behaviors, and it may condition avoidance (Huber, 2006; Skinner, 1974).

Accentuating the positive with plenty of praise and positive feedback may increase the frequency of desired behavior. If, however, a subordinate admits to less than desirable behavior, the manager may respond, "I appreciate your honesty," while reminding the worker of the goal.

When desired results are not obtained, managers should analyze the situation. First, they should assess the working environment for interference. Do the employees have adequate time to complete the task? Does the system allow nurses to maximize their efficiency, or must they spend most of their time running to central supply to gather materials that should have been readily available? If leaders and managers do not locate the cause of the problem in the environment, they must ask themselves if the employees have been properly utilized. Do they have the knowledge and skills necessary to do the job? If not, can they be taught? If they cannot be taught, can they be replaced and assigned other duties?

Equity Theory

"There is no limit to how much good you can do if you don't care who gets the credit." —Anonymous

During the 1960s, Jo Stacy Adams (1965) studied perceptions of equity and inequity. She found that employees assess fairness by considering their input and their psychological, social, and financial rewards in comparison with those of others. Perceived inequity causes tension. The amount of the tension was found to be proportional to the magnitude of the perceived inequity. Tension motivates people to reduce its cause.

BOX 4-4 Equity Theory

A person compares his or her input/output with and perceives relation to a reference person.

$$\left.\begin{array}{l} IP = IRP \\ OP = ORP \end{array}\right\} \quad \text{Equity}$$

$$\left.\begin{array}{l} IP < IRP \\ OP < ORP \end{array}\right\} \quad \text{Inequity}$$

$$\left.\begin{array}{l} IP > IRP \\ OP > ORP \end{array}\right\} \quad \text{Inequity}$$

IP = Inputs of the person
OP = Outputs of the person
IRP = Inputs of reference person
ORP = Outputs of reference person

Accordingly, the strength of the motivation to reduce the perceived inequity is proportional to the cognitive dissonance. To reduce the inequity, people may alter input or output, cognitively distort input or output, change the basis for comparison, or leave. If people feel overworked and underpaid, they are likely to decrease their productivity. Less often, employees feel overrewarded and strive to improve their performance. People resist changing their bases of comparison or distorting their perceptions. People do not usually leave an organization unless there is extreme inequity. If the comparison is equal, people feel that they are treated fairly. If not, they are motivated to take corrective action. Managers should be attentive to the perceived equity of the reward system (Box 4-4).

Intrinsic Motivation

Deci has studied intrinsic motivation and the self-determination theory. He found that some activities are ends in themselves, not just means to ends. There is no apparent reward except the activity itself. Intrinsically motivated behavior seems to be stimulated by people's needs for feeling competent and self-determining. When there is no stimulation, people will seek it. When they are over stimulated, they back away, regroup, and reaffirm competence. People engage in a process of seeking and conquering to feel competent and self-determined. When people's feelings of competence and self-determination are enhanced, their intrinsic motivation will increase. If their perceptions of competence and self-determination are diminished, their intrinsic motivation will decrease. Extrinsic rewards have a controlling aspect that may decrease intrinsic rewards. Insufficient extrinsic rewards tend to increase intrinsic motivation because people try to reduce cognitive dissonance. Based on these findings, managers should foster stimulation through means such as continuing education and special projects (Deci, Guardia, Moller, et al, 2006; Gagné & Deci, 2005).

McGregor's Theory X and Theory Y

Douglas McGregor (1960) has classified traditional management theories as Theory X. They are based on the assumption that people will avoid work if possible because they dislike it; consequently, most people must be directed, controlled, coerced, and threatened. Theory X assumes that people want direction, have little ambition, and avoid responsibility, but want security. A leader or manager with a Theory X philosophy would probably use fear and threats to motivate personnel, supervise closely, delegate little responsibility, and not consider personnel participation in planning.

McGregor maintains that if people behave as described in Theory X it is because of what the system has done to them—not because of their inherent nature. He believes that as long as leader and managerial strategies are based on Theory X, leaders and managers will fail to discover, let alone use, the potentials of their personnel.

McGregor classifies the newer developments in management as Theory Y. In this theory, McGregor makes the assumption that people like and enjoy work, are self-directed, and seek responsibility. It maintains that most people have imagination, ingenuity, creativity, and other intellectual capacities that are only partially utilized. A manager with a Theory Y philosophy will use positive incentives such as praise and recognition, give general supervision, provide opportunities for individual growth, delegate responsibilities, and encourage participation in

TABLE 4-2 McGregor's Theory X and Theory Y

X	Y
People dislike work.	Work is natural.
People must be directed to do work.	People will exercise self-control.
People want to avoid responsibility.	People enjoy responsibility.
People believe that achievement is irrelevant.	People value achievement.
People are dull and uncreative.	People have potential, imagination, and creativity.
Money is the reason for working.	Money is only one reason for working.
People lack desire to improve quality.	People want to improve quality.

problem solving. Job enrichment and decentralization are additional motivational techniques that may stimulate personnel's performance to the extent that it exceeds the requirements stated in the job description (Huber, 2006; McGregor, 1960; Roussel, Swansburg, & Swansburg, 2006) (see Chapter 7) (Table 4-2).

Likert's Participative Management Theory

Rensis Likert believes that effective managers are highly sensitive to their staff associates, use communication to keep the group working as a unit, and foster supportive relationships among all group members. His research indicates that employee-centered supervision is more productive than job-centered–supervision and that more supservision leads to less productivity. Participative management is a human relations theory that may use management by objectives, shared governance councils, and job-enrichment approaches (Huber, 2006; Likert, 1961) (see Chapter 7).

Theory Z

The Japanese form of participative management is known as Theory Z. The major firms of Japan are organized into *zaibatsu*, small groups of 20 to 30 firms representing each important industrial sector. Each firm hosts satellite companies that provide a service or manufacture a subassembly for the host firm. Employees are hired to work for the host firm until retirement. After slow evaluation and promotion in nonspecialized careers, employees retire at age 55 years. They then work on a part-time basis for a satellite company. Women worked temporarily and served as a buffer to the job security of the male work force. Their schedules were flexible so they could care for their families, and they were laid off in slack periods. Those practices are changing.

Concern for the worker is apparent. Japanese companies form inclusive personal and professional relationships and provide social support. Because personnel anticipate lifetime relationships, they are cautious about interpersonal conflicts. Cooperation is stressed. Collective decision making is practiced. Through the ritual *ofringi*, ideas pass from manager to manager for approval. This helps establish trust and cooperation. Objectives and the procedures to achieve them are implicitly described. Quality circles are formed when two to ten employees meet to identify problems, explore options, and make decisions. Quality circles have increased worker productivity, enhanced job satisfaction, and reduced turnover in addition to solving identified problems. Decisions are made by consensus. Because it takes so much time to reach a consensus, only policy and behavior changes are dealt with. Responsibility is also collective. An emphasis is placed on developing all aspects of the employees, and they are rewarded with regular pay bonuses based on the company's performance.

The Japanese Theory Z managers focus on the four soft Ss of management: staff, skills, style, and superordinate goals. Staff is the workers. Skills are the capabilities of the organization or key personnel. Style refers to the cultural style of the organization or how managers achieve goals.

The superordinate goals are the guideposts as determined by the personnel.

Less attention is given to the hard Ss: system, structure, and strategy. The system is the mechanism whereby information circulates through the organization. Structure is the organization, and strategy is the plan of action (Ochi, 1981) (see Chapter 7).

Historical Development of Motivation Theory

Traditional management theory is based on McGregor's Theory X. Traditional theory addresses itself to Maslow's primary physiological and safety needs and employs the monistic theory for reinforcement. The latter, according to Herzberg, helps meet some of the hygiene needs but does not provide motivation.

Newer developments in management are based on McGregor's Theory Y. Maslow's secondary needs of belonging, esteem, and self-actualization are more prepotent than the primary needs for most personnel. Because a satisfied need is no longer a motivator, hygiene factors such as money and working conditions do not serve as motivators. People are more interested in autonomy, responsibility, achievement, recognition, variety in work, and efforts for self-actualization. Argyris has suggested that personnel may become more self-actualized if their personal goals are consistent with the goals of the organization. Talents and interests should be considered when assigning jobs. And then, according to Skinner, positive reinforcement will further increase desired behaviors (Box 4-5).

Participation is a major factor in newer management techniques. Personnel are encouraged to contribute to decisions, goals, and plans. Decentralization is supported to the point of management by objectives, allowing personnel to define their own objectives and to determine how they plan to achieve them. The supervisor approves the goals, makes sure they are consistent with the organization's goals, and evaluates personnel using their own objectives as the standard. Modern leaders and managers delegate duties and assist others to work more effectively. They

---

BOX 4-5 Motivation Theories

PERSONAL NEEDS THEORIES
Taylor's Monistic Theory
Maslow's Hierarchy of Needs
Alderfer's Modified Need Hierarchy
McClelland's Basic Needs Theory
Herzberg's Motivation Hygiene (Two-Factor) Theory
Argyris's Psychological Energy Theory
Vroom's Expectancy Theory
Emotional Intelligence Theory
Genetic Predisposition to Personality

PROCESS THEORIES
Skinner's Positive Reinforcement Theory
Equity Theory
Intrinsic/Extrinsic Motivation Theory
McGregor's Theory X and Theory Y
Likert's Participative Management Theory
Theory Z

---

help each person develop his or her own talents and try to maintain a close relationship between the interests and skills of the individual and the requirements of the job. Job enrichment and job rotation may be used to help develop personnel fully. When personnel are actively striving toward esteem and self-actualization and when their goals are consistent with those of the organization, there is likely to be a noticeable effect on the accomplishment of the organization's goals and productivity.

EMOTIONAL INTELLIGENCE

"You are young only once, but you can stay immature for life." —Anonymous

History of Emotional Intelligence

From 1900 to 1969, intelligence and emotions were viewed as separate narrow fields. However, the renowned psychologist E.L. Thorndike (1935) did write about social intelligence. Wechsler (1955) continued to develop his intelligence quotient (IQ) test but did consider affective capacities as part of the human repertoire of capabilities. The decades from 1970 to 1989 contained precursors to emotional intelligence as the field of cognition and affect emerged to examine how emotions interacted with thoughts. The field of nonverbal communications developed. Gardner (1993) proposed a new theory of multiple intelligences, including an intrapersonal and interpersonal intelligence that included the capacity to perceive and symbolize emotions. Social skills and empathy were studied as social intelligence. Brain research started separating out connections between emotion and cognition. Bar-On (1988) developed attempts to assess emotional intelligence in terms of a measure of well-being. Emotional intelligence emerged during 1990 to 1993, particularly in the brain sciences. Salovey and Mayer published the seminal article "Emotional Intelligence" in 1990. The popularization and broadening occurred from 1994 to 1997, especially with the publication of Goleman's worldwide best-selling book, *Emotional Intelligence*, in 1995. Bar-On (1997) identified the five main domains in his model as intrapersonal skills, interpersonal skills, adaptability, stress management, and general mood. A number of personality scales were developed and published under the name of emotional intelligence. Research on and institutionalization of emotional intelligence have occurred since 1998 (Bar-On & Parker, 2000; Cherniss & Adler, 2000; Cherniss & Goleman, 2001).

Competencies of Emotional Intelligence

Goleman (1995) indicates that how well we handle each other and ourselves is even more important than IQ or advanced degrees for success in organizations. He says star performers have a capacity to work well with individuals and teams as well as have personal achievement, whereas people who are isolated or explosive can be toxic or disruptive to the whole organization. He labels the ability to work with individuals and groups as emotional intelligence and identifies the five components of emotional intelligence as self-awareness, self-regulation, motivation,

empathy, and social skills. These are further divided into personal competence and social competence (Goleman, 1998) (Box 4-6).

Personal competence influences how we manage ourselves. Self-awareness involves doing an accurate self-assessment to know our strengths and weaknesses and an emotional awareness of our emotions and their effects. These help ensure self-confidence about our self-worth and capabilities.

Self-regulation involves keeping our disruptive emotions and impulses under control, maintaining honesty and integrity, taking

---

BOX 4-6 Emotional Intelligence

PERSONAL COMPETENCE

Self-awareness
   Emotional awareness
   Accurate self-assessment
   Self-confidence
Self-regulation
   Self-control
   Trustworthiness
   Conscientiousness
   Adaptability
   Innovation
Motivation
   Achievement drive
   Commitment
   Initiative
   Optimism

SELF-COMPETENCE

Empathy
   Understanding others
   Developing others
   Service orientation
   Leveraging diversity
   Political awareness
Social skills
   Influence
   Communications
   Conflict management
   Leadership
   Change catalyst
   Building bonds
   Collaboration and cooperation
   Team capabilities

From Goleman D: *Working with emotional intelligence,* New York, 1998, Bantam Books.

responsibility for our own performance, being flexible for handling change, and becoming comfortable with new information and approaches.

Motivation can help us reach goals by striving to meet a standard of excellence, aligning our personal goals with the group and organizational goals, taking advantage of opportunities, and keeping a positive attitude about pursuing goals despite obstacles and setbacks.

Social competence determines how we handle relationships. Empathy involves taking an interest in others' concerns and understanding them, developing others' abilities, anticipating and meeting customers' needs, leveraging diversity to cultivate opportunities, and political awareness.

Social skills are an adeptness at inducing desirable responses in people through influence, listening and sending convincing messages, resolving disagreements, inspiring others, managing change, nurturing relationships, collaborating and cooperating toward shared goals, and creating group synergy through team development (Goleman, 1998).

Goleman (1998) reports that there are more similarities between groups of men and women than differences. Although on the average women may be better than men at some emotional skills, some men are better than most women. Women may be able to detect fleeting feelings in others better than men, but the gender gap in reading emotions closes when emotional cues are less easy to control than facial expression, such as tone of voice or body language. There appears to be no gender difference in being able to sense someone's specific thoughts. That empathic accuracy integrates both cognitive and affective skills (Goleman, 1998).

Promoting Emotional Intelligence

Cherniss and Adler (2000) described several model programs for promoting emotional intelligence such as training for conflict management, self-management, stress management, emotional competence, empathy, human relations, achievement motivation, supervising

---

BOX 4-7 Model Training Programs for Developing Emotional Intelligence

Conflict management
Self-management
Stress management
Emotional competence
Empathy
Human relations
Achievement motivation
Supervisory training
Caregiver support program
Executive coaching
Leadership lab

Adapted from Cherniss C, Adler M: *Promoting emotional intelligence in organizations: Make training in emotional intelligence effective*, Alexandria, VA, 2000, American Society for Training & Development.

BOX 4-8 Key Components to Teach for Emotional Intelligence

1. Awareness of self and others
2. Positive attitudes and values
3. Responsible decision making
4. Communication skills
5. Social skills

From Bar-On R, Parker JDA, editors: *The handbook of emotional intelligence: Theory, development, assessment and application at home, school and in the workplace*, San Francisco, 2000, Jossey-Bass, p. 400.

---

and providing a caregiver support program, executive coaching, and leadership lab (Box 4-7). Bar-On and Parker (2000) identified key components to be taught as: (1) awareness of self and others; (2) positive attitudes and values; (3) responsible decision making; (4) communication skills; and (5) social skills (Box 4-8). Segal (1997), Saarni (1997), and Ryback (1998) contributed to the discussion about relevant skills, principles, and related curriculum. Taking care of one's body, reducing stress through healthy fitness habits, being aware of one's and others' feelings, accepting feelings, appreciating self and others, using assertive communications and humor, and using creative innovation through playful openness were themes.

Ciarrochi, Forgas, and Mayer (2001) outlined the history of the emergence of the emotional intelligence concept and discussed the applications of emotional intelligence research to everyday life, while Feldman (1999) provided a hands-on guide to understanding and applying the 10 skills of emotionally intelligent leadership and a 50-question self-assessment. Cherniss and Adler (2000) identified a four-phase model for promoting emotional intelligence-based learning in work organizations.

GENETIC PREDISPOSITIONS TO ATTITUDES/PERSONALITY

There is much in the literature about genetic predisposition to various diseases. Some research has also been done about genetic predisposition to attitudes, personalities, cognitive abilities, and leadership. Studies have shown genetic influences on personality but less for cognitive factors and leadership variables. Environmental factors accounted for most of the remaining variance. Therefore, predisposition is not destiny. We can influence our personality, cognition, and leadership skills (Burchum J, 2006, personal correspondence).

MORALE

"There's nothing either good or bad, but thinking makes it so." —William Shakespeare

Morale is a state of mind related to cheerfulness, confidence, and discipline. A person who works confidently, courageously, and with discipline demonstrates high morale. A person who is apathetic, cowardly, disorderly, devious, fearful, complaintive, or rebellious demonstrates low morale. Morale is related to productivity, quality, job satisfaction, and motivation.

Morale is related to leadership style and the interpersonal and communication skills of the leader. Involving people in decision making, keeping them informed, and helping them know the why and how of their jobs is important to morale. Ensuring social acceptance, treating people as

winners, instilling pride, giving recognition, rewards, praise, and celebrating success contribute to high morale. Being proactive rather than reactive, promoting flexible work schedules, assigning discouraged workers to optimistic workers, and getting rid of morale destroyers and troublemakers help morale.

Replacing competition with an effort to outdo one's own previous accomplishments is helpful. That leads to continuous improvement. One sees others as benchmarks while trying to improve one's own performance and appreciates one's own importance. This replaces the old competitive paradigm of the game where the goal is winning; the others are enemies; and I am separate and better than they. The transformational leader helps others gain enthusiasm from shared accomplishments and permission to take risks. This encourages initiating, asserting, engaging, collaborating, appreciating, and supporting toward a high-focused energy.

Because both the individual worker and the work environment are changing, managers need to constantly monitor the work environment regarding morale and job satisfaction. Organizational morale is the attitudes of the workers toward the quality of their work lives. Each work environment is unique, and each worker's view of the quality of life is uniquely related to how it satisfies one's needs. Increased interpersonal conflict; criticism of policies, procedures, and rules and disregard of rules; decreased productivity; decreased quality of work; and increased lateness, absenteeism, and job turnover are signs of low morale.

Acknowledgement of a morale problem is important as a first step to solving the problem. Managers can observe, listen, and ask related questions to assess morale. Managers should survey workers' perceptions of the importance of job factors and their satisfaction with those factors through such efforts as attitude surveys, employee focus groups, suggestions boxes, telephone hotlines, an ombudsman program, and exit interviews. Even when there is not evidence of low morale, some organizations do periodic attitude surveys (McConnell, 2006).

RESEARCH Perspective 4-1

Data from Yang KP, Huang CK: The effects of staff nurses' morale on patient satisfaction, *J Nurs Res* 13(2):141-151, 2005.

Purpose: The purpose of this survey was to examine staff nurses' morale and its effect on patient satisfaction.

Methods: A structured questionnaire was received from 332 nurses and 265 inpatients in 21 medical-surgical units of a medical center in Taiwan. Litwin and Stringerm's (1968) Work Morale Scale was administered to the registered nurses. Yang's (1997) Nursing-Sensitive Patient Satisfaction-Scale was used to measure patient outcomes for patients who had

been admitted for at least 3 days and were ready to be discharged.

Results/conclusions: The results showed that job position and pay had a significant effect on nurses' work morale, which accounted for 66.7% of the discriminate power to predict nursing-sensitive patient satisfaction. The researchers recommended that nursing leaders put effort into improving nurses' involvement and identification with their organizations because both are significant factors associated with nursing unit morale.

In general, there are age-related differences related to morale. Younger people make commitments to the job more slowly than older adults do. They are concerned about career decisions rather than just working. Because they often have been raised under more permissive conditions than older people have, they respond well to participative leadership styles rather than an autocratic environment. Challenge, opportunity to learn, and involvement are more important to the younger worker, whereas security becomes increasingly important as the worker grows older. Money is important but is not always the most important factor. Automation has eliminated most of the needs for physical labor and endurance that were important in the past.

Young people tend to be loyal to their profession but not necessarily to the job or boss. They tend to want to prove themselves, push for opportunities, and be recognized.

It is natural for older workers to refer to how it was done in the past. They need consistent and frequent feedback to help them through change. They have been through a variety of leadership styles, may be suspicious of new leadership, and need open and direct communication. It is preferable to ask them for what the manager wants and needs specifically. They seem to respect high standards. They respond favorably to having their knowledge and experience used. They like to know that seniority counts. Habits, routines, and

work schedules may be ingrained and difficult to change (Karp, Fuller, & Sirias, 2002; Lancaster & Stillman, 2002; Raines, 2003; Raines & Hunt, 2000; Tulgan, 2000; Tulgan & Martin, 2001).

Manager morale is important too. The first 3 months on a new job are very important for setting an impression. Projecting confidence and enthusiasm and building relationships are important. Each worker should be respected and treated fairly and equally to develop credibility and good working relationships. Managers should act as a buffer for outside stressors, should save time for planning, and should not make changes too quickly. Managers should involve people in decisions and slowly introduce innovations to help maintain good morale. They should get to know the business and the people; communicate the goals and expectations clearly; clarify values and priorities; and motivate, delegate to, and reward people. It is very important for managers to replenish their energy by eating a balanced diet, exercising, resting, and relaxing to help maintain their morale.

WORKPLACE INCIVILITY AND HORIZONTAL VIOLENCE

Workplace incivility contributes to low morale, and low morale may contribute to horizontal violence. The consequences of workplace incivility and horizontal violence have spiraled to a cost of billions of dollars and have resulted in hundreds of deaths (Hutton, 2006). Horizontal violence is dysfunctional behavior that includes antagonism, bullying, criticism, gossiping, innuendo, insubordination, intimidation, passive-aggressive actions, physical aggression, scapegoating, undermining, and withholding information. Nurses are apparently more concerned about aggression from their colleagues than from other sources. Horizontal violence is linked to decreased job performance, morale, and satisfaction (Baltimore, 2006). The abuse of power behavior is related to feelings of discontent, inadequacy, insecurity, and personal envy.

People typically do not see themselves in the same way they see others. When one acts aggressively, one tends to label it as passion and blame external circumstances and having no other options. We often have self-serving views of ourselves and take credit for positive outcomes. Alternatively, we tend to blame others, the environment, and factors out of our control for less desirable outcomes.

There is an incivility spiral. One thoughtless act can be perceived as incivility and injustice, cause a negative effect, create a desire for reciprocation and another uncivil act. That chain keeps repeating itself. When one has been the target of aggression, that person is more likely to engage in future aggressive behavior. In addition, when there is an ambiguous intent to harm, it tends to create collateral damage when co-workers seek retribution for the initial target. That collateral damage creates a toxic work environment. Manager incivility is more detrimental than employee-to-employee incivility. Managers are culpable for incivility when there is no disciplinary action for abusive behavior. Organizational blaming and scapegoating are major barriers to decreasing incivility. Horizontal violence and insidious cannibalism (nurses eating their own) can destroy the nursing profession before outside forces do.

Many practical solutions have been recommended to reduce horizontal violence including but not limited to: socializing new staff members, role modeling professional behaviors, validating assumptions and perceptions before drawing conclusions, using open communication, engaging in conflict resolution, rewarding nurses for supporting each other, and fostering a culture of recognition. However, there is still a need for research to determine the best practices to manage incivility and decrease toxic workplace environments (Baltimore, 2006; Hutton, 2006; Peck, 2006).

BURNOUT

"Obstacles are those frightful things you see when you take your eyes off your goal." —Henry Ford

Burnout is a state of emotional exhaustion primarily caused by stress that leads to negative attitudes and behaviors. It is characterized by depletion of energies, disillusionment, doubts, depersonalization, and frustration, leading to loss of purpose, ideas, and energy. A person with burnout may feel alienated, apathetic, and exhausted. The person is at high risk for developing symptoms of stress, including backaches, headaches, indigestion, and lowered resistance. Family difficulties and social problems may develop. Burnout leads to low morale, excessive absenteeism, and turnover.

Factors contributing to burnout include but are not limited to long hours, dissatisfaction with quality of work, lots of paperwork, lack of appreciation, lack of support, low pay, sense of powerlessness, and few advancement opportunities.

Improving job design, personnel policies, and staff relationships are appropriate. One should appraise the situation, set priorities, and focus on what work needs to be done. Meeting goals can reduce stress. When one is busy doing what one can, achieving goals, feeling comfortable with what one is doing, and getting recognition for work well done, one will probably use less energy for being stressed. Open communications, identifying negative feelings and talking them through, good nutrition, physical exercise, rest and relaxation, and stress management should help prevent burnout.

The manager can help create a pleasant work environment; set realistic goals; make realistic demands on self and others; acknowledge people's good work; prioritize; identify and talk about negative feelings; rotate undesirable, popular, and unpopular tasks; and facilitate good health habits. A stress management workshop including delegation, time management, meditation, relaxation techniques, and yoga could help. A multifaceted worker-support program including exercise programs; nutrition instruction; stress management; health promotion education such as hypertension screening, stop-smoking activities, and weight loss plans; and individual counseling help (Smith, Jaffe-Gill, Segal, & Segal, 2007).

Personal hardiness through commitment, control, and challenge helps prevent burnout. Commitment is a tendency to involve oneself in whatever one does to find purpose and meaning in events, things, and people. Control is influence over the surroundings, events, and people. One believes one can influence life events rather than feel helpless. Challenge is anticipation of change as an opportunity instead of a threat. Stress management techniques help prevent burnout. Exercise, good nutrition, rest, and relaxation are helpful. Setting limits on commitment to work and giving attention to meaningful relationships and satisfying activities are important.

JOB SATISFACTION

"He who seeks only for applause from without has all his happiness in another's keeping." —Oliver Goldsmith

Job dissatisfaction contributes to higher turnover rates and decreased productivity. Considerable time and money are required to recruit and select a replacement for someone who leaves a position. It takes time to socialize the new employee to the organization's norms. This orientation period is expensive because of educational expenses and decreased productivity. Other employees must carry more than their share of the load until the new individual can work to capacity, and group redevelopment is necessary after each change in membership. For all these reasons job satisfaction is a concern for nursing administrators.

Job dissatisfaction has been shown to be correlated with absenteeism and turnover. Herzberg maintains that satisfiers and dissatisfiers are mutually exclusive. He classifies the sense of achievement, recognition for achievement, the work itself, responsibility, advancement potential, and possibility of growth as motivators or satisfiers; matters such as working conditions, policies, supervision, interpersonal relations, salary, status, and job security are classified as hygiene factors or dissatisfiers. He concludes that hygiene factors cannot motivate employees but can only prevent dissatisfaction. Herzberg's work remains controversial.

Maslow's theory shows insight into Herzberg's findings. It suggests that hygiene factors can be motivators and that only when hygiene factors are satisfied do satisfiers such as responsibility become motivators. Several research studies have indicated that people at lower educational, socioeconomic, and occupational levels and minority members tend to place more emphasis on hygiene or extrinsic job factors, whereas people at higher educational, socioeconomic, and occupational levels and Caucasian Americans are more concerned with motivators or intrinsic factors. In accordance with Maslow's theory, physiological and safety needs are apparently prepotent for lower socioeconomic groups, whereas these needs have probably been satisfied for people at higher educational and occupational levels, such as nurses, for whom esteem and self-actualization needs have become prepotent.

The desire for influence in decision making is affected by individual differences. Even though people presumably desire some control over their environment, this desire is not equally strong for all people. Vroom (1960) found that authoritarians are relatively unaffected by participating in decision making but that participation in decision making generally has a favorable effect on job satisfaction. Role ambiguity (the result of a failure to inform an individual of what is needed to do the job) is relatively common. Even if the role is clear, an employee in that role may resign if role conflict is present and persists. Role conflicts may result from a number of factors and are affected by individual differences. Likewise, job satisfaction is multidimensional and subject to individual differences.

Women seem to show more variation than men in their job attitudes. Women emphasize working conditions, hours and ease of work, supervision, and social aspects of the job, whereas men emphasize wages, opportunity for advancement, company management and policies, and task interest. College-educated women rank the importance of motivators such as achievement, recognition, and responsibility significantly higher than female clerical workers without college degrees. People tend to have more job satisfaction before the age of 20 years and after the age of 35 years than during the period between. Younger people tend to be more interested in income, whereas older people are more interested in security.

Nurses surveyed about their sources of satisfaction identify a sense of achievement, recognition,

challenging work, responsibility, advancement potential, autonomy, authority, pleasant work environment, agreeable working hours, and adequate staffing all as satisfiers. Nurses stress the importance of respected hospital administrators, supportive nursing administrators, trustworthy managers, fair evaluations, and adequate feedback. Poor planning, poor communication, inadequate explanations of decisions affecting jobs, unclear rules and regulations, unreasonable pressure, excessive work, workload negatively affecting work quality, understaffing, uncooperative physicians, nonnursing duties, and unqualified managers are all sources of dissatisfaction. Reduced productivity, increased absenteeism, and rapid turnover are expensive consequences of job dissatisfaction but can be reduced if the nursing administrator fosters job satisfaction through organization and management (Best & Thurston, 2004; Ingersoll, Olsan, Drew-Cates, et al, 2002; Ruggiero, 2005).

 RESEARCH Perspective 4-2

Data from Best M, Thurston, N: Measuring nurse job satisfaction. *JONA* 34(6):283-290, 2004.

Purpose: The purpose of this research was to answer the following questions: (1) What is the level of job satisfaction of registered staff nurses employed in four acute care hospitals within one regional health authority, and (2) are there significant relationships between job satisfaction and patient acuity, workload, and staff mix?

Methods: A stratified sample of 20% of approximately 4000 full-time, part-time, and casual (PRN) staff nurses working in one child and three adult acute care hospitals. The Stamps and Piedmonte Index of Work Satisfaction (IWS) was used to measure nurse job satisfaction. The IWS is organized in two parts to measure nurses' expectations (importance) and satisfaction on each of six job components, including pay, autonomy, task requirements, organizational policies, professional status, and interaction. Two added, open-ended questions asked respondents about the most satisfying aspect of their work life and about what one thing they would change. For part A, a frequency matrix was created and components were ranked according to relative

importance. For part B, satisfaction percentages were calculated for each response option in each statement.

Results/conclusions: Factors contributing to the level of job satisfaction in order of importance were autonomy, pay, professional status, interaction, task requirements, and organizational policies. Satisfaction scores were ranked in a different order, which was professional status, interaction, autonomy, task requirements, and organizational policies. Autonomy was the most important component for level of job satisfaction but only third for satisfaction. Although professional status was highest in satisfaction, it was less important than were autonomy and pay. What nurses thought was important was not necessarily what brought them satisfaction. Nurses wanted more staffing, more time to discuss care with colleagues, more recognition for professional abilities from doctors and support from administrators, more time and support to attend workshops, and less paperwork.

CHAPTER SUMMARY

There are numerous theories of motivation including Taylor's monistic theory, Maslow's hierarchy of needs theory, Alderfer's modified need hierarchy, McClelland's basic needs theory, Herzberg's motivation hygiene (two-factor) theory, Argyris's psychological energy theory, Vroom's expectancy theory, Skinner's positive reinforcement theory, equity theory, intrinsic motivation, McGregor's Theory X and Theory Y, Likert's participative management theory, and Theory Z. The historical development of motivation theory progressed from autocratic to more participative and caring about people. Emotional and social intelligence gained attention in the 1990s. Workplace incivility, horizontal violence, and workplace violence affect morale, burnout, and job satisfaction and can contribute to turnover.

CASE STUDY

You have identified that Ann has a high need for achievement, Betty for power, and Carl for affiliation. What assignments will you give them to meet those needs and motivate them?

CRITICAL THINKING ACTIVITY

Reflective Journal: Reflect on several motivation theories, and identify which one explains what motivates you the best. Explain why. Do any not apply to you? If so, which? Ask a nurse manager what he or she does to motivate workers. Ask some staff nurses and colleagues what motivates them.

ONLINE RESOURCES

evolve Additional critical thinking activities, worksheets, and case studies are available online at http://evolve.elsevier.com/Marriner/guide8e.

REFERENCES

Adams JS: Inequity in social exchange. In Berkowitz L, editor, *Advances in experimental social psychology*, New York, 1965, Academic Press.

Argyris C, Schon DA: *Theory in practice: Increasing professional effectiveness*, San Francisco, 1974, Jossey-Bass.

Baltimore JJ: Nurse collegiality: Fact or fiction, *Nursing Management* 37(5):28-36, 2006.

Bar-On R: *Development of a concept of psychological well-being*, Unpublished doctoral dissertation, 1988, Rhodes University, South Africa.

Bar-On R: *The emotional quotient inventory (RQ-I): Technical manual*, Toronto, 1997, Multi-Health Systems.

Bar-On R, Parker JDA, editors: *The handbook of emotional intelligence: Theory, development, assessment and application at home, school and in the workplace*, San Francisco, 2000, Jossey-Bass.

Best MF, Thurston NE: Measuring nurse job satisfaction, *JONA* 34(6):283-290, 2004.

Burchum J: Personal correspondence, 2006.

Cherniss C, Adler M: *Promoting emotional intelligence in organizations: Make training in emotional intelligence effective,* Alexandria, VA, 2000, American Society for Training & Development.

Cherniss C, Goleman D: *The emotionally intelligent workplace: How to select for, measure, and improve emotional intelligence in individuals, groups, and organizations,* San Francisco, 2001, Jossey-Bass.

Ciarrochi J, Forgas JP, Mayer JD, editors: *Emotional intelligence in everyday life: A scientific inquiry*, Philadelphia, 2001, Psychology Press.

Deci EL, La Guardia JG, Moller AC, et al: On the benefits of giving as well as receiving autonomy support: Mutuality in close friendships, *Personality and Social Psychology Bulletin* 32:313-327, 2006.

Feldman DA: *The handbook of emotionally intelligent leadership: Inspiring others to achieve results,* 1999, Falls Church, VA: Leadership Performance Solutions Press.

Gagné M, Deci EL: Self-determination theory and work motivation, *Journal of Organizational Behavior* 26:331-362, 2005.

Gardner H: *Frames of mind: The theory of multiple intelligences,* New York, 1993, Basic Books.

Goleman D: *Emotional intelligence: Why it can matter more than IQ,* New York, 1995, Bantam Books.

Goleman D: *Working with emotional intelligence,* New York, 1998, Bantam Books.

Herzberg F: One more time: How do you motivate employees? In Carroll L, Paine R, Miner A, editor: *The management process,* ed 2, New York, 1977, Macmillan.

Herzberg F, Mausner B, Snyderman BB: *The motivation to work,* ed 2, New York, 1959, John Wiley & Sons.

Huber DL: *Leadership and nursing care management,* ed 3, Philadelphia, 2006, Elsevier.

Hutton S: Workplace incivility: State of the science, *JONA* 36(1):22-27, 2006.

Ingersoll GL, Olsan T, Drew-Cates, et al: Nurses' job satisfaction, organizational commitment, and career intent, *JONA* 32(5):250-263, 2002.

Karp H, Fuller C, Sirias D: *Bridging the boomer Xer gap: Creating authentic teams for high performance at work,* Palo Alto, CA, 2002, Davies-Black Publishing.

Lancaster LC, Stillman D: *When generations collide: Who they are, why they clash, how to solve the generational puzzle at work,* New York, 2002, HarperCollins.

Lewin K: *Field theory in social sciences,* New York, 1951, Harper & Row.

Likert R: *New patterns of management,* New York, 1961, McGraw Hill.

Litwin GH, Stringerm, Jr RA: *Motivation and organizational climate,* Boston, 1968, Division of Research, Harvard University.

Maslow AH II: *Motivation and personality,* ed 3, Upper Saddle River, NJ, 1987, Prentice Hall.

McConnell CR: *Umiker's management skills for the new health care supervisor,* ed 4, Boston, 2006, Jones and Bartlett.

McGregor D: *The human side of enterprise,* New York, 1960, McGraw-Hill.

Ochi WG: *Theory Z: How American business can meet the Japanese challenge,* New York, 1981, Avon Books.

Peck M: Workplace incivility: A nurse executive responds, *JONA* 36(1):27-28, 2006.

Porter L, Bigley GA, Steers RM, editors: *Motivation and work behavior,* Boston, 2003, McGraw-Hill/Irwin.

Porter L, Lawyer E: *Managerial attitudes and performance,* Homewood, IL, 1968, Dorsey Press.

Raines C: *Connecting generations,* Menlo Park, CA, 2003, Crisp Learning.

Raines C, Hunt J: *The Xers & the boomers: From adversaries to allies—A diplomat's guide,* Menlo Park, CA, 2000, Crisp Publications.

Roussel L, Swansburg RC, Swansburg RJ: *Management and leadership for nurse administrators,* ed 4, Boston, 2006, Jones and Bartlett.

Ruggiero J: Health, work variables, and job satisfaction among nurses, *JONA* 35(5):254-263, May 2005.

Ryback D: *Putting emotional intelligence to work: Successful leadership is more than IQ,* Boston, 1998, Butterworth-Heinemann.

Saarni C: Emotional competence and self-regulation in childhood. In Salovey P, Sluyter DJ, editors: *Emotional development and emotional intelligence: Implications for educators*, New York, 1997, Basic Books.

Salovey P, Mayer JD: Emotional intelligence, *Imagination, Cognition, and Personality* 9:185-211, 1989-1990.

Segal J: *Raising your emotional intelligence: A practical guide,* New York, 1997, Henry Holt.

Skinner BF: *About behaviorism,* New York, 1974, Random House.

Smith M, Jaffe-Gill E, Segal J, Segal R: *Burnout: Signs, symptoms, and prevention,* 2007 (website): www. helpguide.org/mental/burnout_signs_symptoms.htm. Accessed January 23, 2007.

Sullivan EJ, Decker PJ: *Effective leadership and management in nursing,* ed 6, Upper Saddle River, NJ, 2005, Pearson/Prentice Hall.

Taylor FW: *Shop management,* New York, 1903, Harper & Bros.

Taylor FW: *The principles of scientific management,* New York, 1911, Harper & Bros.

Thorndike EL: *The psychology of wants, interests, and attitudes,* New York, 1935, Appleton-Century-Crofts.

Tulgan B: *Managing generation X: How to bring out the best in young talent,* New York, 2000, WW Norton.

Tulgan B, Martin CA: *Managing generation Y: Global citizens born in the late seventies and early eighties,* Amherst, MA, 2001, HRD Press.

Vroom VH: *Some personality determinants of the effects of participation,* Englewood Cliffs, NJ, 1960, Prentice-Hall.

Vroom V: *Work and motivation,* New York, 1964, John Wiley & Sons.

Wechsler D: *Wechsler adult intelligence scale,* St. Peters, Australia, 1955, Psychological Corporation.

Yang, KP: A study of correspondence with patient satisfaction between the measurement of magnitude estimation and interval scaling. In the Department of Research (Ed.), *The collective research report of Taichung Veterans General Hospital,* Taichung, Taiwan, 1997, Taichung Veterans General Hospital.

Yang KP, Huang CK: The effects of staff nurses' morale on patient satisfaction, *J Nurs Res* 113(2):141-151, 2005.

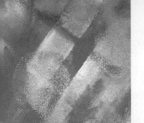

Power, Politics, and Labor Relations

5

"Diplomacy is the art of letting someone else have your way." —Daniele Vare

Chapter Overview

Chapter 5 describes power, sources of power, authority, power and gender, empowerment, politics, labor relations, labor laws, unionization, the nurse leaders' and managers' role in collective bargaining, and advantages and disadvantages of collective bargaining.

Chapter Objectives

- Identify at least five sources of power.
- Describe at least two ways to communicate with legislators.
- Outline the process by which a bill becomes a law.
- Clarify the four phases of unionization.
- Explain the decertification process.
- Identify four advantages and disadvantages of collective bargaining.

Online Resources

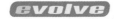

Critical thinking activities, worksheets, and case studies are available online at http://evolve.elsevier.com/Marriner/guide8e.

Major Concepts and Definitions

Power *one's capacity to influence others*
Formal power *power related to position*
Informal power *power related to personal power*
Reward *something given in recompense for a good deed*
Coercive *restraining, constraining, or curbing in nature*
Legitimate *logically correct*
Referent *a type of power based on identification with a leader and what that leader symbolizes*
Expert *skillful, having knowledge and training*
Information *knowledge or access to information*
Connection *coalition*
Authority *legitimate power determined by structure*
Politics *group decision making*
Labor relations *relations between the workers and management*
Unionization *organization of workers*
Collective bargaining *organization of workers to bargain for working conditions*
Synergy *the sum is greater than the individual parts*

POWER, AUTHORITY, AND POLITICS

Power and authority are closely related and often confused. Power is one's capacity to influence others, whereas authority is the right to direct others. One's power may be greater or less than the authority of the position. Authority is obtained through legitimate position power, but there are several sources of power (Box 5-1). Politics is a process for group decision making that uses various sources of power.

Sources of Power

French and Raven (1959) identified a widely accepted power base classification of reward, coercive, expert, referent, and legitimate. Connection and information were added to the list later. Several other sources such as persuasion, charismatic, personal, interpersonal, and position power have also been discussed (Finkelman, 2006; Huber, 2006; Marquis & Huston, 2006; McConnell, 2006; Roussel, Swansburg, & Swansburg, 2006; Sullivan & Decker, 2005; French & Raven, 1959) (Box 5-1).

Reward Power

Much of a leader's or manager's power comes from the ability to reward others for complying. When a staff associate perceives that leaders and managers have the ability to provide something valued, the leader or manager has reward power. Sources of reward power include money, desired schedule, desired assignments, provision of personal space, or the acknowledgment of accomplishments.

Coercive Power

Coercive/punishment power is the opposite of reward power and is based on fear of punishment if one fails to conform. Undesired schedule or assignments, embarrassment in front of others, withheld pay increases, transfer, layoff, demotion, and termination are sources of coercive power.

Legitimate Power

Their official positions in the organizational hierarchy give leaders and managers legitimate power. Legitimate power gives the leader or manager the right to influence and the staff

BOX 5-1 Sources of Power
Reward
Coercive
Legitimate
Referent
Expert
Information
Connection
Persuasion
Charismatic
Personal
Interpersonal
Position

member an obligation to accept that influence. The chief nurse executive, vice president, or director of nursing has more legitimate power than the division manager, who, in turn, has more legitimate power than the unit manager. Cultural values that give a person the right to prescribe appropriate behavior for another (such as parents for children), social structures involving a hierarchy of authority, and election processes to legitimize a person's right to an office are bases for legitimate power.

Referent Power

Referent power is based on identification with a leader and what that leader symbolizes. The leader is admired and exerts influence because the followers desire to be like the leader. Personal feelings of acceptance and approval develop through association with a powerful person. Referent power cannot be enforced through legitimate position power.

Expert Power

People gain expert power through knowledge, skills, information, experience, and competence. Their expertise gains people respect and compliance. Knowledge of the organization and its rules, regulations, and work flow helps one to acquire power over others who need the knowledge to meet their responsibilities. This power is limited to a specific area of expertise.

Information Power

Information power comes from knowledge, access to information, and the sharing of information. It is especially powerful when others need the information (Finkelman, 2006).

Connection Power

Connection power comes from formal or informal coalitions and interpersonal relations and links to prestigious and influential people within and outside of the organization (Sullivan & Decker, 2005).

Persuasion Power

Persuasion power comes from presenting an effective point of view (Finkelman, 2006).

Charismatic Power

Charismatic power is generated by a dynamic, popular, and powerful persona. Those get generated through personal charm.

Personal Power

Informal sources of power are related to one's personal power rather than position power. Some people have situational power because they happen to be in the right place at the right time. Others have personal power because of their unique characteristics.

Education, experience, drive, and decisiveness are viewed positively and help establish credibility through expert, information, and persuasion power. The person with these qualities may be viewed as reliable, and therefore others are willing to cooperate. Attractiveness gains an individual access to people who will help promote a cause, because people enjoy being around others who have a happy temperament, generate a sense of well-being, and foster goodwill in others. Personal appearance, good manners, body language, posture, gestures, eye contact if culturally appropriate, and speech with a firm, confident voice contribute to personal power through connection power.

Location also influences others, because individuals communicate more with people who are located near them in the organization, and communication increases their opportunities to influence.

For instance, full voting membership on powerful committees places one in close proximity for persuading other members and provides the opportunity to confront, negotiate, and solve problems. In general, people are most comfortable with others who have similar values, beliefs, and customs. Social pressure from people who share social norms encourages others to conform to those norms. Coalitions then strengthen one's power base. Consequently, friendships and associations with people can be a source of connection power.

Personal power is gained by having what someone else wants and by being irreplaceable. It can be derived by having the ability to make decisions through expert or information power and by being able to provide resources through reward power.

There are several ways to expand one's personal resources. Start by taking good care of oneself. Eat a well-balanced diet, rest, relax, exercise, and develop relationships to maintain one's personal energy and to project a good image to others. Develop hobbies and interests. Have fun. Use a good sense of humor. Develop and focus on one's goals. Recognize opportunities. Be assertive. Learn how to collect and review accurate information. Be a proactive decision maker. Expand one's personal resources by broadening one's skill base and continuing one's education. Show up to do networking and develop political alliances and coalitions. Ninety percent of success may be showing up and volunteering (Sullivan & Decker, 2005) (Box 5-2).

Interpersonal Power

Interpersonal power comes from connection, information, and group decision-making powers. Relationships provide access to the informal communication network. Doing favors for others so that they owe you favors creates an obligation-based power. One may gain power by default when there is no one else available or by autonomy when the decision is one's own to make. Control of resources, such as information, procedures, equipment, and personnel, also strengthens one's power base. Religion, politics, race, and national origin are bases for establishing power

---

BOX 5-2 Sources of Personal Power

Education
Experience
Drive
Decisiveness
Attractiveness
Happy temperament
Personal appearance
Manners
Body language
Posture
Gestures
Confident voice
Location
Coalitions

---

in some situations but interfere with power bases in others. For example, a nurse of a certain faith may be given priority for a job on the staff of an institute run by that faith, but religion may be held against the person seeking a position at a hospital affiliated with another religion or denomination.

Connection power is based on connections with a powerful person or others as a way to get accurate and reliable information. One can expand the network of communication contacts to increase connection power by joining listservs and professional and community organizations, and volunteering for committee work. One should identify the formal and informal leaders and facilitate the empowerment of others.

Information is power if used strategically. Increase information power through connections, and try to get on routing lists. Learn the language, symbols, and culture of the organization. Seek role models for advice. Assertively let others know your strengths. Work with the organizational priorities.

Group decision-making power can create synergy when people come together to make decisions and go forth as a united front. Increase decision-making power by volunteering for problem-solving committees and task forces. Coaching, counseling, delegating, mentoring, and rewarding are concepts closely related to interpersonal power (Huber, 2006) (Box 5-3).

> **BOX 5-3** Sources of Interpersonal Power
>
> Connections
> Information
> Group decision-making powers

> **BOX 5-4** Sources of Position Power
>
> Centrality
> Criticality
> Flexibility
> Relevance
> Visibility

Position Power

Position power is increased by centrality, criticality, flexibility, relevance, and visibility. Organizational informal power is enhanced by expertise, career goal setting, and communication skills plus understanding the organization, having a sense of unity with the organizational goals, mentoring, networking, coalition building, negotiating, collaborating, fostering collegiality, and using an empowering attitude.

Centrality provides access to information in a communication network and increases position power. One can increase centrality power by getting centrally located and by having information routed through oneself.

Criticality increases position power. It is determined by (1) how dependent others are on the work performed by the position, (2) the number of others performing the same tasks, and (3) the level of knowledge and skills required by the position. General-purpose positions have less power than highly technical and specialized positions, which fewer people can do. One can increase criticality by increasing the technical sophistication of one's job, by making part of one's job responsibilities unique, and by taking on tasks that are critical to the work processing.

Flexibility or discretion allows one to exercise judgment. It is associated with the life cycle of a position. It is more difficult to make new tasks routine than it is to make old tasks routine. The number of rules governing a position increases with the number of people occupying the position over time. Flexibility is associated with novelty and variety. The more routine the work and the fewer tasks assigned to a person the easier it is to establish routines, and the less powerful the position is. One can increase flexibility power by getting involved in new projects, participating in decision-making processes, initiating new ideas,

reducing the percentage of routine activities in one's job, expanding task novelty and variety, and seeking unusual jobs rather than maintenance-oriented, repetitive jobs.

Relevance involves positions related to central objectives and issues of the organization that contribute to more position power. The trainer, mentor, evaluator, advocate, or representative is a relevantly powerful position. Trainers reduce uncertainty for new employees and tend to be appreciated by those who have benefited from the training. Evaluators are powerful by virtue of the dependence on good evaluations for organizational rewards. Advocacy identifies a person with important causes. One can increase relevance power by becoming involved in activities central to the priorities of the organization and by expanding one's work domain.

Visibility is a key to success. Excellent performance is multiplied by visibility. Direct contact with face-to-face communication is a way to have visibility. A good presentation of a report will get more visibility than writing the report. Participating in problem-solving task forces gives one visibility. Name recognition gives visibility and can be addressed by introducing oneself to others, using business cards, sending out information with a signed cover note, sending a note of congratulations or appreciation to colleagues as appropriate, and sharing good ideas with appropriate parties in person with a follow-up memo (Huber, 2006) (Box 5-4).

Authority

Authority is legitimate and position power and in some cases can be expert power. It is determined by structure in an organization and involves rules, roles, and relations. Rules legitimize authority and tend to suspend the subordinate's critical thinking. In autocratic hierarchical structures, subordinates tend to do unquestioningly what the superior with legitimate authority tells them to do. Role is position or office. Authority is inherent in the position. Relations are related to credibility, which is obtained through knowledge and expertise.

Authority is traditionally structured as line authority or staff authority. Line authority refers to levels of authority and superior-subordinate relationships, and it therefore provides the framework for the organization. Staff authority has no command privileges. It has only the right to advise or assist managers in the performance of their duties. Staff members provide assistance when requested, must sell their ideas to the leader or manager over whom they have no authority, and must sell their ideas up the line to leaders and managers who have the line authority to implement the ideas. More recently, functional authority, or authority of the specialist, has emerged. Functional authority is normally limited to the performance of defined duties for a limited period.

It is preferable for a leader's or manager's power to be equal to the authority of the position. The nurse leader's or manager's knowledge of sources of power and authority can help one assess and use them. Nurses have the authority to delegate but remain responsible for what they delegate. (See Chapter 2 regarding delegation.) (Finkelman, 2006; Huber, 2006; Marquis & Huston, 2006; McConnell, 2006; Sullivan & Decker, 2005).

Power and Gender

Gender differences are noted in relation to power. There has been a tendency to socialize women into family and societal roles to facilitate others' success. Men have generally been socialized to relate to hierarchical order of rank, status, income, privilege, and reputation. Women are often more concerned about relating to people. Some women have negative views of power and did not learn to use it constructively. Women may view power as dominance and physical strength instead of accomplishments and skills. Hegyvary (2003) stated that power is not good or evil, but its purpose determines if it is good or bad. There are indications that views of women and men as being powerful have been gradually changing over the 1990s (Lips, 2000), so it is difficult to say if men or women are stereotyped as more powerful in organizations (Leder & Henley, 2000).

Men had limited opportunities in nursing until after World War II. Then nursing education for men was facilitated through financial support from GI bills. Men in nursing have experienced role strain. Female nurses have sometimes expected male nurses to function like orderlies by assisting with lifting and transferring patients and by doing male procedures. Sex is biological and universal while gender is cultural and variable. Gender defines the expectations and norms for males and females. As society has begun to challenge gender-specific occupations, more men are entering nursing (Marquis & Huston, 2006; Roussel, Swansburg, & Swansburg, 2006).

Empowerment

Empowerment is the process of gaining control. Coercive and reward power tend to bring about resistance. Legitimate power tends to bring about compliance. Expert power and referent power tend to bring about commitment. Becker (2005) has said that in the nineteenth century, women were told that their moral virtue was their power. Now power is said to reside in the woman's ability to relate to others and to take better care of herself so she can take care of others. Becker believes that this belief perpetuates the myth that women's problems are more medical than societal and more personal than political (Becker, 2005).

There are several activities men or women can do to empower oneself. One can use physical, psychological, and material resources for empowerment. Maintaining one's physical health provides a basis for personal power. A balanced diet, exercise, rest, and relaxation help one maintain good health, making it easier to become more powerful and giving one the stamina to handle the power.

RESEARCH Perspective 5-1

Data from Finegan JE, Laschinger HKS: The antecedents and consequences of empowerment, *JONA* 31(10):489-497, 2001.

Purpose: The purpose of this study was to explore the possibility of gender differences in empowerment.

Methods: Kanter's conceptualization of empowerment as three separate sources (formal power, informal power, access to certain organizational structures) was used as the theoretical framework. A nonexperimental predictive survey design was used. A questionnaire was mailed to 300 men and 300 women; 412 were usable: 195 (70.1%) from men and 217 (75.6%) from women. Items were summed and averaged on a five-point Likert scale. Structural equation modeling was used to determine whether the model derived from Kanter's work worked equally for men and women. The AMO statistical package within SPSS-PC was used. Independent t-tests were run on all variables used in the mode.

Results/conclusions: Empowerment influenced affective commitment indirectly through its impact on trust in management. The amount of variance explained in affective commitment was 26%. Men's responses were similar to women's responses. Empowerment influenced affective commitment both directly and indirectly through trust. Empowerment did not predict continuance commitment strongly for either men or women. This suggests that the impact of work conditions on continuance commitment is mediated by trust in management. Empowerment might be more important to people with a need for achievement. These people might be more likely to desire and achieve formal and informal power. Both trust and empowerment will lead to increased affective commitment.

Personal psychological resources are also important for gaining control. One should schedule activities to maintain one's mental health and emotional balance. One needs a strong self-concept and a clear understanding of one's strengths and weaknesses. Effective decision making and creative problem solving demonstrate expert power. One needs to be able to admit mistakes and look for solutions instead of someone to blame. Maintaining a positive outlook is important to one's power.

Material resources may include money, clothing, supplies, or personnel. Much power is derived from control of material resources. An awareness of what material resources are needed and how to get them is important to empowerment.

One can help empower oneself by developing expertise through formal education, continuing education, in-service classes, and reading. Joining a professional organization, attending meetings, and reading professional journals help develop both information and connection power. One can seek legitimate power by seeking a position or promotion to a position with greater authority.

Leaders and managers can facilitate empowerment. However, people need to be willing to be empowered. Some people may resist empowerment. People might view delegation as dumping or feel they will be punished for doing the delegated task. Leaders and managers may facilitate empowerment through facilitation of relationships and through delegation by providing freedom that allows people to successfully do what they want to do rather than getting them to do what the managers want them to do. Research results show a positive correlation between participation and acceptance of change, commitment, desire for more work, productivity, and satisfaction. Quality of decisions can be improved through empowered delegation by using more information closer to the problem than the leader or manager alone has. Dimensions of delegated empowerment include choice, sense of competence, value, impact, and security (see Chapter 2 regarding delegation).

Selecting and training employees and creating fair and public organization policies is a start toward empowerment. By removing barriers, controls, and constraints, leaders and managers can design work situations to energize and stimulate intrinsic motivation. People then perform because of intrinsic motivation instead of external rewards. Leaders and managers can facilitate empowerment of employees by letting those closest to the situation do the decision making, and by setting meaningful goals consistent with the goals for the organization. Leaders and managers may provide access to resources, give access to information, encourage personal growth and achievement through staff development, recognize excellence and expertise, and emphasize the importance of contributions of individuals. That may help develop self-confidence and higher self-esteem.

Empowered employees tend to be more satisfied, productive, and innovative. They are likely to produce higher quality products and services than nonempowered employees (see Chapter 4 regarding motivation). Clients and patients can be given decisional control too. They can be informed of what is happening and what is expected in the future. They can be allowed to make decisions based on information and their goals (Finkelman, 2006; Huber, 2006; Lee, 2000; Marquis & Huston, 2006).

The best ways to articulate a vision are through metaphors, real-life examples, stories, and word pictures. SMART goals are specific, measurable, aligned, reachable, and time bound. Vision and goals should be associated with personal values. Success breeds success because it helps develop self-esteem.

Leaders and managers can role model by demonstrating correct and desirable behavior and can give recognition to others' successes. Feedback about good performance by means of praise, thank-you notes, and recognition ceremonies provide support. It is also important to provide social and emotional support.

Leaders and managers may help employees develop an awareness and belief that they can succeed. Finding opportunities for small successes or a small-wins strategy can help build self-confidence and lead to bigger successes. Leaders and managers can divide large problems into smaller ones and delegate simpler tasks before more complex ones.

Counseling and training can help empower people through changes. They can also help replace negative emotions such as anxiety, fear, and complaints with positive emotions such as anticipation, excitement, and passion.

Information is a power tool that helps empower people with self-determination, personal control, and trust to work more productively and in harmony with the organization's goals. If people are given relevant information instead of too much information, overload is less likely to occur.

People need task-related information and the resources necessary to do their jobs. Connecting an individual's work with organizational outcomes helps develop a sense of self-efficacy, personal consequence, and self confidence. Authentic, honorable, and trustworthy behavior contributes to confidence in employees and managers.

Federal Government

It is helpful for nurses to know civics and the rights and duties of citizens. Leaders in professional nursing organizations use their knowledge of the structure of the federal government and the dates events occur to know when and where to be politically active. There are three branches of the federal government: executive, legislative, and judicial. The executive branch contains the office of the president, executive agencies, departments, and numerous independent agencies, boards, committees, and commissions (Mason, Leavitt, & Chaffee, 2006) (Box 5-5).

The Executive Office of the President includes the White House; Cabinet; Council of Economic Advisors; Council on Environmental Quality; Domestic Policy Council; National Economic

BOX 5-5 Branches of the U.S. Government

Executive
Legislative
Judicial

Council; National Security Council; Offices of Administration, Faith-Based and Community Initiatives, Homeland Security, Management and Budgets, National AIDS Policy, National Drug Control Policy, Science and Technology Policy; President's Foreign Intelligence Advisory Board; and Office of the United States Trade Representative.

The Executive Department cabinet agencies include the Departments of Agriculture, Commerce, Defense, Education, Energy, Health and Human Services, Housing and Urban Development, Interior, Justice, Labor, State, Transportation, Treasury, and Veterans Affairs.

The Executive Office includes numerous independent establishments and government corporations including but not limited to the Central Intelligence Agency; Commission on Civil Rights; Consumer Product Safety Commission; Environmental Protection Agency; Equal Employment Opportunity Commission; Federal Housing Finance Board; Federal Trade Commission; Federal Labor Relations Authority; Federal Mediation and Conciliation Service; National Archives and Records Administration; National Education Goals Panel; National Endowment of the Arts; National Labor Relations Board; National Mediation Board; National Science Foundation; Office of Government Ethics; Office of Personnel Management; Office of Special Council; Peace Corps; Securities and Exchange Commission; Selective Service System; Small Business Administration; Social Security Administration; United States International Trade Commission; and the United States Postal Service. In addition, there are dozens of boards, commission, committees, and quasi-official agencies.

The legislative branch is the bicameral Congress composed of the Senate and the House of Representatives. The main purpose of Congress is to make the laws. The Senate is composed of two senators from each state elected for six-year terms, with one third of them up for election every two years. The House of Representatives members are elected for two-year terms. The number representing each state depends of the state's population. The House membership is reapportioned every 10 years based on census results.

The Congressional sessions begin shortly after January 1. The members of the Senate and House choose their own leaders and make committee assignments. The president and president pro tempore of the Senate and the Speaker of the House are elected in accordance with the Constitution. Both the Senate and the House elect majority and minority leaders and assistants to the majority and minority leaders that are not defined in the Constitution.

The vice president serves as the president of the Senate but has little power and does not vote except to break ties. The president pro tempore is elected by the members of the Senate from the majority party and is third in line for the presidency, after the Speaker of the House. The majority and minority leaders support their party's positions.

The Speaker of the House presides over the House of Representatives and is second in line of succession for the presidency if the president or vice president is unable to do those duties. The Speaker is nominated by the majority party and voted on by the entire membership of the House. The Speaker has considerable power over committee assignments, deciding the scheduling of bills to be heard or not, and other procedural maneuvering in the House.

The majority leader is elected by vote of the majority party at the beginning of each session of Congress. The majority party leader assists the Speaker, is the chief strategist, and is spokesperson for the party positions. The minority leader heads the opposition party's contrasting efforts against the majority party's positions. The majority and minority whips or assistants are to lobby members for votes and keep the party members in compliance with the party's positions (Box 5-6).

The duties of Congress are to conduct hearings on topics that may require legislation; draft legislation; determine the impact of the proposed legislation; enact or defeat legislation; levy taxes; determine budget levels for programs; review the success or failures of legislated programs;

BOX 5-6 Legislative Branches

BICAMERAL CONGRESS (MAKES LAWS)
Senate

Two senators for each state for 6-year terms

President of the senate is Vice President of the United States

President pro tempore is elected from the majority party, and is third in line to the U.S. presidency after the president and vice president

Majority leader

Minority leader

Whips assist the majority and minority leaders

House of Representatives

Represent each state, with the number of representatives per state dependent on population figures, for 2-year terms

Speaker of the house is nominated from the majority party, and is fourth in line to the U.S. presidency

Majority leader

Minority leader

Whips assist the majority and minority leaders

BOX 5-7 Congressional Committees

Study issues
Hold hearings
Write bills
Report bills to the floor

---

appropriate funds for federal operations, confirm or reject presidential nominations for some federal positions; and on rare occasions override presidential vetoes.

Congress has organized itself into committees because of the complexity and volume of the work. Each committee has specific legislative jurisdiction and is governed by rules. The committee members study issues, hold hearings, and write bills; they also report the bills to the floor of the Senate or House for a vote unless the bill is defeated in the committee (Box 5-7). Many of the committees are relevant to nurses and health care. It is important for nurses to know which committee deals with the issues they are concerned about and who serves on those committees (Mason, Leavitt, & Chaffee, 2006).

The judicial branch is composed of the U.S. federal court system. According to the Constitution, the Congress is to establish a Supreme Court and inferior courts. The Supreme Court is the highest court in the United States. It is composed of the chief justice and eight associate justices.

The Supreme Court hears cases that at some point originated in local or state courts and involve questions about the Constitution and federal laws. It reviews the decisions of the lower courts and has jurisdiction over treaties. The court system is divided into federal and state courts.

Politics

Politics is the authoritative allocation or the art of influencing allocation of scarce resources and the use of power for change. It requires legitimate power to distribute goods, services, and other resources that are less abundant than desired. A political system is a social system that gets people to do what they would not ordinarily want to do. There are several theories that help explain the dynamics of political systems. According to *game theory*, politics is a fascinating game with rules, referees, and players on opposing sides. *Elite theory* purports that political power is concentrated with people who hold top positions in large, centralized, political, economic, legal, educational, scientific, civic, and cultural institutions. According to the elite theory, it is single elite, not a multiciplicity of competing groups, that makes important decisions. The middle level makes relatively minor decisions, and the common person has almost no input. *Pluralist theory* explains that political life is based on competition between interest groups. The influence of political groups is determined by their political organization, strategies, and leadership. These competitive relationships are unstable because interest groups and related alliances are short-lived and new coalitions and interest groups develop as old ones decline. The power of interest groups is limited by dependence on other groups and the need for compromises. *Exchange theory* states that political behavior is based on the exchange of resources.

People decide what they want, what it will cost, and whether they have the resources to exchange for it (Byrd, 2006; Finkelman, 2006; Huber, 2006; Sullivan & Decker, 2005) (Box 5-8).

Stages of Political Development

Nurses vary from no interest in politics to leadership positions in professional organizations and in the government. There are stages of political development and activism that individual nurses and the profession of nursing use (Mason, Leavitt, & Chaffee, 2006; Yoder-Wise, 2007):

- Apathy—The nurse has little to no interest in politics and does not belong to a professional organization. Nurses were quite inactive in politics before the late 1970s.
- Buy-in—The nurse recognizes the importance of activism within professional organizations and may join a professional organization but is not active. During the 1980s, nursing leaders formed the first political action committee (PAC) and started publishing articles about political action.
- Self-interest—The nurse uses professional organizations for networking to further one's own career and the interests of the profession. Nursing leaders started focusing on education and research and wrote legislation for expanding practice.
- Political sophistication—The nurse moves beyond self-interest to activism on behalf of the public through holding offices in professional organizations at local and state levels. By the mid-1990s, nursing leaders were being recognized for expertise in health policy.
- Leadership—The nurse provides leadership on broad issues, often by serving in elected and appointed positions in professional

organizations and beyond. By the 2000s, nursing leaders were achieving appointments to heads in state and federal government and university presidencies (Mason, Leavitt, & Chaffee, 2006).

Levels of Political Participation

There are levels of political participation ranging from apathetic inactivists who engage in no political activity to complete activists who engage in numerous activities. As nurses become involved in politics, they can expand their influence beyond a single vote. Spectator political activities include gathering political information, displaying bumper stickers or wearing buttons, initiating political discussions, trying to persuade others, and voting. As one becomes increasingly involved, one can make financial contributions, attend political meetings, and contact political leaders. Activists become active members in political parties, attend caucus meetings, contribute time to political campaigns, solicit funds, and run for offices.

Mason, Leavitt, and Chaffee (2006) identified four spheres of political action in which nurses can effect change as follows: (1) workplace, (2) government, (3) professional organizations, and (4) community. Magnet institutions involve nurses at all levels of the organization and give nurses a voice in policy formation. Policy and procedure manuals are common in health care organizations. Important workplace policy issues include but are not limited to working conditions, mandatory overtime, substitution of unlicensed personnel for registered nurses, clinical ladder, smoking areas, family visiting privileges, and referral process for home health care (Box 5-9).

The government sphere is extensive and includes such issues as where alcohol and tobacco products can be advertised and used, reproductive rights, distribution of condoms to prevent the spread of sexually transmitted diseases (STDs), clean needles for drug users to prevent the spread of blood-borne pathogens, treatment for violence, pollution, and low-income housing. Professional organizations develop standards of

BOX 5-9 Spheres of Political Action
Workplace Government Professional organizations Community

Identified by Mason DJ, Leavitt JK, Chaffee MW: *Policy & politics in nursing and health care*, ed 4, St. Louis, 2006, Mosby.

practice, advocate change for health care, and facilitate collective action. The national organization should have a national presence, and the local organization should have visibility in the local community. Organizations should identify issues of health care importance, bring those issues to the attention of the public, and take leadership in the development of related policies. Collective action in a specific direction increases power.

The community can be the workplace, government, professional organization, neighborhood, social unit, or international online group where there is a special interest. There are interrelationships among all four spheres. It takes time and effort to develop influence in all of the spheres, and networking and collaborating with others are critically important to that process.

Nurse managers can encourage others to become more politically active by educating them in issues, posting and circulating information, and encouraging staff discussion of political topics. They can educate and encourage others to work with legislators by providing formal classes on the legislative process, a list of key contacts, and information about voting records. The nurse manager can encourage participation in professional organizations, consumer groups, boards, legislative committee meetings and hearings, and political functions. Staff members can be sent to testify at hearings and be assigned to attend political activities. The manager can generally support political activities, exemplify political involvement, encourage others to vote, and grant release time for political participation.

Communicating with Legislators

Nurse administrators have found that communicating with legislators, building coalitions, being knowledgeable about current issues, providing testimony, solving problems, educating and involving other nurses, and knowing the legislator before needing help are the most successful political strategies. Less effective political strategies include mass mailings, petitions, demonstrations, and reliance on others to protect nurses' interests. Factors that have contributed to unsuccessful political outcomes include emotionalism, lack of preparation, lack of unity among nurses, failure to build an adequate power base, failure to attend political meetings, failure to contact policy makers until too late, lack of publicity, and lack of feedback from politicians, other nurses, and community members.

Legislators spend so much time in sessions and at committee meetings that it can be difficult to reach them by telephone. A letter is a written record that requires a written reply and is more likely to reach the legislator. Messages should be kept brief, preferably one and not more than two pages. A personal letter is more effective than a form letter or a petition. The title and number of the bill one is addressing and a brief interpretation of it should be included. One's position should be stated succinctly. The name and address of the writer should be legible, and when possible writers should identify themselves as nurses and voters in the legislator's district. One must use discretion in selecting a time to discuss an interest with a legislator. One should know the party of which the legislator is a member and address him or her as a representative or senator, as appropriate, to show respect. One should be specific and reasonable about what is wanted and should ask legislators to do only what is within their power.

E-mail is an option. It is direct and immediate, and yet the legislator has flexibility for when to open the message and address the subject. Guidelines for writing letters can be used for e-mails as well. It is possible to send attachments. However, there may be fear of computer viruses, and recipients may refuse to open attachments.

A face-to-face meeting with legislators and their staff is generally an effective lobbying strategy. The guidelines for written messages can be applied to meetings. It is preferable not to talk to legislators who are engrossed in activities related to another bill; one should wait until they can give their full attention to one's concerns. Appointments are set up ahead of time. The nurse should prepare a short, well-written statement of what legislative action is preferred and why, specifying the direct impact it will have on the legislator's constituents. Making a list of talking points can be helpful. The points should be concise and accompanied with news clippings, research reports, and other supportive documentation. It is preferable to deal with one issue at a time, to keep the meeting short, and to end with a specific request. A dialogue can be continued by writing to express gratitude for the meeting and by sending new information as it becomes available (Mason, Leavitt, & Chaffee, 2006).

Organizing Political Meetings

Nurses can take the initiative to organize political meetings. A political meeting could be organized to meet with legislators or to organize for lobbying. It is best to start with a small group with political and organizing experience. The group should include all organizations and important people willing to be involved. One should compile lists of members of organizations, agency directories, officers, names from newspaper articles, and so on. Personal time and money will be needed to type, copy, and mail invitations, as well as for refreshments, room rental, supplies such as name tags and agendas, and follow-up correspondence.

The meeting should be held at a neutral meeting site. A map should be included with the invitation. A self-addressed, stamped response postcard and request for correction of address and telephone number should also be enclosed. Brief handouts and name tags should be prepared in advance of the meeting. A minimum of

food should be served. The atmosphere of the political meeting should be kept comfortable and professional (Yoder-Wise, 2007).

The Legislative Process

Because the legislative process is complex and technical, nurses need to know the process to determine when to intervene. The state legislative process is similar to the national process that follows. First, legislation is drafted and introduced. These legislative proposals originate in a number of ways and may be introduced in either the Senate or the House. Either individuals such as members of Congress or special interest groups may introduce legislation. Any member of Congress can introduce a bill at any time the House is in session by placing the bill in a wooden box known as the hopper, which is located at the side of the rostrum in the House or Senate chamber. The member introducing the bill is known as the primary sponsor. An unlimited number of congresspersons can co-sponsor a bill.

Next, there is committee referral. A bill is considered read for the first time when it is referred to a committee. Only a member of Congress can introduce legislation in the committee. There is no limit to the number of bills a member may introduce. In the House of Representatives and the Senate, a bill is numbered according to its place in the order of introduction, referred to committee, labeled with the sponsor's name, and printed by the Government Printing Office. Bills are prefixed with HR when introduced in the House of Representatives and S when introduced in the Senate. After referral to a standing committee, most legislation is referred to a subcommittee. Most bills go no further. Each bill introduced must pass the House of Representatives and the Senate in identical form within 2 years to become a law.

Standing committees are required to have regular meeting days at least once a month. Three or more committee members may file a written request for the chairperson to call a special meeting, or the chairperson may convene additional meetings. All business meetings of standing committees, except the Committee of

Official Conduct, must be open to the public unless the majority of committee members present determines by recorded vote that all or part of the meeting should be closed to the public. Committees are not to meet during a joint session of the House and Senate or during a recess when a joint meeting of the House and Senate in is progress. Committees may meet during an adjournment or other recesses up to the expiration of the constitutional term.

After referral to a standing committee and a subcommittee, hearings are held by the subcommittee. The chairperson of the committee makes a public announcement of the date, place, and subject matter to be discussed at the hearing at least one week before the hearing unless the chairperson, in concurrence with the ranking minority member, or the committee by majority vote determine there is a reason to meet earlier.

Often only a few members of the subcommittee who have a special interest in the subject will participate in the hearings. The chairperson uses the agenda, funds, and staff to expedite, delay, or modify legislation. The subcommittee usually schedules public hearings and invites testimony from private and public witnesses. Interested individuals submit written requests to testify. Once they are informed of when to testify, rescheduling is not allowed. If one cannot be present at the designated time, one may file a written statement for the record of the hearing. Witnesses who share common positions are urged to consolidate testimony and designate a single spokesperson. Groups with similar concerns that are unwilling to have a single spokesperson may form panels. Panelists are allowed a 6-minute presentation of the key points in their written documents and are urged to avoid repeating other presentations. All witnesses are required to file a written statement with the committee at least one day before the scheduled appearance or the preceding Friday if the testimony is to be on Monday or Tuesday. The statement should be typed on letter-size paper and include a summary of the principal points. Witnesses should not read their written statements but should summarize

the key points in no more than 6 minutes. Once the testimony has been given, each subcommittee member may ask questions.

If, after the hearing, the subcommittee members decide the legislation should go further, they do a markup session and consider the language line by line and section by section to determine the language of the final bill, which is then favorably recommended to the full committee with or without amendment. A bill could also be recommended unfavorably or without recommendation.

When presenting the bill to the floor of the House or Senate, the full committee justifies its actions in a written report that accompanies the bill. Bills that are unanimously voted out of committee have a good chance on the floor. However, dispute is likely to occur on the floor if there has been a divided committee.

After a bill has passed one house, it is sent to the other, where the same process takes place. If the second house approves the bill as it was passed by the first, it is sent to the president for his or her signature. However, if the bill was revised or amendments added, the bill must be returned to the originating chamber for approval of the changes. If that body refuses to approve the revised bill, both versions are sent to a conference committee. The bill is then sent to the president for signature or veto after the differences are reconciled and there is a final vote of acceptance by the conference committee. In the case of a presidential veto, both houses can override the veto to make the bill law.

The process is similar in each state bicameral legislature. However, Nebraska is a unicameral legislature. Specific procedures for each state can be located on the Internet (Johnson, 2003) (Box 5-10).

LABOR RELATIONS

Why Employees Join Unions

Employees join a union essentially to increase their power to get certain responses from management. Management's actions or inactions have probably caused the employees to reach

> **BOX 5-10** How a Bill Becomes a Law
>
> Bill is drafted
> Bill is introduced
> Bill is referred to a committee
> First reading
> Bill is probably referred to a subcommittee
> Public hearing
> Markup
> Final committee action
> Repeat the process from the introduction
>   onward in the other house

their limit of tolerance. Poor working conditions and job inequities in wage increments, promotion, and benefits cause distress. Poor quality of immediate supervision, arbitrary treatment from management, and poor communications between employer and employee are major reasons for unionization. Instead of quitting their jobs and giving up their seniority, security, and friends to move to another job, employees form a union.

Labor Law

In 1935, the *National Labor Relations Act* (NLRA), or the *Wagner Act*, was passed in an effort to end the Depression. It prevented some employers from cutting wages in the hopes that higher worker incomes and increased spending would lessen the severity of the economic depression. Unfortunately, some employers went bankrupt because they could not decrease wages. Employers could not legally fire employees who sought unionization. The NLRA created the National Labor Relations Board (NLRB) to investigate and initiate administrative proceedings against employers who violated a law that listed employer violations only.

In 1887, the Nurses' Associated Alumnae of the United States and Canada was formed, and in 1911 it became the American Nurses Association (ANA). In 1946 the ANA started the Economic Security Program to help state associations bargain collectively.

Because the NLRA was biased toward unions, it was amended in 1947 by the *Taft-Hartley Act*,

or *Labor Management Relations Act*. It listed union restrictions to restore equality between employers and employees. Nonprofit health care institutions, however, were exempted from the law. The unions developed public relations problems when some of them went on strike during the war and when unions were blamed for the postwar inflation.

In 1959 the laws were further modified by the *Landrum-Griffin Act*, or *Labor-Management Reporting and Disclosure Act*, to safeguard against corrupt financial and election procedures used by some unions. The Union Members' Bill of Rights resulted.

The *Equal Pay Act* of 1963 establishes that men and women performing equal work should receive equal compensation.

The *Civil Rights Act* of 1964 prohibits discrimination and promotes employment based on ability and merit. It specifically mentions race, color, religion, gender, and national origin. Equal employment opportunity legislation is to prevent discrimination while affirmative action plans are to actively seek to correct past injustices.

The *Age Discrimination in Employment Act* (ADEA) of 1967 promotes employment of older people based on their ability rather than age, and the 1978 amendment increased the protected age to 70 years. Although statistics show a trend toward earlier retirement, Congress voted to remove the age restriction except in certain categories in 1987.

The Rehabilitation Act of 1973 provides affirmative action to recruit, hire, and advance qualified handicapped people. Congress passed the *Americans With Disabilities Act* (ADA) in 1990 to eliminate discrimination against people with physical or mental impairments, including physical disabilities, cancer, diabetes, and human immunodeficiency virus, and persons recovering from alcoholism and drug use.

The *Vietnam Veterans Act* of 1973/1974 addresses employment rights and privileges for veterans. It has also allowed some nurses to get reemployed after serving in the Persian Gulf War even though there was a nursing surplus at the time.

In 1974, Public Law 93-360, the *Nonprofit Health Care Amendments to the Taft-Hartley Act*, extended federal collective bargaining rights to private sector employees. It created notification procedures that must precede a strike and ensured employees of the right to join, or refrain from joining, a union. The 1974 amendments to the NLRA resulted in the following changes:

- Required unions to give a 10-day prestrike notice
- Did not permit a strike or lockout during the notice period
- Required unions to give advance written notice of contract termination or modification to the employer and to a federal mediator and conciliation service
- Required mediation by a federal mediator and conciliation service
- Allowed a board of inquiry to be established to settle disputes
- Allowed employees to be held exempt from a requirement to join or financially support a union for bona fide religious grounds

This extended the legal protection of nurses for collective bargaining. Because of declining union membership in manufacturing industries, unions welcomed the expanded market. The shift from manufacturing to service industries, increase in nonstandard work like part-time jobs, technology, globalization, capital mobility, worker attitudes, employer resistance, and hostile legislation have challenged unions.

The Taft-Hartley Amendment gives the NLRB the responsibility to determine the composition and size of bargaining units. However, all NLRB decisions are subject to review by several federal circuit courts of appeal, which did reject separate bargaining units for registered nurses. In 1984 the NLRB made a landmark decision to recognize two broad units of professional and nonprofessional employees (St. Francis Hospital II NLRB 948, 1984), which the federal court of appeals overturned in 1987. In 1987 the NLRB designated eight bargaining units: registered nurses, employed physicians, all other professionals, technical employees, skilled maintenance employees, business office

and clerical staff, security guards, and all other nonprofessional employees. Nursing homes, psychiatric hospitals, and rehabilitation facilities were exempt. The NLRB had never used its rule-making power to establish bargaining units before. In May 1989 the American Hospital got injunctive relief against the rules, and the Chicago Federal District Court issued a permanent injunction against the rule in July 1989. However, in April 1990 the U.S. Court of Appeals for the Seventh Circuit reversed the lower court's decision. In 1991 the U.S. Supreme Court upheld the NLRB ruling that unions can organize eight separate groups of hospital employees. This opened the market of the minimally unionized health care industry to unions (Grohar-Murray & DiCroce, 2003; National Labor Relations Act, 1935).

The *Family and Medical Leave Act* (FMLA) of 1993 was intended to cover pregnancy and maternity leave but became very broad. The act requires employers with 50 or more employees to provide up to 12 weeks per year of unpaid, job-protected leave. Eligible workers must be employed for at least 12 months and completed 1250 hours of service during the 12 months immediately preceding the leave. A worker is entitled to a leave for the following circumstances: (1) for the birth of the worker's child, (2) for adoption or foster placement of a child with the worker, (3) to provide care for a child, spouse, or parent with a serious health condition, and (4) when the worker is unable to perform functions of the job position because of a serious health condition. The worker then has the right to return to work in the same or an equivalent position with equivalent benefits, compensation, and conditions of employment and to take leave on a reduced time or intermittent basis if medically necessary for a serious health condition of the worker, child, spouse, or parent. The employer can require the worker to use accrued paid vacation and sick leave time in lieu of part of the 12 weeks of unpaid leave. The employer must continue to pay health benefits for the duration of the leave. Records are to be maintained with the medical information and kept confidential and separate from the personnel file (Grohar-Murray & DiCroce, 2003).

In 1994, the U.S. Supreme Court decision in *National Labor Relations Board (NLRB) v. Health Care and Retirement Corporation of America* was that licensed practical nurses employed by Heartland Nursing Home in Urbana, Ohio, were considered "supervisors" who acted in the interest of their employer when performing patient care duties, and were consequently not eligible for protection under the amended NLRA. In 1996 the NLRB reinterpreted the NLRA and issued a decision containing a detailed analysis of nursing duties, defining true supervisory work according to labor law. In the NLRB decision (not the Supreme Court decision), nonsupervisory employees continue to have the right to organize for collective bargaining purposes.

NLRA Section 7 about employee rights states the following:

> Employees shall have the right to self-organization, to form, join, or assist labor organizations, to bargain collectively through activities for the purpose of collective bargaining or other mutual aid or protection, and shall also have the right to refrain from any or all such activities except to the extent that such right may be affected by an agreement requiring membership in a labor organization as a condition of employment as authorized in section 8(a)(3).

NLRA Section 2(11) defines supervisor as follows:

> The term "Supervisor" means any individual having authority, in the interest of the employer, to hire, transfer, suspend, lay off, recall, promote, discharge, assign, reward or discipline other employees, or responsibility to direct them, or to adjust their grievances, or effectively to recommend such action, if in connection with the foregoing the exercise of such authority is not of a merely routine clerical nature, but requires the use of independent judgment.

This section has implications for nursing, particularly since registered nurses are supervising more and more unlicensed personnel. This definition of supervision eliminates many nurses from bargaining units.

Title VII prohibits an employer from engaging in conduct that creates a hostile or offensive working environment on the basis of race, religion, gender, or national origin. To state a claim of harassment or discrimination, plaintiffs must establish that the behavior endured by them at their place of work was severe and pervasive enough to alter the conditions of their employment and to create an abusive working environment. The behavior reported to be harassment or discrimination usually is an action or inaction by a supervisor. The U.S. Supreme Court placed vicarious liability on employers for the actions or inactions of their supervisors in the context of sexual harassment. If an employee is being harassed by anyone who is a supervisor, the employer is vicariously liable for the harassment. This is true whether the harassment is in the form of sexual favors or jokes or tangible job detriment, such as a cut in pay, termination, or demotion. The only defense the employer will have is claiming an effective antiharassment policy was in place and that the employees failed to use the policy to avoid harm otherwise. These rulings have not been extended beyond the areas of sexual discrimination as of 1999. Supervisors are not individually liable for Title VII, ADA, or ADEA violations because they are not "employers" as that term is defined in Title VII, ADA, or ADEA (McCrory, 2003).

The 1999 ANA House of Delegates supported affiliation with the American Federation of Labor Congress of Industrial Organizations (AFL-CIO), a federation of trade and professional unions. The AFL-CIO's constitution requires that federation members do not raid other federation unions. That would provide the state nurses associations (SNAs) some protection and allow more time and resources for educating, organizing, and representing registered nurses instead of fending off other unions. The 1999 ANA House of Delegates also recommended establishment and funding of a Task Force on Workplace Advocacy to develop and evaluate models by which the ANA and SNAs could ensure that nurses not represented by a collective bargaining unit will have access to workplace advocacy (ANA House of Delegates conference materials, 1999). The United American Nurses replaced the Institute of Constituent Members Collective Bargaining Programs (Marquis & Huston, 2006; Roussel, Swansburg, & Swansburg, 2006) (Table 5-1).

Unfair Labor Practices by Management

The NLRA's section 8(a) prohibitions on management are known as the unfair labor practices. They include interference, 8(a)(1); domination, 8(a)(2); discrimination, 8(a)(3); discrimination, 8(a)(4); and refusal to bargain, 8(a)(5). Restraining, coercing, or otherwise interfering with employees during the exercise of their right to organize is an unfair labor practice. Management

may not contribute financial or other support or otherwise dominate or interfere during the development or administration of a labor organization. The employer may not discriminate in hiring or tenure or other terms of employment to encourage or discourage membership in a labor organization. Nor can the employer discriminate against an employee for filing charges or giving testimony. The employer is also forbidden to refuse to bargain with representatives of the employees.

Unfair Labor Practices by Unions

Before 1935, management's power had few limitations. From 1935 to 1947, managers had to contend with unfair labor practice limitations,

TABLE 5-1 Labor Laws

Date	Act	Action
1935	National Labor Relations Act (NLRB)/Wagner Act	Created the National Labor Relations Board (NLRB) Was biased toward unions
1947	Taft-Harley Act/Labor Management Relations Act	Amended the NLRB Listed union restrictions Nonprofit health care institutions were exempt
1959	Landrum-Griffin Act/Labor-Management Reporting and Disclosure Act	Union Members Bill of Rights/Safeguard against corrupt financial and election procedures
1963	Equal Pay Act	Establishes that men and women performing equal work should receive equal compensation
1964	Civil Rights Act	Prohibits discrimination and promotes employment based on ability
1967 1978 amendment 1987	Age Discrimination in Employment Act (ADEA)	Promotes employment of older people based on ability rather than age (1967) Increased protection to age 70 years (1978) Congress voted to remove the age restriction except in certain categories (1987)
1970 many amendments	Occupational Safety & Health Act (OSHA)	Requires employers to provide a safe place to work
1973	Rehabilitation Act	Provides affirmative action to recruit, hire, and advance qualified handicapped people
1973/1974	Vietnam Veterans Act	Addressed employment rights and privileges for veterans
1974	Nonprofit Health Care	Extended federal collective
1974	Amendments to the NLRA	Created many requirements for striking
1993	Family and Medical Leave Act (FMLA)	Covered pregnancy, maternity leaves, and more
1994	U.S. Supreme Court Decision	Supervisors who acted in the interest of their employers when performing patient care duties are not eligible for protection under the NLRA; this disqualifies many nurses from bargaining

but no such unfair labor practices were defined for labor organizations. In 1947 the Labor Management Relations Act amended the NLRA and added restrictions for labor organizations. These include interference, 8(b)(1); induced discrimination, 8(b)(2); refusal to bargain, 8(b)(3); strikes and boycotts, 8(b)(4); initiation fee, 8(b)(5); featherbedding, 8(b)(6); and recognition picketing, 8(b)(7). Labor organizations may not restrain or coerce an employer in the selection of a representative for collective bargaining. The union may not cause an employer to discriminate against an employee who is not a member of the union. Nor can a union representative of the employees refuse to bargain with the employer. With adherence to required notification procedures, an employee organization may strike against the employer when negotiations have failed. A primary boycott is a strike action taken by union members against their employer. The illegal or protected status of strikes or boycotts depends on the union objectives and the tactics used.

Labor unions may not force an employer to join any organization, or to cease using specific products or doing business with someone, thus making "hot cargo" clauses illegal. Hot cargo agreements are stipulations on the employer's use of products that give the union power over other organizations. A secondary boycott that is directed at a customer or supplier of the employer is also illegal. An employee group may not force an employer to bargain with them if the employees are represented by another bargaining agent. Labor organizations may not force "any employer to assign particular work to employees in a particular labor organization...rather than to employees in another labor organization," (National Labor Relations Act, 1935) and they may not honor strike lines against other employers by refusing to cross the picket lines. Informational picketing is not barred because it does not disrupt the employer's operation. Recognition picketing to get an employer to recognize an employee group is lawful except when the employer has recognized another labor organization, when it is within 12 months preceding a valid election, and when picketing has been conducted without a petition. The union may not charge discriminatory or excessive initiation fees or cause an employer to pay for services not performed, a practice called featherbedding.

UNIONIZATION

A labor union consists of wage earners organized to bargain with employers to serve the members' interests regarding wages and working conditions. Advantages of unionization include a contribution to a high standard of living and potentially a way to secure justice in the workplace through the opportunity to share power with employers. Contracts have allowed nurses input regarding policies, procedures, and nursing care standards. Working conditions that may be negotiated include but are not limited to staffing, posting of vacancies, shift rotations, floating, flexible staffing, nonnursing duties, meal breaks, rest breaks, continuing education, tuition reimbursement, educational leaves, time away from work, maternity/paternity leave, discipline, peer review, career ladders, and joint committees. Disadvantages are: the labor unions cost money, can cause adversarial relationships between labor and management, and can encourage dependence while discouraging work (Roussel, Swansburg, & Swansburg, 2006). Phases of unionization are listed in Box 5-11.

Organizing Phase

To form a union, an organizer must establish internal contacts. In a hospital or other health care agency, the organizer needs at least one nurse on each shift to assist with unionization.

BOX 5-11 Phases of Unionization

Organizing
Recognition
Contract negotiation
Contract administration
Decertification

BOX 5-12 Questions to Help Determine Whether Staff Are in the Organizing Phase

A "yes" answer to the following questions may indicate that personnel are in the organizing phase:

- Have you seen union authorization cards anywhere on the agency premises?
- Have you heard of any union-sponsored meetings outside the organization?
- Have you heard of any employee meetings being held at an employee's home?
- Has there been an increase in the number of peer work social activities?
- Have you noticed a repeated presence of strangers or ex-employees mingling with employees outside the agency as employees are coming to and going from work?
- Have employees been forming into groups that include people who do not normally associate with one another?
- Are you finding employees in work areas where they do not/should not visit normally?
- Have you seen employees talking together in small groups and either breaking up their conversation and walking away or becoming silent as you or other members of management approach?

- Have employees who are usually friendly toward supervisors become "cool" toward them?
- Has there been any significant increase in the number of employee complaints about wages or conditions of employment?
- Has there been an increase in employee complaints regarding schedules, staffing levels, content or frequency of in-service education programs, or unclear and overlapping job classifications?
- Has there been an increase in the number of argumentative questions asked during meetings?
- Has there been an increase in graffiti or cartoons that direct humorous hostility toward management?
- Are local or national news items about unions or union settlements put up on bulletin boards?
- Has there been a change in the rate of turnover?
- Are you aware of any other factors that appear to be out of the ordinary and seem to be separating administration from employees?

The organizer should be known by a majority of the nurses, be knowledgeable about related laws, and be able to use free time for organizing. The organizers ascertain the level of interest informally by listening, asking questions, and supplying information. After an assessment period, the organizers meet, discuss the prevailing climate, identify the frustration level, enumerate the kinds and extent of employment problems, and assess the nurses' interest in unionization. If interest is minimal, further organizing efforts should be postponed. If nurses show interest in organizing, the campaign is planned.

There must be commitment from the nurses before a formal organization can be established. To achieve this, the organizers hold informational meetings. Coordination of efforts, development of unity, identification of problems and concerns, education about collective bargaining, and active participation of nurses are the tasks to be accomplished in the organizing meetings. The organizers should work in nonwork areas

on their own time. The organizers contact the labor organization that they want to represent them for information and authorization cards. An organizing committee can research facets of the institution, prepare a timetable, anticipate employer tactics, and identify ways to deal with them, and develop a system for communication with nurses. The labor organization can send a letter to the employer informing management that the nurses within that agency are organizing and that the activity is protected by law. The union petitions the NLRB for an election. Box 5-12 lists questions that the manager can ask to help determine whether staff members are in the organizing phase.

Recognition Phase

The organizers must get at least 30% of the nurses to be represented to sign individual authorization cards before the labor organization can act on behalf of the group. Handing out authorization cards is solicitation but cannot be prohibited by management anywhere in the agency during nonworking time. Recognition of the labor organization by the employer is necessary before collective bargaining can begin. Some employers will recognize the labor organization on a voluntary basis when given proof of the majority representative status. However, employers often refuse to recognize the labor organization voluntarily on the basis of a good faith doubt of majority representation. Thus it becomes necessary to obtain certification from the NLRB.

The NLRB does not start an election until requested to do so by an employee organization. A *petition* for an election must be accompanied by designation cards signed by 30% of the employees in the bargaining group to indicate a substantial show of interest. Labor organizations usually obtain signatures from at least 50% of the potential members before they file a petition.

A *preliminary hearing* is held before an election is scheduled. This provides participants an opportunity to express their opinions. The regional director of the NLRB assesses that the employer is under the board's jurisdiction; determines that other criteria are met; determines the bargaining unit and voter eligibility; and sets the date, hours, and place for the election and informs workers of the date, time, and place of the *election*. The election usually takes place during working hours on the employer's premises about one month after the hearing. All employees in the bargaining unit who were on the employer's payroll during a given payroll period in the recent past are allowed to vote. This rule prevents hiring people to vote in the election.

The number of bargaining units within an agency is held to a minimum. Appropriate bargaining units include the following: (1) technical employees, such as x-ray technicians, surgical technicians, and licensed practical nurses; (2) service and maintenance employees, such as employees doing kitchen work, laundry, and housekeeping; (3) business office clerical employees, such as receptionists, clerks, and switchboard operators; and (4) professional employees, such as nurses.

Spouses and children of the employers, temporary employees, and managerial employees are not eligible to vote. People who have the authority to hire, fire, and direct others are considered managers. This may include nurse managers, head nurses, and charge nurses. As a member of management, the vice president or director of nursing is ineligible to vote.

During the preelection period, the employer is required to post NLRB election notices stating the time, date, and place of the election. On election day, the field examiner from the regional board sets up the election machinery and does not allow electioneering around the polling place. Eligible employees cast secret ballots. Ballots are counted in the regional office. The tabulation of votes is forwarded to the office of the General Counsel in Washington, DC, and the General Counsel decides the election. If employees no longer want to be represented by the labor organization, they can initiate a decertification election with a requisite 30% show of interest. If a bargaining unit is denied because of the vote tabulation, the labor organization is not permitted to seek certification among the same people until after a 12-month moratorium, and the management group should rectify the problems identified during the organization phase. If a union wins the election, both parties prepare to negotiate.

Contract Negotiation Phase

The piecemeal, total, and combination approaches can be used for contract negotiations. The piecemeal is a step-by-step approach that tries to settle the issues one by one. The total approach considers nothing settled until everything is settled. This allows for calculation of the effects of the interdependent variables on each other. The combination method uses both approaches. The step-by-step method is used to progress from the easy to the hard issues. The decisions are not irrevocable, trading takes place, and decisions are reworked until negotiations are acceptable to both parties. The union representatives present the solutions to the members for a ratification vote to accept or reject the offer. If the solutions are accepted, the employee and management representatives sign the agreement, and it becomes binding. If they are rejected, the representatives reassemble to continue negotiating the contract.

During contract negotiations, the union is on the offensive and management is on the defensive. The union makes most of the demands, whereas management defends itself against them and prepares for a strike. The threat of a strike strengthens the union negotiator's position.

Strikes in the health care field require more special and elaborate notification procedures than those in other industries. This allows for the delay of new admissions or referral to other facilities. Alternative health care plans are made for ambulatory patients. Some hospitalized patients may be transferred to other agencies, and supervisory personnel are scheduled to care for the remaining patients.

The NLRB categorizes collective bargaining types into three groups: illegal, voluntary, and mandatory. Illegal topics violate the NLRA and other laws. Voluntary subjects need not be negotiated unless both sides consent to do so. Voluntary issues include size of the bargaining team, union dues, management salaries, and patient charges. Mandatory subjects are related to conditions of employment, work hours, and remuneration.

Contracts often start with a preamble that states both parties' objectives and a pledge of cooperation. Near the beginning there is a statement of the employer's recognition of the union as the bargaining representative for specific employees with specification of employees who are excluded.

A union security clause requires new workers to join the union. Union security is protected by establishing a closed shop, union shop, agency shop, or maintenance-of-membership arrangement in the contract. The closed shop requires the employer to hire and retain only union members in good standing. However, this is prohibited by the Labor Management Relations Act of 1947 for employers and employees in industries affecting interstate commerce. A union shop requires all employees to become members of the union within a specific time after hiring (usually 30 to 60 days) and to maintain membership as a condition of employment.

An agency shop requires all employees in the negotiating unit who do not join the union to pay a fixed amount equivalent to organization dues on a regular basis as a condition of employment. The money may go to the organization's welfare fund or to a charity. The maintenance-of-membership clause requires union members to maintain their membership during a specific period, such as the duration of the contract.

Financial remuneration—including wages and salaries, shift differentials, overtime rates, holiday pay, cost-of-living adjustment, longevity, and merit increases—receives considerable attention. Nonfinancial remuneration—including insurance, retirement plans, employee services such as free lunches and parking, vacations, holidays, leaves, and educational assistance—also receives considerable attention. The union usually strives to have rewards made on the basis of seniority. Guidelines for discipline, grievance procedures, and professional standards are also negotiated. After acceptance of the contract by the union members through a ratification vote, the contract is signed by employee and employer representatives and becomes binding (Roussel, Swansburg, & Swansburg, 2006).

Contract Administration

Implementation of the agreement, the final phase of the unionization process, interprets and enforces the agreement developed during negotiations. When one of the parties involved does not abide by the terms of the contract, a grievance may result. Grievances are most commonly filed against management because management has a more active role than the union in the administration of the contract. The grievance procedure is usually addressed in the contract.

Underlying causes of grievances should be identified and corrected so that future grievances will be prevented. Different types of grievances require different reactions from managers and union leaders. A legitimate grievance results when one party violates the agreement between parties. Managers' ignorance of the agreement and lack of commitment are the major causes. It is not uncommon for first-line managers to function without having read the contract and with the attitude that labor relations are a chore. On the other hand, union stewards are more motivated to understand the agreement and must have an interest in labor relations to obtain their positions. Consequently, most legitimate grievances are against management. It is advisable to develop training programs to familiarize managers with the contract and to set labor relations objectives as priorities for managers.

Imagined grievances occur when a party incorrectly believes that there has been a violation. Employees sometimes imagine a grievance because they do not understand their rights. The steward should correct the misunderstanding before it becomes a formal grievance.

Political grievances occur for reasons other than the concern itself. Management may want to appear supportive to subordinate managers and stewards to union members, so they do not adequately advise the complainant about available information. A cooperative atmosphere between labor and management is the best way to avoid political grievances.

Harassment grievances are sometimes fabricated to distress the other side. They are most commonly used by unions in connection with negotiations. Management usually denies the grievances, forcing the union to drop the grievance or request arbitration. If the contract indicates that both sides share arbitration expenses, harassment grievances are usually dropped.

Organizations should have a grievance procedure even if they are not unionized. This allows employees access to management regarding issues of concern to them and conveys management's intent to be fair. Grievances should be handled quickly through the use of a grievance procedure. Grievances may be handled in a decentralized or centralized manner. In a decentralized process, the immediate supervisor tries to resolve as many problems as possible, and grievances rarely progress further. This encourages a close working relationship between manager and staff members. Unfortunately, there may be inconsistent decisions because of the number of different people involved in the process.

In a centralized grievance procedure, the immediate manager denies the validity of the grievance, and it is handled by the next level of management or by a personnel department. Thus, decisions are made consistently among units because of the few people involved in the decision making. Unfortunately, cooperation between the manager and staff associate is not fostered.

Arbitration

Most contracts allow either side to seek arbitration when a grievance is not satisfactorily resolved, but both parties must agree on the arbitrator. The American Arbitration Association and the Federal Mediation and Conciliation Service are primary sources for professional arbitrators. The payment of costs involved is specified in the contract. Commonly, both parties share the costs, but some contracts specify that the loser must pay.

In any case, arbitration is not automatic and must be requested by the dissatisfied party. Both sides select a representative, the grievance is reviewed, fact finding is done, and witnesses are interviewed. Preparation of one's case from the opponent's view encourages one to consider both sides and develop a stronger case. Presenting one's case to a friend who will act as an advocate helps further identify weaknesses in one's presentation and further strengthens the case. Documents should be prepared in triplicate for the hearing so that the arbitrator, opponent, and presenter can each have a copy. When witnesses are being used for the hearing, their availability should be confirmed. Witnesses should also be informed of where and when to attend the hearing and what will be expected of them.

A hearing is similar to courtroom proceedings. The arbitrator makes opening remarks, and the initiating party comments on the purpose of the hearing and outcomes desired. The responding side may respond then or wait until later. Witnesses are presented and cross-examined in an alternating pattern. First, a witness testifies for the initiator, and then one for the responding party testifies and is cross-examined. The initiating party makes closing remarks, followed by the responding party's closing statement, each pointing out evidence to support that side. The arbitrator studies the evidence and makes a decision. The arbitrator may issue a summary judgment shortly after the proceedings or a written decision to both parties within 1 month. The decision of the arbitrator is enforceable in court (Cherry & Jacob, 2002; Roussel, Swansburg, & Swansburg, 2006; Sullivan & Decker, 2005).

Decertification

When employees no longer want to be represented by their present union, they can request a decertification election. Management may also request an election if it is in good faith, doubting that the union is representing the majority of employees. The decertification election is similar to the certification process. First, a decertification petition must be signed by at least 30% of the bargaining unit to file a show of interest. In reality, more than 50% and probably closer to 75% need to show interest to guarantee a successful election. The petition is filed with the NLRB by the employer. It can be filed on the expiration date of a contract or ideally during the 30-day period before the 90-day period preceding expiration of the contract.

After receiving the decertification petition, the NLRB distributes a notice about it to the union, the petitioners, and the employer. The employer is asked to submit the following to the NLRB: (1) names and addresses of other interested unions, (2) copies of current and recent contracts covering the employees petitioning for decertification, and (3) names and job classifications of all employees in the bargaining unit.

A preelection hearing may be scheduled if there are questions regarding representation. If neither the union nor the employer requests a hearing, an election date and time are set. The selection of the date is extremely important to the success of the election. Campaigning is limited to 24 hours before the election so that the decertification process momentum is not disrupted by a weekend. Wednesday, Thursday, and Friday are preferable days for the election. A day that will ensure maximal turnout, such as payday, is desirable. The election should be held within three weeks of confirmation of the election by the NLRB.

Decertification campaigns are similar to certification efforts. Managers should have various meetings, including individual meetings, small group meetings, and entire unit meetings, to assure personnel that they are in good hands with management and that they will be better off without a union. However, decertification cannot be accomplished just by holding meetings during the campaign. Management needs to have earned the confidence of the employees over time through the use of good management techniques.

The NLRB conducts the election on the specified date. If the union loses the election, management stops negotiating with the union. If not, the next contract is negotiated (Sullivan & Decker, 2005). Key terms used in collective bargaining are defined in Box 5-13.

STRIKES

A strike is an organized work stoppage by union members or the withholding of labor to bring economic pressure on the employers to coerce the employer to meet the union members' demands. It is usually used as a last resort. Firing striking employees is illegal, but it is legal to hire premanent replacements. Then the managers only have to hire back former strikers as there are openings available. Nurses have historically not done much striking. If they do, a 10-day notice must be given by law to allow the facilities the opportunity to prepare for striking nurses' absences (Roussel, Swansburg, & Swansburg, 2006; Sullivan & Decker, 2005).

NURSE LEADERS' AND MANAGERS' ROLE IN COLLECTIVE BARGAINING

Nurse managers should evaluate their management skills and take continuing education courses to improve their skills. Motivational techniques are particularly important for nurse administrators to possess because they work through others. They must listen carefully to staff concerns and represent staff associates' wishes to top management. Nurse administrators also need to know about labor relations.

BOX 5-13 Key Terms Used in Collective Bargaining

Agency shop: A business where nonmembers are required to join the union as a condition of employment

Arbitration: Procedures for using the services of a third party to settle labor disputes

Arbitrator: The person chosen by agreement of both parties to decide the dispute between them

Authorization cards: Cards the employees sign to authorize representation by a specific union

Bargaining agent: A person or group accepted by an employer and chosen by members of the bargaining unit to represent them in collective bargaining

Bargaining unit: An employee group that the state or National Labor Relations Board recognizes as an appropriate division for collective bargaining

Certification: The official recognition of a labor organization as the exclusive bargaining agent for employees of a specific bargaining unit

Collective bargaining: A legal process used by organized employees to negotiate with an employer about wages and related concerns resulting in an employment contract

Contract violations: Acts that break the terms of a contract

Deadlock: A stall in negotiations when neither party is willing to compromise about an issue

Decertification: The withdrawal of official recognition of a union as the exclusive bargaining agent for a bargaining unit

Grievance: Any complaint by an employer or union concerning an aspect of employment

Grievance procedures: Steps both sides have agreed to follow to settle disputes

Mediation: A process for settling labor disputes where a mediator helps the parties reach their own agreements

Open shop: A business where employees are not required to belong to the bargaining unit

From Foley M, Center for Labor Relations: *Key terms used in collective bargaining,* Washington, DC, nd, American Nurses Association.

RESEARCH Perspective 5-2

Data from Matthews S, Spencer Laschinger HK, Johnstone L: Staff nurse empowerment in line and staff organizational structures for chief nurse executives, *JONA* 36(11):526-533, 2006.

Purpose: Kanter's theoretical constructs of empowerment (access to information, support, resources and opportunity, and formal and informal power) was used to link chief nurse executives line and staff organizational structures to staff nurse perceptions of workplace empowerment.

Methods: Two hundred fifty-six staff nurses were surveyed in two large teaching hospitals; one was a line structure and the other a staff structure. Multiple regression analysis was used to test the proposed model.

Results/conclusions: The nurses in the line structure felt significantly more empowered in their access to resources than nurses in a staff structure. Access to information, resources, and formal power were important predictors of nurses' global empowerment in the line hospital. Only access to support was a significant predictor in the staff hospital. Support for the model tested suggest the importance for the chief nurse executive to create and sustain healthy work environments for nurses.

The vice president or director of nursing should not serve as the chief negotiator during collective bargaining because it would put the director in an adversary role. The agency's legal representative is usually the negotiator. During negotiations the vice president or director of nursing defines what is best for the nursing care of patients. Once the contract has been negotiated, nurse managers must learn the terms of the contract and have copies of the contract available to them. Problems should be solved through problem-solving techniques as they

TABLE 5-2 Advantages and Disadvantages of Collective Bargaining

Advantages	Disadvantages
Equalization of power	Adversary relationship
Viable grievance procedures	Strikes may not be prevented
Equitable distribution of work	Leadership may be difficult to obtain
Professionalism promoted	Unprofessional behavior
Nurses control practice	Interference with management

arise. Nurse leaders and managers can facilitate interest based bargaining and such strategies as participative management and governing councils that stimulate more satisfying relationships than collective bargaining.

ADVANTAGES AND DISADVANTAGES OF COLLECTIVE BARGAINING

There are advantages and disadvantages to collective bargaining. Some equalization of power between administrators and staff associates can be obtained because of the staff associates' strength in numbers. Professionalism can be promoted. Nurses can gain control of practice. Grievance procedures become viable, and staffing for systematic and equitable distribution of work can be established. Unfair treatment of employees can be reduced. The quality of services can be influenced while economic security can be increased.

Unfortunately, unions cost money; an adversarial relationship may develop between administration and staff associates; and strikes may not be prevented. Unionization is considered unprofessional by many nurses and many nurses do not actively participate by attending unit meetings or attending conventions. Unions can interfere with the management of the organization. Leadership for unions may be difficult to obtain because many professional nurses are not experienced in positions of authority. Many women tend to view employment as a job instead of a career, minimizing interest in leadership positions, and if the bargaining unit and the professional association are the same, top administrators may have to drop membership in the professional organization, further depleting the

leadership (Roussel, Swansburg, & Swansburg, 2006) (Table 5-2).

CHAPTER SUMMARY

There are several sources of personal power, informal power, and power in general. Gender differences have been noted in relation to power. Authority is legitimate position power. Empowerment is the process of gaining control. Coercive and reward power tend to bring about resistance. Legitimate power tends to bring about compliance. Expert power and referent power tend to bring about commitment.

There are stages of political development and levels of political participation. One can communicate with legislators through face-to-face meetings, letters, e-mails, and phone calls. It is helpful for nurses to understand the legislative process and to have negotiation skills to be able to intervene in timely and appropriate ways. Nurse leaders and managers are responsible for knowing and implementing labor law. Unions are a last resort to equalize power between labor and management. Nurse leaders and managers can use assertive communications, problem solving, and participative management to decrease felt needs to unionize.

CASE STUDY In the hospital where you work, patients' length of stay is greatly reduced and the patient census is down. Nurses' time has been cut back. Nurses are increasingly dissatisfied, and there is some talk of unionizing. As a manager, what can you do to reduce the felt need to unionize?

CRITICAL THINKING ACTIVITY

Reflective Journal: Make observations in a clinical setting, or reflect on past experiences. What is your major source of power? What is the major source of power for someone else you know? Have you ever communicated with a legislator? If so, how? How might you get more involved in politics? Have you observed aspects of collective bargaining? What happened?

ONLINE RESOURCES

evolve Additional critical thinking activities, worksheets, and case studies are available online at http://evolve.elsevier.com/Marriner/guide8e.

REFERENCES

ANA House of Delegates conference materials, Washington, DC, June 1999.

Becker D: *Myth of empowerment: Women and the therapeutic culture in America,* New York, 2005, New York University Press.

Byrd ME: Social exchange as a framework for client-nurse interaction during public health nursing maternal-child home visits, *Public Health Nursing* 23(3):271, 2006.

Cherry B, Jacob SR: *Contemporary nursing issues, trends, & management,* ed 2, St. Louis, 2002, Mosby.

Finegan JE, Laschinger HKS: The antecedents and consequences of empowerment, *JONA* 31(10): 489-497, 2001.

Finkelman AW: *Leadership and management in nursing*, Upper Saddle River, NJ, 2006, Pearson/ Prentice Hall.

French J, Raven B: The bases of social power. In Cartwright D, editor: *Studies in social power, (150-167)* Ann Arbor, MI, 1959, University of Michigan. Institute for Social Research.

Grohar-Murray ME, DiCroce HR: *Leadership and management in nursing*, Stamford, CT, 2003, Appleton & Lange.

Hegyvary ST: Foundations of professional power, *Journal of Nursing Scholarship* 24(1):104, 2003.

Huber DL: *Leadership and nursing care management,* ed 3, St. Louis, 2006, Elsevier.

Johnson CW: *How our laws are made,* Washington, DC, 2003, U.S. Government Printing Office.

Leder LM, Henley TB: Perceptions of women's power as a function of position within an organization, *Journal of Psychology* 134(5):515-527, 2000.

Lee L: Buzzwords with a basis. Motivation, mentoring, and empowerment aren't just management jargon—they're resources you use every day, *Nursing Management* 31(10):25-27, 2000.

Lips HM: College students' visions of power and possibility as moderated by gender, *Psychology of Women Quarterly* 24(1):39-44, 2000.

Marquis BL, Huston CJ: *Leadership roles and management functions in nursing,* ed 5, Philadelphia, 2006, Lippincott Williams & Wilkins.

Mason DJ, Leavitt JK, Chaffee MW: *Policy & politics in nursing and health care,* ed 4, St. Louis, 2006, Mosby.

Matthews S, Spencer Laschinger HK, Johnstone L: Staff nurse empowerment in line and staff organizational structures for chief nurse executives, *JONA* 36(11):526-533, 2006.

McConnell CR: *Umiker's management skills for the new health care suprervisor,* ed 4, Boston, 2006, Jones and Bartlett.

McCrory JL, Ivers W of Steward and Irwin, PC in Indianapolis. Personal communication, 2003.

National Labor Relations Act, 1935, 29 U.S.C. §§ 151-169.

Roussel L, Swansburg RC, Swansburg RJ: *Management and leadership for nurse administrators,* ed 4, Boston, 2006, Jones & Bartlett.

St. Francis Hospital #NLRB 948, 1984.

Sullivan EJ, Decker PJ: *Effective leadership and management in nursing,* ed 6, Upper Saddle River, NJ, 2005, Prentice Hall.

Yoder-Wise PS: *Leading and managing in nursing,* ed 4, St. Louis, 2007, Mosby.

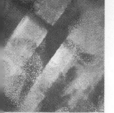

Conflict Management and Negotiation

"Build your adversary a golden bridge to retreat across." —Sun Tzu

Chapter Overview

Chapter 6 presents sources of conflict, types of conflict, reactions to conflict, escalation techniques, stages of conflict, approaches to conflict management, deescalation tactics, mediation, arbitration, and strategies for managing intrapersonal, interpersonal, group, intergroup, and organizational conflict. Nominal group technique, role negotiations, and decision charting and negotiations in general are discussed in detail. Sexual harassment, workplace violence, and how to handle a hostage situation are also addressed.

Chapter Objectives

- Identify at least five sources of conflict.
- Name at least five kinds of conflict.
- Describe at least five reactions to conflict.
- Explain five approaches to conflict resolution.
- Assess appropriate times to use each approach to conflict resolution.
- Identify at least five deescalation techniques.
- Outline nominal group technique.
- Explain role negotiations.
- Describe principled negotiations.
- Compare hard and soft negotiation tactics.
- Describe how to handle sexual harassment.
- Identify what to do in a hostage situation.

Online Resources

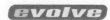

Critical thinking activities, worksheets, and case studies are available online at http://evolve.elsevier.com/Marriner/guide8e.

Major Concepts and Definitions

Conflict *clash, fight, battle, struggle*

Role ambiguity *person does not know what is expected*

Role overload *person is unable to accomplish what is expected within the allotted time frame*

Nominal group technique *a group participation method for making decisions*

Role negotiations *the process of preventing role conflicts, role ambiguities, and role overload*

Negotiation *bargaining process*

Sexual harassment *intimidation or tormenting of a sexual nature*

Hostage situation *the situation of holding a person or persons in a restricted state against their will*

CONFLICT THEORY

Conflict, which is closely related to power and political issues, is inevitable and can be constructive or destructive. It may offer an individual personal gain, provide prestige to the winner, be an incentive for creativity, increase interest, serve as a powerful motivator, improve quality of decisions, and foster change. It can also have destructive outcomes by diminishing communication and cohesiveness and by fighting and hindering performance. Indeed, there seems to be an optimal level of conflict or anxiety necessary for effective functioning. Too little conflict lacks stimulation and motivation, while too much is immobilizing. Some conflict and anxiety stimulates interest and creativity, can improve decision quality, and can facilitate change. Conflict that is managed instead of avoided, ignored, or suppressed can be used effectively. If conflict goes beyond the invigorating stage, it becomes debilitating. That can hinder performance, constrict communications, decrease cohesiveness, and increase fighting. Conflict is a warning to management that something is amiss, and it should stimulate a search for new solutions through problem solving, clarification of objectives, establishment of group norms, and determination of group boundaries. However, eliminating conflict is not always necessary. If leaders and managers learn the sources and types of conflict and how to manage them,

they can minimize stress on individuals and the organization and maximize effectiveness (Huber, 2006) (Box 6-1).

Sources of Conflict

Cultural differences may contribute to differing attitudes, values, beliefs, and behaviors. Conflict can arise because the individuals involved do not have the same facts. They define the problem differently, have different pieces of information, place more or less importance on various aspects, or have divergent views of their own power and authority. Varying goals and objectives or contrasting procedural strategies for accomplishing mutually acceptable goals produce conflict. Variations in personal value systems or in perceptions of ethical responsibilities can lead to divergence in choices of both goals and methods, thus producing conflict.

When people work together in a complex organization, there are numerous sources of conflict. Conflict increases with both the number of organizational levels and the number of disciplines and specialties. It is greater as the degree of association increases and when some parties depend on others. Ambiguous jurisdictions, competition for scarce resources, and the need for consensus all contribute to conflict. Communication barriers impede understanding, and separations in time (working different days or shifts) and space (working on different floors or in different buildings) foster factionalism rather than mutual cooperation. Although standardized policies, rules, and procedures regulate behavior, make relationships more predictable, and decrease the number of arbitrary decisions, they impose added controls over the individual. Men and women who value autonomy are likely to resist such control. Clearly, the sources of conflict seem endless, and the number of conflicts increases with the number of unresolved differences (Finkelman, 2006; Huber, 2006; McConnell, 2006; Roussel, Swansburg, & Swansburg, 2006; Sullivan & Decker, 2005).

BOX 6-1 Model for Managing Conflict

Determine the basis of the conflict:
  Intrapersonal
  Interpersonal
  Group
  Intergroup
  Organizational
Analyze the sources of the conflict:
  Cultural differences
  Different facts
  Separate pieces of information
  Different perceptions of the event
  Defining the problem differently
  Divergent views of power and authority
  Role conflicts
  Number of organizational levels
  Degree of association
  Parties dependent on others
  Competition for scarce resources
  Ambiguous jurisdictions
  Need for consensus
  Communication barriers
  Separation in time and space
  Accumulation of unresolved conflict
Consider alternative approaches to conflict management:
  Avoiding
  Accommodating
  Compromising
  Collaborating
  Competing
Choose the most appropriate approach.
Implement the conflict management strategy.
Evaluate the results.

Types of Conflict

Structurally based conflict can be thought of as either vertical or horizontal, based on a hierarchical model. Differences between managers and staff members (vertical conflict) are often related to inadequate communication, opposing interests, and lack of shared perceptions and attitudes. In vertical situations, managers often attempt to control staff associates' behavior, and the staff associates resist, often leading managers to apply position power through impersonal bureaucratic rules. Manager and staff conflict may be intradepartmental strife. Line-staff conflict, which is usually horizontal, is commonly a struggle among domains related to activities, expertise, and authority and may be related to interdepartmental strife.

Interdepartmental differences are related to the degree of interdependence among departments. Interdependence demands collaboration, and the latter provides the occasion for conflict. The need for consensus, work sequence, and use of shared facilities or services are potential areas of conflict aggravated by differing departmental goals. Both the personalities and status of individuals involved affect trust and cooperation, which are as important as the communication and interaction structures.

There are several types of role conflict (Box 6-2). Intrasender conflict originates in the sender who gives conflicting instructions or expects conflicting or mutually exclusive behavioral responses. For example, the same supervisor may demand a higher quality of nursing care, refuse to allow the head nurse to fire incompetent

---

BOX 6-2 Types of Conflict

Intrasender
Intersender
Interrole
Person-role
Interperson
Intragroup
Intergroup
Role ambiguity
Role overload

help, and, in an effort to cut costs, refuse to increase an inadequate staff or to permit overtime.

Intersender conflict arises when an individual receives conflicting messages from two or more sources. For example, leaders or managers may implement an incentive plan to stimulate production, yet peer pressure may discourage "rate busting," which is doing more than the accepted norm. In university settings, the dean may expect department chairpersons to function as administrators, yet the faculty may expect them to act as their faculty advocates. The matrix organization that imposes project management on a functional structure creates intersender role conflict. The project managers may want the worker to do something that conflicts with what the functional manager wants. Anytime one is responsible to more than one person, one can anticipate intersender role conflict.

Interrole conflict can occur when an individual belongs to more than one group. Simultaneous, multiple roles within the same organization or the conflicting expectations that result from being a member of more than one organization are sources of such conflict. For example, a person may be expected to attend two different committee meetings at the same time. Job expectations can easily interfere with one's family life. The individual has to develop a system of trade-offs to determine how to behave at certain times.

Person-role conflict is the result of disparity between internal and external roles. An individual has perceived roles and expectations based on one's values and perceptions of oneself. When one's values, needs, or capabilities are incompatible with the role requirement, person-role conflict is created. Behavioral expectations that exceed one's current level of knowledge and skill set are also stressful. If the nurse believes that people are important but must process patients through a large clinic in a relatively impersonal manner, the nurse may experience person-role conflict.

Interperson conflict is common among people whose positions require interaction with other persons who fill various roles in the same organization or other organizations. Interperson conflict is usually not personal but rather the result of each person's acting as a protagonist for that person's department. For example, the nurse executive competes with other departmental heads for resources. Occasionally the conflict arising from the nature of the roles involved is complicated by personal animosity.

Intragroup conflict occurs when the group faces a new problem, when new values are imposed on the group from outside, or when one's extragroup role conflicts with one's intragroup role. In an academic setting, pressures to have baccalaureate nursing students prepared by

 RESEARCH Perspective 6-1

Data from Grzywacz JG, Frone MR, Brewer CS, Kover CT: Quantifying work-family conflict among registered nurses, *Research in Nursing & Health* 29(5): 414-426, 2006.

Purpose: The purpose of this study was to identify the frequency with which nurses experience work-family conflict and which nurses experience it most frequently.

Methods: Researchers documented the prevalence and frequency of work-family conflict and described the demographic predictors of frequent work-family conflict.

Results/conclusions: Nurses reported greater work interference with family than family interference with work. Fifty percent of nurses reported chronic work interference with family occurring at least once a week. Forty-one percent reported episodic work interference with family occurring less than three days per month. Fifty-two percent of nurses surveyed reported episodic family interference with work, and eleven percent reported chronic family interference with work. Demographic variables did not predict work interference with family or family interference with work.

faculty with master's degrees and graduate students prepared by faculty with doctoral degrees produces intragroup conflict. Faculty members are caught in a conflict over their teaching responsibilities, continuation of their own education, and fulfillment of expectations for service and scholarly work. A group facing a new problem may require a change in role relationships that requires role negotiations. When intragroup conflict becomes intense, two new groups may form and give rise to intergroup conflict.

Intergroup conflict is common where two groups have different goals and can achieve their goals only at the other's expense. The conflict may be between groups on the same level or between groups on different levels within an organization. This could potentially include management and staff, physicians and nurses, staff and patients, or staff and community members. Competition between groups also produces conflict. For example, two or more groups may compete to win a contest or to receive some specific resource that only one group can have. Resolution may be reached by the dominance of one group over the other, by a compromise that rarely satisfies either group, or by an integration of goals attained when each group recognizes the role of the other group in the system. Intergroup conflict need not be dysfunctional. It can stimulate creativity, innovation, and progress. A conflict-free organization suggests stasis, a situation that offers little challenge for group members. The organization may seem free of conflict only because people are not identifying problems or are ignoring them rather than dealing with them. That diminishes opportunity for improvement.

Role ambiguity, a condition in which individuals do not know what is expected of them, frequently occurs in organizations. Inadequate job descriptions, incomplete explanations of assigned tasks, rapid technological change, and the increasing complexity of organizations contribute to role ambiguity and produce uncertainty and frustration.

If individuals cannot meet the expectations placed on them, they will experience role overload. This does not involve a questioning of the legitimacy of the request or of what is expected.

Rather, the person is simply unable to accomplish so much within a limited time period. As a result, quality is sacrificed for quantity, the ego is threatened, and frustration develops (Roussel, Swansburg, & Swansburg, 2006).

Reactions to Conflict

"Better bend than break." —Scottish saying

Numerous psychological mechanisms exist for coping with one's own behavioral reactions to conflict, but such stress can contribute to somatic reactions like cardiovascular diseases and gastric disorders (Box 6-3).

Sublimation is one of the most constructive psychological mechanisms whereby unacceptable feelings are repressed and channeled into socially acceptable activities. Energy from hostility and anger that would be destructive if expressed directly is diverted with positive results into other activities, such as jogging, tennis, community service, aiding the sick, or caring for children. Vigorous physical activity often reduces interpersonal aggression.

People who are displeased with the results of their behavior may increase their efforts. Working

---

BOX 6-3 Reactions to Conflict

Sublimation
Vigorous physical exercise
Increased efforts
Identification
Reinterpreting goals
Substituting goals
Rationalization
Attention getting
Reaction formation
Flight into fantasy
Projection
Displacement
Fixation
Withdrawal
Repression
Regression
Conversion

longer and harder is likely to increase productivity. Flight into activity, a defense mechanism whereby a person keeps busy to avoid thinking about problems, provides some temporary relief but does not solve the problems.

Identification is the practice of enhancing one's self-esteem by imitating another's behavior. The values and beliefs of the other person are internalized, and both achievements and suffering are experienced vicariously. This illustrates the adage, "If you can't beat them, join them." An individual may compensate for a real or imagined inadequacy in one area by substituting a high degree of proficiency in another area. For example, one who lacks social skills may excel academically.

Goals may be reinterpreted to attain an unmet goal, or the goal may be lowered or another goal substituted. A person promoted to vice president with little hope of becoming president may decide that the vice presidency is a satisfactory position. A rejected job applicant may find another job the applicant enjoys more.

Rationalization provides acceptable explanations for undesirable beliefs or behaviors. Managers may find reasons to fire someone they do not like or pad the expense account because "everyone does it."

Attention getting may involve seeking highly visible jobs, engaging in loud or excessive talking, wearing bright or sexy clothing and unusual hair styles, or driving flashy cars. These displays are destructive only if they divert attention from problem solving.

When individuals repress unacceptable behaviors and values and substitute the opposite attitudes and behaviors, they are using a coping mechanism called reaction formation. For example, an employee who was denied a merit pay increase may defend the manager and vigorously support the related policies.

Another mechanism people use to cope with stress is flight into fantasy. Flight into fantasy allows one to think about something else. For example, the nurse's aide may daydream about being the charge nurse. Although daydreaming, watching television, and going to the movies are constructive forms of relaxation, engaging in excessive fantasy interferes with one's productivity.

People may protect themselves from their undesirable feelings and traits by attributing them to others. This defense mechanism is called projection. For example, a student who is unable to answer a test question may claim that the question is unclear. An unsuccessful person who wants to block another's success claims that the colleague is hostile and uncooperative. Projection is a destructive way to meet needs.

Displacement redirects emotions toward ideas, people, or objects other than the source of the emotions. For example, after the director corrects the nurse manager, the nurse manager may displace aggression by snapping at the staff. Some individuals reacting to conflict may resort to negativism, picking apart every idea and action and putting everything in the worst light.

Fixation is the maintenance of a certain maladaptive behavior even though it is obvious that it is not effective in this situation. One who depends on this escape mechanism will make the same mistake repeatedly.

Withdrawal or escape removes one from the area of frustration. For example, a staff nurse who is frustrated by hospital working conditions may go into teaching. This mechanism can be constructive if the person withdraws from a dangerous situation.

Repression or denial pushes painful information and memories into the subconscious, but the material is not truly forgotten. Sometimes people who have been sexually abused do not remember this until later in life when they begin to develop strange symptoms.

With regression, an individual may revert to earlier, even childish behavior. When regressing, staff members may transfer their attitudes toward their parents to their manager and expect the manager to act like a parent. Some people may even have temper tantrums. Regression moves one away from the present and is rarely constructive.

An individual may unconsciously convert an emotional conflict into physical symptoms (somatization), such as the common tension headache. Paralysis of an arm to avoid writing a report or losing one's voice to avoid discussing an unpleasant topic is an extreme form of the coping mechanism called conversion.

Everyone uses psychological mechanisms. They are our unconscious defenses against impaired self-esteem, anxiety, guilt, and other threatening or uncomfortable feelings. Defense mechanisms serve a purpose. They become harmful only when excessive.

In addition to defense mechanisms, people may frame or define problems by confusing interests with positions, confusing material interests with fundamental human needs, de-humanizing opponents, and by being very competitive. People may fail to identify some of the other parties, all the issues, the opponent's options, or the conflict history; do inadequate information collecting; and may have differing definitions of justice. In addition, there could be language differences, misinterpreted motives and communication, poor listening, secrecy, deception, and inflammatory statements. Among other problems, there could be conflicts of interest, inability to deal with uncertainty or complexity, or analysis paralysis.

Escalation-of-Conflict Tactics

Competition can escalate conflict. One tries to outdo the other and often vice versa. When one feels one is righteous, one may stop listening, thus losing an opportunity to learn. Labeling, such as calling someone lazy, escalates the conflict. Identifying the behavior and the negative outcomes can assist with problem solving; for example, "You are often late. That means you do not get the change-of-shift report in a timely way, and patients do not get the care they deserve at the beginning of the shift. People have to tell you what you missed, and we all seem to get off to a bad start." Dealing with personalities escalates conflict and is not appropriate. One should separate the person from the problem. Issue expansion includes issues from other times and rehashing "old baggage." "I am mad about this today. Last week you... Last month you did something else..., and two years ago..." One should stay focused on the current issue.

Bickering often makes conflict worse unless one identifies the problem causing the discomfort and takes a problem-solving approach. Coalition formation gets other people involved and is a power strategy. Constricting others and making threats escalates conflict. Avoidance and the chilling effect by not speaking to someone is not helpful and can lead to decreased commitment and the end of a relationship. One of the most difficult situations to handle is intentional hurt. That may lead to revenge (McConnell, 2006) (Box 6-4).

Stages of Conflict

Conflict usually goes through stages, which may start as latent conflict that then emerges, escalates, then hopefully deescalates and gets resolved permanently, but sometimes only temporarily until it emerges and escalates again. Conflict may be divided into four progressive stages (Box 6-5): latent, perceived, felt, and manifest. Latent conflict is a phase of anticipation in which antecedent conditions, such as different values and beliefs, incompatible goals, role conflicts, structural conflicts, and/or scarcity of resources can predict conflict behavior. When change is required, the manager anticipates differences of opinion about the desirability of the change, how it should be implemented, and how the consequences should be handled.

Perceived conflict, which may or may not be discussed, indicates a cognitive awareness of a stressful situation. One's personal perceptions

---

BOX 6-4 Escalation-of-Conflict Tactics

Competition
Righteousness
Stop listening
Labeling
Dealing with personalities
Issue expansion
Bickering
Coalition formation
Threats
Constricting others
Avoidance
Intentional hurt

BOX 6-5 Stages of Conflict

Latent: Antecedent conditions predict conflict behavior.
Perceived: Cognitive awareness of stressful situation exists.
Felt: Feelings and attitudes are present and affect the conflict.
Manifest: Overt behavior results from three earlier stages.
Resolution: Tension is decreased, negotiation is done, and problem solving is done to find beneficial and mutually agreeable solutions.
Aftermath: Negotiation, peacebuilding, and reconciliation may prevent the reoccurrence of the conflict, or the conflict could reoccur and escalate again.

---

and selective perceptions can contribute to either an accurate or inaccurate assessment of the situation and affect the amount of threat and potential loss the individual anticipates. Conflicts can be perceived when antecedent conditions do not exist, such as when individuals have a limited knowledge of the facts or do not know others' opinions and values. For instance, a manager may think there are limited resources or that someone else wants to use the same materials when, in fact, there is plenty for everyone or no one else is interested anyway. Personal perceptions also can help to avoid conflict. A suppression mechanism may be used to ignore conflict that involves low potential loss or is only minimally threatening. Someone may ignore an insult or even twist it and thank someone for the compliment. An attention-focus mechanism helps the individual select which conditions to change and which to ignore.

Affective states such as stress, tension, anxiety, fear, mistrust, anger, and hostility are present during the felt conflict. Feelings and attitudes may create or avoid conflict. Trust, for example, is a significant factor in the development of a manifest conflict. If the individuals involved possess trusting attitudes, they share information and control and recognize their mutual vulnerability. In the absence of trust, individuals may withhold

information so it cannot be used against them or distort communications to their advantage. They may scheme to increase their control over others and strive to decrease others' control over them. Clearly, trusting attitudes may prevent potential conflict, and the lack of them may actually create conflict. Two self-serving individuals are more likely to have manifest conflict than a dominant and submissive pair.

The personalization or depersonalization of the situation affects the evolution of conflict. When the situation is personalized, the individual is threatened or judged negatively. With a depersonalized approach, the behavior rather than the individual is identified as creating the problem. "You are wrong" is personalized, whereas "your views are very different from mine" is depersonalized. Personalized comments increase anxiety; a depersonalized approach is conducive to problem solving.

Manifest conflict is overt behavior resulting from the latent, perceived, and felt conflict. It is the escalation of conflict when the tensions become active conflict. It can be either constructive or destructive to problem solving. Escalating conflicts can become a spiral when each side provokes the other and seeks revenge. Unfortunately, aggression, competition, and other defenses are learned almost unconsciously through examples, whereas problem solving requires a more deliberate, conscious effort.

Resolution can occur when tension is decreased, and negotiation and problem solving are done to find beneficial and mutually agreeable solutions. The aftermath can be negotiation, peacebuilding, or reconciliation that prevents the reoccurance of the conflict, or the conflict could reoccur and escalate again (Finkelman, 2006; Huber, 2006; Sullivan & Decker, 2005).

CONFLICT MANAGEMENT

"The gem cannot be polished without friction, nor man perfected without trials." —Confucius

Approaches to Managing Conflict

Some common approaches to handling conflict are avoiding, accommodating, compromising, collaborating, and competing (Box 6-6). Avoiding is never acknowledging the conflict and consequently not addressing the problem to solve it. It is reflected in the comment, "Leave well enough alone." Avoiding creates "lose-lose" situations through unassertive and uncooperative means. It may be appropriate to not address the conflict when the other party is more powerful, the issue is unimportant, one has no chance of meeting the goals, or the cost of dealing with the conflict is higher than the benefit of the resolution. It may also be used when it is more appropriate for others to solve a problem, when more information is needed, or when one wishes to reduce tension and gain composure. Withdrawing from a conflict does not resolve it, and the individual who retreats may harbor a gnawing anger over a situation that drains energy needed for more constructive purposes.

Accommodating is cooperative but unassertive. It is self-sacrificing—the opposite of competing. One neglects one's own needs to meet the goals of the other party. It is appropriate when the opponent is right or more powerful, or the issue is more important to someone else. It can be used when preserving harmony is important or when collecting social credits is necessary for later, more important issues. By complimenting one's opponent and accentuating points of agreement, one may smooth out an agreement on minor issues, but the real problems still have to be dealt with. One might try to "kill the enemy with kindness."

Compromising moderates both assertiveness and cooperation. It addresses a problem more effectively than avoidance but less effectively than collaboration. Compromisers are willing to yield less than accommodators but more than competitors as they seek expedient, mutually acceptable answers. Because both parties feel that they are sacrificing something, they are only partially satisfied, and a "lose-lose" atmosphere results. Compromising is useful for reaching expedient answers for limited periods when the goals are only moderately important and the parties have equivalent power. It is a "splitting the difference" strategy.

Collaborating is assertive and cooperative. It is a "win-win" strategy and contributes to effective problem solving because both parties try to find mutually satisfying solutions. This method integrates insights from different perspectives with the commitment developed through participation and the resolution of hard feelings. Problems are identified, alternatives explored, and ramifications considered until difficulties are resolved. Unfortunately, it may take more time than the results are worth. Generally this is a most effective method of conflict resolution. It should be used for important issues and can be used to find creative solutions to interpersonal problems because "two heads are better than one."

Competing is a power-oriented mode that is assertive but uncooperative. In competition one is aggressive and pursues one's own goals at another's expense. This creates a "win-lose" situation reflecting "might makes right." Nevertheless, it is appropriate when a quick or unpopular decision is needed, when the person is very knowledgeable about the situation and able to make a sound decision, or when one must protect oneself from other aggressive people. If this strategy is used too often, colleagues may become afraid to admit mistakes and may simply say what they think the aggressor wants to hear. A manager can always fall back on authority and give orders to staff, but because resolution is forced, it almost certainly will be unsatisfactory (Finkelman, 2006; Huber, 2006; Marquis & Huston, 2006; Roussel, Swansburg, & Swansburg, 2006; Thomas & Kilmann, 1974, 2002).

BOX 6-6 Approaches to Conflict Resolution

Avoiding: unassertive and uncooperative
Accommodating: cooperative but unassertive
Compromising: assertive and cooperative
Collaborating: assertive and cooperative
Competing: assertive but uncooperative

A foundation of mutual trust must underlie any attempt to understand alternative views and to actively seek solutions that will allow each party to achieve its goals. This trust creates an atmosphere conducive to successful conflict resolution.

Deescalation-of-Conflict Tactics

Listening is a good way to deescalate conflict. It shows that one cares about the person by taking one's time to listen to them. The other person may be able to talk through the problem and solve it, particularly if one asks questions that lead one through problem solving, such as the following: What is the problem? What are your options? What will happen if you do that? What do you think is the best way to handle this situation? What are you going to do? Showing tact and concern for others is important. Acknowledging the other person's point of view in soft voice tones is comforting. Appealing to deescalation by saying something such as "I don't want to fight about this" can help. Goodwill gestures such as "Let's get a cup of coffee and discuss this" and allowing the airing of feelings are good. Our feelings often dissipate after we talk about how we are feeling. We usually feel better after talking about our feelings, but talking can also increase anger and stress. Negative inquiry is an assertive technique of asking for more information and trying to resolve the problem. When one is criticized, one tends to get defensive, which escalates the conflict. Then the other person has to work harder to get a person to understand where that person went wrong. When one asks for more information, the criticizer may end up defending the accused.

Using metacommunications, one discusses the communication as it is occurring. "I am trying to talk to you, and you are walking away from me." It is important to respond to all levels of communications, the facts and the feelings. "I know that it is my weekend to work, but I am angry that I have to work." Expressing the feelings helps dissipate the anger. Focusing on the facts helps with reality testing and problem solving. Fractionalization breaks the problem down into more manageable components. Position papers help move people

from opposite poles to a more middle-of-the-road stance. People will often follow flat statements with qualifiers. Problem solving is a very effective deescalator. When all else fails, establishment of outside criteria may be used (Box 6-7).

Strategies for Management of Conflict

Based on one model, there are three ways of dealing with conflict: the "win-lose", "lose-lose", or "win-win" strategy (Box 6-8). "Win-lose" methods include the use of force, competition, position power, mental or physical power, failure to respond, majority rule, and railroading a minority position over the majority. "Lose-lose" strategies include bribes for accomplishing disagreeable tasks, arbitration by a neutral third party, and resorting to the use of general rules instead of considering the merits of individual cases. Both parties often feel they've lost in a compromise. In "win-lose" and "lose-lose" strategies, the parties often personalize the issues by focusing on each other instead of on the problem. Intent on their personal differences, they avoid the more important matter of how to mutually solve their problem. Solutions are emphasized instead of goals and values. Rather than identifying mutual needs, planning activities for resolution, and solving the problem, the parties involved look at the issue from their own point of view and strive for total victory.

By contrast, "win-win" strategies focus on goals. They emphasize consensus and integrative approaches to decision making. The consensus

---

BOX 6-7 Deescalation-of-Conflict Tactics

Listening
Showing tact and concern for others
Appealing to deescalation
Goodwill gestures
Airing feelings
Negative inquiry
Metacommunications
Responding to all levels of communication
Fractionalization
Position paper
Problem solving
Establishing outside criteria

BOX 6-8 Strategies for Conflict Resolution

WIN-LOSE

Competing
Position power
Mental or physical power
Failure to respond
Majority rule
Railroading

LOSE-LOSE

Compromise
Bribes
Arbitration
General rules

WIN-WIN

Consensus
Problem-solving
Collaborating

process demands a focus on the problem (instead of on each other), on the collection of facts, on the acceptance of the useful aspects of conflict, and on the avoidance of averaging and self-oriented behavior. The goal is collaboration that is agreeable to all parties. Thus the group decision is often better than the best individual decision (Huber, 2006; Sullivan & Decker, 2005).

Problem-solving strategies include identifying both the problem and each party's needs, exploring alternatives, choosing the most acceptable alternative, planning, defining roles, implementing, and evaluating the decision.

Mediation

Mediation is a friendly intervention by consent and invitation for settling differences between parties. It is not binding. It is negotiation that involves a third party who is knowledgeable about negotiation procedures and can help the parties do their bargaining. A mediator plays several roles. The mediator serves as a housekeeper who reviews the ground rules and keeps the records; serves as a ringmaster who chairs the meeting and determines when to recess, when to adjourn, and when to have separate meetings; and helps the parties define the problems,

identify the issues, and prioritize multiple issues. The mediator is an educator who facilitates the bargaining process and helps each party consider how to achieve his or her objectives while accommodating the opponent to create a "win-win" solution. The mediator is a communicator and an innovator. Innovation can come about by making suggestions, but the suggestions should be explored in separate meetings because the mediator should never raise questions in the presence of both sides that could be embarrassing for either side. If one party opposes the suggestion, it can be dropped. The mediator is a problem explorer who helps analyze issues from a variety of viewpoints; a resource expander who links parties to outside resources; and an agent of reality who helps create a reasonable and implementable settlement. The mediator helps both parties focus on the issue instead of each other, emphasize shared interests, explore options, stress peaceful resolution, and come to consensus. The mediator is a leader who takes initiative to advance negotiations forward procedurally and may at times offer suggestions for consideration. The mediator may also serve as a scapegoat and take some responsibility and blame for an unpopular decision (Finkelman, 2006; Kheel, 2001; Roussel, Swansburg, & Swansburg, 2006; Sullivan & Decker, 2005) (Box 6-9).

The mediator starts by (1) creating a positive climate and introducing the mediator and parties; (2) commending the parties for their willingness to cooperate in seeking a solution to their problems; (3) defining mediation and the mediator's impartial role; (4) describing the mediation process; (5) defining the parameters of confidentiality; (6) describing the logistics; (7) suggesting behavioral guidelines; (8) answering questions about process; and (9) getting a joint commitment to begin (Mayer, 2000) (Box 6-10).

After bringing the disputants together and creating the effective atmosphere, the mediator clarifies perceptions by helping parties feel heard, hearing each other, and focusing on individual and shared needs. The biggest and most dangerous disputant is to be seated in the deepest and softest chair available. The mediator tries to keep

BOX 6-9 Conflict Interventions

MEDIATOR
Friendly intervener by consent
Housekeeper
Ringmaster
Educator
Communicator
Innovator

PROBLEM EXPLORER
Helps define the problem
Identifies problems
Prioritizes issues
Facilitates bargaining process
Helps create win-win situation
Makes suggestions

ARBITRATOR
Renders binding decision

BOX 6-10 Mediator Actions

Creates positive climate
Defines mediator's role
Describes mediation process
Defines parameters of confidentiality
Describes logistics
Suggests behavioral guidelines
Answers questions
Gets joint commitment

the disputants' eyes on the mediator and the disputants talking to the mediator instead of each other. If the disputants get out of control, the mediator can stand up between them, hold hands out to separate them, and restate the ground rules of listening to one person at a time. The mediator can hold a hand out at the disputant who is not to be talking while looking at the other party. The mediator starts with a low level of force but can escalate to match the disputants' level. Each disputant is to tell only his or her own views of the situation one problem at a time. The mediator frames and reframes issues, concerns, and suggestions to develop shared positive power and an atmosphere of safety. The mediator helps parties learn from the past and focus on the future to generate options and realistic doable actions.

The mediator helps manage communications and emotions and works across cultural, gender, class, and other differences to come to a mutual-benefit agreement. Parties decide who does what by when and set a time for follow-up. To wrap up, the mediator completes all paperwork, writes a written memorandum confirming the understanding, arranges for any necessary follow-up, holds people accountable for their promises, and keeps essential information only (Mayer, 2000; Patterson, Grenny, McMillan, et al, 2002).

In order to come to resolution, the parties should be encouraged to share facts because facts are less controversial and more persuasive. Then they should each tell their stories, talking tentatively and encouraging testing. Parties should disentangle impact and intent; describe feelings carefully instead of venting; share their story rather than evaluating it; describe feelings without judging, attributing, or blaming; and acknowledge the other person's feelings. Exaggerations such as "always" and "never" should be avoided. Open-ended questions should be asked. Listening transforms conversations and encourages others to listen in return. Parties should share where their conclusions come from and not present them as the truth. The mediator asks parties what they think and feel, helps them solve their own problems while teaching the problem-solving process, and then reviews and sums up (Patterson, Grenny, McMillan, et al, 2002; Stone, Patton, Heen, & Fisher 2000).

Arbitration

Arbitration is a structured method of dispute resolution outside the court system that is usually but not always binding. The arbitrator is an impartial third party that does not usually interact with the parties but renders a decision based on a formal presentation of information. The arbitrator uses the law, provisions of contracts, and past practices to examine the facts and make a decision. Union rights include areas of working conditions, wages, and benefits. Management rights include direction of the work force and methods of operation not covered in agreements. Long-standing practices that have been accepted by both parties are as binding as written agreements. Unchallenged customs and practices are considered to be accepted by both parties (Goodman, 2004; Huber, 2006; Roussel, Swansburg, & Swansburg, 2006).

NEGOTIATION

Two ways of negotiating have been identified: 'hard" and "soft." The hard negotiator wants to win and believes that the side that takes an extreme position and holds out longer benefits more. Unfortunately, hard negotiators often exhaust themselves and their resources and harm relationships. On the other hand, the soft negotiator prevents conflict and makes concessions quickly to reach an agreement. The soft negotiator ultimately feels exploited and bitter. The hard bargainer always wins over the soft bargainer (Box 6-11).

Hard negotiation and soft negotiation are similar to distributive and integrative bargaining. Distributive bargaining is comparable to hard bargaining, which tries to divide something up and to get the biggest piece of the pie. It may use dirty tricks, deception, making threats, giving ultimatums, and overpowering and outsmarting the other party. In contrast, interest-based bargaining or integrative bargaining tries to make more of something and shares a larger pie. It is cooperative and starts by focusing on interests instead of positions. Then it uses problem-solving techniques like brainstorming and consensus decision making (Barrett & Dowd, 2005).

Positional bargaining is typical; each side takes a position and argues for it. Negotiations then involve taking and giving up positions successively. The more one defends a position, the more committed one becomes to it and the more difficult it becomes to revise the position. Egos become involved, and "saving face" is an issue. Besides producing unwise agreements, positional bargaining is inefficient. The more extreme the opening position and the smaller the concessions, the longer it takes to reach an agreement. Positional bargaining also damages ongoing relationships.

Principled negotiation, or interest-based/integrative bargaining is a "win-win" option for negotiation that is neither hard nor soft. This method decides issues on their merits, looks for mutual gains, and insists on fair standards. It is hard on merits and soft on people. There are four basic points to principled negotiations: (1) separate the people from the problem, (2) focus on interests instead of positions, (3) generate a variety of options before deciding what to do, and (4) insist that the result be based on an objective (Fisher, Ury, & Patton, 2004; Barrett & Dowd, 2005; Finkelman, 2006; Huber, 2006) (Box 6-11).

During the analysis phase one tries to gather and organize data and to diagnose the situation. One notes the people problems, hostile emotions, unclear communications, interests, and options and standards already identified. During the planning phase each of the four principles is again considered and additional options and criteria are generated. During discussions, differences in perceptions, feelings such as frustration and anger, and difficulties in communication can be identified and addressed. There can be mutual exploration of how to meet each party's concerns by using objective standards. Negotiations that focus on interests, mutually satisfying options, and fair standards are likely to reach sound agreements.

When separating the people from the problem, understanding others' thinking is critical because that thinking is the problem. Activities include discussing each other's perceptions, trying to put yourself in others' shoes, avoiding blaming them for your problem, getting them involved and committed through participation, and making your proposal consistent with their

---

BOX 6-11 Principled Negotiation

- Separate the people from the problem.
- Focus on interests instead of positions.
- Generate a variety of options before deciding what to do.
- Insist that the result be based on an objective standard.

values. It is also important to understand both your and their emotions; make the emotions explicit and acknowledge them as legitimate; let them vent; do not react to their emotional outbursts; and use symbolic gestures of friendship, such as shaking hands, embracing, eating together, apologizing, and sending a note of congratulations or sympathy.

Communications are critical to negotiations. Listen actively, and acknowledge what is being said. Speak calmly to be understood. Speak about yourself instead of about them. Speak with a purpose. Build working relationships, and face the problem, not the people.

Focus on interests instead of positions, because the conflicts among needs, desires, concerns, and fears are the problem. Look for shared and compatible interests, as well as conflicting ones. Realize that each side has multiple interests and that the most powerful interests are the basic human needs for security, belonging, recognition, and control.

Next, invent options for mutual gain. Separate inventing options from judging them. During brainstorming, generate as many ideas as possible without judging them. After brainstorming, note the most promising ideas and invent improvements on them. Later, evaluate the ideas and the ramifications of implementing them. Then decide on the best options. Each side may want different things from the same item, so look for ways to dovetail differing interests. Try to make the desired option so appealing that the decision is easy.

Finally, insist on objective criteria for reaching wise agreements amicably and efficiently. Look for fair standards and fair procedures, such as parliamentary procedure (Fisher, Ury, & Patton, 2004).

Some players will not play fairly. Some assert their position, attack ideas, and even attack others. First, do not attack the idea; look behind it to see what the person's interest is. Second, do not defend the idea; invite criticism and advice instead. Third, reframe the attack as an attack on the problem. When attacked, do not counterattack. Break the vicious cycle by refusing to attack. Avoid pitting one's strength against theirs

directly. Instead of resisting their force, channel their energy into exploring interests, generating options that are mutually acceptable, and finding independent standards. Some people use dirty tricks such as deliberate deception by misrepresenting the facts, using ambiguous authority, and seeking dubious intentions. They employ psychological warfare by using stressful situations, personal attacks, and threats.

Positional pressure tactics, such as refusal to negotiate, extreme demands, escalating demands, and calculated delay, are also common devices. Other dirty tricks include ridicule to undermine the psychological space of others. To counter ridicule, try to keep a relaxed body posture, pleasant smile, and steady gaze. *Smoke screen* uses ambiguous or inappropriate questioning. Simply state that the question is irrelevant to the issue. *Over the barrel* is when one uses the weaknesses of the other to force concessions. Attempt to hide weak spots and desensitize areas of vulnerability. *Seduction* implies future promises that something good will happen. *Flattery* is a form of seduction that causes a loss of power. However, exchanging pleasant opening statements before negotiating is acceptable. Gender is sometimes used as a weapon. Illness and helplessness bring out an impulse to help. Guilt causes discomfort. A definitive statement such as "I know you are an intelligent person" limits the freedom of another person. Self-definition, such as "I am an abused person," is an excuse for not taking responsibility for one's own behavior. *Paternalism* is an attempt to convince the other party that the action will be for that person's good. Favors, flattery, and gifts are forms of ingratiation. *Aggressive takeover* is when someone assumes authority and rapidly makes a decision. Saying "I need time to think about this" helps stop an aggressive takeover. Pacifists win because they refuse to fight (Marquis & Huston, 2006).

There are three steps in negotiating the rules when the other side uses dirty tricks: (1) recognize the tactic, (2) raise the issue explicitly, and (3) question the tactic's legitimacy and desirability by using principled negotiations. Again, separate the people from the problem. Focus on interests instead of positions. Invent options for mutual gain, and insist on objective criteria (Fisher & Ertel, 1995; Fisher, Ury, & Patton, 2004).

Ury (1991) described a five-step method of breakthrough negotiation. The breakthrough strategy is counterintuitive because it requires one to do the opposite of what one might naturally do in difficult situations. Natural reactions are to strike back, give in, or break off. The five steps listed for breakthrough negotiations are (1) do not react, (2) disarm them, (3) change the game, (4) build them a golden bridge, and (5) make it hard to say no. The first step is to control one's own behavior. One needs to break through one's own defensiveness, fear, suspicion, and hostility so one can listen to the other party and break the vicious cycle of action and reaction. One needs to identify one's own interests and one's "best alternative to a negotiated agreement" (BATNA) without the other's agreement. That can be used to evaluate any potential agreements. If one's BATNA is better than anything that can be negotiated, one may decide not to negotiate. Stay focused on the goal, recognize the tactic being used, and name it. Dirty tricks are often obstructive, similar to stone walls that refuse to budge; offensive, such as attackers using pressure tactics to intimidate; and deceptive, such as manipulating data, assuming more legitimate power than one has, and adding on a last-minute demand after one thought the agreement had been reached. Know your hot buttons, buy time to think, pause and say nothing, rewind the tape and review the discussion, take time-outs to cool off, do not make important decisions on the spot, and do not get mad or get even, get what you want.

In step two, disarm your opponent by listening, paraphrasing, and asking for corrections; acknowledge points made and the opponent's feelings; offer an apology when appropriate; and project confidence. Agree when you can without conceding. Send a subtle message of "I am like you" by imitating your opponent's communicative manner—speed of speech, loudness or softness, and body position. Acknowledge the opponent's authority and competence to build

a working relationship. Express your views without provoking by saying "yes and" instead of "but" and using "I" statements instead of "you" statements; and acknowledge the differences with optimism to create a favorable climate for negotiation.

In step three, change the game by reframing instead of rejecting. Ask why, why not, and what if; and ask for the opponent's advice to facilitate problem solving. Ask open-ended questions such as "What makes that fair?" Reframe tactics. You can go around a stone wall by ignoring it (keep talking like you did not hear the comment or change the subject), reinterpreting it (reinterpret an ultimatum as a target), or testing it (ask questions to look for flexibility, or turn it to your advantage: "I'd like to work this out but I can't in that time frame." Deflect attacks by ignoring the attack (pretend you did not hear the attack and continue discussing the problem); reframe the personal attack as an attack on the problem, such as "How would you deal with the situation?" One can reframe a personal attack in a friendly manner with "Thank you for your concern." It is also possible to reframe past wrongs to future remedies by changing the blame to joint responsibility to deal with the problem: "How can we make sure that never happens again?" "You" and "me" can be reframed to "we."

Reframing is challenging but can be done by asking clarifying questions about the opponent's assertions; for example, "You must have good reasons for concluding that. I'd be interested in knowing why you believe that." When you identify a contradiction you can appear confused and say, "I don't understand. Could you explain how that relates to what you said?" Clarify authority early by asking, "Am I correct in assuming that you have the authority to make this decision?" Be sure to get a specific answer, and find out who else must agree and how long it will take to get a decision. When given a last-minute demand after you thought an agreement had been reached, ask, "Are you suggesting that we reopen the negotiation? If not, I think we should just stick to the agreement we reached." Do a reasonable request test by requesting that the opponent live up to his or her pretense of cooperation or drop the sham. One can also use the sham to one's advantage by stipulating consequences. It is appropriate to name the trick or sham and negotiate about negotiations. The turning point of the breakthrough strategy is when players change from positional bargaining to problem-solving negotiation.

Step four is to make it easy to say yes. Some obstacles to agreement include that it is not the opponent's idea, interests are unmet, there is fear of losing face, and the decision seems overwhelming. It is important that both parties develop an agreement together rather than for one to announce the plan. The opponent can be asked for ideas. You can acknowledge and build on those ideas, ask for constructive criticism, and offer a recommendation. Try to identify your opponent's unmet needs without considering the person irrational. Do not assume a "zero sum fixed pie" (the more one person gets, the less for the other party). Look for low-cost, high-benefit solutions. Ask "if then, what" questions. Help your opponent save face by backing away without backing down. One can indicate how circumstances have changed, ask for a third-party mediator's recommendation, or point to a standard of fairness. Then one can help one's opponent write a victory speech. Go slow to go fast. If one goes at a slow pace to think through issues and come to consensus, superior results may be reached more quickly than if one rushes to a finish that is not a consensus. When the situation seems overwhelming, break the agreement into smaller parts and proceed step by step. Do not rush to the finish, and do not ask for a final agreement until the end.

Step five is to make it hard to say no by bringing the opponents to their senses, not to their knees. Use your power to educate the opponent about the consequences of decisions. You can help opponents educate themselves by asking reality-testing questions such as "What do you think will happen if we reach agreement?" "What do you think I will do?" "What do you think you will do?" Warn, but do not threaten. The more power you use, the more resistance you are likely to get. Legitimate power depersonalizes the use of power and gets less resistance. Rather than counterattacking the opponent's power, try to neutralize the attack without striking back. Keep sharpening your opponent's choice. Let opponents know they have a way out. Let your opponents choose from options and potential consequences. Craft a lasting agreement, keeping implementation in mind. Design the agreement to minimize risks. Build in a dispute resolution procedure, reaffirm the relationship, and aim for mutual satisfaction, not victory (Ury, 1991).

Fisher and Brown (1988) indicate that a balance of reason and emotion, understanding, good communication, reliability, and persuasion rather than coercion helps parties deal with differences. Approval and shared values are not necessary. We need to develop an awareness of others and our emotions. Taking a break and counting to 10 before acting is wise. It is appropriate to accept responsibility for our emotions and apologize for them rather than to blame others. Assertive communications would say, "I am feeling angry" instead of "You made me mad." We cannot solve differences without understanding them, so it is important to explore the opponent's views. What does the adversary want? What is the adversary's perceived choice? Consult to promote two-way communication, to be more reliable, and to establish acceptance instead of coercion before making a decision. Be wholly trustworthy but not wholly trusting.

Peter Block (1991) describes negotiating with allies and adversaries. He presents a grid with agreement increasing up the vertical axis and trust increasing to the right along the horizontal axis (Figure 6-1). Adversaries are represented by low agreement and low trust in the lower left quadrant; opponents are represented by low agreement and high trust in the lower right quadrant. Allies are indicated by high agreement and high trust in the upper right quadrant, and bedfellows are indicated by high agreement and low trust in the upper left quadrant. Fence-sitters are represented by low trust and medium agreement between adversaries and bedfellows on the left side of the grid.

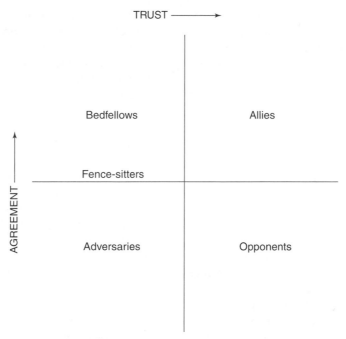

Figure 6-1 • Negotiating with allies and adversaries.

Adversaries, with whom one has low agreement and low trust, use much of one's time and psychic energy. They become adversaries only after one's attempts to negotiate agreement and trust have failed. Steps in dealing with adversaries include the following: (1) state one's vision of the project; (2) state in a neutral way one's best understanding of the adversary's position; (3) identify one's own contribution to the problem, such as having lobbied against the adversary, discounted the adversary's position, gone around the adversary, or talked to a higher authority; and (4) end the meeting with one's plans and no demand.

Opponents are people whom one trusts but who disagree with one's goals and purposes. Opponents can bring out the best in one by challenging and making one clarify one's beliefs and strategies. The steps for dealing with opponents are as follows: (1) reaffirm the quality of one's relationship and mutual trust; (2) state one's position; (3) state in a neutral way what one thinks the opponent's position is; and (4) do problem solving.

One has high agreement and high trust with allies. The allies should be treated as friends; one can discuss doubts and vulnerabilities with them. The basic strategy when dealing with allies is to bring them into the organization and treat them as members. Steps include the following: (1) affirm agreement; (2) reaffirm the quality of the trusting relationship; (3) acknowledge doubts and vulnerabilities related to the project; and (4) ask for advice and support.

One has high agreement and low trust with bedfellows. A person may become manipulative toward people for whom one has little trust. One is careful about how much information to share. The issue is trust, not agreement. To work with bedfellows, (1) reaffirm the agreement; (2) acknowledge caution; (3) be clear about what one wants from the bedfellow, such as keeping one informed; (4) ask what the bedfellow wants and expects; and (5) try to agree about how to work together.

Fence-sitters do not take a stand for or against one; they exhibit doubt, risk, and uncertainty.

To deal with fence-sitters, (1) state your position; (2) ask for the fence-sitter's position; (3) apply gentle pressure to get a decision and express frustration with neutrality; and (4) ask what it would take to get the fence-sitter's support (Block, 1991). Using one's power in organizations and politics through principled negotiations with people with whom one has more or less agreement and trust can advance nursing.

"Speak when you are angry and you will make the best speech you will ever regret." —Ambrose Bierce

Negotiation Process

Negotiations may result around emotional issues such as anxiety, fear of rejection, need for recognition or status, and personal need deprivation as well as substantive issues like policies, rules, and regulations. To do negotiations, parties must recognize that a conflict of interest or incompatibility exists. The relationship should be voluntary, and both parties should desire an agreement that satisfies both parties.

One starts negotiations by creating a dialogue. Exchanging ideas and information helps make the negotiating process a collaborative problem-solving process, allowing parties to communicate openly, seek to understand each other, and identify mutually agreeable solutions. Even though it may be impossible to reach total agreement, dialogue increases the chances of producing productive and viable options. To create the dialogue, one needs to probe, offer ideas, build on ideas, and constructively criticize. Probing is asking questions to get information from the other party, determine the other party's ideas and needs, ensure understanding, and respond to the concerns. By discovering and understanding the needs of the other party, it becomes possible to work toward mutually acceptable solutions instead of becoming locked into a fixed position. Probing helps avoid miscommunications and is useful when one needs to verify or uncover information or to make a decision based on what was said. A probe is a statement or question used to get more information. Open probes encourage people to speak freely. They are often who, what, when, where, why, or how questions, or "explain to me" or "tell me" statements. Closed probes elicit a yes or no response and often include words such as could, would, are, is, or will. Open probes are better for identifying others' needs and ideas and clarifying when one is not sure what the other person means. Closed probes can be used to ensure comprehension by stating your understanding and then using a closed probe to ask for confirmation.

There are two steps involved in offering ideas so that they will more likely be heard. First, indicate one's intent, and then present one's reasons before one's conclusions. The intent may be that one wants to present or support an idea. Indicating intent gives one time to prepare what one wants to say before saying it and prepares the other person for what one is about to say. One might say, "I have a question" or "I would like to make a suggestion." However, do not state an intent if planning to offer a criticism or opposing idea because that would greatly reduce the chances of the other person listening. Because most people stop listening when they hear the bottom line, one should give one's reasons before one's conclusions. That way the other person is more likely to hear one's rationale for one's opinions.

There are two steps involved in building on another person's idea when one wants to increase its usefulness. First, acknowledge the connection, and then add value. One might say, "Your comment made me think about..." Then one can add value by suggesting a modification or different approach to the other person's idea. One retains a significant part of the content or intent of the other person's idea rather than dismissing it.

When one disagrees with the other person's idea or opinion, one may want to constructively criticize. First, state the merits of the idea. Next, state one's concerns. Last, ask for ways to retain the merits and eliminate the concerns. For example, if one was negotiating the redecorating of a wing of a building or a room in one's home and liked the decorator's ideas but thought the cost was too high, one might say, "I love the color scheme and the furnishings. However, the price estimates are about 20% over the budget. Can you think of ways to cut back on the costs?"

It is not uncommon to encounter obstacles, impasses, and even counterproductive tactics. One should break an impasse by stating one's desire to continue and by initiating a change of pace; for example, one can say, "Let's take a 5-minute break and then continue trying to resolve this problem," or "Let's meet again after lunch." Maintain a positive and collaborative tone.

Counterproductive tactics should be confronted. Counterproductive tactics or dirty tricks are underhanded and adversarial to negotiation. They are attempts to strengthen one's position while weakening the other person's position. They undermine the relationship between the parties and the agreement. They are numerous and have been previously discussed. When confronting counterproductive tactics, first confirm the behavior, and then express the impact on you or the negotiation. Make sure one is confirming the person's behavior, not one's judgment of that behavior. Express how the behavior makes one feel. Speak to how it affects the negotiation process. Express the impact in ways that allow the other person to change without losing face.

To plan strategy, analyze the situation. Identify the who, what, when, and where. Determine the facts about the issue, and consider the relationship. Next, organize the information by anticipating the needs and identifying the common ground and options. Then synthesize the approach by examining consequences of options and planning the discussion.

When negotiating, state the purpose and review the situation. Then explore the ideas and needs. Examine ideas from both points of view. Combine ideas. Rework solutions. Reverse perspectives. Uncover dissatisfactions. Restate the desire to satisfy needs. Determine the best alternative. Set terms and conditions. Summarize the agreement, and confirm the next steps (Negotiating self-taught, 1984). Then write a follow-up letter specifying your understanding of the agreement.

Essential Rules of Negotiation

Steinberg and D'Orso (1998, p. 225) identified 12 essential rules of negotiation:

1. Align yourself with people who share your values.
2. Learn all you can about the other party.
3. Convince the other party that you have an option.
4. Set your limits before the negotiation begins.
5. Establish a climate of cooperation, not conflict.
6. In the face of intimidation, show no fear.
7. Learn to listen.
8. Be comfortable.
9. Avoid playing split-the-difference.
10. Emphasize your concessions; minimize the other party's concessions.
11. Never push a losing argument to the end.
12. Develop relationships, not conquests.

Cleary (2001) reminds us that everything is negotiable and negotiations are a process. One needs to be patient and persistent. There is a lot of noise in the process. "No" does not mean "no", and "final" does not mean "final." We should be aware that our actions speak louder than our words, be aware of what is going on away from the table, and take a long view of the negotiations for a continuing relationship. We should probe our counterpart's priorities, ask "what if's," ask "whose interest is this?", clarify interests, and pick up points by making concessions.

"Know when to hold them, known when to fold them, know when to walk away and know when to run." —Don Schlitz (sung by Kenny Rogers)

Intrapersonal Conflict

Intrapersonal conflict occurs within the person and usually involves a struggle over values, desires, or incompatible activities. The conflict is internalized. One should set personal goals and priorities and do problem solving. Becoming self-aware and working to resolve the conflict as soon as possible are important steps for the manager to take to remain physically and psychologically well. The manager should help associates be self-aware and do problem solving too (Marquis & Huston, 2006; Wywialowski, 2004).

Interpersonal Conflict

Interpersonal conflict is inevitable, but the manager can lessen its impact by coaching staff associates in assertive communication and fair fighting. Engaging in a fair fight demands that individuals with a complaint first ask their opponent for a meeting. Once a time and place are agreed on, both parties should determine if their manager should be present. Moreover, a fair fight demands that both parties know the purpose of the meeting so neither will be caught off guard—each can be prepared. The encounter should begin with a statement of the problem. The leader or manager, if present, should act as a mediator and ask the complainer to explain the perceived problem to the opponent. The opponent then should relate his or her understanding of how the complainer perceives the problem. After each has spoken, each can clarify any differences over the statement of the problem. Next, the opponent describes his or her perception of the problem; this description should be followed by the complainer's repeating his or her understanding of how the opponent perceives the problem. Again, there is a pause for clarification.

A clear statement of the problem helps shed light on the negative effects of each person's behavior. This feedback process, which requires each party to repeat what the other has just said, forces each to listen carefully. Were it not for such interaction, one might be so busy thinking of what one is going to say next that one fails to hear what is being said. Feedback does not imply parroting, because an understanding of meaning is more important than sheer memorization of words. Differences often begin to disappear when both parties really hear each other for the first time.

By exploring the alternatives to the problem and the ramifications of their options, the parties can identify and request changes in each other's behavior and respond to the other's requests. The discussion should close with an agreement on whether to change and the establishment of the accompanying conditions. A follow-up engagement should be set to discuss the success or failure of the agreement.

Helpful strategies for mediating interpersonal conflict include the following (Loveridge & Cummings, 1996):
- Do not blame anyone for the problem.
- Focus on the issues, not the personalities.
- Protect each party's self-respect.
- Facilitate open and complete discussion of the issues.
- Give equal time to each party.
- Encourage the expression of both positive and negative feelings.
- Encourage each party to listen actively and try to understand the other person's point of view.
- Help develop alternative solutions.
- Summarize key points and plans.
- Later follow up on the plans and give positive reinforcement as appropriate.
- Facilitate further problem solving as necessary.

Sexual Harassment

Interpersonal conflict can result from sexual harassment. Sexual harassment is an unwelcome verbal, visual, or physical conduct of a sexual nature that creates a hostile environment. The employer is vicariously liable for harassment. The only defense the employer will have is an effective and enforced antiharassment policy in place and a grievance procedure. When there is a complaint, leaders and managers need to investigate and take appropriate actions that could include transferring or reassigning someone. Recirculating the antidiscrimination policy and holding in-service classes about sexual harassment are appropriate actions.

Thousands of sexual harassment complaints are filed each year in the United States. Women seem more likely to be sexually harassed than men, but the victim may be a man or a woman

RESEARCH Perspective 6-2

Data from Fiedler A, Hamby E: Sexual harassment in the workplace, *JONA* 30(10):497-503, 2000.

Purpose: The purpose of this study was to examine the perceptions of nurses and nursing administrators of various types of sexual harassment.

Methods: Surveys were sent to a random sample of 423 nurse administrators and 802 registered nurses licensed in Florida. The researchers received 303 usable responses, including 103 nursing administrators and 200 registered nurses. A total of 24 scenarios were given in a scrambled order in the Sexual Harassment Scale. The scale included four subscales: male-female, female-male, male-male, and female-female. There were also demographic questions.

Results/conclusions: Just over one half of the female registered nurses and nursing administrators and almost one third of the male registered nurses and nursing administrators believed they had been sexually harassed. They were significantly more sensitive to opposite-gender harassment than to same-gender harassment. They were more sensitive to men harassing other men than to women harassing other women. Nursing administrators were significantly more sensitive to sexual harassment than nonadministrative nurses. There were no significant differences between the perceptions of female nursing administrators and male nursing administrators on the total harassment scale. Nurses who had been victims of opposite-gender harassment were more sensitive to all types of harassment. Nurses who had been victims of same-gender harassment showed no increased sensitivity on any of the scales. Nurses did not find all types of sexual harassment equally disturbing.

and of the same or opposite sex. There seems to be a high prevalence of sexual harassment in the hospital setting. Nurses are often harassed by physicians, patients, and co-workers, and could be harassed by the employer, supervisor, subordinate, or a nonemployee like a patient's family member or drug or equipment representative.

Harassment may be verbal or written such as comments about the person's body, clothing, personal behavior, repeated requests for dates, sexual teasing, sexual jokes, sexual innuendos, telling rumors about a person, or threats. It can also be physical with actual touching, stroking, patting, kissing, hugging, fondling, trapping, leaning over a worker, and blocking movement. Nonverbal sexual harassment includes giving suggestive looks, looking up and down a person's body, following a person, and making derogatory gestures or facial expressions. Visual screensavers, drawings, pictures, posters, or e-mails of a sexual nature may also be forms of sexual harassment. These can lead to low morale, inefficiency, and decreased productivity resulting from embarrassment and anger related to sexual harassment.

Women have been advised by other women to trust their instincts. If they feel harassed, they probably are. Then they have to assess their risk/reward situation, decide how to stop the harassment, and decide whether to deal with it informally or to file a formal complaint. Women have been advised to choose an option to stop harassment that feels right to them. One may be able to handle the harassment privately by dealing directly with the offending individual or may need to go public. One may write a letter to the harasser, even if it is never sent. That will help organize thoughts for a confrontation. Role playing how to approach the offender with a friend will help build confidence. If one wants to be less direct, one can send a highlighted version of the company's sexual harassment statement to the offender. Copies of the policy can be posted on bulletin boards. One can send a clear, anonymous, generic message or have an intermediary help confront the harasser directly.

It is advisable to record the dates and details of the harassment—noting in particular incidents that can be substantiated by others—if only for one's private files. If harassment continues, this will be historical documentation for taking formal action. Other than that, one may read the account later to find assurance that nothing was done to encourage the harassment and to help relieve self-blame and embarrassment.

If the risk is not too high, a direct approach can be assertive. Allowing the harasser to save face when the harassment has stopped will decrease the likelihood of damage to one's career. If the offender harasses women, makes explicit threats if sexual favors are not granted, or uses physical contact, a formal complaint is appropriate. It is advisable to have contingency plans such as the following: "If confronting the harasser does not work, I will discuss the situation with my boss. If my boss is not responsive, I will discuss the situation with the personnel officer or other appropriate official." People are encouraged to discuss the harassment with a friend. Otherwise, the harassment may be an emotional drain that causes a decrease in self-confidence.

Women often do nothing but try to avoid the harasser because of guilt from thinking one must have done something to cause the other's behavior or fear of retaliation. Sexual harassment is a legal issue that should be confronted immediately. Because sexual harassment is an unwanted behavior, the harassed person, whether female or male, needs to be very clear that the behavior is offensive. Be assertive, confront the issue, and be clear that the harasser's behavior is unwelcome: "I want to be very clear that I will not tolerate this sexual harassment. I do not want you telling me dirty jokes, brushing against me, and asking me out with an offer of serving me breakfast in bed." Then listen to the harasser's response, hope for an apology, and accept it, making your position clear. "I accept your apology, but I will follow the sexual harassment policies and report this to my supervisor. I will take action on any further harassment. Sexual harassment is illegal." That way one has made one's position clear and implied legal action. Write down what happened and start a paper trail. File a report of the harassment using the grievance procedure. Involve the union if appropriate. If a situation occurs again, confront the behavior immediately and follow the policies of the agency (Equal Rights Advocates, 2007).

Group Conflict

Team development can help prevent and resolve conflict. Planning, goal setting, and rating goals represent the first step in team development. The statement of the core mission of the team is developed by brainstorming and sharing individual mission statements.

The *nominal group technique* is very effective for developing team-performance goals and priorities (Box 6-12). First, individual group members list on separate pieces of paper what they think team-performance goals should be. The group leader helps keep the group problem centered by presenting the question and prevents interruptions of thoughts by asking participants to work silently and independently. This step allows time for thinking, avoids status and conformity pressures, prevents focusing on a particular idea because of a vocal person, and helps avoid choosing among ideas prematurely.

Second, during a "round-robin" session, each person in turn states one team-performance goal, which is then written on a chalkboard or paper for all to see. It is probable that equalization of participation and sharing of all ideas foster group creativity. By citing one goal, each member is encouraged to participate equally. By the second round, each member has participated and the precedent is set, and thus competition from aggressive or high-status members is minimized.

If all of an individual's listed goals have been cited, that individual passes, and other members continue to offer listed goals in turn until all are

---

BOX 6-12 Nominal Group Technique

Listing ideas on paper
Round-robin session
Serial discussion for clarification
Preliminary vote
Analysis of votes
Discussion of preliminary vote
Revote

exhausted. Ideas are not repeated. However, "hitchhiking" may occur. An idea listed by one member may stimulate another member to have an idea not previously listed. That idea can be added to the member's list and cited during the round-robin session.

It is common for many of an individual's ideas about a problem to remain unspoken because of fear of self-disclosure and embarrassment. When one person states several ideas at once, those ideas tend to be associated with that person. However, with the round-robin method, it is difficult to remember who presented what ideas and full disclosure is encouraged.

The written list can be the basis of recorded minutes and serve as a source of information from which the group continues to work. During this step the group leader should see that ideas are recorded as rapidly as possible and in the words used by the contributor. The entire list should be made visible to all group members. Tearing completed sheets from a flip chart and taping them on the walls work well, and they are an early reward in that the group can see the array of ideas generated. The written ideas are more objective and less personal than oral comments because the personality and position of the contributors are separated from the written statement. The group leader should encourage the simple listing of ideas by explaining that a discussion period will follow. Discussion of the ideas, arguments about them, and side conversations while the list is being made should not be allowed.

The third step is a serial discussion for clarification. During this step, each listed idea is discussed in order. This provides an opportunity to clarify ideas, state differences of opinion, provide the logic behind ideas, and prevent undue focusing on one idea. The group leader's responsibility is to clarify the purpose of this step and to pace the group. Arguments can be curtailed by stating that both points of view have been noted and then moving on to the next point. It is better not to ask the contributors to clarify their own items, because such a request can put them on the spot. Instead, the group members can be

asked what the items mean to them. The contributor can clarify when appropriate. This method helps reduce identification of items with specific individuals.

The preliminary vote on item importance is the fourth step. In the nominal group process individuals make independent judgments, express their judgments mathematically by ranking items, use the mean value of the independent judgments for the group's decision, talk over the results, and revote (Delbecq, Van de Ven, & Gustafson, 1975).

Alternative ways to determine a group decision are consensus, majority rule, and independent listing. When using consensus, group members may distort their judgments to maintain group cohesion, and consequently a regression toward the mean may occur. A showing of hands for majority rule is subject to social pressure, and minority positions do not count. Consequently, it may not truly reflect group preference. Independent listing, however, overcomes status, personality, and conformity pressures but does not indicate degree of importance. For example, an item listing might look like the one shown in Table 6-1. An analysis of the votes in Table 6-1 suggests that items 1, 4, 5, and 6 are considered the most important by frequency. Information about degree of importance can be obtained by having the items ranked. Ranking of the list might look like the one shown in Table 6-2. Using a scale of 5 as most important and 1 as least important, an analysis of the votes reveals that items 6, 4, 1, 5, and 8 are considered most important in descending order from 6 to 8.

TABLE 6-1 Analysis by Frequency

Item	Votes
1	5
2	1
3	2
4	5
5	5
6	5
7	1
8	2

TABLE 6-2 Analysis by Ranking

Item	Votes	Totals
1	1-2-5-5-1	14
2	2	2
3	3-2	5
4	4-3-2-4-2	15
5	1-2-1-3-1	8
6	5-5-4-5-4	23
7	1	1
8	3-3	6

This method is more likely to reflect the true group preference.

The group leader asks each individual to select a specific number of most important items from the list; individuals seem most able to accurately list that person's five to nine items. Each member is asked to take that specific number of 3 x 5 index cards, identify that number of items from the list, place the item number in the upper left-hand corner, and write some identifying words in the middle of the card (Figure 6-2). Then the participants are asked to spread out the cards, choose the item they consider most important, and put the high number in the lower right-hand corner of the card and underline it. If five items are being selected, 5 would be the high number. For nine items, 9 would be the high number. That card is turned over, the remaining cards are assessed, and a 1 is put in the lower right-hand corner and underlined for the least important card. That card is turned over, and the next most important item is selected and rated as one less than the highest number, For example, eight for nine items or four for five items. Then the next-to-the-lowest item is chosen and marked as two, and so on, until the middle item is left and numbered. This process encourages careful decisions.

When the card ranking is complete, the group leader collects and shuffles the cards and records the votes on the written list of items.

The fifth step is an analysis of the preliminary vote. Inconsistent voting patterns can be examined, and items receiving many or few votes can be discussed. The sixth step, discussion, will probably allow for corrections of misinformation, misunderstandings, and unequal information, thereby offering a more accurate indication of preferences than voting only. The final step is the revote, which determines the outcome of the process, documents the group judgment, and closes the nominal group process (Delbecq, Van de Ven, & Gustafson, 1975; Huber, 2006; Roussel, Swansburg, & Swansburg, 2006).

Role negotiations—the process of preventing role conflicts, role ambiguities, and role overload—become important once priorities have been set. During this process, group members clarify each individual's role on the team and help resolve any disagreements over the team members' roles. Members initially send one written message to each team member indicating that for them to act, they need the other team member to do more, to do less, or to continue his or her previous performance (Figure 6-3). To whom and from whom are essential parts of the message. The number of role messages sent to any one individual should be limited to prevent an information overload. The message must clearly state how the sender wants the receiver to behave and how a change will help the sender. Each role message must indicate the need for more, less, or the same of some activity. More than one message in the "same" category indicates support for the other person.

Receivers respond by indicating what they can or cannot do, explaining why, and offering alternative solutions, for example, "I can't do x, but I can do y, which should help solve your problem," or "If I do x, I would like you to do y." Receivers analyze the role messages they receive in the "do more, do less, and do the same" categories according to who sent the message and their response to that message. Do the receivers know what is expected of them? Do different people want them to do more and less of the same activity at the same time? Do the receivers have time to meet all the demands made of them? Role definition helps identify role ambiguity, role conflict, and role overload. After roles are negotiated, a contract (Figure 6-4) is written that defines the problem, identifies what each involved person will do, and sets a date for a follow-up check.

6 (item number from original list)

Setting goals for the unit
(identifying words)

2
(rank order number)

Figure 6-2 • Index card illustrating rank order.

ROLE MESSAGE FORM

To:_____
From:_____

In order for me to _____, I need you to do

Less of:

Same of:

More of:

Figure 6-3 • Role message form.

Negotiating involves good communication skills. One can identify needs, ideas, and information by using open-ended probes to clarify. Closed probes can be used to pinpoint specifications and to confirm understanding. One should indicate one's intent ("I support your idea") when one offers ideas of information. It is preferable to present reasons before conclusions, because they seem to be heard better that way, and the speaker is more likely to be considered reasonable. To build on ideas, one should acknowledge the connection ("Bill's comment made me think of...") and then add value. To criticize constructively, merits should be stated before concerns. One should then ask for ways to retain merits and eliminate concerns. One should confront counterproductive tactics by confirming the behavior and expressing its impact. ("That seemed like a personal attack. Is that what you intended? I feel angry when I am treated that way.") To break an impasse, one can indicate one's desire to continue and then initiate a change of pace ("Let's go get a cup of coffee and then try to solve this problem").

```
                          ROLE CONTRACT
  1. Problem:


  2. Person x agrees to:


  3. Person y agrees to:


  4. Others agree to:


  We agree that a follow-up check will be done by _____.
                                                    (date)

                                         Signatures

                                         _____
                                         x
                                         _____
                                         y
                                         _____
                                         others
```

Figure 6-4 • Role contract.

To come to an agreement, the purpose of the meeting and a review of the situation should be discussed. Identify the needs and restrictions, examine ideas from both points of view, and determine the best alternative. The discussion can be closed by summarizing the agreement and confirming the next steps (Negotiating self-taught, 1984).

Decision charting is the next major phase of team development and is concerned with who should be involved in decision making and with the nature of that involvement. To determine who should be involved in decision making, one should assess who has the information necessary to make a sound decision and who is responsible for implementing that decision. The person who will be responsible for implementing the decision needs to understand the decision and be committed to it.

People can be involved in decision making in a variety of ways. Some are directly involved because they have the necessary information and are responsible for implementing the decision. The involvement of some may be limited to input or consultation. Others need to be informed about the decision, and someone must be responsible for managing the overall decision-making process.

A decision chart helps one visualize the decision-making process (Figure 6-5). Decisions to be made are listed down the side of the page, and the involved people are listed across the top in a grid pattern. Placing an M in a square indicates who manages the process; D indicates who is directly involved; C indicates who should be consulted; and I indicates who should be informed. Anyone who is expected to implement the decision obviously must be informed (Rubin, Plovnick, & Fry, 1975, 1978).

Names

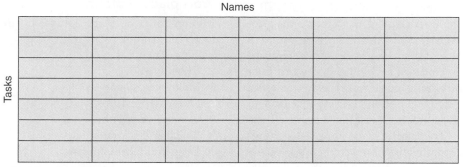

Tasks

Figure 6-5 • Decision chart. M, Manages the process; C, consulted before the decision; D, makes the decision; I, informed of the decision.

Intergroup Conflict

Intergroup conflict is common and can be dysfunctional. As with interpersonal conflict, intergroup resistance may result from low trust, poor communications, and false assumptions. People resist what they perceive as threatening. Intergroup actions may threaten territorial rights and contribute to role overload and conflict. By preventing win-lose situations, emphasizing the organization's goals and effectiveness, rotating personnel among groups to facilitate understanding, and increasing interaction and communication among groups, one can help reduce intergroup conflict.

When a group recognizes its need to solve some intergroup conflict, it must first decide how to begin. A study of the organizational chart will determine who should be involved. Who should represent the group—a person or a committee? Someone who is already friendly with members of the other group? Someone with strong or moderate feelings about the position? What is the group's position, and how much negotiation is acceptable? It helps to emphasize common goals and discuss constraints. The same process used in interpersonal conflict should be used in group conflict situations: setting and rating goals, negotiating roles, and making decisions.

"An open enemy is better than a false friend." —*Greek saying*

Organizational Conflict

Organizations in conflict display the collective symptoms of their members. Personnel feel frustration at work. If they do not think their skills are being used, they experience a loss of self-esteem and a sense of powerlessness, both of which lead to withdrawal from the situation instead of an attempt to solve the problems. Group members also engage in backbiting and blame others for the problems. Subgroups commonly form. Members of the organization identify the same task and group maintenance problems but act contrary to the information, thereby increasing their frustrations. However, personnel do not have the same frustrations or exhibit the same dysfunctional behavior outside the organization.

Organizational factors that may increase conflict include the number of organizational levels, number of specialties, degree of association, and some parties' dependency on others. The higher the number of levels and specialties, the more opportunities for conflict. When there are higher numbers of levels and specialties, more persons need to associate with others and greater dependency of one on another increase the risk of conflict. Competition for scarce resources, ambiguous jurisdictions, and need for consensus increase conflict. Communication barriers, including separation in time and space (as previously discussed) and differing values, increase conflict. An accumulation of unresolved conflict increases the challenge for conflict management.

A leader or manager may soothe a party during organizational conflict to facilitate the process and then deal with the underlying problem later. Leaders and managers should encourage personnel to confront each other and work their problems out themselves. Appropriate behavior change should be expected and may require sensitivity training, team development, and educational tools. The manager should assess things such as the organizational structure, titles, job descriptions, policies, and procedures as related to the apparent conflict. Responsibility charting can help clarify jurisdictional conflicts (Marquis & Huston, 2006).

A consultant may be appointed to assess the situation and make recommendations. The consultant must analyze the organization's structure, the leadership and authority of the institution, the communication patterns, the amount of intergroup cooperation and competition, the group's norms and goals, the group's problem-solving and decision-making processes, and various individual roles and functions within the group. Organizational research can help provide the information necessary to solve the problem.

After data have been collected and analyzed, the consultant offers feedback. Members of the organization can publicly vote on whether they agree with the consultant's views. A public vote facilitates ownership of ideas. If there is disagreement, the consultant helps the group clarify the reasons for the differences and modifies the statement until it reflects the group's thinking.

The consultant then asks all members to write a few sentences about how they contribute to the situation so that they can recognize their own part in the problem. Individuals are likely to maintain the status quo for fear of serious consequences if they confront the issues. The consultant shares his or her theory with the group, helps develop an awareness of dysfunctional behavior, helps individuals cope with their feelings, encourages fantasy and reality testing, and coaches group members toward new behaviors.

Workplace Violence

Millions of people are harassed, threatened, or attacked at their work each year. Unacceptable behavior includes:

- Excessive noise
- Malicious allegation
- Offensive gestures
- General verbal abuse
- Racial and sexual abuse
- Drug and alcohol abuse
- Damage
- Theft
- Threats
- Violence

A number of factors may increase a worker's risk for workplace assault. Health care workers face increased risk in poorly lit parking areas and where there is a prevalence of handguns or other weapons, drugs, or money. Solo work in remote locations, isolated work with patients during examinations and treatments, low staffing levels during increased activity time such as mealtimes and visiting hours, and unrestricted movement of the public are increasing the presence of drug and alcohol abusers, gang members, trauma patients, and patients and families distraught and frustrated from long waits. Lack of training of staff for recognizing and managing assaultive and hostile behavior also increases risk (Reich & Dean, 1996) (Box 6-13).

There are numerous bullying behaviors displayed in the workplace such as undermining, manipulation of reputation, social isolation, intimidation, abuse, aggressiveness, offensive jokes, stalking, and unreasonable assignments. There are also many warning signs of impending violence (Box 6-14) (Gates & Kroeger, 2003).

The U.S. Department of Occupational Safety and Health Administration (Gates & Kroeger, 2003) has recommended eight essential components to a violence prevention plan that is recommended for all workplaces to develop and implement. They include (1) management commitment, (2) employee involvement, (3) work site analysis, (4) prevention of hazards, (5) training and education, (6) prompt recognition, control, and monitoring, (7) record keeping, and (8) evaluation.

BOX 6-13 Risks for Workplace Assault	**BOX 6-14** Warning Signs of Violence
Poorly lit parking areas Contact with the public Exchange of money Delivery of passengers, goods, or services Having a mobile workplace Working with unstable or volatile persons Working alone or in small numbers Working late at night or during early-morning hours Working in high-crime areas Guarding valuable property or possessions Working in community-based settings Lack of training to deal with assault	Attendance problems Carelessness at work History of physical violence Performance problems Personality changes Poor hygiene Substance abuse Social isolation Sudden change in behavior Clenched jaws or fists Increased movement Increased respirations Pacing Shouting threats Staring or pointing Use of profanity

See Box 6-15 for what management commitment should include and Box 6-16 for what employee involvement should include. Worksite analysis includes record analysis and tracking; monitoring trends and analyzing incidents; screening surveys; and workplace security analysis. See Box 6-17 for what engineering controls for hazard prevention include and Box 6-18 for what administrative and work practice controls include.

Training should cover topics listed in Box 6-19. Record keeping is essential to the success of a work place violence prevention program. Good records help determine the severity of the problem, evaluate methods of hazard control, and identify training needs; they include the following: (1) a U.S. Occupational Safety and Health Administration (OSHA) Log of Injury should be filled out; (2) medical reports of work injury and a supervisor's report for each recorded assault should be kept; (3) incidents of abuse, verbal attacks, or aggressive behavior should be part of an assault incident report; (4) information on patients with a history of past violence, drug abuse, or criminal activity should be on the patient's chart; (5) minutes of safety meetings, records of hazard analysis, and corrective actions recommended are to be documented; and (6) records of all training programs, attendees, and qualifications of trainers should be maintained. See Box 6-20 for what the evaluation program committee members should do (Reich & Dean, 1996). OSHA consultation services are available.

The National Institute for Occupational Safety and Health (NIOSH) is the federal agency responsible for research and recommendations for the prevention of work-related illness and injury. Job stress consists of harmful physical and emotional responses that occur because the requirements of the job do not match the capabilities, resources, or needs of the worker. It can lead to poor health, injury, and workplace violence. Interventions could include the following: (1) target source of stress for change, (2) propose and prioritize intervention strategies, (3) communicate planned interventions to employees, and (4) implement interventions. To do evaluations of interventions (1) conduct both short- and long-term evaluations, (2) measure employee perceptions of job conditions, stress, health, and satisfaction, (3) include objective measures, and (4) refine the intervention strategy.

The following can reduce the effects of stressful working conditions:
- Balance between work and family or personal life
- A support network of friends and co-workers
- A relaxed and positive outlook

(United States Department of Agriculture, 1998).

BOX 6-15 Management Commitment

The endorsement and visible involvement of top management
Assigned responsibility for the various aspects of the workplace violence prevention program
Appropriate allocation of authority and resources to responsible parties
A system of accountability
A comprehensive program of medical and psychological counseling
Debriefing for employees witnessing violent incidents
Commitment to support and implement appropriate recommendations from the safety and health department

---

BOX 6-16 Employee Involvement

Understanding and complying with the workplace violence prevention program and other safety measures
Participation in an employee complaint or suggestion procedure
Prompt and accurate reporting of violent incidents
Participation on safety and health committees
Taking part in a continuing education program

BOX 6-17 Engineering Controls for Hazard Prevention

Assess new construction plans to eliminate security hazards.
Install and regularly maintain alarm systems.
Provide metal detectors.
Use a closed-circuit video for high-risk areas.
Place curved mirrors at hallway intersections.
Enclose nurses' station and install deep service counters or bullet-resistant, shatterproof glass.
Provide employee "safe rooms."
Establish "time-out" or seclusion areas.
Provide patient waiting rooms designed to maximize comfort and minimize stress.
Ensure that counseling or patient care rooms have two exits.
Limit access to staff counseling rooms and treatment rooms controlled by using locked doors.
Arrange furniture to prevent entrapment of staff.
Provide lockable and secure bathrooms for staff members separate from patient/client and visitor bathrooms.
Lock all unused doors to limit access.
Install bright, effective lighting indoors and outdoors.
Replace burned-out lights and broken windows and locks.
Keep automobiles well maintained and locked.

Hostage Situations

Mentally disturbed people, criminals, prisoners, and terrorists are the common categories of hostage takers. Hostage situations may involve workplace violence, intoxicated co-workers, angry-client-on-employee, family-member-on-employee, family-member-on-member, domestic violence, or angry-employee-on-client.

The major choices of the hostage taker are to choose martyrdom, kill hostages, and commit suicide; lessen demands and continue negotiations; and to surrender to the police. The two major objectives in handling a hostage situation are to preserve life and to recover property. The hostage as a person is of no value to the hostage taker except as a tool to get what he or she wants. The hostage cannot negotiate for his or her own survival, but a trained hostage negotiator can. Only the trained hostage negotiator should talk to the press.

Time is the most critical element in determining the outcome of a hostage situation. The more time passes, the more likely it is that the situation can be resolved without loss of life. Time can reduce anxiety and stress and increase the rationality of the hostage taker. It also increases the need for food and drink. Time increases the opportunities for hostages to escape. Unfortunately it can also increase exhaustion and boredom.

The first hour "chaotic stage" is the most dangerous time. There may be loud noises and throwing things to scare the hostages. The danger to the hostage of being attacked, shot, or slashed

---

BOX 6-18 Administrative and Work Practice Controls

State clearly to patients, clients, and employees that violence is not permitted or tolerated.

Establish liaison with local police and state prosecutors. Report all incidents of violence. Provide physical layouts of facilities to expedite investigations.

Require employees to report all assaults or threats. Keep logbooks and reports of such incidents.

Advise and assist employees requesting police assistance when assaulted.

Provide management support during emergencies.

Set up a trained response team.

Use properly trained security officers.

Ensure adequate and properly trained staff for restraining patients or clients.

Ensure adequate and qualified staff coverage at all times.

Institute a sign-in procedure for everyone, with additional passes for visitors.

Establish a list of restricted visitors for patients with a history of violence.

Supervise the movement of psychiatric clients and patients throughout the facility.

Control access to facilities other than waiting rooms, particularly drug storage or pharmacy areas.

Prohibit employees from working alone.

Establish policies and procedures for secured areas.

Ascertain the behavioral history of new and transferred patients.

Treat and/or interview aggressive or agitated patients in relatively open areas.

Use case management conferences.

Prepare contingency plans to treat patients who are "acting out."

Transfer assaultive patients to acute care units.

Make sure that nurses and/or physicians are not alone when performing intimate physical examinations.

Discourage employees from wearing necklaces to prevent possible strangulation.

Periodically survey the facility to remove tools or possessions left by visitors.

Provide staff with identification badges.

Discourage employees from carrying keys, pens, or other items that could be used as weapons.

Provide staff members with security escorts to parking areas.

Use the buddy system, especially when personal safety may be threatened.

Develop policies and procedures covering home health care providers.

Establish a daily work plan.

Conduct a comprehensive postincident evaluation.

---

is greatest at this time. Try to be quiet and unobvious. Do not speak unless spoken to. Do look at the hostage taker if he is looking at you when asking a question; it is more difficult to hurt a person when looking into that person's eyes. Do not make suggestions. Don't be argumentative. Get rid of any items that could single you out to your capturers. Be patient. Try to rest. Be observant. Be careful about making any attempt to escape as that may anger the hostage taker. Others may be punished and the person attempting the escape could be killed. If rescuers come, be prepared to "hit the deck." Try to stay low.

When it is necessary to speak, speak in a voice softer and slower than the suspect. Adapt your conversation to the level of education and vocabulary of the suspect. Listen to clues to the suspect's emotional state and willingness to negotiate.

If engaged in a conversation with the hostage taker, try to take time by asking open-ended questions that cannot be answered quickly with "yes" or "no." Elaborating on responses takes more time, may allow the ventilation of anger and frustration the suspect is experiencing, and may provide important information. Be supportive when the subject is expressing rational thoughts and show understanding through words and tone of voice. Encourage the suspect to keep talking by encouraging through such comments as, "Could you tell me more about that?" "I would like to hear your views," "And then?" "Uh-huh," "I see." Ask for details. Stall some more by paraphrasing or restating the hostage taker's comments to see if you understand and that your understanding is correct. This may encourage the suspect to elaborate some more on what has been said. Have the

---

BOX 6-19 Training Topics

The workplace violence prevention policy

Risk factors that cause or contribute to assaults

Early recognition of escalating behavior or recognition of warning signs or situations

Ways of preventing or diffusing volatile situations or aggressive behavior, managing anger, and using medications as chemical restraints

Information on multicultural diversity to develop sensitivity to racial and ethnic issues and differences

A standard response action plan for violent situations, including availability of assistance, response systems, and communication procedures

How to deal with hostile persons

Progressive behavior control methods and safe methods of restraint application or escape

The location and operation of safety devices such as alarm systems, along with the required schedules and procedures

Ways to protect oneself and co-workers, including use of the buddy system

Policies and procedures for reporting and record keeping

Policies and procedures for obtaining medical care, counseling, workers' compensation, or legal assistance for a violent episode or injury

---

BOX 6-20 What an Evaluation Program Should Include

Establishing a uniform violence reporting system and regular review of reports

Reviewing reports and minutes from staff meetings on safety and security issues

Analyzing trends and rates in illnesses/injuries or fatalities caused by violence or workplace violence

Keeping up-to-date records of administrative and work practice changes to prevent workplace violence and evaluate their effectiveness

Surveying employees before and after making job or work-site changes or installing security measures

Keeping abreast of new strategies available to deal with violence

Surveying employees who experience hostile situations about the medical treatment they received, several weeks afterward and then several months later

Requesting periodic law enforcement or outside consultant review of the work site for recommendations for improving employee safety

---

suspect reflect on his or her feelings. You might be able to say something like "I understand that you are angry. Have you felt this way before? How did you handle your feelings then? Why do you think this has you so upset?" Keep the hostage taker in a constant decision mode. Is he or she hungry? Does he or she want a sandwich? What does he or she want on the sandwich? What kind of bread does he or she want? Don't interrupt. Be careful not to annoy. Change your tactic if the hostage taker gets more aggravated. Be observant and collect information. Where is the activity? What has occurred? When? Who is involved? How many hostages are there? How long have they been held? What are their physical descriptions? What are their physical conditions? Are there injuries? What are the hostage taker's demands? Does he or she have weapons and if so, what types? What is the layout of the area? Are there escape routes? Where are telephones located? What is background information of the hostage taker: emotional state, intelligence, problems he or she is facing, goals? Food, fluids, media coverage, and help related to the hostage taker's problems are negotiable. Introduction of weapons, alcohol, illegal drugs, amnesty, freedom, money, and exchange of hostages are nonnegotiable. Giving in increases the hostage taker's behavior (Law enforcement exploring, 2003; Thompson Rivers University, 2005).

Prevention of Conflict

"The best general is the one who never fights." —Sun Tzu

Careful development of an organization's structure, strategic and comprehensive planning, management and organizational development, and careful selection and placement of personnel help prevent organizational conflict. The same strategies also prevent intergroup, group, and interpersonal conflict. Although conflict can be reduced, it cannot be totally avoided. Conflict can be constructive or destructive depending on how it is handled. By capitalizing on the positive aspects of conflict, the negative features can seem more bearable.

CHAPTER SUMMARY

There are many sources of conflict and numerous ways individuals and groups can respond to the conflict. There are also many ways to escalate the conflict. Fortunately, there are also ways to deescalate it. Open assertive communications and problem solving are particularly good approaches to dealing with conflict. Mediation can be used when parties want to come to an agreement, and arbitration can be used when a third, neutral party makes a decision that is based on laws and contracts; arbitration is usually binding. Nominal group technique, role negotiations, and decision charting are formal techniques used to diminish conflict. Leaders, managers, and others may also have to deal with workplace violence and hostage situations.

CASE STUDY   Two staff nurses on the team want the same weekend off. You need someone to work. How are you going to go about resolving the conflict?

CRITICAL THINKING ACTIVITY

Reflective Journal: Reflect on an organizational setting. What are the most common sources of conflict in that setting? How do people respond to the conflict? What kind of conflict do you have in your life? How do you handle it? What might you do differently to get even better results?

ONLINE RESOURCES

evolve Additional critical thinking activities, worksheets, and case studies are available online at http://evolve.elsevier.com/Marriner/guide8e.

REFERENCES

Barrett J, Dowd JO: *Interest-based bargaining: A user's guide,* Cheshire, UK, 2005, Trafford Publishing.

Block P: *The empowered manager,* rep ed, San Francisco, 1991, Jossey-Bass.

Cleary PJ: *The negotiation handbook,* Armonk, NY, 2001, ME Sharp.

Delbecq AL, Van de Ven AH, Gustafson DH: *Group techniques for program planning: A guide to nominal group and Delphi processes,* Glenview, IL, 1975, Scott Foresman.

Equal Rights Advocates: *Know your rights: Sexual harassment at work,* 2007 (website): www.equalrights.org/publications/kyr/shwork.asp. Accessed August 12, 2007.

Fiedler A, Hamby E : Sexual harassment in the workplace, *JONA* 30(10):497-503, 2000.

Finkelman AW: *Leadership and management in nursing,* Upper Saddle River, NJ, 2006, Pearson/Prentice Hall.

Fisher R, Brown S: *Getting together: Building relationships as we negotiate,* New York, 1988, Penguin Books.

Fisher R, Ertel D: *Getting ready to negotiate,* New York, 1995, Penguin Books.

Fisher R, Ury RY, Patton WY: *Getting to yes: Negotiating agreement without giving in,* Boston, 2004, Houghton Mifflin.

Gates DM, Kroeger D: Violence against nurses: The silent epidemic, *ISNA Bulletin* (1) 29:25-29, 2003.

Goodman AH: *Basic skills for the new mediator,* ed 2, Rockville, MD, 2004, Solomon Publications.

Grzywacz JG, Frone MR, Brewer CS, Kover CT: Quantifying work-family conflict among registered nurses, *Research in Nursing & Health* 29(5):414-426, 2006.

Huber DL: *Leadership and nursing care management,* ed 3, Philadelphia, 2006, Saunders/Elsevier.

Kheel TW: *The keys to conflict resolution,* New York, 2001, Four Walls Eight Windows.

Law enforcement exploring: *Hostage negotiation study guide,* 2003 (website): www.nicic.org/Library/019490. Accessed August 12, 2007.

Loveridge CE, Cummings SH: *Nursing management in the new paradigm,* Gaithersburg, MD, 1996, Aspen.

Marquis BL, Huston CJ: *Leadership roles and management functions in nursing,* Philadelphia, 2006, Lippincott.

Mayer B: *The dynamics of conflict resolution: A practitioner's guide,* San Francisco, 2000, Jossey-Bass.

McConnell CR: *Umiker's management skills for the new health care supervisor,* ed 4, Boston, 2006, Jones and Bartlett Publishers.

Negotiating self-taught, Stamford, CT, 1984, Learning International.

Patterson K, Grenny J, McMillan R, et al: *Crucial conversations: Tools for talking when stakes are high,* New York, 2002, McGraw-Hill.

Reich R, Dean J: Guidelines for preventing workplace violence for health care and social service workers, Washington, DC, 1996, U.S. Department of Labor.

Roussel L, Swansburg FC, Swansburg RJ: *Management and leadership for nurse administrators,* ed 4, Boston, 2006, Jones and Bartlett.

Rubin IM, Plovnick MS, Fry RE: *Improving the coordination of care: A program for health team development,* Cambridge, MA, 1975, Ballinger.

Rubin IM, Plovnick MS, Fry RE: *Managing human resources in health care organizations: An applied approach,* Reston, VA, 1978, Reston.

Steinberg L, D'Orso M: *Winning with integrity: Getting what you're worth without selling your soul,* New York, 1998, Villard.

Stone D, Patton B, Heen S, Fisher R: *Difficult conversations: How to discuss what matters most,* New York, 2000, Penguin Books.

Sullivan EJ, Decker PJ: *Effective leadership management in nursing,* ed 6, Upper Saddle River, NJ, 2005, Pearson/Prentice Hall.

Thomas KW, Kilmann RH: *Thomas-Kilmann conflict mode instrument,* Sterling Forest, Tuxedo, NY, 1974, XICOM.

Thomas KW, Kilmann RH: *Thomas-Kilmann conflict mode instrument,* Sterling Forest, Tuxedo, NY, 2002, XICOM.

Thompson Rivers University: *Hostage situations,* 2005 (website): www.tru.ca/hsafety/emergency/incident_response_procedures/hostage.html. Accessed August 12, 2007.

United States Department of Agriculture: *The USDA handbook on workplace violence prevention and response,* 1998 (website): www.usda.gov/news/pubs/violence/wpv.htm. Accessed August 12, 2007.

Ury W: *Getting past no: Negotiating with difficult people,* New York, 1991, Bantam Books.

Wywialowski EF: *Managing client care,* ed 3, St Louis, 2004, Mosby.

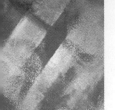

Theories of Leadership and Management Development

"Lead, follow, or get out of the way."   —Anonymous

Chapter Overview

Chapter 7 discusses several theories of leadership and management, the development of management thought, diversity among leaders, followership, and character development.

Chapter Objectives

- Identify the two dimensions of leadership behavior and at least three activities in each dimension.
- List the three aspects of a situation that structure the leader's role as identified by Fiedler in contingency theory.
- Identify the variable from which Hersey and Blanchard's situational leadership theory predicts the most appropriate leadership style.
- Differentiate the differences between transactional and transformational leadership.
- Select at least two theorists in each of the following management eras: scientific management, classic organization, human relations, and behavioral science.
- Indicate at least three of the concepts stressed in scientific management, classic organization, human relations, and behavioral science.
- Choose a major thinker regarding transformational leadership, servant leadership, learning organizations, emotional intelligence, and results-based leadership.
- Select a major idea regarding transformational leadership, servant leadership, learning organizations, emotional intelligence, and results-based leadership.
- Compare Maslow's, Herzberg's, and McGregor's theories.
- Describe each of Likert's four types of management systems.
- Classify at least three types of diversity among leaders.
- Identify at least five characteristics of a good character.

Online Resources

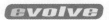 Critical thinking activities, worksheets, and case studies are available online at http://evolve.elsevier.com/Marriner/guide8e.

Major Concepts and Definitions

Lead *to show, mark the way, guide the course*

Transaction *the negotiation of business*

Transformation *a change in the nature of someone or something*

Charisma *an inspirational quality that some leaders possess*

Situational *appropriate to the requirements of different situations*

Contingency *the uncertainty of an event's occurrence*

Management *act of planning, organizing, staffing, directing, and controlling*

Scientific management *focused on the best way to do a task*

Classic organization *focused on planning, organizing, and controlling of the organization as a whole*

Human relations *focused on the effect individuals have on the success of the organization*

Behavioral science *focused on scientific validation*

Servant leadership *tending to people's highest priority needs*

Learning organizations *shared vision, systems thinking, and team learning*

Emotional intelligence *self-awareness and self-regulation*

Diversity *differences such as gender, racial, sexual orientation, and disability*

Follower *one who subscribes to the methods of another*

Character *qualities that distinguish one person from another*

THEORIES OF LEADERSHIP

Theories of leadership are numerous. The following survey covers the alternatives, beginning with the oldest notion and advancing to ideas currently in vogue. By familiarizing themselves with these theories, nurses can select and adapt the most suitable approach for dealing with different situations. As a role model, the nursing leader can reduce the autocratic atmosphere and, hence, some of the role conflicts (Box 7-1).

Leaders need to do the right things, are challenged by change, focus on purposes, and have a future time frame. They ask why and use strategies on their journeys to achieve human potential. On the other hand, managers do things right, are challenged by continuity, and focus on structures and procedures in a present time frame. They ask who, what, when, where, and how as they use schedules to get to destinations and evaluate human performance (Bennis & Nanus, 1985, 2007) (Table 7-1).

BOX 7-1 Theories of Leadership

Great Man Theory
Charismatic Theory
Trait Theory
Situational Theory
Contingency Theory
Path-Goal Theory
Situational Leadership Theory
Transactional Leadership
Transformational Leadership
Integrative Leadership Model

Drucker (2006) has observed over the past seven decades that leader attitudes, personalities, strengths, and weaknesses varied from nearly reclusive to extroverted, from controlling to easygoing, and from parsimonious to generous. However, he did observe common practices among them, including that they focused on what needed to be done, developed action plans,

TABLE 7-1 Comparison of Leadership and Management

	Leadership	Management
Motto	Do the right things	Do things right
Challenge	Change	Continuity
Focus	Purposes	Structures and procedures
Time frame	Future	Present
Methods	Strategies	Schedules
Questions	Why?	Who, what, when, where, and how?
Outcomes	Journeys	Destinations
Human	Potential	Performance

From Bennis W, Nanus B: *Leaders: The strategies for taking charge*, New York, 1985, Harper & Row.

took responsibility for communicating, listened before speaking, ran productive meetings, used "we" instead of "I", took responsibility for decisions, and focused on opportunities rather than problems (Drucker, 2006).

Great Man Theory

The great man theory argues that a few people are born with the necessary characteristics to be great. Early research about leadership was based on the study of men who were already considered great leaders and were usually from the aristocracy.

Leaders may be well rounded and simultaneously display both instrumental and supportive leadership behavior. Instrumental activities include planning, organizing, and controlling the activities of subordinates to accomplish the organization's goals. Obtaining and allocating resources such as people, equipment, materials, funds, and space are particularly important. Supportive leadership is socially oriented and allows for participation and consultation from subordinates for decisions that affect them. Men who used both instrumental and supportive leadership behaviors were considered "great men" and supposedly can be effective leaders in any situation. Contrary contemporary thought is that leadership skills can be developed even when they are not inborn (Marquis & Huston, 2006).

Charismatic Theory

People may be leaders because they are charismatic, but relatively little is known about this intangible characteristic. What constitutes charisma? Most agree that it is an inspirational quality possessed by some people that makes others feel better in their presence. The charismatic leader inspires others by obtaining emotional commitment from followers and by arousing strong feelings of loyalty and enthusiasm. Under charismatic leadership one may overcome obstacles not thought possible. However, because charisma is so elusive, some may sense it while others do not.

Charismatic leaders have a strong conviction in their own beliefs, high self-confidence, and a need for power. They are likely to set an example by their behavior, communicate high expectations to followers and express confidence in them, and arouse motives for the group's mission.

Charisma is more likely attributed to a leader who advocates a vision discrepant from the status quo, emerges during a crisis, accurately assesses the situation, communicates self-confidence, uses personal power, makes self-sacrifices, and uses unconventional strategies. Followers may idolize and worship charismatic leaders as spiritual figures or superhumans. This blind obedience can lead to good or bad outcomes, such as group suicide. Both Mahatma Gandhi and Adolf Hitler can be classified as charasmatic leaders. Transformational leaders use charisma for good (Bass, 1998; Conger & Kanungo, 1998; Sullivan & Decker, 2005; Yukl, 1994).

Trait Theory

Until the mid-1940s, the trait theory was the basis for most leadership research. Early work in this area maintained that traits are inherited,

RESEARCH Perspective 7-1

Data from Stanley D: Role conflict: Leaders and managers, *Nursing Management* 13(5):31-37, 2006.

Purpose: The purpose of this study was to identify the differences between leadership and management.

Methods: This was a qualitative study that used grounded theory in three phases: (1) Results from 830 questionnaires with general information about clinical leadership; (2) 42 focused, in-depth interviews with a random selection of nurses; (3) Eight further interviews with nurses nominated as clinical leaders during the 42 initial interviews.

Results/conclusions: Those interviewed indicated that managerial responsibilities often were detrimental to nurses' clinical leadership.

but later theories suggested that traits could be obtained through learning and experience. Researchers identified the leadership traits as energy, drive, enthusiasm, ambition, aggressiveness, decisiveness, self-assurance, self-confidence, friendliness, affection, honesty, fairness, loyalty, dependability, technical mastery, and teaching skill. Asking themselves what traits leaders possess, various researchers arrived at different conclusions but identified some common leadership traits: intelligence, initiative, creativity, emotional maturity, communication skills, persuasiveness, perceptiveness, sociability, and visualization skills (Maxwell, 1999; Sullivan & Decker, 2005).

Tourangeau and McGilton (2004) studied nursing leadership practices. They worked from Kouzes and Posner's (1995, rev 2007) and Posner and Kouzes' (1988, 1994) pattern of five leadership practices and associated leadership strategies; from these they derived a pattern of three leadership practices. They condensed Posner and Kouzes' (1) challenging the process by (a) searching for opportunities and (b) experimenting and taking risks, and (2) inspiring a shared vision by (a) envisioning the future and enlisting the support of others into their newly derived cognitive leadership practice. They also condensed Posner and Kouzes' (3) enabling others to act by (a) fostering collaboration and (b) strengthening others; (4) modeling the way by (a) setting the example and (b) planning small wins into behavioral leadership behavior, and (5) encouraging the heart by

(a) recognizing contributions and (b) celebrating accomplishments.

The authoritarian leader maintains strong control, does the planning, makes the decisions, and gives the orders. Autocratic leaders tend to be directive, critical, and punitive. They may make decisions that are not in the best interest of the group. They give themselves a higher status than the group members, which reduces open communications and trust. They tend to get good quantity and quality of output but little autonomy, creativity, or self-motivation. This can be appropriate for an emergency situation when the leader knows what to do, but it does not develop people (Table 7-2).

Democratic leaders maintain less control; ask questions and make suggestions rather than issue orders; and get the group involved in planning, problem solving, and decision making. The participation tends to increase motivation and creativity. It works when people have knowledge and skills and work well together over time. It can be cumbersome. It is often less efficient than autocratic control.

Laissez-faire is very permissive, nondirective, passive, and inactive. Members may work independently and possibly at cross purposes because there is no planning or coordination and little cooperation. Chaos is likely to develop unless an informal leader emerges. This style can work with very mature, autonomous workers, but it is more likely to be inefficient and unproductive (Marquis & Huston, 2006).

TABLE 7-2 Comparison of Autocratic, Democratic, and Laissez-Faire Leadership

Autocratic	Democratic	Laissez-Faire
Strong control	Less control	No control
Gives orders	Offers suggestions	Nondirective
Does decision making	Makes suggestions	Abdicates decision making
Leader does planning	Group does planning	No planning
Directive	Participative	Uninvolved
Fosters dependency	Fosters independence	Fosters chaos

The bureaucratic style is more characteristic of a manager than a leader. The leader or manager uses rules and policies with an autocratic approach to directions and expects compliance. It works best with people who are externally motivated (Finkelman, 2006; Sullivan & Decker, 2005).

The trait theory expanded knowledge about leadership, but it was not without its flaws. Few if any traits are identified in all trait theory research. They are not mutually exclusive, and there is considerable overlap between categories or definitions of the characteristics. It is not clear which traits are most important, which traits are needed to acquire leadership, and which traits are needed to maintain it. Trait theory does not view personality as an integrated whole, does not deal with subordinates, and avoids environmental influences and situational factors.

Ohio State Leadership Studies researchers compiled a list of about 1800 examples of leadership behavior that factored out two dimensions: consideration and initiating structure. Consideration involves behaving in a friendly and supportive way, looking out for others' welfare, showing concern, treating others as equals, taking time to listen, consulting others on important matters, being willing to accept suggestions, and doing personal favors. Initiating structure is the way the leader structures roles to attain the goals. It includes assigning tasks, defining procedures, setting deadlines, maintaining standards, suggesting new approaches, and coordinating activities (Huber, 2006; Roussel, Swansburg, & Swansburg, 2006).

Researchers at the University of Michigan focused on identification of relationships among leader behavior, group process, and group performance. They found that three types of leadership behavior marked the difference between effective and ineffective leaders: (1) task-oriented behavior, (2) relationship-oriented behavior, and (3) participative leadership. Task-oriented behavior includes planning, scheduling, and coordinating activities. Relationship-oriented behavior includes acting friendly and considerate, showing trust and confidence, expressing appreciation, and providing recognition. Participative leadership uses group meetings to enlist associate participation in decision making, improve communications, promote cooperation, and facilitate conflict resolution (Huber, 2006).

Maxwell (1999) discussed 21 qualities of a leader as character, charisma, commitment, communication, competence, courage, discernment, focus, generosity, initiative, listening, passion, positive attitude, problem solving, relationships, responsibility, security, self- discipline, servanthood, teachability, and vision, while Blank (2001) provided self-assessment tools for 108 leadership skills.

Situational Theory

Situational theories became popular during the 1950s. These theories suggest that the traits required of a leader differ according to varying situations. Among the variables that determine the effectiveness of leadership style are factors such as the personality of the leader; the performance requirements of both the leader and followers; the attitudes, needs, and expectations of the leader and followers; the degree of interpersonal contact possible; time pressures; physical

---

BOX 7-2 Group-Atmosphere Scale

Describe the atmosphere of your group by checking the following items:

	8	7	6	5	4	3	2	1	
1. Friendly	:_____	:_____	:_____	:_____	:_____	:_____	:_____	:_____	: Unfriendly
2. Accepting	:_____	:_____	:_____	:_____	:_____	:_____	:_____	:_____	: Rejecting
3. Satisfying	:_____	:_____	:_____	:_____	:_____	:_____	:_____	:_____	: Frustrating
4. Enthusiastic	:_____	:_____	:_____	:_____	:_____	:_____	:_____	:_____	: Unenthusiastic
5. Productive	:_____	:_____	:_____	:_____	:_____	:_____	:_____	:_____	: Nonproductive
6. Warm	:_____	:_____	:_____	:_____	:_____	:_____	:_____	:_____	: Cold
7. Cooperative	:_____	:_____	:_____	:_____	:_____	:_____	:_____	:_____	: Uncooperative
8. Supportive	:_____	:_____	:_____	:_____	:_____	:_____	:_____	:_____	: Hostile
9. Interesting	:_____	:_____	:_____	:_____	:_____	:_____	:_____	:_____	: Boring
10. Successful	:_____	:_____	:_____	:_____	:_____	:_____	:_____	:_____	: Unsuccessful

From Fiedler FE: *A theory of leadership effectiveness*, New York, 1967, McGraw-Hill, p 269.

---

environment; organizational structure; the nature of the organization; the state of the organization's development; and the influence of the leader outside the group. A person may be a leader in one situation and a follower in another, or a leader at one time and a follower at other times because the type of leadership needed depends on the situation (Marquis & Huston, 2006).

Contingency Theory

During the 1960s, Fred Fiedler introduced the contingency model of leadership. Refuting the ideal leadership style theory, he argued that a leadership style will be effective or ineffective depending on the situation. He identified three aspects of a situation that structure the leader's role: (1) leader-member relations, (2) task structure, and (3) position power.

Leader-member relations involve the amount of confidence and loyalty the followers have with regard to their leader. Leadership is assessed by a group-atmosphere scale (Box 7-2). Fiedler also used a sociometric index of the least-preferred co-worker (LPC) score. Followers were asked to think of everyone with whom they have ever worked and to rate the least-preferred co-worker on an eight-point bipolar adjective scale, which included adjectives such as friendly and cooperative. A high score described the person in favorable terms, and a low score was a negative rating. Although the LPC scores are difficult to interpret and it is hard to say what they measure, Fiedler suggests that high scorers are relationship oriented and low scorers are mostly task oriented.

Task structure is high if it is easy to define and measure a task. The structure is low if it is difficult to define the task and to measure progress toward its completion. Fiedler used four criteria to determine the degree of task structure: (1) goal clarity: extent to which a goal is understood by followers; (2) extent to which a decision can be verified: knowing who is responsible for what; (3) multiplicity of goal paths: number of solutions; and (4) specificity of solution: number of correct answers. Technical nursing, which focuses on procedures, may have a high task structure, but situations involving human relations and value judgments may have numerous solutions with no specific correct answer and consequently have a low task structure.

Position power refers to the authority inherent in a position, the power to use rewards and punishment, and the organization's support of one's decisions. Directors of nursing, managers, and sometimes patient care coordinators have high position power with the right to hire and fire, promote, and adjust salaries. People with low position power may be elected, function in an acting position, or be subject to removal by peers or subordinates. Elected committee chairpersons have low position power. Team leaders and staff nurses

TABLE 7-3 Summary of Fiedler Investigations of Leadership Group Situation

Condition	Leader-Member Relations	Task Structure	Position Power	Leadership Style Correlation with Productivity
1	Good	Structured	Strong	Directive
2	Good	Structured	Weak	Directive
3	Good	Unstructured	Strong	Directive
4	Good	Unstructured	Weak	Permissive
5	Moderately poor	Structured	Strong	Permissive
6	Moderately poor	Structured	Weak	No data
7	Moderately poor	Unstructured	Strong	No relationship level
8	Moderately poor	Unstructured	Weak	Directive

From Donnelly JH Jr, Gibson JL, Ivancevich JM: *Fundamentals of management functions, behavior, models*, Dallas, 1981, Business Publications. Copyright 1981 by Business Publications, Inc.

usually have low position power. Given the critical conditions, Fiedler argues that one can predict the most productive leadership style (Table 7-3).

If a task is structured but the leader is disliked and therefore needs to be diplomatic, or if the task is ambiguous and the leader is liked and therefore seeks the cooperation of the workers, the considerate, accepting leadership style probably will be most productive. When a disliked leader faces ambiguous tasks, a directive style is more productive. The most productive leadership style is contingent on the situational variables.

Empirical findings have not provided conclusive evidence for the contingency model. It is difficult to say what the psychologically distant manager and psychologically closer manager measures are really recording. Correlations were used for predicted direction even when they were not statistically significant. The model is primarily academic in that it has not been used in management development for improving group performance and organizational effectiveness. However, Fiedler's complex, three-dimensional contingency model has contributed to some leadership theory development (Fiedler, 1967; Fiedler & Chemers, 1974; Fiedler, Chemers, & Mahar, 1976; Huber, 2006; Roussel, Swansburg, & Swansburg, 2006; Sullivan & Decker, 2005).

Path-Goal Theory

House derived the path-goal theory from the expectancy theory. The expectancy theory argues that people act as they do because they expect

their behavior to produce satisfactory results. In the path-goal relationship, the leader facilitates task accomplishment by minimizing obstructions to the goals and by rewarding followers for completing their tasks. The leader helps staff associates assess needs, explores alternatives, helps associates make the most beneficial decisions, rewards personnel for task achievement, and provides additional opportunities for satisfying goal accomplishment.

House noted that studies done during the 1950s revealed that leaders who structured activities for staff associates generally had more productive work groups and got higher performance evaluations from superiors. Structure includes planning, organizing, directing, and controlling through activities such as clarifying expectations of staff associates, scheduling work, making assignments, determining procedures, and setting standards. Structured activity can increase motivation by reducing role ambiguity and allowing for externally imposed controls. In contrast, considerate leaders had more satisfied workers. They created an atmosphere of friendliness, warmth, and support by tending to the personal welfare of their subordinates. Leader consideration seems particularly important for routine jobs. People who perform a variety of tasks may find their jobs more satisfying and have less need for social support.

House recognized that individual differences will affect the staff members' perception of leader behavior. For instance, experienced staff members may prefer a task-oriented style, whereas less mature, less experienced, and consequently less secure individuals may prefer a considerate leader. Staff members with a high need for achievement probably will prefer a task-oriented leader, but people with a high need for affiliation will prefer a considerate leader. The path-goal theory introduced staff members as a variable (House, 1971; Sullivan & Decker, 2005; Yoder-Wise & Kowalski, 2006).

> *"Instruction does much, but encouragement does everything."* —Johann Wolfgang von Goethe

Situational Leadership Theory

In situational leadership theory, the leader looks at the different variables surrounding the situation to make the best choice in terms of leadership style. Paul Hersey and Kenneth Blanchard developed the Situational Leadership Model with four quadrants depicting leadership styles (Figure 7-1). The vertical axis indicates relationship behavior from low supportive behavior to high supportive behavior; the horizontal axis depicts directive behavior from low (left) to high (right). The relationship behavior and the directive behavior are used in response to the follower's readiness, as illustrated beneath the four-quadrant model.

In the lower right quadrant (S1), the follower lacks both the ability to perform the task and the willingness to do so. The leader should appropriately then make the decisions and supervise the follower closely. In the upper right quadrant (S2), the follower shows increasing ability but still is not performing at a sustained and acceptable level. The follower may also be committed to the project and/or really want to do a good job and so should receive a high amount of supportive behavior and direction from the leader. The leader makes the decisions but incorporates suggestions from the follower into the process. The upper left quadrant (S3) shows the follower who has the ability and skill necessary for a project but lacks the confidence to perform. Thus, the follower requires a high amount of supportive behavior from the leader to bolster confidence. The lower left quadrant (S4) is the delegating style where the follower has the ability and commitment to sustain a project with minimal directives from the leader. The leader is still involved in the decision-making process, but the follower is in charge of the project. To determine the most appropriate leadership style, the leader must assess the follower's readiness on each task and adapt each style to correspond to the follower's readiness level.

Chris Argyris's immaturity-maturity continuum indicates that as people mature, they progress from a passive to an active state and from dependence to independence. With maturity, they pass from a need for structure and little relationship, through a decreasing need for structure and increasing need for relationship, and to little need for either. The progression is not always smooth. Stress may cause members of the group to regress, and leaders must adjust their behavior accordingly. Situational theories therefore emphasize the importance of the maturity level of individuals or the group, and the leader needs to adapt leadership styles accordingly (Hersey, 1984; Hersey & Blanchard, 1969; Hersey, Blanchard, & Johnson, 2007; Hersey & Duldt, 1989; Huber, 2006; Yoder-Wise & Kowalski, 2006).

Transactional Leadership

Transactional leadership focuses on management tasks and trade-offs to meet goals. It is an exchange posture that identifies the needs of followers and provides rewards to meet those needs in exchange for expected performance. It is a contract for mutual benefits that has contingent rewards. The leader or manager is a caretaker who sets goals for employees, focuses on day-to-day operations, and uses management by exception. It is a competitive, task-focused approach that takes place in a hierarchy. It tends to maintain the status quo through policies, procedures, routinized performance, self-interests, and interpersonal dependence (Bass, 1990; Huber, 2006;

Situational Leadership®
LEADER BEHAVIORS

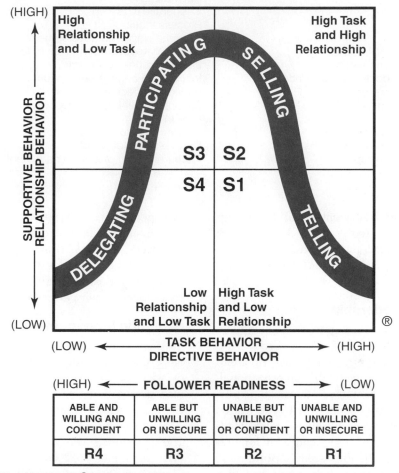

Figure 7-1 • Situational Leadership® Model. (Reprinted with permission of the Center for Leadership Studies, Inc., Escondido, CA 92025. Copyright 2006.)

Marquis & Huston, 2006; Sullivan & Decker, 2005; Yoder-Wise & Kowalski, 2006).

Transformational Leadership

Transformational leadership is inspirational leadership that promotes employee development, attends to needs and motives of followers, inspires through optimism, influences changes in perception, provides intellectual stimulation, and encourages follower creativity. The leader is a role model who uses individualized consideration, provides a sense of direction, and encourages self-management. Transformational leadership is a cooperative, process-focused networking that is led by valuing, visioning, coaching, empowering, team building, and promoting quality. Attributes essential for leadership are identity, independence, authenticity, responsibility, courage, and integrity. Table 7-4 summarizes the key points of several views of

TABLE 7-4 Comparison of Transactional and Transformational Leadership

Transactional	Transformational
Hierarchy	Networking
Competitive	Cooperative
Task focus	Process focus
Exchange posture	Promote employee development
Identify needs of followers	Attend to needs and motives of followers
Provide rewards to meet needs	Inspire through optimism
Exchange for expected performance	Influence change in perception
Contract for mutual benefits	Provide intellectual stimulation
Contingent rewards	Encouragement of follower creativity
Caretaker	Role model
Set goals for employees	Individualize consideration
Focus on day-to-day operations	Provide sense of direction
Management by exception	Encouragement of self-management

transactional and transformational leadership (Bass, 1985; Bass, Avolio, 1993; Burns, 1978; Kouzes & Posner, 2007; Posner & Kouzes, 1988; Huber, 2006; Marquis & Huston, 2006; Sullivan & Decker, 2005).

Integrative Leadership Model

From a review of leadership theories, obviously there is no one best leadership style. Leaders are rarely totally people oriented or task oriented. Intrapersonal, interpersonal, organizational, cultural, physical, mental, emotional, and spiritual perspectives are all important. The leader, the follower, the situation—all influence leadership effectiveness. Consequently, an integration of leadership theories seems appropriate. Leaders need to be aware of their own behavior and influence on others, individual differences of followers, group characteristics, motivation, task structures, environmental factors, and situational variables and adjust their leadership style accordingly. Integrative leadership is a wholistic approach to oneself and others that requires adaptive behavior.

DEVELOPMENT OF MANAGEMENT THOUGHT

A familiarity with the development of management thought can be useful to nursing leaders in creating their own management styles. No single management theory is sufficient in itself to guide the nursing leader's every action, but through an eclectic approach, drawing from the best and most applicable theories in each situation, nurse administrators can create individual management styles to meet their particular needs (Table 7-5).

Scientific Management

Theories of management do not remain static. Since the introduction of the earliest principles of scientific management over a century ago, management thought has been marked by constant change. Scientific management started around 1900 with stopwatch studies to identify efficiency. The key theorists were Taylor, Gilbreths, and Gantt (Marquis & Huston, 2006: Roussel, Swansburg, & Swansburg, 2006; Sullivan & Decker, 2005).

Taylor

Frederick Taylor (1856-1915) is generally recognized as the father of scientific management. Through the use of stopwatch studies, he applied the principles of observation, measurement, and scientific comparison to determine the most efficient way to accomplish a task (Taylor, 1903, 1911).

Gilbreth

Frank Gilbreth (1868-1924) and Lillian Gilbreth (1878-1972) also did pioneering work in time-and-motion studies. They emphasized the benefits of job simplification and the establishment

TABLE 7-5 Development of Management Thought

Scientific Management 1900-	Classic Organization 1930-	Human Relations 1940-	Behavioral Science 1950-	Transformational 1980-	Servant Leadership 1990-	Learning Organizations 1990-	Emotional Intelligence 1995-	Results-Based Leadership 1995-	Chaos or Quantum Leadership 2000-
Taylor *Father of Scientific Management*	Fayol *Father of Management Process*	Hawthorne studies *Work Norms*	Maslow *Hierarchy of Needs*	Bass *Transformational Leadership*	Robert Green-leaf and others	Sange and others	Goleman and others	Welch and others	Porter-O'Grady Wheatley and others
Gilbreths *Time motion studies*	Weber *Father of Organizational Theory*	Lewin *Group Dynamics*	Herzberg *Two Factory Theory*	Bennis, Nanus, and Goldsmith *Lead vs. Manage*					
Gantt *Gantt chart*	Conceptualized *Bureaucracy*	Moreno *Sociogram*	McGregor *Theory X & Y*						
			Ouchi, Pascale, and Athos *Japanese Management, Theory Z*						
			Argis *Personal & Organizational Needs*						
			Likert *Likert Scale and Participative Management, Linking Pin Concept*						
			Blake and Mouton *Managerial Grid*						
			Fiedler *Contingency Theory*						
			Hersey and Blanchard *Situational Leadership Model*						
			Drucker *Management by Objectives*						
			Peters *Manage Ambiguity*						
			Kotter *Leadership and Change*						

of work standards, as well as the effects of incentive wage plans and fatigue on work performance.

The Gilbreths also developed the flow diagram and the process chart to record their observations. The work process was diagrammed to indicate operations, delays, inspection, transportation, and storage, and the process was then studied to shorten, combine, or eliminate steps. The Gilbreths recommended written instructions to prevent misunderstandings and started a merit-rating system for workers (Gilbreth, 1909, 1911; Gilbreth & Gilbreth, 1917).

Lillian Gilbreth is known as the first lady of management. Her doctoral dissertation was published with the author listed as L.M. Gilbreth, thus obscuring the fact that she was a woman. It was one of the first contributions toward understanding human factors in industry. Her work on the effects of fatigue complemented her husband's efforts (Gilbreth, 1914; Gilbreth & Gilbreth, 1919). The Gilbreths and their 12 children are the subjects of the popular book *Cheaper by the Dozen* (Gilbreth, Carey, & McKay, 1984).

Gantt

Henry Gantt (1861-1919), a disciple of Taylor, also was concerned with problems of efficiency. He contributed to scientific management by refining previous work rather than introducing new concepts. The Gantt chart, a forerunner of the PERT (program evaluation and review technique) chart, depicts the relationship of the work planned or completed on one axis to the amount of time needed or used on the other. Gantt also developed a task and bonus remuneration plan whereby workers received a guaranteed day's wage plus a bonus for production above the standard to stimulate higher performance. Gantt recommended that workers be selected scientifically and provided with detailed instructions for their tasks. He argued for a more humanitarian approach by management, placing emphasis on service rather than profit objectives, recognizing useful nonmonetary incentives such as job security, and encouraging staff development (Gantt, 1916, 1919).

Classic Organization

Classic administration-organization thinking began to receive attention in 1930. Deductive rather than inductive, it views the organization as a whole rather than focusing solely on production. Managerial activities are classified as planning, organizing, and controlling. The concepts of scalar levels, span of control, balance of authority with responsibility, accountability, unity of control, line-staff relationships, decentralization, and departmentalization became prevalent. Key theorists of the classic organization era were Fayol and Weber (Marquis & Huston, 2006; Roussel, Swansburg, & Swansburg, 2006; Sullivan & Decker, 2005).

Fayol

Henri Fayol (1841-1925) studied the functions of managers and concluded that management is universal. All managers, regardless of the type of organization or their level in the organization, have essentially the same tasks: planning, organizing, issuing orders, coordinating, and controlling.

He believed in the division of work and argued that specialization increases efficiency. Fayol recommended centralization through the use of a scalar chain or levels of authority, responsibility accompanied by authority, and unity of command and direction so that each employee receives orders from only one superior. He believed that although individual interests should be subordinated to agency interest, workers should be allowed to think through and implement plans and should be adequately remunerated for their services. Fayol encouraged development of group harmony through equal treatment and stability of tenure of personnel. A firm believer in order, he advocated "a place for everything and everything in its place." He also urged that management be taught in the colleges (Fayol, 1925).

Weber

Max Weber (1864-1920) earned the title of "father of organization theory" by his conceptualization of bureaucracy with emphasis on rules instead of individuals and on competence over favoritism as the most efficient basis for organization. He conceptualized a structure of authority that would facilitate the accomplishment of the organizational objectives.

Human Relations

"There is something that is much more scarce, something finer far, something rarer than ability. It is the ability to recognize ability." —Anonymous

The human relations movement began in the 1940s with attention focused on the effect individuals have on the success or failure of an organization. Classic organization and management theory concentrates on the physical environment and fails to analyze the human element; human relations theory stresses the social environment. The chief concerns of the human relations movement are individuals, group process, interpersonal relations, leadership, and communication. Instead of concentrating on the organization's structure, managers encourage workers to develop their potential and help them meet their needs for recognition, accomplishment, and sense of belonging. Mayo, Lewin, and Moreno were the leaders for the human relations era (Marquis & Huston, 2006; Roussel, Swansburg, & Swansburg, 2006; Sullivan & Decker, 2005).

The Hawthorne Studies

The Hawthorne studies, done 1924 to 1932, although criticized for poor research methods, stimulated considerable interest in human problems on the job. Conducted at the Chicago Hawthorne plant of Western Electric by Elton Mayo and researchers from Harvard University, the studies investigated the effects of changes in illumination on productivity. Lighting was changed for the experimental group but remained constant for the control group. As the illumination was increased for the experimental group, the production of both groups increased. When it was decreased for the experimental group, production continued to increase for both groups until the level of illumination reached

moonlight, at which point there was a significant decrease in output for both groups. The researchers concluded that lighting had little effect on production. The effects of the number and length of work breaks, refreshments, length of workdays and workweeks, temperature, and humidity were observed on five volunteers with little or no effects shown. A group piecework incentive plan was studied. The researchers anticipated that fast workers would pressure slow workers to increase their output. However, they found that group norms were set and workers were pressured not to be rate busters by overproducing or chiselers by underproducing. Workers slacked off when it became apparent that they could meet the rate for the day. Work norms obviously had more influence than wage incentive plans. The Hawthorne studies gave the human relations movement its thrust (Mayo, 1953; Marquis & Huston, 2006; Roussel, Swansburg, & Swansburg, 2006; Sullivan & Decker, 2005).

Lewin

In the early 1930s, Kurt Lewin (1890-1947) revived the study of group dynamics. Lewin maintained that groups have personalities of their own: composites of the members' personalities. He showed that group forces can overcome individual interests. He confirmed the importance of group control over output, coined the terms *life space, space of free movement,* and *field forces* to describe group pressures on individuals, and became known as the founder of modern social psychology.

Lewin advocated democratic supervision. His research indicated that democratic groups in which participants solve their own problems and have the opportunity to consult with the leader are most effective. Autocratic leadership, on the other hand, tends to promote hostility and aggression or apathy and to decrease initiative. Conducting experiments during World War II to change people's eating habits to include consumption of more organ meats, he found that only 3% of the women who attended lectures (autocratic method) changed their behavior, but 32% of the women who participated in a discussion after the lecture (democratic method) started eating more organ meats (Lewin, 1951; Sullivan & Decker, 2005).

Moreno

Jacob Moreno (1889-1974) developed sociometry to analyze group behavior. Claiming that people are attracted to, repulsed by, or indifferent toward others, he developed the sociogram to chart pairings and rankings of preferences for others. This process of classification can be used to calculate which workers are capable of harmonious interpersonal relationships. With this knowledge, work groups can be organized with a predicted minimum of disruptive tendencies for maximal efficiency and for promotion of high morale. Moreno also contributed to psychodrama (individual therapy), sociodrama (related to social and cultural roles), and role-playing techniques for the analysis of interpersonal relations.

Behavioral Science

During the 1950s, advocates of the behavioral sciences became concerned that much scientific, classic, and human relations management theory had been accepted without scientific validation. Behavioral science emphasizes the use of scientific procedures to study the psychological, sociological, and anthropological aspects of human behavior in organizations. Behavioral scientists indicate that management is not strictly a technical process, that it cannot be haphazard, and that it should not be executed through authority. Rather, they stress the importance of maintaining a positive attitude toward people, training managers, fitting supervisory actions to the situation, meeting employees' needs, promoting employees' sense of achievement, and obtaining commitment through participation in planning and decision making.

Maslow

Abraham Maslow (1908-1970) initiated the human behavioral school in 1943 with his development of a hierarchy-of-needs theory. He outlined a hierarchical structure for human needs classified into five categories: (1) physiological, (2) safety, (3) belonging, (4) esteem, and (5) self-actualization. The physiological needs are the most important and the most necessary for survival. They include the needs for oxygen, water, food, sleep, sex, and activity. Safety includes freedom from various kinds of danger, threat, and deprivation, such as physical harm, economic distress, ill health, and unnecessary, unexpected occurrences. Belonging needs are composed of affectionate relations with others, acceptance by one's peers, recognition as a group member, and companionship. Esteem comprises self-respect, positive self-evaluation, and regard by others. Self-actualization is composed of self-fulfillment and achievement of one's full capacity. In Maslow's hierarchy, physical needs must be met before other needs become prepotent and so on, and the satisfaction of self-actualization needs is possible only after all other needs are met. Once a need is satisfied, it is no longer a motivator and the next need becomes prepotent. As a need begins to be satisfied, it decreases in importance as a motivator in relation to other needs, some of which are never completely satisfied and never completely cease to motivate.

Maslow's work has been very influential in management and has stimulated subsequent research. Although Maslow's outline is correct in general, human needs are more complex than a simple listing would indicate. Because no two people are alike, needs vary in type and intensity from one person to another. People differ in the amount of gratification needed before the next goal becomes prepotent. For example, some people do well with 6 hours of sleep per day, but others need 10 hours to function. Varying degrees of importance may be placed on the needs dependent on cultural and individual differences. One person may desire recognition, whereas a sense of belonging to a group may be more important to someone else. People do tend to attach importance to what they do not have. It is socially more acceptable to request that physical needs be met than that social or psychological goals receive attention. The process of motivation is complicated by the fact that one's needs change.

When one accepts a job, the pay, work hours, and geographical location may be prepotent. Soon after, the social needs and need for achievement and recognition may become prepotent. People also meet their needs in different ways. Some people may get recognition for the quantity and quality of work they produce, whereas others may get even more attention through negative behavior such as inferior work and tardiness. There are some situations that seem to defy Maslow's theory. Although most of us will eat if we are hungry, some people fast to achieve higher-level needs, or creativity may seemingly override all other needs for some time. Maslow's work marked the beginning of behavioral science. Much subsequent work has been based on his theory (Maslow, 1970; Huber, 2006; Marquis & Huston, 2006; Roussel, Swansburg, & Swansburg, 2006; Sullivan & Decker, 2005) (see Figure 4-1).

Herzberg

Frederick Herzberg (1923-2000) and his colleagues used the critical-incident method in 1959 to interview 200 Pittsburgh-area engineers and accountants about job situations that they had found satisfying or dissatisfying. The stories were analyzed according to content and classified according to the job factors each contained. The researchers found that job factors in situations associated with satisfaction were different from job factors in situations associated with dissatisfaction. The motivators or satisfiers identified were achievement, recognition, work itself, responsibility, advancement, and the potential for growth. These job-content factors (factors in the job) can raise the level of performance and meet the higher-order needs (see Figure 4-2). In Maslow's hierarchy-of-needs model, the hygiene factors or dissatisfiers identified were supervision; company policy; working conditions; interpersonal relations with superiors, peers, and subordinates; status; job security; and effect on one's personal life. These job-context factors (surrounding environmental factors) cannot motivate but can lower performance and cause job dissatisfaction. They meet lower-order needs in Maslow's model (see Figure 4-3).

Herzberg's theory is very controversial and has stimulated considerable research, some of which supports the theory and some of which does not. His work has been the subject of much criticism. For example, he studied only two jobs and used only one measure of job attitude. No validity or reliability data were reported. Statements of critical incidents were subject to memory loss and selective perception. The mere fact that one is more likely to blame others than oneself when asked about an unpleasant experience but is willing to assume the responsibility when something good happens could explain Herzberg's findings. No observations or measurement of job behavior were taken, and Herzberg could have identified wrong categories and misclassified highly subjective stories. Herzberg did, however, develop a taxonomy of job situations based on research that has contributed to a better understanding of human motivation. His work complements Maslow's (Herzberg, 1977; Herzberg, Mausner, & Snyderman, 1959; Huber, 2006; Marquis & Huston, 2006, Roussel, Swansburg, & Swansburg, 2006; Sullivan & Decker, 2005).

McGregor

Douglas McGregor (1906-1964) developed the managerial implications of Maslow's theory. He notes that one's style of management depends on one's philosophy of humans and categorizes those assumptions as Theory X and Theory Y. In Theory X the manager's emphasis is on the goal of the organization. The theory assumes that people dislike work and will avoid it; consequently, workers must be directed, controlled, coerced, and threatened so that organizational goals can be met. According to Theory X, most people want to be directed and to avoid responsibility because they have little ambition. They desire security. Managers who accept the assumptions of Theory X will do the thinking and planning with little input from staff associates. They will delegate little, supervise closely, and motivate workers through fear and threats, failing to make use of their potentials.

In Theory Y the emphasis is on the goal of the individual. It is the manager's assumption that people do not inherently dislike work and that work can be a source of satisfaction. Theory Y managers assume that workers have the self-direction and self-control necessary for meeting their objectives and will respond to rewards for the accomplishment of those goals. They believe that under favorable conditions people seek responsibility and display imagination, ingenuity, and creativity. According to Theory Y, human potentials are only partially used. Managers who believe the assumptions of Theory Y will allow participation. They will delegate, give general rather than close supervision, support job enlargement, and use positive incentives such as praise and recognition (see Table 4-2).

McGregor suggests that when people are unable to satisfy their higher-level needs, they experience personal frustrations resulting in negative behaviors. Some managers have responded to the consequences of the personal frustration with punitive measures without determining the cause. Managers with a human relations orientation have made working conditions pleasant and have provided rewards unrelated to job performance. McGregor believes that both approaches are ineffective and recommends that the work situation be structured so that workers can meet their personal goals while working toward the goals of the organization. He suggests collaboration between the manager and the worker for integration of goals. Table 7-6 shows the relationships among the Maslow, Herzberg, and McGregor theories (McGregor, 1960; Huber, 2006; Marquis & Huston, 2006; Roussel, Swansburg, & Swansburg, 2006; Yoder-Wise & Kowalski, 2006).

Ouchi, Pascale, and Athos

William Ouchi (1943-) contrasts Japanese organizations with organizations in the United States. The Japanese organizations have "lifetime employment; slow evaluation and promotion; nonspecialized career paths; implicit control mechanisms; collective decision making; collective responsibility; and wholistic concern," whereas the organizations in the United States have "short-term employment;

TABLE 7-6 Relationships among the Maslow, Herzberg, and McGregor Theories

Maslow	Herzberg	McGregor
Physiological needs	Hygiene factors	Theory X
Safety needs	Motivators	Theory Y
Belonging needs		
Esteem needs		
Self-actualization needs		

Modified from Kelly J: *Organizational behaviour*, rev ed, Homewood, IL, 1980, Irwin, p. 220. Copyright by Richard D. Irwin.

rapid evaluation and promotion; specialized career paths; explicit control mechanisms; individual decision making; individual responsibility; and segmented concern" (Ouchi, 1981, pp. 48-49; Marquis & Huston, 2006; Roussel, Swansburg, & Swansburg, 2006). Pascale and Athos explain that organizations in the United States tend to favor strategy, structure, and systems, whereas the Japanese organizations focus on staff, skills, style, and superordinate goals (Pascale & Athos, 1981).

Argyris

Chris Argyris (1923-), focusing his research on the coexistence of personal and organizational needs, found that individuals give priority to meeting their own needs. He found that the greater the disparity between individual and organizational needs, the more tension, conflict, dissatisfaction, and subversion result. Argyris recommends that leaders help workers achieve self-actualization by implementing a Theory Y philosophy, and he maintains that this will help one's personality to grow from passivity and dependence to activity and independence. Incongruency between the mature personality and management based on classic principles makes workers subordinate, dependent, and passive, thereby causing psychological failure and job dissatisfaction. Managers can make jobs more meaningful by taking advantage of people's talents and letting them participate in planning, goal setting, and problem solving, thus creating learning organizations (Argyris, 1953, 1957, 1964, 1993, 1999, 2006;

Argyris, Putnam, & Smith, 1985; Argyris & Schon, 1978; Marquis & Houston, 2006).

Likert

Rensis Likert's (1903-1981) theory of management is based on his work at the University of Michigan's Institute for Social Research. He identified three types of variables in organizations: (1) causal, (2) intervening, and (3) end result. The causal variables include leadership behavior, organizational structure, policies, and controls. Intervening variables are perceptions, attitudes, and motivations. The end-result variables are measures of profits, costs, and productivity. Likert believed that managers may act in ways harmful to the organization because they evaluate end results to the exclusion of intervening variables. Consequently, he developed a Likert scale questionnaire that includes measures of causal and intervening variables. The Likert scale measures several factors related to leadership behavior process, motivation, managerial influence, communication, decision-making processes, goal setting, and staff development.

Likert also identified four types of management systems: (1) exploitative-authoritative, (2) benevolent-authoritative, (3) consultative, and (4) participative group. He associated the first system with the least effective performance. Managers show little confidence in staff associates and ignore their ideas. Consequently, staff associates do not feel free to discuss their jobs with their managers. Responsibility for the organization's goals is at the top; goals are established through orders. What little communication is used is directed downward, is often inaccurate, and is accepted with suspicion. Although managers do not know about their staff members' problems, they make decisions without input from below. Policing and punishment are used as control functions by top administration. Allowed no input, the workers strongly resist the organization's goals and develop an informal organization of their own.

In the benevolent-authoritative system, the second type of system, the manager is condescending to staff. Staffs' ideas are sometimes sought, but they do not feel very free to discuss their jobs with their manager. Top management and middle management are responsible for setting goals. There is little communication, and it is mostly directed downward after being censored by the manager and is received with some suspicion. Decisions are made at the top with some delegation. Managers do have some knowledge of the staffs' situation, and staff members are occasionally consulted for problem solving. Goals are established through orders with some comment invited and moderate resistance received. Rewards and punishment are used as control functions by top administration. There is usually an informal organization resisting the formal one.

In the third system, the consultative system, the manager has substantial confidence in staff members. Their ideas are usually sought, and they feel free to discuss their work with the manager. Responsibility for setting goals is fairly general. Although there is considerable communication, both upward and downward, it has limited accuracy and is accepted with some caution. Managers are quite familiar with the problems faced by their staff associates. Broad policy is set at the top with delegation; goals are set after discussion; and there is decision making throughout the organization. Control functions are delegated to lower levels, where reward and self-guidance are used. Sometimes an informal organization resists the formal goals.

Participative management, the fourth system, is associated with the most effective performance. Managers have complete confidence in their staff associates. Staff associates' ideas are always sought, and they feel completely free to discuss their jobs with the manager. Goals are set at all levels. There is a great deal of communication—upward, downward, and sideways—that is accurate and received with an open mind. Managers are very well informed about the problems faced by their staff associates, and the decision making is well integrated throughout the organization with full involvement of staff members. Because goals are established through group action, there is little or no resistance to them. There is not an informal organization resisting the goals of the formal organization because the goals of both are the same. Control is widely shared through the use of self-guidance and problem solving.

Likert was a strong proponent of participative management and supportive relationships. His linking-pin concept is based on studies about the differences between good and poor managers as measured by their level of productivity. Good managers were found to have more influence on their own managers than did poor managers, and their managerial procedures were better received by their staff members. Consequently, Likert suggested that managers form groups for supportive relationships and that those groups be linked by overlapping groups of managers. This facilitates three-way communications—upward, downward, and sideways. When middle managers have the opportunity for interaction with their manager, workers can have input, and there is a chance for the individual's and the organization's goals to become similar (Likert, 1961; Likert & Likert, 1976; Huber, 2006; Roussel, Swansburg, & Swansburg, 2006) (Figure 7-2).

Blake and Mouton

Robert Blake (1918-) and Jane Mouton (1930-1987) maintain that there are two critical dimensions of leadership: (1) concern for people and (2) concern for production. They depict these on a 9 × 9 or 81-square managerial grid (Figure 7-3). The two dimensions are independent, so a manager can be high on both, low on both, or high on one and low on the other. The vertical axis represents the manager's concern for people, and the horizontal axis represents concern for production. Each axis is on a 1 to 9 scale, from a minimal concern for people or production to a maximal concern. The five basic styles are located at each corner and in the middle.

The task manager at 9,1 has the highest regard for production and the lowest concern for people. This manager stresses operating efficiency through controls and views people as tools of production. Workers are paid to do what they are told without questioning.

As reflected on the grid, 1,1 management is impoverished. The manager has a lack of concern for both production and people. This style may be found in some managers who feel they have been repeatedly denied promotion or otherwise mistreated and who have consequently compensated through a low level of involvement with their jobs. The organization man management at 5,5 represents a moderate concern for both people and production but not necessarily at the same time. The manager's emphasis shifts. The country club manager, 1,9, is thoughtful and friendly but has little concern for production.

Blake and Mouton consider team management, 9,9, the optimal managerial style. These managers integrate their concern for people and production. Problems are confronted directly, and mutual trust, respect, and interdependence are fostered (Blake & Mouton, 1964, 1978; Blake & McCanse, 1991; Huber, 2006; Marquis & Huston, 2006; Roussel, Swansburg, & Swansburg, 2006; Yoder-Wise & Kowalski, 2006).

Hersey and Blanchard

Paul Hersey (1930-) and Kenneth Blanchard (1939-) extended the work of Blake and Mouton by considering the readiness of the followers in more detail. As the readiness of one's followers increases, the leadership style requires less structure and emotional support. Groups with below-average readiness function best under leaders with high task–low relationship orientations. Groups with average readiness function best under leaders with high task–high relationship or high relationship–low task orientations. The most effective leadership style depends on the readiness of the group (Hersey, 1984; Hersey & Blanchard, 1969; Hersey, Blanchard, & Johnson, 2007; Hersey & Duldt, 1989; Huber, 2006; Marquis & Huston, 2006; Roussel, Swansburg, & Swansburg, 2006) (see Situational Leadership Theory in this chapter).

Drucker

In his prolific writings about management, Peter Drucker (1909-2005) maintains that the only way for management to justify its existence is through economic results. He introduced

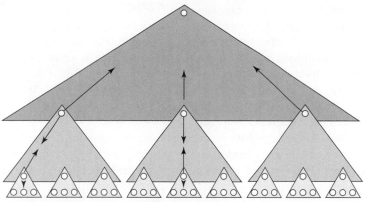

Figure 7-2 • Linking pin concept. Arrows indicate linking-pin function. (From Likert R, Likert JG: *New ways of managing conflict.* New York, 1976, McGraw-Hill.)

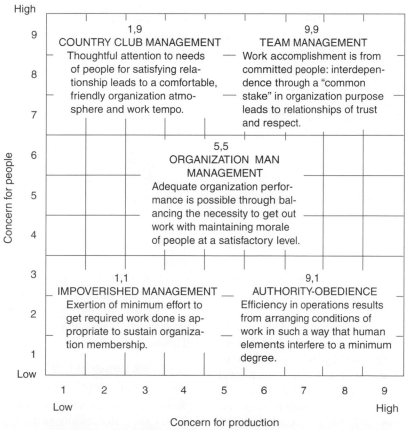

Figure 7-3 • Managerial grid. (From Blake RR, Mouton JS: *The new managerial grid.* Houston, 1978, Scientific Methods, Inc.)

management by objectives as a way to manage managers. Relying on self-control instead of control from above, managers are directed by objectives of performance rather than by their manager. For management by objectives, the manager develops the framework, and the staff associate supplies the goals, which are agreed on by both. The staff associate gives progress reports to the manager. Objectives are developed for every level of management in the hierarchy and each unit in the organization. The manager checks objectives for compatibility with other units and contribution to the objectives at the next level of the hierarchy. Drucker maintains that it is more productive for workers to set their own norms and measure their own performance than for minimal standards to be set.

Drucker recommends that jobs be designed to fit the worker, that workers be given more control over their jobs, and that the worker be considered the most vital resource in the agency. He has stressed the importance of managing for the future. He believes it is pointless to predict the future. By the late 1990s he was indicating the importance of managing society's knowledge resources (Drucker, 1964, 1974, 1980, 1985, 1986, 1992, 1995, 1998, 2001, 2003, 2005; Marquis & Huston, 2006; Roussel, Swansburg, & Swansburg, 2006).

Peters

Tom Peters has been provocative during the 1980s and 1990s through seminars and several books. He and others have stressed the importance of managing ambiguity and paradox, having a bias for action to get things done, remaining close to the customer to know his or her needs and anticipate wants, fostering autonomy and entrepreneurship, reinforcing shared values by celebrating heroes, getting productivity through people, demonstrating values through direct interventions, keeping to what you know instead of widely diversifying, keeping a simple form and lean staff, and the importance of having a passion and searching for excellence through team-based innovations (Peters 1987, 1992, 1994, 1997; Peters & Austin, 1985; Peters & Waterman, 1982).

Kotter

John Kotter has reported his research about topics related to leadership in a number of books. His research is primarily about traits, management, change, and transactional issues (Kotter, 1982, 1985, 1988, 1990, 1996, 2002).

Transformational Leadership

Transformational leadership became popular during the 1980s and 1990s with stress on the need for leadership versus management, the importance of values, and a commitment to service (Huber, 2006; Marquis & Huston, 2006; Roussel, Swansburg, & Swansburg, 2006; Sullivan & Decker, 2005).

Bass

Bernard Bass identified the need for charisma, inspirational leadership, individualized consideration, and intellectual stimulation to have transformational leadership instead of just transactional or a contingent reinforcement leadership. He indicated that women are more inclined to transformational leadership than men (Bass, 1985, 1998; Bass & Avolio, 1993).

Bennis, Nanus, and Goldsmith

Warren Bennis has stressed the importance of leading rather than just managing, described how people become leaders, and described characteristics of great groups. He and Burt Nanus lead a paradigm shift to transformative leadership. They discussed the need to manage oneself to lead others, attention through vision, meaning through communication, trust through positioning, deployment of self, and empowerment (Bennis, 1989, 1997; Bennis & Goldsmith 1997; Bennis & Nanus, 1985) (see the Bibliography located on the Evolve site for the work of Anderson, Black, Blanchard, Collins, Kouzes, Posner, and Tichy).

Servant Leadership
Greenleaf and Others

Robert Greenleaf wrote *Servant Leadership* (1977, 1991). He conceptualized the idea of the servant as leader from Hermann Hesse's *The Journey to the East* (1956), in which the servant who does the menial chores also sustained the party's spirits through his extraordinary presence. When the servant left the group, the group fell into disarray and the journey was abandoned. Servant leadership puts serving first, takes a holistic approach, shares decision making, and builds community.

> The servant leader is servant first.... It begins with the natural feeling that one wants to serve, to serve first. Then conscious choice brings one to aspire to lead... The difference manifests itself in the care taken by the servant—first to make sure that other people's highest priority needs are being served (Greenleaf, 1991).

Larry Spears has identified 10 characteristics of the servant-leader by studying Greenleaf's work: (1) listening, (2) empathy, (3) healing, (4) awareness, (5) persuasion, (6) conceptualization, (7) foresight, (8) stewardship, (9) commitment to the growth of people, and (10) building community. Spears has edited several anthologies about servant leadership (Spears, 1995, 1998a, 1998b, 2002; Huber, 2006; Marquis & Huston, 2006; Sullivan & Decker, 2005) (see the Bibliography located on the Evolve site for related work by Autry, Block, Covey, DePree, Jeffries, Jaworski, McGee-Cooper, McKee, Moxley, Northouse, Palmer, Peck, Pohlman & Gardiner, Rinehart, and Vaill) (Box 7-3).

Greenleaf says the test of servant leadership is "Do those served grow as persons; do they, while being served, become healthier, wiser, freer, more autonomous, more likely themselves to become servants? And, what is the effect on the least privileged in society; will he benefit, or, at least, will he not be further deprived?" (Greenleaf, 1991 p. 7).

Learning Organizations

> *As for the best leaders, the people do not notice their existence. The next best, the people honor and praise. The next the people fear; and the next, the people hate. When the best leader's work is done, the people say, "We did it ourselves"* —Lao tzu

---

BOX 7-3 Characteristics of Servant Leaders

Listening
Empathy
Healing
Awareness
Persuasion
Conceptualization
Foresight
Stewardship
Commitment to the growth of people
Building community

BOX 7-4 Five Disciplines of a Learning Organization

Systems thinking
Personal mastery
Mental models
Shared vision
Team learning

Senge and Others

Peter Senge discusses five disciplines: (1) systems thinking, (2) personal mastery, (3) mental models, (4) shared vision, and (5) team learning and tools and strategies to build a learning organization (Senge, 1990; Senge, Kleiner, Roberts, et al, 1994; Marquis & Huston, 2006) (Box 7-4). They address participation as a basis of learning to prevent organizational learning disabilities instead of participation as an entitlement. Senge's beliefs about systems thinking have been influenced by many people and books (see the Bibliography located on the Evolve website for related books by Belasen, Capra, Chapel, Conger, Gray, Harvey, Miller, Schaffer, Schein, Sims, Tannen, and Wheatley).

Emotional Intelligence
Goleman and Others

Daniel Goleman's emotional competence framework identifies self-awareness, self-regulation, and motivation as important to personal competence, and empathy and social skills as important to social competence. He stresses the importance of teaching emotional competence and gives guidelines for training, including how to assess the job, assess the individual, deliver assessments with care, gauge readiness, motivate, make change self-directed, focus on clear and manageable goals, prevent relapse, give performance feedback, encourage practice, arrange support, provide models, encourage, reinforce change, and evaluate (Goleman, 1995, 1998; Goleman, Boyatzis, & McKee, 2002; Huber, 2006). Emotional intelligence is more important than intelligence quotient (IQ) or technical expertise for success in organizations (Ryback, 1998).

Goleman, Boyatzis, and McKee (2002) identified the necessary emotional intelligence competencies as (1) visionary to mobilize others to follow a vision through self-confidence, empathy, change catalyst, and visionary leadership; (2) affiliative to create harmony through empathy, building bonds, and conflict management; (3) democratic to build commitment through participation; (4) coaching to build strengths for the future through developing others, empathy, and emotional self-awareness; (5) coercive for immediate compliance to kick start a turnaround through achievement, drive, initiative, and emotional self-control; and (6) pace setting to perform tasks to a high standard through conscientiousness, achievement drive, and initiative (Box 7-5).

Feldman (1999) indicated that leaders need core skills for effective individual contribution plus higher-order skills. He identified the five core skills as (1) knowing yourself (recognizing your emotions, differentiating between emotions, knowing the reason behind the emotion), (2) maintaining control (resisting or delaying an impulse, drive, or temptation to act; controlling aggression, hostility, and irresponsible behavior; managing emotions in a flexible and adaptable way), (3) reading others (being aware of the emotions of others, appreciating the emotions of others, understanding how and why people feel and act as they do), (4) perceiving accurately (accurately assessing a situation, having clear vision, keeping a broad perspective, being objective), and (5) communicating with flexibility (having a full range of emotional expression, being authentic, addressing your

---

BOX 7-5 Emotional Intelligence Competencies

Visionary: To mobilize others to follow a vision through self-confidence, empathy, change catalyst, and visionary leadership

Affiliative: To create harmony through empathy, building bonds, and conflict management

Democratic: To build commitment through participation

Coaching: To build strengths for the future through developing others, empathy, and emotional self-awareness

Coercive: For immediate compliance to kick-start a turnaround through achievement, drive, initiative, and emotional self-control

Pacesetting: To perform tasks to a high standard through conscientiousness, achievement, drive, and initiative

---

needs as well as the needs of others) (Box 7-6). In the 1990s, attention turned to action management, results-based leadership, and the accountability revolution.

Results-Based Leadership
Welch and Others

Under Jack Welch's (1935-) leadership, General Electric became a benchmark for excellence. He did it in three stages: destruction, creation, and quality. During the 1980s he globalized the company, especially into Europe and Japan. During the late 1980s, he introduced "work out." He had workers tell managers what was wrong and make suggestions for improvements. The goals were to build trust, empower employees, eliminate unnecessary work, and create a boundaryless culture by tearing down the walls between management and workers and between functions such as marketing and production. He started with relatively short-lived change instead of incremental change. To create the boundarylessness, he (1) listened to the people closest to the customers; (2) gave people who did the work a say in how the work could be done better; (3) lowered boundaries among vertical (hierarchical relationships), horizontal (between functions), external (suppliers and customers), and geographic (different countries) structures,

> ### BOX 7-6 Emotional Intelligence Core Skills
>
> Knowing yourself (recognizing your emotions, differentiating between emotions, knowing the reason behind the emotion)
>
> Maintaining control (resisting or delaying an impulse, drive, or temptation to act; controlling aggression, hostility, and irresponsible behavior; managing emotions in a flexible and adaptable way)
>
> Reading others (being aware of the emotions of others, appreciating the emotions of others, understanding how and why people feel and act as they do)
>
> Perceiving accurately (accurately assessing a situation, having clear vision, keeping a broad perspective, being objective)
>
> Communicating with flexibility (having a full range of emotional expressions, being authentic, addressing your needs as well as the needs of others)

realizing that not all the answers were within the company walls; and (4) implemented the best ideas no matter where they originated. He hired "A" leaders who could articulate a vision and rally workers to take responsibility to make the vision a reality. Those "A" leaders had "Four E's": energy, edge, energizer, and execution. He did not tolerate managers who used intimidation. He nurtured only those leaders who shared the company's vision and harnessed the power of change. He searched out confident managers who put the customer first. They used learning to build confidence, moved decision making down the hierarchy, and let employees know that their ideas were valued. He met with his managers on a regular basis. They used story boards to give attention to the best practices. Welch fired 10% of the least productive workers each year. He recommended simplifying practices and procedures. Limiting the number of approvals needed and the number of pages in forms streamlined processes.

In the mid-1990s, Welch started the product services focus that generated revenues and Six Sigma, an employee-driven quality movement. Quality became an issue for everyone in the organization. The six ingredients in Six Sigma were as follows: (1) a genuine focus on the customers, (2) a data-driven management, (3) a management- and improvement-focused process, (4) a proactive management, (5) boundaryless collaboration, and (6) a drive for perfection with a tolerance for failure. The four-step process included measuring, analyzing, improving, and rigorously controlling each process and transaction once it had been improved. People learned that strategy cannot be reduced to a formula, and that long-range plans should not be followed blindly. In the late 1990s after watching his employees order Christmas presents online, Welch got the company into the e-business movement.

Recurring themes from Welch's leadership include the following: (1) leaders who live the values are more important than those who make the numbers; (2) command and control are not the best ways to run an organization; (3) ideas should rule over tradition and hierarchy; (4) involving everyone is a key to enhancing productivity; (5) developing a learning community creates a competitive enterprise; and (6) market-leading business can ensure long-term growth (Crainer, 1999; Kramer, 2001; Pande, Neuman, & Cavanaugh, 2002; Slater, 1999, 2000; Welch & Byrne, 2001; Welch & Welch, 2005). Others had similar ideas about results based leadership (see the Bibliography located on the Evolve website for related books by Bossidy, Buckingham, Perkins, Redwood, Samuel, and Ulrich) (Box 7-7).

Chaos or Quantum Leadership

Proponents of chaos theory believe that the universe is not orderly and that things do not progress in a linear fashion. Much of nature moves in a circular and ebbing manner. Disturbances create disequilibrium that can lead to growth. Nature is self-organizing and self-renewing. A distinguishing feature of a self-renewing organization is that it has resiliency instead of stability (Wheatley, 1992). Life tries to find what works and uses messes to arrive at better solutions because messes can be opportunities. It is good for us to be authentic, support each other, and to thrive on our differences (Wheatley & Keller-Rogers, 1996).

Quantum leadership is about using curiosity to ask questions and discover the process. It requires creativity, flexibility, and breakthrough thinking to solve problems. Leadership is about the journey and helping others deal with changes. Leaders need to do horizontal thinking and develop relationships. We need to create more fluid boundaries. The system works from the point of service outward. Each worker should add value to the activities. Leaders should plan for error, and manage risks and relationships. Leaders should notice changes through interacting with others. Anticipating the next step and helping others understand it is important (Porter-O'Grady & Malloch, 2003) (Box 7-8).

DIVERSITY AMONG LEADERS

Diversity

Diversity should be defined in a broad and inclusive way to prevent widespread opposition. Employees should understand that everyone's diversity is valued. Diversity can affect individuals' values, perceptions of self and others, and opportunities at work. Primary dimensions include age, ethnicity, gender, mental and physical abilities, race, and sexual orientation. Secondary dimensions include communication style, education, family status, first language, geographical location, income, military experience, organizational role, religion, work experience, and work style. Organizations should value primary and secondary diversity.

At first, organizations focus on expectations, norms, and operating assumptions. As the organization moves up the continuum of diversity implementation, diversity in styles, communications, and problem solving gains greater acceptance. Marilyn Loden (1996) identified five segments of a diversity adoption curve: innovators, change agents, pragmatists, skeptics, and traditionalists. Adoption is sped up by compatibility, high relative advantage, observability, simplicity, and testability. Adoption is slowed down by complexity, incompatibility, little or no relative advantage, little observability, and little or no testability. The different concerns and

---

BOX 7-7 Recurring Themes of Results-Based Leadership

Leaders who live the values are more important than those who make the numbers.
Command and control are not the best ways to run an organization.
Ideas should rule over tradition and hierarchy.
Involving everyone is a key to enhancing productivity.
Developing a learning community creates a competitive enterprise.
Market-leading business can ensure long-term growth.

BOX 7-8 Activities of Quantum Leaders

Ask questions.
Discover the process.
Have creativity.
Have flexibility.
Do breakthrough thinking to solve problems.
Take the journey.
Help others deal with changes.
Do horizontal thinking.
Develop relationships.
Create more fluid boundaries.
Work from the point of service outward.
Add value to the activities.
Plan for error.
Manage risks and relationships.
Notice changes through interacting with others.
Anticipate the next step.
Help others understand.

---

needs of all segments of the diversity should be considered in a plan to ensure a rapid and successful adoption.

It seems to be the diversity mind-set that separates effective facilitators from those who merely pay lip service to the need to implement diversity. The valuing diversity mind-set includes the idea that diversity benefits all and is good for individuals as well as the company.

Diversity must be inclusive, requires investment of time and human resources, and requires a long-term culture change. Building support among those who are willing to adopt change while minimizing involvement of resistant people helps minimize backlash. Building a business case of the strategic and financial arguments for valuing diversity will help strengthen the adoption. Although excellent training will not ensure cultural change, inappropriate training can harm diversity efforts. Focusing on the common needs for inclusion, opportunity, and respect can help close the gaps among diverse employee groups. Administrative support is the single most important factor for predicting implementation success (Box 7-9).

Segmentation helps adoption occur more quickly with less confusion and less conflict. Innovators generally look for opportunities to create. Change agents are among the first to try out new ideas and are interested in self-learning. Pragmatists are suspicious about the practicality of change and tend to wait rather than move quickly. They want to know that something is "good for the people." Skeptics are predisposed to delay implementation of change. They start considering change when they find themselves out of sync with mainstream values. Traditionalists tend to totally avoid involvement. They need ongoing repetitive endorsements from leaders about the strategic importance and adoption of change as less painful than continued resistance (Box 7-10).

The timing and content of training should differ for different segments. Loden identifies best practices across organizations as follows: (1) setting the context for change, (2) providing ongoing communication, (3) focusing on data-driven change, (4) providing awareness and skill-based training, (5) encouraging ongoing learning, (6) multicultural mentoring, (7) providing flexible benefits and scheduling, (8) linking rewards to effective diversity management, and (9) building common ground.

Gender Differences

In the classic book *The Managerial Woman*, Hennig and Jardim (1966, 1977) discussed why women are at a comparative disadvantage to men for advancement in companies; how they are socialized to be a nurse, not a doctor, or a secretary, not a boss; and how "queen bees," women who have

> **BOX 7-9** Common Needs Regarding Diversity
>
> Inclusion
> Opportunity
> Respect

> **BOX 7-10** Segmentation for Adoption
>
> Innovators
> Change agents
> Pragmatists
> Skeptics
> Traditionalists

made it to the top, do not want to share their power with other women. Harragan (1977) described games that still exist, making it difficult for women to advance in business. Ashley (1976) spoke specifically to hospitals, paternalism, and the role of the nurse. Melia (1986) indicated that it was women keeping women out of the boardroom because men stab each other in the back for gain, but women do it just to do it.

With the help of Equal Opportunity Employment legislation, women have been able to make an impact in business. Morrison, White, and Van Velsor (1987) did a 3-year study to determine success or derailment factors in breaking the glass ceiling. The glass ceiling is a transparent barrier that few women had been able to break. They found that men and women did not score differently on most factors measured.

There are differences in male and female leadership styles. Women tend to be more democratic and participative by sharing enlightened power and information, encouraging consultation, creating connections, enhancing group members' self-worth, and boosting emotional well-being. They use their interpersonal skills, authenticity, charisma, and networking to influence others toward the accomplishment of goals (Coughlin, Wingard, & Hollihan, 2005). Many women prefer to discuss while most men prefer to make decisions (Gray, 1992).

Anecdotal information suggested that stages of motherhood may teach people about qualities of leadership. Traits of maternal leadership demonstrated by 50 successful business women included sensitivity, warmth, patience, full attentiveness, adaptability, tolerance, and staying positive (Grzelakowski, 2005).

Men tend to be more direct and autocratic. They use the organization's formal authority structure and their positions as their power base. With the organizational trends from competitive individualism, secrecy, and control toward trust, teamwork, and information sharing, women seem well equipped for leadership beyond the 2000s.

To know how women manage differently from men, Helgesen needed to know how men manage. She referred to Mintzberg's 1968 dissertation, which was published in 1973 as *The Nature of Managerial Work*. Mintzberg followed five male executives through their days and found that they worked at a relentless pace without breaks. Their days were filled with interruptions, discontinuity, and fragmentation. They had little time for activities not directly related to their work. They had a preference for live action encounters and maintained a complex network of relationships with people outside the organization. They immersed themselves in their jobs, had little time for reflection, had difficulty sharing information, and identified with the job.

Helgesen (1990) did diary studies on four women, two of whom are entrepreneurs. She found that women worked at a steady pace with small breaks throughout the day. The pace was steady and fast but not frantic. The subjects did not view unscheduled tasks as interruptions. They made time for activities not directly related to their work. They did not sacrifice important family time or restrict their reading to work-related items. They preferred live action but did schedule time to read the mail. They too maintained a complex network of relationships with people outside the organization. They focused on the ecology of leadership, scheduled time to share information, and saw their identities as complex and multifaceted. Men have been socialized to work sun up to sun down, whereas women know their work is never done. Women's

work is cyclical and unending. They are process oriented and get pleasure from doing the work instead of getting it done. Women repeatedly used the metaphor of voice. They lead with voice. Helgesen found that the most successful women executives knew they had complex identities with various roles in both public and private life.

Entry of women into the public arena has been occurring at the same time as rapid economic and technological change. The postindustrial economy has been influenced by women who are pioneers in new ways of learning and who improvise their own lives instead of just conform to the needs of large organizations (Helgesen, 1998).

Rosener (1995) telephone interviewed executive men across the United States. A content analysis revealed four working relationships: supervising women, working with women as peers, competing with women, and working for women. The major issues of concern for the men were loss of power and control, loss of male identity and self-esteem, and increasing discomfort or sexual static. Faludi (1991) chronicled the resentment of women's accomplishments that is characterized by antagonism and scapegoating. She found that some angry white men believe that women's growing presence in the workforce is depriving them of well-paying jobs and job security.

She also found that women have some of the same career aspirations and receive challenging assignments, but taking time off for family reasons continues to be a problem for them. The men thought that women bring attention to detail, compassion, different perspectives, sensitivity, and a willingness to work hard to the job. Black men felt differently about working with women. They are sympathetic about the underutilization of women in the workforce but also think women have taken jobs away from them. There is a need for corporations to increase gender awareness through specific training, including role playing, videos, case studies, and skill development. The female underutilization is worldwide. The number of Japanese women with career aspirations is quite small, and there is an increase in Japanese women requesting to be assigned abroad. American and British women, especially married women, feel underutilized. Some believe that women are the greatest undeveloped natural resource in the world.

One can provide bosses with what they need, study leaders in the organization, read profiles and biographies of achievers, develop one's own talents into expertise, make one's self visible, and work in a safe environment by joining professional and civic organizations (Rosener, 1995). Brooks and Brooks (1997) indicated that successful people (1) realize the importance of a mentor/advocate/cheerleader/coach, (2) know how to increase their visibility, (3) know how to develop an effective network, (4) have learned to communicate effectively, (5) know how to balance work and home, (6) know when to take smart risks, and (7) understand the politics of the organization. O'Brien, O'Brien, and Martin (1998) say a key to success is finding a culture that matches one's values.

Catalyst (1998) indicates that efforts to maximize women's talents will probably be successful only if an organization takes a comprehensive, problem-solving approach. Both internal and external benchmarking of women's advancement should be done. Internal research allows companies to establish the current status of women in the organization by reviewing recruitment, retention, and advancement data; develop short- and long-term goals for improvement after the baseline has been determined; and evaluate the effectiveness of the initiatives that were generated from the benchmarking by measuring and reporting the progress toward specific goals (see the Bibliography located on the Evolve site for related work by Enkles, Giberd, Hochschild, Kanter, Nichols, and Scheele).

Racial Differences

William Wilson (1994) identifies three stages of race relations in the United States: (1) plantation economy and racial-caste oppression; (2) industrial expansion, class conflict, and racial oppression; and (3) progressive transition from racial inequalities to class irregularities. Racial

diversity is visible and subject to stereotyping (in which the person is viewed as a member of a group and the images others have about that group are ascribed to the person), and prejudice (when predetermined negative attitudes toward people are based on a group identity).

Taylor Cox and Ruby Beale (1997) identify numerous ways of developing competency to manage diversity, including providing awareness training; providing opportunities for in-house trainers; creating interorganizational relationships with organizations with different dominant groups; providing some support for on- and off-site dialogue meetings; providing a reading list on diversity; sponsoring cultural diversity celebrations; sponsoring events to facilitate mentor-protege matchups; providing overseas assignments; allowing time for travel or sponsoring travel for career development; providing financial support for college courses about diversity, foreign language courses, and national conferences on diversity; sponsoring cultural social events; creating diversity task forces; sponsoring educational activities and diversity roundtables; integrating cultural diversity issues into staff meetings; and helping employees obtain requested job assignments.

The working environment is often lonely and unfriendly for nontraditional managers. Sometimes people of color and women have information withheld from them to sabotage them. They may have trouble finding role models and mentors. They may lack organizational savvy, take comfort in working with persons in similar situations, have difficulty balancing career and family, get a backlash from threatened white males, have infighting from the oppressed group, and have to deal with prejudice. Agencies should give management training. Helping new managers get acquainted with key workers so they will feel comfortable dealing with them later is important (Morrison, 1992).

Sexual Orientation Differences

Same sex (lesbian, gay), and both sexes (bisexual) orientations are more invisible from opposite sex (heterosexual) orientations than some other minorities. The law protects against sexual orientation discrimination including recruitment, hiring, training, promotion, status, pay, benefits, transfer opportunities, and dismissal. Indirect discrimination such as having a conference in a country where homosexuality is illegal is unlawful even if it was not done intentionally. One is also protected against harassment by association with another person such as a gay or lesbian friend. Same-sex couples in some states can register a civil union that entitles the same benefits as a married couple for such benefits as insurance and survivor benefits in a company policy. Some employers may ask for sexual orientation information to monitor policies or as part of an equal opportunities questionnaire, but one is not required to give that information (Schwartz & Conley, 2001).

Disabilities

Many disabilities are visible and affect people at different chronological ages with a variety of physical disabilities. The Rehabilitation Act of 1973, required all government-contracted employers granted more than $25,000 funding to take affirmative action to recruit, hire, and advance qualified disabled people. There was slow progress in getting companies to hire people with disabilities, but there has been steady progress. In 1990, Congress passed the Americans with Disabilities Act to eliminate discrimination against people with physical or mental disabilities in the work place. The act is closely related to the Civil Rights Act of 1964 and incorporates the antidiscrimination principles of the Rehabilitation Act of 1973. This law includes people with cancer, diabetes, human immunodeficiency virus (HIV), and acquired immunodeficiency (AIDS), as well as recovering substance abusers and people with obvious physical disabilities. The law protects persons with disabilities unless they are not qualified or are unable to do a job.

Defining disability eligibility has been an issue and has stimulated a number of lawsuits. Conditions that have not been found to constitute a disability have included (1) pregnancy, *Jessie v. Carter Health Care Centers, Inc., 1996*; (2) erratic behavior, *Webb v. Mercy Hospital, 1996*; (3) lifting disability, *Thompson v. Holy Family Hospital, 1997*; (4) medicated for depression, *Wilking v. County of Ramsey, 1997*; and (5) depression and anxiety, *Cody v. Cigna Healthcare of St. Louis, Inc., 1998*. The court did not require job restructuring for a person who qualified for other jobs not requiring the accommodations, *Mauro v. Borgess Medical Center, 1995*. The person must be able to meet the qualifications for employment like the ability to work rotating shifts, *Laurin v. Providence Hospital and Massachusetts Nurses Associaton, 1998*, and ability to restrain psychiatric patients, *Jones v. Kerrville State Hospital, 1998*. The employer is required to inform a disabled person when a person is qualified by making reasonable accommodations but is not required to hire the disabled person before fully qualified, nondisabled people, *Zamudio v. Patia, 1997* (Finkelman, 2006; Marquis & Huston, 2006; Sullivan & Decker, 2006; Yoder-Wise & Kowalski, 2006).

Disability is quite common, at about 20% of Americans. Blindness, deafness, learning disabilities, and mobility impairment are common. While about two thirds of unemployed people with disabilities say they would like to work, only about a third of disabled people ages 18 to 64 work full or part time. Over 80% of nondisabled people ages 18 to 64 are employed. Applicants with disabilities have indicated that they have been refused job interviews, turned down for jobs for which they are qualified, given lesser responsibilities than others, passed over for promotions, and denied health insurance. When people come to onsite interviews, they should be asked if they need any accommodations with the understanding that outward manifestations of disability do not mean there is diminished human capacity. People can do much work through computer conferencing, electronic mail, and by telephone without revealing their disabilities (Rothman, 2003; Schwartz & Conley, 2001; Szymanski & Parker, 2003).

FOLLOWERSHIP

"If you think you are leading and no one is following you, then you are just taking a nice walk." —*John Maxwell*

One cannot lead without followers, and followers need leaders. Great followers as well as great leaders are needed, and team efforts are often highly valued. People may be leaders at times and followers at other times. Leaders get work done through others and may be better leaders because they also know how to follow. Leaders contribute only about 20% to the success of organizations. Followers contribute the remaining 80%. People spend more time reporting to others than having others report to them. Some leaders became leaders by having been such good followers by volunteering for tasks, willingly accepting assignments, voicing differences of opinions, and making suggestions, (but supporting the group's decision and displaying loyalty to the group) that their peers have asked them to take on leadership responsibilities.

Effective followers view themselves as equals of the leaders and work for the common good. Conformist followers believe they must always please the boss, and alienated followers tend to snipe at leaders. Less effective followers have a limited worldview, mainly considering their own needs and rarely considering the pressures the leader has. Excellent followers work cooperatively with leaders rather than as adversaries (Frisina, 2005).

Effective followers do not always agree with the leader but are likely to use the following guidelines: When disagreeing with the leader, discuss the disagreement privately rather than in a public forum. Do not approach the leader during a crisis or deadline. Present the situation as a joint problem, not as the leader's stupid idea. Go to the meeting with potential solutions. Take the leader's point of view into consideration when brainstorming alternatives. Do not go to the leader while angry, because that is likely to escalate conflict (Box 7-11).

BOX 7-11 Guidelines for Followers

Discuss the disagreement privately rather than in a public forum.
Do not approach the leader during a crisis or deadline.
Present the situation as a joint problem, not as the leader's stupid idea.
Go to the meeting with potential solutions.
Take the leader's point of view into consideration when brainstorming alternatives.
Do not go to the leader while angry.

Followers do maintain independent and critical thinking. They may be vigilant about unchecked leaders by: (1) being proactive, (2) gathering the facts, (3) seeking wise counsel and listening before taking a stand, (4) building one's fortitude by focusing, (5) working within the system, following channels of communications and responsibilities, identifying one's expectations of the leader and one's own responsibilities and positions, (6) framing one's position so it can be heard, (7) educating others on how one's view serves others' best interests, (8) supporting and challenging one's leader and the group, (9) taking collective action; if one meets leader resistance, one may seek higher authority, and (10) having the financial and emotional cushions to exercise other alternatives (Ellis & Hartley, 2004; Finkelman, 2006; Huber, 2006).

CHARACTER DEVELOPMENT

"Always do right. That will gratify some of the people, and astonish the rest." —*Mark Twain*

There is an increased focus on ethics and the need for character development resulting from a rise in violence; increasing lying, cheating, and stealing; growing disrespect for authority figures; increasing peer cruelty; a rise in prejudice and hate crimes; a deterioration of language; a decline in the work ethic; declining personal and civic responsibility; increasing self-destructive behaviors such as premature sexual activity, substance abuse, and suicide; and the growing ethical illiteracy (Center for the 4th and 5th Rs, 2007a).

There are a variety of approaches to moral and character education. First, some ignore it. Second, some take a value-neutral approach and assume that no values or character traits are more valid than others. Third, some assume that moral and character decisions are made rationally and teach a decision-making process. Fourth, some use the approach that changing thinking will lead to changes in behavior and engage students and professionals in discussion of moral issues. It is the change in behavior that differentiates values education from character education. Fifth, some teach students and professionals are given a set of values and accompanying appropriate actions. Sixth, some use the inculcation, values education, analysis, and moral development approaches and have students and professionals put their thoughts and feelings into actions through a variety of social actions. This approach involves action learning, service learning, and community service. The combination of approaches includes the volition and action aspects of character development that are not present in values education (Huitt, 2004).

Character Education Partnership's 11 principles of effective character education could be modified for health care as: (1) character development promotes core ethical values as the basis of good character, (2) character must be comprehensively defined to include thinking, feeling, and behavior, (3) effective character development requires an intentional, proactive, and comprehensive approach that promotes the core values in all phases of life, (4) the organization must be a caring community, (5) to develop character, staff need opportunities for moral action, (6) effective character development includes a meaningful and challenging curriculum staff development program that respects all learners and helps them succeed, (7) character development should strive to develop peoples' intrinsic motivation, (8) the organization must become a learning and moral community in which all share responsibility for character development and attempt to adhere to the same core values that guide the organization, (9) character development requires moral leadership from both management and staff, (10) the organization must recruit staff and community members as full partners in the character-building effort, and (11) evaluation of character development should assess the character of the organization, the staff's functioning as character factors, and the extent to which staff manifest good character (Character Education Partnership, 2005).

Allen Elementary School is an inner-city school in Dayton, Ohio, where more than 60% of the students lived in single-parent families and more than 70% of the families received public assistance. The faculty had trouble teaching because of the discipline problems. The faculty started a word of the week program to promote a different value each week. Values promoted included cheerfulness, citizenship, cleanliness, courage, courtesy, helpfulness, honesty, kindness, loyalty, patience, punctuality, respect, responsibility, self-control, self-reliance, sportsmanship, thrift, and tolerance. Students brainstormed examples of the behaviors and had short homeroom discussions about the word of the week. Teachers tried to connect classroom activities to the word. Students were sent to the principal's office for compliments about their exemplary ways. A newsletter was sent to parents with discussion topics and bedtime story suggestions to promote the week's value. Within 2 years, student respect and other behaviors had markedly improved, suspensions dropped, teacher absenteeism decreased, PTA funding increased, and faculty relationships improved through staff development and trust building (Center for the 4th and 5th Rs, 2007b). Other words that have been associated with character development include accountability, caring, compassion, cooperation, excellence, integrity, perseverance, promise keeping, loyalty, self-discipline, truthfulness, fairness, faith, friendship, justice, and citizenship. The education examples can be adapted to nursing. The organization's mission, philosophy, values, and goals help visualize the values and can help structure a character development atmosphere. Rules and procedures help clarify expected behaviors. Staff can learn together by brainstorming and discussing virtues periodically through staff meetings and staff development programs. Bennett's (1993) *The Book of Virtues* is a collection of moral stories. Short selections could be selected and discussed. Staff can also be encouraged to do community service through the health care organization's outreach to the community (Yoder-Wise & Kowalski, 2006) (Box 7-12).

NURSING ADMINISTRATION TODAY

Several documents are very influential for forming nursing administration today. Nursing's Social Policy Statement (American Nurses Association [ANA], 2003) addresses the social context of nursing, values and assumptions of nursing's social contract, the knowledge base for nursing practice, and self-, professional-, and legal regulation of nursing practice (Nursing Power. Net, 2007). The Code of Ethics for Nurses (ANA, 2001) presents nine provisions related to respect for human dignity, primacy of the patient's interest, confidentiality, accountability and responsibility, moral behavior and responsibility, advancing the profession, responsibilities to the public, and assertion of values. It makes clear that a nurse's primary responsibility is to the patient and secondly to the institution. All nurses but especially nursing leaders have a responsibility to improve health care environments and working conditions (American Nurses Association, 2001).

The American Nurses Association (1996) leaders identified scope and standards for nurse administrators. The American Organization of Nurse Executives (AONE) developed a list of competencies needed by executive leaders. The document defined major competencies including communication, relationships building, health care environment, business skills, and leadership (AONE, 2005). The American Association of Colleges of Nursing (AACN) and AONE

BOX 7-12 Characteristics for Moral Development
Cheerfulness
Citizenship
Cleanliness
Courage
Courtesy
Helpfulness
Honesty
Kindness
Loyalty
Patience
Punctuality
Respect
Responsibility
Self-control
Self-reliance
Sportsmanship
Thrift
Tolerance

(1997) leaders did a joint position statement that addressed educational context for nurse administrators. It supported interdisciplinary work, augmenting nursing core courses with courses from other fields such as business, economics, sociology, psychology, or health services administration. It specified the need for information about information systems, leadership, marketing, negotiations, policy development, and strategic planning. The Council on Graduate Education for Administration in Nursing Education in Nursing's Essentials for Master's Education also addressed graduate education preparation for nursing administration.

AACN leaders have published *Hallmarks of the Professional Nursing Practice Environment*, which outlines characteristics of the practice setting that best supports professional nursing practices (American Association of Colleges of Nursing, 2002). AACN leaders, in partnership with practice partners, initiated the concept of a lateral integrator of care for coordinating a group of patients and providing direct care in complex situations (American Association of Colleges of Nursing, 2007; Tornabeni, 2006). Many colleges and schools of nursing have started clinical nurse leader education in masters programs.

One agency has implemented a modified version of the clinical nurse leader and evaluated the pilot using nurse-sensitive indications such as nurse recruitment and retention, nurse job satisfaction, patient and physician satisfaction, and patient length of stay. The results showed positive trends for all of the nurse sensitive indicators (Smith, Manfredi, Hagos, Drummong-Huth, Moore, 2006). Another agency has also done a pilot project and has made some adaptations to enhance outcomes. Filling clinical nurse leadership positions with nurse practitioners is a consideration (Bowcutt, Wall, & Goolsby, 2006).

Sigma Theta Tau International leaders have suggested four different categories for education and scope of practice reflecting the level of education and practice. A level would be for unlicensed care providers, B for a post-licensure with an internship, C for a residency, and D for graduate education. B and C are recommended to have distinctively different registered nurse licenses. One is to be able to advance from C to D by getting graduate education (Robert Wood Johnson Foundation, 2002). This discussion is ongoing. Regulatory agencies and state boards of nursing greatly influence the education and practice of nursing and would have to approve of the changes for licensing and scope of practice before they could be implemented (Yoder-Wise & Kowalski, 2006).

Leadership and management are both components of nursing administration. Nursing leadership is broader than management and is inspirational for doing the right things. It does overlap some with management, which is more process oriented for doing things right. Management is transforming from a more step-by-step approach to an interactive process type of leadership (Angelucci, 2005; Huber, 2006). George, Sims, McLean, and Mayer (2007) have addressed the importance of authentic leadership that emerges when leaders use their own life stories and find their own voices. Amcona, Malone, Orlikowski, and Senge (2007) praise incomplete leaders who make up for their own weaknesses by surrounding themselves with people who have the skills the leaders are lacking. Ibarra and Hunter (2007) discuss the importance of creating and using networks, and the importance of who one knows as well as what one knows to get desired outcomes. Managers do need to spend some time away from the analytical tasks to develop relationships with people who can help implement the organizational strategies. Evidence-based practice and the use of intuition are also important for leadership and management (see Chapter 8). Health care economics (see Chapter 9), globalization (see Chapter 10), innovation (see Chapter 11), succession (see Chapter 12), and safety as related to the nursing shortage and getting magnet status (see Chapters 13 and 15) are major topics of discussion in the 2000s.

RESEARCH Perspective 7-2

Data from Sherman R: Growing our future nursing leaders. *Nurs Admin Q* 29(2):125-132, 2005.

Purpose: The purpose of this study was to learn which factors influence young nurses to accept or reject nursing leadership positions. There is a need for leadership succession.

Methods: This qualitative research study used focus groups with 48 nurses under age 40 that were not in nursing leadership positions. A consensus process was used to identify and prioritize the factors that influence their decisions to accept or reject leadership positions.

Results/conclusions: Adequate compensation and decision-making power were issues of concern for these younger nurses. Feedback they received from current nursing leaders was not positive. It is important to recruit younger nurses into leadership positions to replace older nursing leaders who will be retiring.

CHAPTER SUMMARY

Theories can be very practical, and a good theory can be universal and applied in numerous situations. Some of the research done by people in various disciplines over the past few decades can still provide a basis for evidence-based nursing leadership and management. By surveying the history of the development of management thought, one can see that there has been a trend from autocratic to democratic management and from a focus on efficiency to a greater regard for the well-being of personnel. Although the focus has changed, elements from each era maintain their validity and can be used by the nurse administrator. Leaders cannot lead without followers. People may be leaders at times and followers at other times. A leader may be a better leader for knowing how to be a good follower. Leaders are diverse, but all are responsible for creating desirable working conditions. Character development activities may be used to facilitate a supportive environment.

By studying leadership theories and the development of management thought, a nurse administrator can define one's leadership role, develop one's philosophy of management, learn tools and techniques for implementation of one's responsibilities, and gain an increased understanding of how to work with others to accomplish goals through evidence-based practice.

CRITICAL THINKING ACTIVITY

Reflective Journal: Make observations in a clinical setting, or reflect on past experiences. Answer the following questions: How would you describe your leadership style? What are some leadership styles you have observed? Did they seem appropriate to the situation, and why? To what styles do you respond best? How could you become a more transformational leader?

CASE STUDY

You are a new patient care coordinator. The previous one was very autocratic. How will you begin changing from the autocratic atmosphere to a participative style?

ONLINE RESOURCES

evolve Additional critical thinking activities, worksheets, and case studies are available online at http://evolve.elsevier.com/Marriner/guide8e.

REFERENCES

Amcona D, Malone TW, Orlikowski WJ, Senge PM: In praise of the incomplete leader, *Harvard Business Review* 85(2):92-100, 2007.

American Nurses Association: *Code of ethics for nurses with interpretive statements*, 2001 (on-line publication): www.nursingworld.org/ethics/chcode. htm. Accessed February 2, 2007.

American Association of Colleges of Nursing: *Hallmarks of the professional nursing practice environment*, 2002 (website): www.aacn.nche.edu/Publications/ positions/hallmarks.htm. Accessed August 12, 2007.

American Association of Colleges of Nursing: *The clinical nurse leader*, 2007 (website): www.aacn.nche.edu/ CNL. Accessed August 12, 2007.

American Association of Colleges of Nursing, American Organization of Nurse Executives: *Joint position statement on nursing administration education*, Washington, DC, 1997, AACN.

American Nurses Association: *Scope and standards for nurse administrators*, Washington, DC, 1996, The Association.

American Nurses Association: *Code of ethics for nurses with interpretative statements*, Washington, DC, 2001, The Association.

American Nurses Association: *Nursing's social policy statement*, ed 2, Washington, DC, 2003, The Association.

American Organization of Nurse Executives: AONE nurse executive competencies, *Nurse Leader* 3(1):15-21, 2005.

Angelucci P: For leadership effectiveness, look inside, *Nursing Management* 36(11):12-15, 2005.

Argyris C: *Executive leadership*, New York, 1953, Harper & Bros.

Argyris C: *Personality and organization*, New York, 1957, Harper & Bros.

Argyris C: *Integrating the individual and the organization*, New York, 1964, John Wiley & Sons.

Argyris C: *Knowledge for action*, San Francisco, 1993, Jossey-Bass.

Argyris C: *On organizational learning*, Malden, MA, 1999, Blackwell Publishers.

Argyris C: *Reasons and rationalizations: The limits to organizational knowledge*, United Kingdom, 2006, Oxford Press.

Argyris C, Putnam R, Smith DM: *Action science*, San Francisco, 1985, Jossey-Bass.

Argyris C, Schon DA: *Organizational learning: A theory of action perspective*, Reading, MA, 1978, Addison-Wesley.

Ashley JA: *Hospitals, paternalism, and the role of the nurse*, New York, 1976, Teachers College Press.

Bass BM: *Leadership and performance beyond expectations*, New York, 1985, Free Press.

Bass BM: From transactional to transformational leadership: Learning to share the vision, *Organizational Dynamics Winter:*19-31, 1990.

Bass BM: *Transformational leadership: Industry, military, and educational impact*, Mahwah, NJ, 1998, Lawrence Erlbaum Associates, Publishers.

Bass BM, Avolio BJ: Transformational leadership and organizational culture, *Publ Admin Q* 17:112-121. Spring, 1993.

Bennett WG: *The book of virtues*, NY, 1993, Simon & Schuster.

Bennis W: *On becoming a leader*, Reading, MA, 1989, Addison-Wesley.

Bennis W: *Organizing genius*, Reading, MA, 1997, Perseus Books.

Bennis W, Goldsmith J: *Learning to lead: A workbook on becoming a leader*, Reading, MA, 1997, Perseus Books.

Bennis W, Nanus B: *Leaders: The strategies for taking charge*, New York, 1985, Harper & Row.

Bennis W, Nanus B: *Leaders: The strategies for taking charge*, London, 2007, Collins.

Blake RR, McCanse AA: *Leadership dilemmas—Good solutions*, Houston, 1991, Gulf.

Blake RR, Mouton JS: *The new managerial grid*, Houston, 1964, Gulf.

Blake RR, Mouton JS: *The new managerial grid*, Houston, 1978, Gulf.

Blank W: *The 108 skills of natural born leaders*, New York, 2001, AMACOM.

Bowcutt M, Wall J, Goolsby MJ: The clinical nurse leader: Promoting patient-centered outcomes, *Nursing Administration Quarterly* 30(2):156-161, 2006.

Brooks DL, Brooks LM: *Seven secrets of successful women*, New York, 1997, McGraw Hill.

Burns J: *Leadership*, New York, 1978, Harper & Row.

Burns JM: *Transforming leadership: A new pursuit of happiness*, New York, 2004, reprint, Grove Press.

Catalyst: *Advancing women in business—The catalyst guide*, San Francisco, 1998, Jossey-Bass.

Center for the 4th and 5th Rs, 2007a (website): www.cortland.edu. Accessed August 12, 2007.

Center for the 4th and 5th Rs: *Word of the week*, 2007b (website): www.cortland.edu/character/success/success04.htm. Accessed June 6, 2007.

Character Education Partnership: *Eleven Principles of Effective Character Education*, 2005 (website): www.character.org. Accessed August 12, 2007.

Cody v. Cigna Healthcare of St. Louis, Inc, 139F. 3d 595 (8th Cir. 1998).

Conger J, Kanungo R: *Charismatic leadership in organizations*, Newbury Park, CA, 1998, Sage.

Coughlin L, Wingard E, Hollihan K, editors: *Enlightened power: How women are transforming the practice of leadership*, San Francisco, 2005, Jossey-Bass.

Cox T, Beale RL: *Developing competency to manage diversity*, San Francisco, 1997, Berrett-Koehler.

Crainer S: *Business the Jack Welch way: 10 secrets of the world's greatest turnaround king*, New York, 1999, AMACOM.

Donnelly JH Jr, Gibson JL, Ivancevich JM: *Fundamentals of management functions, behavior, models*, Dallas, 1981, Business Publications.

Drucker P: *Managing for results: Economic tasks and risk-taking decisions*, New York, 1964, Harper & Row.

Drucker P: *Innovation and entrepreneurship: Practice and principles*, New York, 1985, Harper & Row.

Drucker P: *The frontiers of management*, New York, 1986, EP Dutton.

Drucker P: *The essential Drucker: The best of sixty years of Peter Drucker's essential wriring on management*, New York, 2003, Collins.

Drucker P: *The daily Drucker: 336 days of insight and motivation for getting the right things done*, New York, 2005, Collins.

Drucker PF: *The essential Drucker: Selections from the management works of Peter F. Drucker*, New York, 2001, Harper Business.

Drucker PF: *Management: Tasks, responsibilities, practices*, New York, 1974, Harper & Row.

Drucker PF: *Managing in turbulent times*, New York, 1980, Harper & Row.

Drucker PF: *Managing for the future: The 1990s and beyond*, New York, 1992, Truman Talley Books/Plume.

Drucker PF: *Managing in a time of great change*, New York, 1995, Truman Talley Books/Dutton.

Drucker PF: *On the profession of management*, Boston, 1998, Harvard Business.

Drucker PF: What executives should remember, *Harvard Business Review* 84(2):144–152, 2006.

Ellis JR, Hartley CL: *Managing and coordinating nursing care*, Philadelphia, 2004, JB Lippincott.

Faludi S: *Backlash: The undeclared war against women*, New York, 1991, Anchor Books/Doubleday.

Fayol H: *Administration industrielle et generale*, Paris, 1925, Dunod.

Feldman D: *The handbook of emotional intelligent leadership: Inspiring others to achieve results*, Falls Church, VA, 1999, Leadership Performance Solutions Press.

Fiedler FE: *A theory of leadership effectiveness*, New York, 1967, McGraw-Hill.

Fiedler FE, Chemers MM: *Leadership and effective management*, Glenview, IL, 1974, Scott, Foresman.

Fiedler FE, Chemers MM, Mahar L: *Improving leadership effectiveness: The leader match concept*, New York, 1976, John Wiley & Sons.

Finkelman AW: *Leadership and management in nursing*, Upper Saddle River, NJ, 2006, Pearson/Prentice Hall.

Frisina M: Learn to lead by following, *Nursing Management* 36(3):13, 2005.

Gantt HL: *Industrial leadership*, New Haven, CT, 1916, Yale University Press.

Gantt HL: *Organizing for work*, New York, 1919, Harcourt, Brace and Howe.

George B, Sims P, McLean AN, Mayer D: Discovering your authentic leadership, *Harvard Business Review* 85(2):129-138, 2007.

Gilbreth FB: *Bricklaying system*, New York, 1909, Myron C Clark.

Gilbreth FB: *Motion study*, New York, 1911, D Van Nostrand.

Gilbreth FB, Carey EG, McKay D: *Cheaper by the dozen*, New York, 1984, Bantam Books.

Gilbreth FB, Gilbreth LM: *Applied motion study*, New York, 1917, Sturgis and Walton.

Gilbreth FB, Gilbreth LM: *Fatigue study*, ed 2, New York, 1919, Macmillan.

Gilbreth LM: *The psychology of management*, New York, 1914, Sturgis and Walton.

Goleman D: *Emotional intelligence*, New York, 1995, Bantam Books.

Goleman D: *Working with emotional intelligence*, New York, 1998, Bantam Books.

Goleman D, Boyatzis R, McKee A: *Primal leadership: Realizing the power of emotional intelligence*, Boston, 2002, Harvard Business School Press.

Gray J: *Men are from Mars, women are from Venus*, New York, 1992, Harper Collins.

Greenleaf RK: *Servant leadership*, New York, 1977, Paulist Press.

Greenleaf RK: *Servant leadership*, New York, 1991, Paulist Press.

Grzelakowski M: *Mothers lead best: 50 women who are changing the way organizations define leadership*, Chicago, 2005, Kaplan Business.

Harragan BL: *Games Mother never taught you: Corporate gamesmanship for women*, New York, 1977, Warner Books.

Helgesen S: *Everyday revolutionaries*, New York, 1998, Doubleday.

Helgesen S: *The female advantage: Women's ways of leadership*, New York, 1990, Bantam Doubleday Dell.

Hennig MM, Jardim A: *The managerial woman*, Garden City, NY, 1966, Anchor Press/Doubleday.

Hennig MM, Jardim A: *The managerial woman*, Garden City, NY, 1977, Anchor Press/Doubleday.

Hersey P: *The situational leader*, New York, 1984, Warner Books.

Hersey P, Blanchard KH: *Management of organizational behavior: Utilizing human resources*, Paramus, NJ, 1969, PrenticeHall.

Hersey P, Blanchard KH, Johnson DE: *Management of organizational behavior ed 9*, Upper Saddle River, NJ, 2007, Prentice Hall.

Hersey P, Duldt BW: *Situational leadership in nursing*, Norwalk, CT, 1989, Appleton & Lange.

Herzberg F: One more time: How do you motivate employees?. In Carroll L, Paine R, Miner A, editors: *The management process*, ed 2, New York, 1977, Macmillan.

Herzberg F, Mausner B, Snyderman BB: *The motivation to work*, ed 2, New York, 1959, John Wiley & Sons.

Hesse H: *The journey to the east*, New York, 1956, Noonday Press.

House RJ: A path-goal theory of leader effectiveness, *Adm Sci Q* 16:321-339, 1971.

Huber DL: *Leadership and nursing care management*, ed 3, St. Louis, 2006, Elsevier.

Huitt WL: *Moral and character development*, Educational Psychology Interactive, Valdosta State University, 2004 (website): http://chiron.valdosta.edu/whuitt/col/morchr/morchr.html. Accessed August 12, 2007.

Ibarra H, Hunter M: How leaders create and use networks, *Harvard Business Review* 859(1):40-47, 2007.

Jessie v. Carter Health Care Center Inc. 926 F. Supp. 613 (E.D. Ken., 1996).

Jones v Kerrville State Hospital, 142 F. 3d 263 (5th Cir., 1998).

Kotter JP: *The general managers*, New York, 1982, Free Press.

Kotter JP: *Power and influence*, New York, 1985, Free Press.

Kotter JP: *The leadership factor*, New York, 1988, Free Press.

Kotter JP: *A force for change*, New York, 1990, Free Press.

Kotter JP: *Leading change*, Boston, 1996, Harvard Business School Press.

Kotter JP: *The heart of change: Real-life stories of how people change their organizations*, Boston, 2002, Harvard Business School Press.

Kramer JA: *The Jack Welch lexicon of leadership*, New York, 2001, McGraw-Hill.

Kouzes JM, Posner BZ: *The leadership challenge,* ed 4, San Francisco, 2007, Jossey-Bass.

Laurin v. Providence Hospital and Massachusetts Nurses Association, 150 F. 3d 52 (1st Cir., 1998).

Lewin K: *Field theory in social sciences ed n/a*, New York, 1951, Harper & Row.

Likert R: *New patterns of management*, New York, 1961, McGraw-Hill.

Likert R, Likert JG: *New ways of managinag conflict*, New York, 1976, McGraw-Hill.

Loden M: *Implementing diversity*, Chicago, 1996, Irwin.

Marquis BL, Huston CJ: *Leadership roles and management functions in nursing*, ed 5, Philadelphia, 2006, Lippincott Williams & Wilkins.

Maslow A: *Motivation and personality*, ed 2, New York, 1970, Harper & Row.

Mauro v. Borgess Medical Center, 494 CV 05 (Michigan, 1995).

Maxwell JC: *The 21 indispensable qualities of a leader: Becoming the person others will want to follow*, Nashville, 1999, Thomas Nelson Publishers.

Mayo E: *The human problems of an industrialized civilization*, New York, 1953, Macmillan.

McGregor D: *The human side of enterprise*, New York, 1960, McGraw-Hill.

Melia J: *Breaking into the boardroom: What every woman needs to know*, New York, 1986, GP Putnam's Sons.

Mintzberg H: *The nature of managerial work*, New York, 1973, Harper & Row.

Morrison AM: *The new leaders*, San Francisco, 1992, Jossey-Bass.

Morrison AM, White R, Van Velsor E: *Breaking the glass ceiling: Can women reach the top of America's largest corporations?* Reading, MA, 1987, Addison-Wesley.

Nursing Power: *Nursing's social policy statement* (summary outline), 2007 (website): www.nursingpower.net/nursing/sps.html. Accessed February 2, 2007.

O'Brien V, O'Brien V, Martin L: *Success on our own terms*, New York, 1998, John Wiley & Sons.

Ouchi WG: *Theory Z: How American business can meet the Japanese challenge*, New York, 1981, Avon Books.

Pande PS, Neuman RP, Cavanaugh RR: *The six sigma way team fieldbook: An implementation guide for project improvement teams*, New York, 2002, McGraw-Hill.

Pascale RT, Athos AG: *The art of Japanese management: Applications for American executives*, New York, 1981, Warner Books.

Peters T: *Thriving on chaos*, New York, 1987, Harper & Row.

Peters T: *Liberation management*, New York, 1992, Fawcett Columbine.

Peters T: *The Tom Peters Seminar*, New York, 1994, Vintage Books.

Peters T: *The circle of innovation*, New York, 1997, Alfred A Knopf.

Peters T, Austin N: *A passion for excellence*, New York, 1985, Warner Books.

Peters T, Waterman RH: *In search of excellence*, New York, 1982, Harper & Row.

Porter-O'Grady T, Malloch K: *Quantum leadership: A textbook of new leadership*, Boston, 2003, Jones and Bartlett.

Posner BZ, Kouzes JM: Development and validation of the leadership practices inventory, *Educational and Psychological Measurement* 53:483-496, 1988.

Posner BZ, Kouzes JM: An extension of the leadership practices inventory to individual contributors, *Educational and psychological measurement* 54: 959-966, 1994.

Robert Wood Johnson Foundation: Radical changes proposed for nursing profession, from licensing to scope of practice, 2002 (website): www.rwjf.org/reports/grr/038622.htm. Accessed August 12, 2007.

Rosener JB: *America's competitive secret: Utilizing women as a management strategy*, New York, 1995, Oxford University Press.

Rothman JC: *Social work practice across disabilty*, Boston, 2003, Allyn & Bacon.

Roussel L, Swansburg FC, Swansburg RJ: *Management and leadership for Nurse Administrators*, ed 4, Boston, 2006, Jones and Bartlett Publishers.

Ryback D: *Putting emotional intelligence to work: Successful leadership is more than IQ*, Boston, 1998, Butterworth-Heinemann.

Schwartz S, Conley C: *Human diversity: A guide for understanding*, New York, 2001, McGraw-Hill Primis Custom Publishing.

Senge PM: *The fifth discipline: The art and practice of the learning organization*, New York, 1990, Doubleday.

Senge PM, Kleiner A, Roberts C, et al: *The fifth discipline fieldbook*, New York, 1994, Doubleday.

Sherman R: Growing our future nursing leaders, *Nursing Admin Q* 29(2):125-132, 2005.

Slater R: *Jack Welch and the GE way: Management insights and leadership secrets of the legendary CEO*, New York, 1999, McGraw-Hill.

Slater R: *The GE way fieldbook: Jack Welch's battle plan for corporate revolution*, New York, 2000, McGraw-Hill.

Smith SL, Manfredi T, Hagos O, Drummond-Huth B, Moore P: Application of the clinical nurse leader role in an acute care delivery model, *Journal of Nursing Administration* 36(1):29-33, 2006.

Spears LC, editor: *Insights on leadership: Service, stewardship, spirit, and servant leadership*, New York, 1998a, John Wiley & Sons.

Spears LC, editor: *The power of servant leadership*, San Francisco, 1998b, Berrett Koehler.

Spears LC, editor: *Reflections on leadership: How Robert K. Greenleaf's theory on servant leadership influenced today's top management thinkers*, New York, 1995, John Wiley & Sons.

Spears LC, Lawrence M, editors: *Focus on leadership: Servant leadership for the 21st century*, New York, 2002, John Wiley & Sons.

Stanley D: Role conflict: Leaders and managers, *Nursing Management* 13(5):31-37, 2006.

Sullivan EJ, Decker PJ: *Effective leadership management in nursing*, ed 6, Upper Saddle River, NJ, 2005, Pearson/Prentice Hall.

Szymanski EM, Parker RM: *Work and disability: Issues and strategies in career development and job placement*, ed 2, Austin, TX, 2003, pro-Ed.

Taylor FW: *Shop management*, New York, 1903, Harper & Bros.

Taylor FW: *The principles of scientific management*, New York, 1911, Harper & Bros.

Thompson v. Holy Family Hospital, 122 F. 3d 357 (9th Cir., 1997).

Tornabeni J: The evolution of a revolution in nursing, *JONA* 36(1):3-6, 2006.

Tourangeau AE, McGilton K: Measuring leadership practices of nurses using the leadership practices inventory, *Nursing Research* 53(3):182-189, 2004.

Webb v. Mercy Hospital, 102 F. 3d 958 (8th Cir., 1996).

Welch J, Byrne JA: *Jack: Straight from the gut*, New York, 2001, Warner Books.

Welch J, Welch S: *Winning*, Scranton, PA, 2005, Collins.

Wheatley M: *Leadership and the new science*, San Francisco, 1992, Berrett-Koehler.

Wheatley MJ, Keller-Rogers M: *A simpler way*, San Francisco, 1996, Berrett-Koehler.

Wilking v. County of Ramsey, 983 F. Supp. 848 (D. Kan., 1997).

Wilson WJ: *The declining significance of race: Blacks and changing American institutions. In Grusky DB: Social stratification*, Boulder, CO, 1994, Westview Press.

Yoder-Wise PS, Kowalski KE: *Beyond leading and managing: Nursing administration for the future*, St. Louis, 2006, Mosby/Elsevier.

Yukl GA: *Leadership in organizations*, ed 3, Gaithersburg, MD, 1994, Aspen.

Zamudio v. Patia, 956 T. Supp. 803 (N.D. Ill., 1997).

PART
TWO

MANAGEMENT

Managers deal with structures, procedures, schedules, performance, and continuity. They may manage a budget, help select and develop personnel, manage a staffing schedule, evaluate and discipline personnel, and assist with continuous quality improvement and evidence-based practice. First-level managers work with nonmanagerial staff and the day-to-day activities, as well as operational planning. Middle-level managers supervise several first-level managers and are the link between them and upper-level management. Upper-level managers are the organizational executives that are responsible for establishing strategic plans and goals for the organization. Managers are responsible for interpreting and enforcing the agency's policies, procedures, and mandates. They need to be outcome oriented through problem solving and team development.

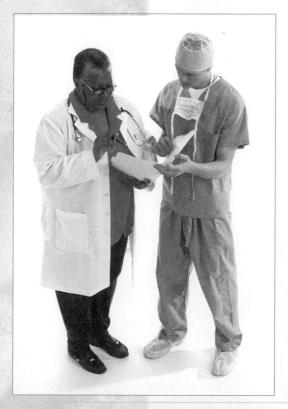

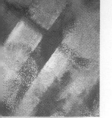

Strategic and Operational Planning

8

"The greatest thing in this world is not so much where we are, but in what direction we are moving." —*Oliver Wendell Holmes*

Chapter Overview

Chapter 8 illustrates the planning process, history of strategic planning, strategic planning process, vision, values, mission, philosophy, goals, objectives, strategies, policies, procedures, and evidence-based practice.

Chapter Objectives

- Identify at least two differences between strategic and operational planning.
- Describe at least five changes in health care delivery systems that should be taken into account in strategic planning.
- Identify at least five benefits of strategic planning.
- Explain the relationships among purpose, philosophy, goals, and objectives.
- Explain the relationship between policy and procedure.
- Summarize the development of evidence-based practice.

Online Resources

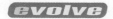 Critical thinking activities, worksheets, and case studies are available online at http://evolve.elsevier.com/Marriner/guide8e.

Major Concepts and Definitions

Strategic planning *long-range planning usually extending 3 to 5 years into the future*

Operational planning *short-range planning that deals with day-to-day maintenance activities*

Belief *conviction that certain things are true*

Vision *mental image of something not actually visible*

Value *the worth, usefulness, or importance of something*

Mission/purpose *an aim to be accomplished; mission statement*

Philosophy *statement of beliefs and values that directs behavior*

Goal *the end or outcome to be accomplished*

Objective *something aimed at or striven for; things done to achieve the goal*

Policy *a governing plan for accomplishing goals and objectives*

Procedure *chronological sequence of steps within a process*

Protocols *documents of agreement*

Business *plan for new ventures, such as new products or services*

Evidence-based practice *the integration of patient values, clinical expertise, and the research evidence applied to one's practice*

PLANNING PROCESS

There are two major types of organizational planning: long-range, or strategic planning, and short-range, or operational planning. Strategic planning extends 3 to 5 years into the future. It begins with in-depth analysis of the internal environment's strengths and weaknesses and the external opportunities and threats so that realistic goals can be set for the preferred future. It determines the direction of the organization, allocates resources, assigns responsibilities, and determines time frames. Strategic planning goals are more generic and less specific than operational planning.

Nurse managers are more likely to be involved in the operational planning. Operational planning is done in conjunction with budgeting, usually a few months before the new fiscal year. It develops the departmental maintenance and improvement goals for the coming year.

History of Strategic Planning

"Keep your eyes on the stars, and your feet on the ground." —Anonymous

---

Private business started using strategic planning in the mid-1950s when the demand for products began to level off and decline, and competitive products became available from foreign businesses. The health care industry started strategic planning during the mid-1970s when the federal government established restricted payment regulations. Third-party payers also developed restrictions, and payment shifted from the federal government to individuals and other payers. These reimbursement changes increased price sensitivity and competition. Alternative delivery systems, such as preferred provider arrangements, health maintenance organizations, self-help and wellness programs, and ambulatory services, proliferated. Chief executive officers considered these alternatives to maximize bargaining and negotiation strength for contracting as mergers, acquisitions, joint ventures, and informal networking increased.

High-cost technology responded to the competitive environment with greater acuity of care in acute-care settings, tertiary settings, and homes. At the same time the population was aging, increasing numbers of the population were underinsured or uninsured. Quality of life and ethics also became important issues. Consequently, strategic planning became prevalent in health care settings and literature during the 1980s (Table 8-1).

During the 2000s, trends from the 1990s continued. Medicare spending increased as the population continued to grow older. Declining numbers of people with private insurance, increasing numbers of uninsured people, and the declining ability of health care providers to deliver uncompensated care increased. Violence had increased. Health care spending was growing. Technology continued to increase costs through new products and services. Increased use of technology also increased productivity and contributed to less pain with treatments and shorter recovery times with less loss of work time. There was a greater focus on prevention and management of disease. A larger proportion of the population was seeking alternative therapies. International and comprehensive health care systems were enlarging. It became increasingly important to be cost-efficient, seek out partnerships, share resources, decrease duplications, and provide high quality care. There is still a need for risk-adjusted outcome data for improving health care quality and efficiency.

Purpose of Strategic Planning

Strategic planning clarifies beliefs and values: What are the organization's strengths and weaknesses? What are the potential opportunities and threats? Where is the organization going? How is it going to get there? Executives using the strategic planning process give direction to the organization, improve efficiency, weed out poor or underused programs, eliminate duplication of efforts, concentrate resources on important services, improve communications and coordination of activities, provide a mind-expanding opportunity, allow adaptation to the changing environment, set realistic and attainable yet challenging goals, and help ensure goal achievement.

Leaders need vision that is realistic and feasible. Development of a strategic vision involves analysis of the agency's environment, capabilities, and resources; development and articulation of a conceptual image; clarification of values; development of a mission statement; identification of goals and objectives; and identification of strategies for reaching the goals. The strategic vision should be clear, cohesive, consistent, and flexible (Huber, 2006; Marquis & Huston, 2006; McConnell, 2006; Roussel, Swansburg, & Swansburg, 2006; Sullivan & Decker, 2005).

Strategic Planning Process

"Decision makers can turn opportunities into realities." —Anonymous

It is important that top-level administrators be committed to strategic planning. Otherwise such planning may be viewed as mere busywork. Managers need to be taught the importance of strategic planning and the way to do it. The process

TABLE 8-1 Trends during the 1990s

Moving from	Moving to
Individual provider	Team provider
Physician's needs	Payer's/customer's needs
Specialties	Primary care
Reliance on physician care	Use of physician extenders
Hospital episodic care	Ambulatory continuum of care
Institutional care	Alternative care
Individual-based treatment	Population-based treatment
Curative care	Preventative care
Acute care	Chronic care
Technologically oriented	Humanistically oriented
Younger population	Older population
Content mastery	Process mastery
Governed professionally	Governed managerially
Competitive	Cooperative
Cost unaware	Cost aware
Fee for service	Capitation
Paper health record	Computerized health record
No data on best practices	Emerging data on best practices

BOX 8-1 Strategic Planning Process

External assessment
  Opportunities and threats
Internal assessment
  Strengths and weaknesses
Priority strategic issues and programs
Vision
Values
Mission
Philosophy
Goals
  Strategic
    Organization
Operational
  Division
    Unit
Objectives
Strategies
  Timelines and responsibility matrix
  Plans
Policies
Procedures
Implementation
Evaluation
  Production/operations
  Finance
  Marketing

should involve many people and gives planners a sense of direction. That inclusive process allows unexpected crises to be addressed and enables unexpected opportunities to be used. The process may be more important than the plan itself (Roussel, Swansburg, & Swansburg, 2006) (Box 8-1).

An external assessment looks at opportunities and threats, whereas an internal assessment checks for strengths and weaknesses. A situation audit, or environmental assessment, analyzes the past, current, and future forces that affect the organization. Expectations of outside interests such as opinion leaders, governmental officials, insurance companies, and consumers are sought. Expectations of inside interests such as physicians, staff, administrators, and patients are collected (David, 2006; Hitt, Ireland, & Hoskisson, 2006).

The management team can use a grid to visualize the situation audit. The past, present, and future are represented on the horizontal axis. Criteria for areas such as clients, competition, market share, environment, demographics, economics, laws, politics, technology, resources and facilities, finances, and human resources are represented on the vertical axis.

 RESEARCH Perspective 8-1

Data from Arnold L, Drenkard K, Ela S, et al: Strategic positioning for nursing excellence in health systems: Insights from chief nurse executives, *Nursing Administration Quarterly* 30(1):11, 2006.

Purpose: The purpose of this research was to answer the following questions: (1) What are the principal nursing intergration strategies deployed by a sample of health system chief nurse executives? (2) What is the top priority of a sample of health system chief nurse executives in areas of strategic focus? (3) What are the critical success factors for a health system chief nurse role, as perceived by a sample of health system chief nurse executives?

Methods: Thirty-five chief nurse executive members of the Health Management Academy were surveyed to elicit nonstructured responses to questions. The survey findings were reviewed during an interview with each chief nurse executive to verify responses and gather more detailed information. The findings were compiled, themes were identified, and data was collapsed into categories. The researchers and each chief nurse executive did presentations. Then there was a discussion by the entire group to identify gaps and misinterpretations of findings.

Results/conclusions: Chief nursing executives reported that their initial integration strategies were typically mapped to the integration strategies established for the health system. Chief nurse executives reported that their health systems were focused on achieving financial stability through efficiency-related cost reductions; establishing clinical standardization and integration; and expanding market share by leveraging quality brands. The clinical nursing executive strategies were collapsed into four categories: (1) financial performance, (2) clinical integration, (3) quality, patient safety, and compliance, and (4) nursing practice and professionalism.

A SWOT (strengths, weaknesses, opportunities, threats) analysis worksheet is also helpful. Each quadrant of a paper is labeled as one of the four categories, and appropriate factors are listed in each quadrant for a bird's-eye view of the situation audit (Box 8-2). Internal strengths or weaknesses may include management development, qualifications of staff, medical staff expertise, abundance or scarcity of staff, financial situation, cash flow position, marketing efforts, market share, facilities, location, and quality of services. Opportunities include nurse and physician recruitment, referral patterns, new programs, new markets, diversification, population growth, improved technology, and new facilities.

Threats may be shortage of nurses, decrease in patient satisfaction, decrease in insured patients, increase in accounts receivable, decrease in demand for services, competition, regulations, litigation, legislative changes, unionization, and loss of accreditation (Yoder-Wise & Kowalski, 2006).

After the situation audit is done, the management team reviews the philosophy, identifies vision and values, writes a purpose or mission statement, identifies organizational goals and objectives, plans strategies to accomplish the objectives, identifies required resources, determines priorities, sets time frames, and determines accountability (Huber, 2006; Marquis & Huston, 2006; McConnell, 2006; Roussel, Swansburg, & Swansburg, 2006; Sullivan & Decker, 2005; Yoder-Wise, 2007).

Business plans are plans for new ventures, such as new products or services that meet many of the standards for strategic plans and resemble grant proposals (Box 8-3). They integrate strategic, operational, and financial planning. The cover page notes the name of the company, the business plan and year, and names and phone numbers of the contact person or persons. The executive summary, which is about two pages long, is a brief overview of the entire plan. The table of contents should identify at least each major section of the report. The introduction describes

---

BOX 8-2 SWOT Analysis

STRENGTHS
Management development
Qualifications of staff
Medical staff expertise
Facilities
Location
Quality of services

WEAKNESSES
Scarcity of staff
Financial situation
Cash flow position
Marketing efforts
Marketing share

OPPORTUNITIES
Nurse recruitment
Physician recruitment
Referral patterns
New programs
New markets
Diversification
Population growth
Improved technology
New facilities

THREATS
Shortage of nurses
Decrease in patient satisfaction
Increase in accounts receivable
Decrease in demands for services
Competition
Regulations
Litigation
Unionization
Loss of accreditation

BOX 8-3 Business Plan

Cover page
Executive summary
Table of contents
Introduction
Description of the business
Analysis of the market
Analysis of customers
Analysis of the competition
Product or service development
Strategy
Operational plan
Marketing plan
Organizational plan
Development schedule
Financial plan
Contingency plans

the nature of the organization and identifies the business plan's philosophy, goals, objectives, and projected outcomes. The market analysis identifies the product, price, place, and promotions for the new product or service and describes the market characteristics, market trends, and market environment. The market analysis includes a customer, competitor, and resource analysis. The customer analysis describes potential customers and changing characteristics of customers. The analysis of the competition describes the competition and identifies the competitive edge. Product or service development identifies the resources needed and a time frame for the development of the new product or service and presents a quality control plan. The strategy includes the objectives, customer targets, competitor targets, and value proposition. The operational plan and tactics identify the program or product design, desired location, and the needed facilities, equipment, and personnel. The marketing plan describes the mission, goals, strategies, staffing, and financial plans for marketing and branding, pricing, sales/distribution programs, communications and advertising programs, public relations and publicity programs, and customer service. The organizational plan presents an organizational chart with job descriptions and short resumes. The development schedule identifies tasks, required training, and milestone dates. The financial plan identifies developmental costs of projects, income goals, and expenditures. The contingency plans identify alternative assumptions, and alternative strategies (Fralic & Morjikian, 2006; Roussel, Swansburg, & Swansburg 2006). There are computer programs for preparing business plans and samples on the Web (Austin & Boxerman, 2002).

Top-level managers, such as chief executive officers, chief nurse officers, and chief financial officers, do strategic planning for 3 to 5 years. They are responsible for the whole organization and need an awareness of external influences.

Middle-level managers, such as directors, unit supervisors, department heads, and clinical specialists, do intermediate planning for 6 months to 2 years. They are responsible for integrating organizational and unit planning. They may develop and monitor tactics, develop and monitor control plans, and develop and control evaluation plans.

Lower-level managers, such as managers of nursing units, patient care coordinators, charge nurses, team leaders, case managers, and primary care nurses, do operational planning of daily, weekly, and monthly activities that support the other plans. They assess, plan, implement, and evaluate care (Huber, 2006; Marquis, Huston, 2006) (Table 8-2).

"Look upon the present as the past of your future." —Anonymous

VISION

A vision is a mental image or the power of imagination to see something that is not actually visible. When doing strategic planning or business plans, the vision should be the preferred future (Sullivan & Decker, 2005; McConnell, 2006) (Boxes 8-4 and 8-5).

"A vision is an image without great detail. It acts as a flag around which the troops will rally." —Michael Hammer

VALUES

Value is the worth, usefulness, or importance of something. Core values do not change. They are the anchors for the mission even as operation strategies change. Leadership, management, and personnel should determine what their values are and keep their plans and actions consistent with their values. A values statement is a planning tool (Huber, 2006) (Box 8-6).

"Good customer service springs from individuals within the organization. It requires compassion, and the rare ability to understand that only by routinely putting the needs of the customer first can we hope to be first as an organization." —Unknown

TABLE 8-2 Leadership and Management Related to Planning

Leader	Manager
Strategic planning	Operational planning
Positions may include: Chief Executive Officer Chief Nursing Officer Chief Financial Officer	Middle management positions may include: Director Unit supervisor Department head Clinical specialist Lower level management positions may include: Patient Care Coordinator Charge nurse Team leader Case manager Primary nurse Staff nurse
Responsible for the whole organization and awareness of external influences	Middle management is responsible for integrating organizational and unit planning Lower level management is responsible for short-term daily and weekly planning
Focus is on strategic planning Creates innovative products and services Assesses the market Sets priorities Forecasts resource requirements	Middle managers participate in long- and short-range planning Develop and monitor tactics Develop and monitor control plans Develop and monitor evaluation plans Lower level managers do short range operational planning Assess, plan, implement, and evaluate care

BOX 8-4 Planning Tools

Vision
Values
Mission
Philosophy
Goals
Objectives
Policies
Procedures

BOX 8-5 Sample Vision

GENERAL HOSPITAL VISION STATEMENT

The vision for General Hospital is to be the preeminent health care provider in the region by doing the following:

Being the premier full-service, integrated health care delivery network that provides a continuum of health services to diverse people

Creating an environment that exceeds the expectations of our customers

Developing creative solutions to the challenges facing us

Providing economically viable, cost-effective services to our customers

Working in partnership with other leading health care organizations

Promoting wellness and healthy lifestyles through community health education programs in partnership with community efforts

BOX 8-6 Sample Values Statement

The guiding values for General Hospital are as follows:
Quality
Compassion
Fairness
Integrity
Innovation
Fiscal responsibility

PURPOSE OR MISSION STATEMENT

Organizations exist for a purpose. Clarification of the mission or purpose is a high priority for planning. Most nursing services exist to provide high-quality nursing care to clients. Some also encourage teaching and research. Each specialty area, with its own specific purposes, contributes to the overall purpose of the institution. For example, the purpose of the in-service education department is to orient staff to the job and to provide educational programs to improve the quality of the staff work; the burn unit exists to provide good-quality nursing service to patients with burns.

The mission or purpose influences the philosophy, goals, and objectives. For example, if a progressive care unit exists to help patients adjust to their diseases, it should be staffed with professional nurses particularly skilled in teaching and counseling. If, however, the unit's purpose is to cut hospital and patient expenses, it may be a minimal care unit with reduced services given by nonprofessional workers. The relationships among the mission, philosophy, goals, and objectives should be examined periodically for consistency (Ingersoll, Widzel, & Smith, 2005) (Box 8-7).

"Empowering mission statements focus on contributions, on worthwhile purposes that create a collective deep burning 'Yes!' They come from the hearts and minds of everyone involved—not as an executive decree from 'Mount Olympus'." —Stephen Covey

---

PHILOSOPHY

The philosophy articulates a vision and provides a statement of beliefs and values that direct one's practice. It should be written, included in appropriate documents such as the staff handbook and annual reports, and reviewed periodically. If the philosophy is stated in vague, abstract terms that are not easily understood, it is useless. Conflicting philosophies between overlapping units cause confusion and should be avoided. Workers are most likely to interpret the philosophy from the pronouncements and actions of the leaders in the institution. Therefore conformity of action to belief is important.

When developing or reevaluating a philosophy, the manager should consider theory, education, practice, research, and nursing's role in the total organization. Approaches that can be used to incorporate nursing theory into the philosophy include an eclectic approach that selects ideas from various nursing theories and incorporates them into the philosophy statements or a theory might be adopted and integrated into the philosophy. Attaching an explanation of the theory to the philosophy would also be useful. Secondary sources give an overview of various nursing

BOX 8-7 Sample Mission Statement

The mission of General Hospital is to deliver comprehensive health care services to promote physical and mental health; to prevent disease, injury, and disability; and to promote healing of the body, mind, and spirit. Related instruction, public service programs, and research will facilitate high-quality health care.

theorists' work, reference the theorists extensive publications, and address work related to the theorists' work (Marriner Tomey & Alligood, 2006).

Levine and Orem focus on nursing therapeutics. Wholism, holism, integrity, and conservation are major concepts in Levine's conservation principles. Orem's theories of self-care and self-care deficits are particularly useful in community health and promotion of health situations. Johnson and Roy emphasize the client. Johnson used a behavioral model and identified six subsystems as (1) attachment-affiliation, (2) achievement, (3) sexual, (4) ingestive-eliminative, (5) aggressive, and (6) dependency. Sister Callista Roy's adaptation model is particularly useful in acute care settings.

King, Newman, Orlando, Patterson, Zderad, Travelbee, and Wiedebach discuss interaction. King's conceptual framework specified personal, interpersonal, and social system interactions. Her theory of goal attainment is particularly useful for nursing care and nursing administration. Newman stressed purposeful interventions and a total person approach. Orlando addressed deliberative nursing actions that purposefully identify and meet the patient's needs. She maintained that automatic actions may not meet the patient's needs. Patterson and Zderad developed a humanistic nursing theory and indicated that the defining event in nursing is the interaction between the patient and the nurse. Wiedebach developed a philosophy of nursing and a flow chart that identifies a need-for-help.

Rogers focused on the environment and interactions of human beings. Her conceptual model of unitary human beings is very abstract and thought provoking. Middle-range theories that are specific to a particular aspect of nursing practice may be useful for specific agency units. Middle-range theories of nursing are proliferating (Marriner Tomey & Alligood, 2006).

It is appropriate to comment on skill levels needed, advanced preparation for certain positions, need for continuing education, provision of educational opportunities for students, and specific practice modalities. The value of applying research findings to practice, supporting research efforts, and acknowledging nursing's role in the overall organization could also be clarified in the philosophy (Box 8-8).

GOALS AND OBJECTIVES

"Wishing consumes as much energy as planning." —Anonymous

Goals and objectives state actions for achieving the mission and philosophy. In fact, if the mission or purpose and philosophy are to be more than good intentions, they must be translated into explicit goals. The more quantitative the goal, the more likely its achievement is to receive attention and the less likely it is to be distorted. Goals are central to the whole management process—planning, organizing, staffing, directing, and controlling/evaluating. Planning defines the goals; the institution is organized and staffed to accomplish the goals. Direction

stimulates personnel toward accomplishment of the objectives, and control compares the results with the objectives to evaluate accomplishments.

Goals and objectives may address services rendered, economics, use of resources—people, funds, facilities—innovations, and social responsibilities. Objectives are selective rather than global, are multiple, and cover a wide range of activities. The immediate, short-term, and long-term goals should be balanced, interdependent, and ranked in order of importance. It is common to have more short-term than long-term goals.

Classic theory contends that the board of directors and top administration should determine institutional goals. Behavioral scientists are interested in having workers involved in setting goals. Empowered staffs often focus on goals that relate to their work environment or patient care that are very relevant to them. Those goals are more likely to be addressed by staff than goals set by others. Competitive or external data should drive strategic goals to position the organization for success. Service interest, profit motives, governmental regulations, union representation, and personal goals all influence decision making.

It is appropriate for the board of directors and top administrators, including the chief nurse executive, to set institutional goals and objectives; for the vice presidents for nursing, directors of nurses, and patient care coordinators to set the goals and objectives for the nursing service; for the staff members to determine the unit goals and objectives; and for the nurses to determine their goals and objectives with their

RESEARCH Perspective 8-2

Data from Tuck I, Harris LH, Baliko B: Values expressed in philosophies of nursing services. *JONA* 30(4):180-184, 2000.

Purpose: The purpose of this study was to identify the values that are evident in philosophies of nursing services.

Methods: Ten community hospitals and medical centers within a southeastern state submitted their philosophies of nursing services for content analysis.

Results/conclusions: The most frequently cited value was caring. Professionalism was the second most frequently found value. Individualism was the third reported value. The remaining categories of need fulfillment, culture, well-being or health, and adaptation were distributed selectively across the philosophies.

BOX 8-8 Sample Philosophy

PHILOSOPHY OF GENERAL HOSPITAL

General Hospital is committed to assessing and meeting the physical, emotional, spiritual, environmental, social, and rehabilitative health needs of the citizens in the region. The worth, dignity, and autonomy of individuals (customers, employees, and others) are recognized, as is each individual's right to self-direction and responsibility for one's own life. Individual uniqueness will be considered when assessing needs and delivering quality care. Educational pursuits, research, and public service programs will be used toward innovations and improvement of health care in the region. General Hospital personnel will work in collaboration with customers and in partnership with other organizations to provide cost-effective services.

BOX 8-9 Sample Goal and Objectives

GOAL

Develop and implement staff development programs to meet the need for increased knowledge

OBJECTIVE

Develop and implement at least 12 staff development programs by the end of the fiscal year

STRATEGIES

Continue to develop, implement, and evaluate continuing education programs for personnel

Evaluate, revise, and implement the orientation program for new personnel

Develop, implement, and evaluate in-service programs regarding new products

Investigate the feasibility of a mentorship program for less experienced nurses

---

immediate manager. The overlap created by the chief nurse executive's, vice president's, and director's working on institutional and nursing service goals and the patient care coordinator's contributing to nursing service and the unit's goals helps facilitate continuity and compatibility of goals. Participation in the determination of goals and objectives increases commitment, transforming them from stated to implemented goals.

Because goals are dynamic, they change over time. They should be reviewed periodically so that they can be changed in an evolutionary rather than a radical manner. Goals should be specific rather than vague, and challenging yet reachable. Necessary support elements should be available (Box 8-9).

Goals help focus attention on what is important and are broader statements than objectives. Objectives are more specific ways to reach the goal. It is recommended that objectives be achievable, specific, measurable, and outcome oriented, starting with "to" followed by a verb. Each objective should be about a single result with a target date. Strategies identify how the organization will attain the vision. The development of long- and short-term objectives is appropriate. A form with four columns (one for goals/objectives, one for strategies/actions, one for target dates and person or persons responsible, one for accomplishments) can be a helpful planning tool (Table 8-3).

Policies

"Honesty is a question of right and wrong, not a matter of policy." —Anonymous

Policies and procedures are means for accomplishing goals and objectives. Policies explain how goals will be achieved and serve as guides that define the general course and scope of activities permissible for goal accomplishment. They serve as a basis for future decisions and actions, help coordinate plans, control performance, and increase consistency of action by increasing the probability that different managers will make similar decisions when independently facing similar situations. Consequently, morale is increased when personnel perceive that they are being treated equally. Policies also serve as a means by which authority can be delegated.

Policies should be comprehensive in scope, stable, and flexible so they can be applied to different conditions that are not so diverse that

TABLE 8-3 Planning Tool

Goals/Objectives	Strategies/Actions	Target Dates/Person(s) Responsible	Accomplishments
1. To develop and implement at least 12 staff development programs by the end of the fiscal year	A. Develop class regarding performance appraisal for middle managers.	January 2008/nurse manager educator	Collect materials first week; write lesson plans second week; develop course teaching tools third week; print course packet fourth week.
	B. Implement performance appraisal class for middle managers.	February 2008/nurse manager educator	Class taught February.
	C. Evaluate class regarding performance appraisal.	February 2008/nurse manager educator	Pass out evaluation form at end of class; tabulate data within week.

they require separate sets of policies. Consistency is important because inconsistency introduces uncertainty and contributes to feelings of bias, preferential treatment, and unfairness. Fairness is an important characteristic that is attributed to the consistent application of the policy. Policies should be written and understandable.

Policies can be implied or expressed. Implied policies are not directly voiced or written but are established by patterns of decisions. They may have either favorable or unfavorable effects and represent an interpretation of observed behavior. Courteous treatment of clients may be implied versus expressed. Sometimes policies are implied simply because no one has ever bothered to state them. The presence or absence of workers who are over 50 years of age, minority members, women, or pregnant women may lead to an interpretation of implied policies of hiring or not hiring those categories of people. At times, policies may deliberately be implied because they are illegal or reflect questionable ethics. Sometimes implied policy conflicts with expressed policy; these double standards should be prevented.

Expressed policies may be oral or written. Oral policies are more flexible than written ones and can be easily adjusted to changing circumstances. However, they are less desirable than written ones because they may not be known by some staff members.

The process of writing policies reveals discrepancies and omissions and can cause the manager to think critically about the policy, thus contributing to clarity. Once written, they are readily available to all in the same form; their meaning cannot be changed by word of mouth; misunderstandings can be referred to the written words; the chance of misinterpretation is decreased; policy statements can be sent to all affected by them; they can be referred to whoever wishes to check the policy; and they can be used for orientation purposes. Written policies indicate the integrity of the organization's intention and generate confidence in management.

A disadvantage of written policies is the reluctance to revise them when they become outdated. However, even oral policies become obsolete. Managers should review policies periodically, and if that fails, personnel can appeal for a revision.

Policies can emerge in several ways—originated, appealed, or imposed (Box 8-10). The originated, or internal, policies are usually the responsibility of top management to guide subordinates in their functions. Strategy for originated policy flows from the objectives of the organization as defined by top management and may be broad in scope, allowing staff associates to develop supplemental policies, or well defined with little room for interpretation. Lower managerial decisions should implement the broader policy defined by top management.

BOX 8-10 Emergence of Policies

Originated
Appealed
Imposed

Sometimes policies are generated at the operating and first-line manager levels and imposed upward. The extent to which this happens is influenced by the organizational atmosphere and adequacy of policies generated by top management. At times policies may be formulated simultaneously from both directions or by a policy and procedures committee.

When staff members do not know how to solve a problem, disagree with a previous decision, or otherwise want a question reviewed, they appeal to the manager for a decision. As appeals are taken up the hierarchy and decisions are made, precedents known as appealed policy develop and guide future managerial actions.

Policies developed from appeals are likely to be incomplete, uncoordinated, and unclear. Unintended precedents can be set when decisions are made for a given situation without consideration for possible effects on other dimensions of the organization. This aimless formation of policy makes it difficult to know what policies exist. Sometimes managers dislike facing issues until forced to do so and consequently delay policy making until precedents have been set. Appealed policies can be foresighted and consistent, especially when the manager knows that the decision constitutes policy. Nevertheless, when a number of policies are being appealed, it is time to assess policies for gaps and needs for updating and clarification so originated policies can dominate. One can expect health care agencies to require policies about patient care assignments, noting physicians' orders, administration of medications, patient safety, charting, and infection control.

Imposed, or external, policies are thrust on an organization by external forces, such as government or labor unions. Policies of the organization must conform to local, state, and federal laws.

Collective bargaining and union contracts direct labor policies. Professional and social groups—such as the American Nurses Association, the National League for Nursing, churches, schools, and charitable organizations—mold policy.

The planning process involves defining, communicating, applying, and maintaining policies. The development of a policy can originate anywhere in an organization and should involve personnel who will be affected by the policy. They have valuable information for sound policy formation and can ensure that the policy will be implemented. Before writing a policy, one must consider whether there are specific, recurring problems, how frequently they occur, whether they are temporary or permanent in nature, and whether a policy statement would clarify thinking and promote efficiency.

When policies are written, the purpose, philosophy, goals, and objectives should serve as guides. Policies should be consistent and help solve or prevent specific problems. Clear, concise statements that establish areas of authority and perhaps include reference to supporting policies minimize exceptions. Managers need sufficient guidance with accompanying freedom for action. It is advisable to have the policy statement reviewed and approved by leaders and the affected managers before the policy is formalized.

Policies are of no use if no one knows of their existence. Oral communication is appropriate to introduce and explain new policies. It is appropriate to send a letter of purpose and a copy of policies to personnel affected by them. The written policies can then be referred to later. Policies should be written in a specific, concise, and complete manner and stored in a policy manual, which may be a hard copy or a computer document that is easily accessible to all personnel to whom the policies apply. The manual will be well organized if policies are classified, noted in the table of contents, and indexed by topic. Policies should be easily replaceable when revised.

Once a policy has been stated and approved, it is applied. Policy formation is a continuous process; the policy is continually reappraised and restated as necessary (Figure 8-1). Continuing

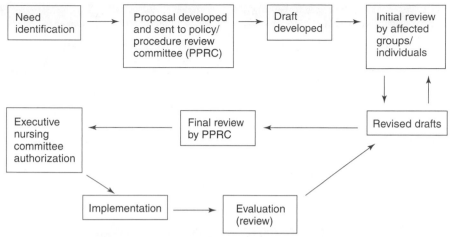

Figure 8-1 • Flowchart for policies/procedures/protocols.

surveillance to determine that the policy is understood and applied is important. Periodic analysis and evaluation of existing policies can suggest the need for revision. Personnel should be encouraged to help formulate, review, and revise policies. Boxes 8-11 through 8-15 present sample policies for generating and reviewing nursing policies, procedures, and protocols.

Procedures

Procedures supply a more specific guide to action than policy does. They help achieve a high degree of regularity by enumerating the chronological sequence of steps. Procedures are intradepartmental or interdepartmental and consequently do not affect the entire organization to the extent that policy statements do.

Procedure manuals provide a basis for orientation and staff development and are a ready reference for all personnel. They standardize procedures and equipment and can provide a basis for evaluation. Good procedures can result in time and labor savings. Box 8-16 presents a sample procedure for ambulating a patient with one assistant.

Improvement in operating procedures increases productivity and reduces cost. Waste in performing work can be decreased by applying work simplification that strives to make each part of a procedure productive. First, one decides

what work requires simplification by identifying problem areas. Next, the work selected is analyzed carefully and in detail. Charts that depict the components of the work and the work flow are useful for motion or procedural analysis.

A questioning attitude helps determine why work is done, by whom, when, where, and how. What is the purpose of the procedure? Does it need to be done? Can it be eliminated? For example, are "closed" beds and "surgical" beds really necessary, or could "open" beds be used for all purposes? Who does the work? Can someone else do it better, or can it be assigned to someone with less skill? Is there duplication of efforts? Can two or more activities be combined? Will changing the time sequence improve the procedure? Can changing the location reduce transportation? Once these questions have been answered, rearranging, combining, or eliminating components should simplify work. Then the improved methods must be communicated so they can be implemented.

Written procedures may use a consistent format that considers the definition; purpose; materials needed and how to locate, requisition, and dispose of them; steps in the procedure; expected results; precautions; legal implications; nurse, patient, and physician responsibilities; and appropriate charting. Each step in the procedure leading to the accomplishment of a goal should

---

BOX 8-11 Process for Generation of Policy/Procedure/Protocol

Issue Date July 1989		**Policy No.** A/O QA.08
Review Dates Annually		**Subject** Quality Assurance

POLICY

Written policies, procedures, and protocols that reflect optimal standards of nursing practice will guide the provision of nursing care.

SCOPE

This policy applies to all of Nursing Services.

PURPOSE

To provide a consistent format for the writing and processing of policies/procedures/protocols (P/P/P); to identify resources for creating, reviewing, and changing P/P/P General Hospital Nursing Services; to eliminate duplication of efforts and ensure current and consistent practice.

PROCESS

1. Any nurse with approval of the unit director or associate director when appropriate may initiate a written P/P/P. A self-study packet is available to assist with this process.
2. A proposal for all new P/P/Ps will be sent to the Nursing Service Policy/Procedure Review Committee (PPRC). (See attached form.) The proposal includes the topic/title, patients affected by the procedure, why it is needed, resource persons who will be used to write or consult, and appropriate signature(s). In some cases a proposal may not be necessary, but the intent to write a P/P/P should be communicated to the PPRC. The committee will then serve as a resource for format, for other resources, and for distribution. Exceptions for the initial proposal might be direction from the Executive Nursing Council or the hospital system.
3. Approval/disapproval to write will then be communicated to the initiating individual(s) by the PPRC after considering the possible overall need, already existent P/P/P, and additional resources. A member of the PPRC will be assigned to each approved proposal to ensure consistency of format. (See attached format guidelines.)

Associate Director of Hospitals for Nursing Joy Plesant	Date 10/10/07

---

be necessary and in proper relationship to the other steps. Balance between flexibility and stability should be maintained. At times there are best ways to do something. At other times, any numbers of ways are acceptable. As with the policy manual, the procedure manual should be easily accessible, well organized with a table of contents, and indexed. Each procedure should be easily replaceable when revised. Because there is a tendency to add new procedures instead of revising existing ones, it is important to review and revise the procedure manual periodically. In reviewing, one should check the effectiveness

and workability with personnel to determine whether the procedure has been followed. Procedures should be realistic and written in simple language that is easy to understand. Changes should be dated and provided to all appropriate personnel.

Before spending valuable time writing procedures, one must consider whether a procedure is actually needed. With preservice and on-the-job preparation, is there really a need to have on each unit procedures on how to feed a patient and how to make a bed? Goals can be reached in a variety of ways, and consequently nursing

BOX 8-12 Proposal for Policy/Procedure

PROPOSAL FOR POLICY/PROCEDURE

This form is submitted to the Policy/Procedure Committee of Nursing Services to request a written Policy/Procedure designed to implement policy and maintain policy standards in regard to the following nursing care:

Topic: _____

Patients affected by the policy/procedure: _____

Explanation of the policy/procedure: _____
_____

Problems that arise as a result of not having a written policy/procedure: _____
_____

Resources that you will use to write and document the validity of this policy/procedure: _____
_____

Name _____

Unit director _____

Associate director _____

****

For Use by Policy/Procedure Committee

Date received: _____

Approval for writing of policy/procedure: Yes   No

Contacts within Nursing Services and Medicine that must be made for coordination of the writing of this procedure: _____
_____

Committee member assigned to supervise project: _____

Guidelines for Procedure Format

Title
Policy statement
Scope
Purpose (optional)
Assessment and planning
    Nursing considerations
    Cautions
    Resources
Implementation
    Sequence of interventions/rationale
    Cautions
Evaluation
Documentation
Authorization signature
Reference:
Written by:
Date of revision(s):
Date of review(s):

BOX 8-13 Review Process for Policies/Procedures/Protocols		

Issue Date November 2007		**Policy No.** A/O QA.07
Review Dates Annually		**Subject** Quality Assurance

POLICY

All policies, procedures, and protocols (P/P/Ps) will be reviewed annually and revised as necessary.

SCOPE

This policy applies to all Nursing Service policies, procedures, and protocols.

PROCESS

1. Reviews of P/P/Ps will be conducted in quarterly periods (Jan-Mar, Apr-Jun, Jul-Sept, Oct-Dec).
2. Before the beginning of the upcoming quarter, the Policy/Procedure Review Committee (PPRC) will receive notice of which P/P/Ps are due for review. Members of the PPRC will be assigned accountability for the review of specific P/P/Ps.
3. The accountable PPRC member will review the P/P/P and will solicit feedback from appropriate content experts, using the appropriate Policy or Procedure Review Questionnaire. (See attached.)
4. The content experts will complete the Review Questionnaire after obtaining input from most affected groups or individuals. The completed questionnaire and a draft of the revised P/P/P will be returned to the accountable PPRC member by the deadline date indicated.
5. On receipt of the questionnaire and draft, the accountable PPRC member will submit the final draft of the revised P/P/P to the PPRC.
6. Upon approval by the PPRC, the final draft will be submitted to the Executive Nursing Council for authorization and signature.
7. Revised P/P/Ps will then be distributed to all holders of Nursing Service Policy/Procedure Manuals.
8. Requests to review P/P/Ps can be made at any time during the year to the PPRC.*

Date of Revision(s): 7/06
Date of Review(s): 7/9/07

Associate Director of Hospitals for Nursing	Date

*See Figure 8-1.

students are taught principles rather than procedures. There are textbooks with bedside nursing procedures, and many disposable products with directions are available. It seems most important for the procedure manual to contain information that may vary from institution to institution. Not all parts of the procedure format may be necessary for each procedure. New personnel and float nurses can serve as valuable resources for nursing managers to consult when they are determining what contents are important for the procedure manual. A shared governance organization can use a policy and procedure committee to develop and update policies and procedures (Hudson, 2006).

The planning process is a critical element of management. Nurse administrators must learn it because it will not happen by accident. Planning is largely conceptual, but its results are clearly visible. The statement of the purpose or mission, philosophy, goals, objectives, policies, and procedures are all consequences of planning and set the stage for smooth operations.

Evidence-Based Practice

Evidence-based practice information is useful for developing policies and procedures as well as for making other management decisions (Boswell, 2007). Nurses have been known to use obsolete information that they learned in

---

BOX 8-14 Procedure Review Questionnaire

PROCEDURE REVIEW QUESTIONNAIRE

Name of procedure _____

Date of review _____

Reviewer(s) _____

(Name)	(Title)	(Service/Unit)

(Name)	(Title)	(Service/Unit)

(Note: The reviewer may wish to carry out the procedure exactly as written before addressing the questions below.)

Please circle the number that most accurately reflects your response to the following.

Where procedure differs from practice, please note discrepancies on separate sheet of paper. Please write recommended revision on separate sheet of paper and return to _____ by _____.

	YES	NO	UNCERTAIN	COMMENTS
1. Does the procedure accurately reflect all equipment/ materials necessary to carry out the procedure				
a. safely?	1	2	3	
b. competently?	1	2	3	
2. Does the procedure reflect equipment used?	1	2	3	
3. Is the sequence of steps correct?	1	2	3	
4. Is the sequence of steps complete?	1	2	3	
5. Are the contraindications, if any, clearly identified?	1	2	3	
6. Does the scientific rationale provide a meaningful reason for each intervention?	1	2	3	
7. Does the procedure reflect results of current research and state-of-the-art clinical nursing practice?	1	2	3	
8. Does the procedure reflect current clinical practice at GH?	1	2	3	
9. Is the procedure in conflict with any other hospital or Nursing Services' policies/procedures? If so, please list.	1	2	3	

Additional Comments:

RECOMMENDED ACTION

_____ The procedure is correct as written. Recommend adoption of procedure   _____ Discrepancies noted. Recommend revision attached   _____ Recommend procedure not be adopted

12/07

---

nursing school long ago, long-standing but unproven traditions, methods they find comfortable, ways learned from experience, and vendor information. Evidence-based practice has gained attention since the 1970s as medical advances proliferated and health care consumers became better informed and developed higher expectations of their health care providers. More nurses became educated at the masters and doctoral levels and influenced nursing education and practice with research. The American Nurses Association Cabinet on Nursing Research and the National Center for Nursing Research at the National Institutes of Health were formed and promoted nursing research. British and Canadian movements such as the Best Evidence Database, The Cochrane Library, and Bandolier developed databases for systematic reviews,

---

BOX 8-15 Policy Review Form

POLICY REVIEW FORM

Name of policy _____

Date of review _____

Reviewer _____

          (Name)   (Service)

INSTRUCTIONS: Please circle the number that most accurately reflects your response to the following questions. Please check at the bottom your recommended action.

	Yes	No	Comments
1. Is there a need for the policy?	1	2	
2. Is the policy relevant to this institution and staff?	1	2	
3. Is the policy consistent with General Hospital's Nursing Services philosophy?	1	2	
4. Is the policy in conflict with any other hospital or nursing policies?	1	2	
5. Does the policy create any inequities between hospital staff or patients?	1	2	
6. Is the policy reasonable (i.e., can compliance be enforced)?	1	2	
7. Is the policy clearly written so that anyone unfamiliar with the subject can understand it?	1	2	
8. Is the information accurate?	1	2	
9. Is the policy complete (i.e., does it include the scope, purpose, and any related information)?	1	2	

Additional Comments:

RECOMMENDED ACTION:

_____ No action required   _____ Revision required   _____ Remove from manual

      Approved as written   (Changes attached)   (Justification attached)

---

meta-analysis, and clinical guidelines for best practices (Malloch & Porter-O'Grady, 2006; Pfeffer & Sutton, 2006).

The movement for total quality management and continuous quality improvement during the 1980s stimulated a debate about the differences between research and evaluation. Research was more generalizable while evaluation was more specific to a situation. Evidence-based practice started to appear in the literature by the mid-1990s and has been associated with quantative and qualitative research methods (Dawes, Davies, & Grey, 2005; Meinyk & Fineout-Overholt, 2004; Smith, James, Lorentzon, & Pope, 2004) (see Chapter 15 for the research process). Some problems associated with trying to use

research to guide practice are: it may be difficult to locate related research; the research findings might not apply to the situation in question; there could be several related research studies with conflicting and confusing findings; people may not be able to understand the implications for practice; it took time and energy to critique the research; and even institutions with good research infrastructures could not generate rigorous data for most of the needed decisions. However, leaders could learn from small experiments, pilot programs, and qualitative data. So the traditional research to generate knowledge was noticeably different from evaluating concrete practices that could produce evidence (Malloch & Porter-O'Grady, 2006; Pfeffer & Sutton, 2006).

BOX 8-16 Procedure

PROCEDURE

Ambulating with One Assistant

1. Definition: to walk or move about with help from one person
2. Purpose
   a. Prevent complications of immobility.
   b. Improve balance and muscle tone.
   c. Increase feelings of physical and mental well-being.
   d. Progress from needing assistance to becoming independent in ambulation.
3. Materials needed
   a. Robe or hospital gown to put on backwards to prevent exposure of patient's back
   b. Slippers or shoes that have nonslip soles and fit well
   c. Safety belt if indicated
4. Steps in procedure
   a. Check patient's chart regarding ambulation.
   b. Wash hands.
   c. Explain the procedure and rationale to the patient.
   d. Place the bed in a low position, and help the patient sit on the edge of the bed.
   e. Assess the patient for faintness or dizziness.
      (1) Rationale: Having the patient sit on the edge of the bed before standing to reduce faintness and dizziness will reduce the risk of falling.
   f. Apply safety belt if the patient is unsteady.
      (1) Rationale: The safety belt helps support the patient and decreases the risk of injury.
   g. Help the patient to stand and observe the patient for balance.
   h. Grasp the patient around the waist to stabilize, and grasp the arm near the assistant with the other hand to guide the patient.
   i. Stand by the weaker side except when with cerebrovascular accident patient; then stand on the stronger unaffected side.
      (1) Rationale: Flaccid muscles on the affected side do not provide enough muscle strength for the assistant to grasp and support the patient.
   j. Encourage the patient to look straight ahead and to use good posture.
      (1) Rationale: There is a tendency for the patient to look down, and that may increase vertigo.
   k. Instruct the patient to lift each foot to take a step instead of shuffling.
   l. Remember the patient has to walk back, and pace the distance to the patient's ability.
   m. Chart the activity and the patient's tolerance.

Modified from Smith SF, Duell DJ, Martin BC: *Clinical nursing skills: Basic to advanced skills*, ed 5, Upper Saddle River, NJ, 2004, Prentice Hall Health.

An Institute of Medicine (IOM, 2001) report addressed evidence-based practice as the integration of patient values, clinical expertise, and the best research evidence. The evidence-based clinical system means include electronic data, clinical research, medical records, clinical conferencing, national protocols, disciplinary data, protocols, practice, experience, and patients (Craig & Smyth, 2002; Malloch & Porter-O'Grady, 2006; Meinyk & Fineout-Overholt, 2006; Pearson, Field, & Jordan, 2007). Malloch and Porter-O'Grady (2006) identified the evidence-based clinical system processes as collect data, link information, construct protocols, test practices, aggregate results, evaluate outcomes, and establish best practices. The Malloch and Porter-O'Grady disciplined clinical inquiry model has five phases: (1) needs assessment and environmental scan, (2) learning and knowledge generation, (3) knowledge assimilation, (4) knowledge application, and (5) appraisal/evaluation. They indicate that one can develop one's learning inquiry by becoming a reflective nurse clinician; identifying clinical issues and establishing priorities;

identifying practice standards and establishing priorities; translating clinical issues into a researchable problem/focused question; accessing the best evidence; evaluating research studies; utilizing the best evidence; and then doing strategic thinking and action planning.

Malloch and Porter-O'Grady (2006) identified disciplined clinical inquiry and evidence-based nursing practice pathways. First nurses develop evidence-based practice standards by accessing and utilizing current sources of best evidence. Nurses should conduct research about valued practice issues that have institutional significance. It is useful to then prepare notes for other nurses in a concise, evidence-based fact sheet. Journal clubs provide opportunities to critique research and determine its applicability to the practice setting. Clinical inquiry sessions foster reflections on actual care, the problems encountered, and the successes achieved. Peer mentors can provide leadership for helping peers develop their disciplined clinical inquiry and evidence-based nursing practice.

Still there are times when research data or evidence-based information is not available. Martelli (2006) said that leaders seldom make decisions based on evidence that meets the classical standards of research. They need to use accessible, accurate, actionable, and applicable information. Some people make decisions based on their gut instinct or intuition. Intuition is a knowing or sensing without deductive reasoning or rational processes. It is a perceptive insight and instinctive knowing. Hosszu (2006) said people may need to make on-the-spot decisions without first considering available information. Intuition may make the right decision under those circumstances. He believed that people develop a knowledge based on prior decisions that can be used to make decisions. Humer (2007) believes that executives acquire judgment by being hyperaware of the environment.

Benner (2001) identified five levels of competency in clinical nursing practice: novice, advanced beginner, competent, proficient, and expert. The novice stage of skill acquisition is when the person has no background experience for the current situation. That could be a nursing student or a professional nurse out of his or her area of expertise. The advanced beginner stage is when the person can do a marginally acceptable performance by having enough experience to grasp some aspects of the situation. That nurse is usually guided by rules and focuses on task completion. The advanced beginner moves to the competent level when the beginner has learned from practice situations and by following the actions of others. At the competent level, the nurse perceives the situation as a whole and has an intuitive grasp of the situation based on previous understanding. The expert has an intuitive grasp of the situation and is able to take action without needing to consider alternative solutions (Benner, 1998).

Nurse executives are needed to help create an infrastructure and environment for evidence-based practice (Simpson, 2006). Clinical nurse leaders, clinical nurse educators, and nurse researchers can provide leadership for evidence-based practice if allowed the time (Penz & Bassendowski, 2006). They tend to be early adapters and have the necessary research skills. They can help staff nurses become reflective clinicians and brainstorm to identify clinical issues and priorities to be studied. They can help staff nurses focus questions and state researchable problems.

Institutional technology is important for collecting available sources of information, analyzing data, and getting the evidence-based findings as evidence-based fact sheets to the point of care (Matter, 2006). Practice information sheets, clinical guidelines, and clinical audits to evaluate evidence-based practice facilitate implementation (Craig & Smyth, 2002). Journal clubs and discussion groups to review and critique research and reflect on its application to actual care and its economic feasibility can facilitate the diffusion of evidence-based practice (Shirey, 2006; Stone, Curran, & Bakken, 2002). Multisite evidence-based research can further contribute to excellence (Kramer, Maguire, & Schmalenberg, 2006). Global multi sites may become increasingly important.

CHAPTER SUMMARY

Strategic planning, or the long-range planning process, includes the development of vision, values, mission, philosophy, goals, objectives, strategies, policies, and procedures. They are all interactive. The mission influences the philosophy, goals, and objectives. The philosophy articulates the vision and values that direct the mission and practice. The organizational long-range goals are set by top administration with input from others. Middle managers set goals and objectives for the nursing service, while first-line staff members determine the unit goals and objectives and do the short-range or operational planning. Policies and procedures are means for accomplishing the goals and objectives. Evidence-based information can be used to develop the policies and procedures and to provide excellent care. It is important to do the financial management to be able to implement the plans.

CRITICAL THINKING ACTIVITY

Reflective Journal: Make observations in a clinical setting or reflect on past experiences. Answer the following questions. What is the agency's vision? Is a vision statement document visible to staff and visitors? What values are supported? What is the agency's philosophy? Does the organization have a strategic plan?

CASE STUDY

Lake View Hospital is a 98-bed general hospital. It is one of two hospitals serving an industrial community with a population of about 90,000. Patients are being discharged earlier, so there is an increasing vacancy rate on the medical-surgical units. At the same time there is an increasing demand for geriatric services and ambulatory care. Demands for home health have also increased. Consider current trends. Identify a needed new unit to meet the community needs. Write the goals and objectives for that new unit.

ONLINE RESOURCES

evolve Additional critical thinking activities, worksheets, and case studies are available online at http://evolve.elsevier.com/Marriner/guide8e.

REFERENCES

Arnold L, Drenkard K, Ela S, et al: Strategic positioning for nursing excellence in health systems: Insights from executives, *Nursing Administration Quarterly* 30(1):11, 2006.

Austin C, Boxerman SB: *Information systems for healthcare management*, ed 6, Chicago, 2002, Health Administration Press.

Benner P: *From novice to expert*, Upper Saddle River, NJ, 2001, Prentice Hall.

Benner P: *Experience in nursing practice: Caring, clinical judgment, and ethics*, New York, 1998, Springer.

Boswell C: *Introduction to nursing research: Incorporating evidence-based practice*, Sudbury, NJ, 2007, Jones and Bartlett Publishers.

Craig JV, Smyth RL: *The evidence-based practice manual for nurses*, St. Louis, 2002, Churchill Livingstone.

David E: *Strategic management: Concepts and cases*, Upper Saddle River, NJ, 2006, Prentice Hall.

Dawes M, Davies P, Gray A: *Evidence-based practice: A primer for health care professionals*, St. Louis, 2005, Churchill Livingstone.

Fralic M, Morjikian R: The RWJ executive nurse fellows program, Part 3: Making the business case, *JONA* 36(2):96-102, 2006.

Hitt MA, Ireland RD, Hoskisson RE: *Strategic management: Concepts and Cases*, ed 7, Lakeland, CO, 2006, South-Western College Pub.

Hosszu T: Evidence-based management, *Harvard Business Review* 84(4):142-143, 2006.

Huber DL: *Leadership and nursing care management*, ed 3, Philadelphia, 2006, Saunders/Elsevier.

Hudson K: Policy and procedure management, *Nursing Management* 37(6):34-38, 2006.

Humer F: Intuition, *Harvard Business Review* 85(1):17-18, 2007.

Ingersoll G, Widzel P, Smith T: Using organizational mission, vision and values to guide professional practice model of development and measurement of nurse performance, *JONA* 35(2):86-93, February 2005.

Institute of Medicine (IOM): *Crossing the quality chasm: A new health system for the 21st century*, Washington, DC, 2001, National Academy Press.

Kramer M, Maguire P, Schmalenberg CE: Excellence through evidence: The what, when, and where of clinical autonomy, *JONA* 36(10):479, 2006.

Malloch K, Porter-O'Grady T: *Introduction to evidence-based practice in nursing and health care*, Boston, 2006, Jones and Bartlett Publishers.

Marquis BL, Huston CJ: *Leadership roles and management functions in nursing*, ed 5, Philadelphia, 2006, Lippincott Williams & Wilkins.

Marriner Tomey A, Alligood MR: *Nursing theorists and their work*, St. Louis, 2006, Mosby.

Martelli P: Evidence based management, Harvard Business Review 84(7/8):184, 2006.

Matter S: Empower nurses with evidence-based knowledge, *Nursing Management* 37(12):34, 2006.

McConnell CR: *Umiker's management skills for the new health care supervisor*, Boston, 2006, Jones and Bartlett Publishers.

Meinyk BM, Fineout-Overholt E: Consumer preferences and values as an integral key to evidence-based practice, *JONA* 30(2):123-127, 2006.

Meinyk M, Fineout-Overholt E: *Evidence-based practice in nursing and healthcare: A guide to best practice*, Philadelphia, 2004, Lippincott Williams & Wilkins.

Pearson A, Field J, Jordon A: *Evidence-based clinical practice in nursing and healthcare: Assimilating research, experience and expertise*, Ames, IA, 2007, Blackwell Publishing Professional.

Penz KL, Bassendowski SL: Evidence-based nursing in clinical practice: Implication for nurse educators, *The Journal of Continuing Education in Nursing* 37(6): 250-255, 2006.

Pfeffer J, Sutton R: Evidence-based management, *Harvard Business Review* 84(1):62-74, 2006.

Roussel L, Swansburg RC, Swansburg RJ: *Introductory management and leadership for nurses*, ed 4, Boston, 2006, Jones & Bartlett.

Shirey MR: Evidence-based practice: How nurse leaders can facilitate innovation, *Nursing Administration Quarterly* 30(3):252, 2006.

Simpson RL: Evidence-based practice: How nursing administration makes it happen, *Nursing Administration Quarterly* 30(3):291, 2006.

Smith P, James T, Lorentzon M, Pope R: *Shaping the facts: Evidence-based nursing and health care*, St. Louis, 2004, Churchill Livingstone.

Smith SF, Duell DJ, Martin BC: *Clinical nursing skills: Basic to advanced skills*, ed 5, Upper Saddle River, NJ, 2004, Prentice Hall.

Stone PW, Curran CR, Bakken S: Economic evidence for evidence-based practice, *Journal of Nursing Scholarship* 34(3):277-282, 2002.

Sullivan EJ, Decker PJ: *Effective leadership management in nursing*, ed 6, Upper Saddle River, NJ, 2005, Pearson/Prentice Hall.

Tuck L, Harris LH, Baliko B: Values expressed in philosophies of nursing service, *JONA* 30(4):180-184, 2000.

Yoder-Wise PS, Kowalski KE: *Beyond leading and managing: Nursing administration for the future*, St. Louis, 2006, Mosby/Elsevier.

Yoder-Wise PS: *Leading and managing in nursing*, ed 4, St. Louis, 2007, Mosby.

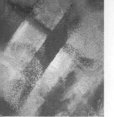

Financial Management, Cost Containment, and Marketing

9

"Money is a terrible master, but an excellent servant." —Anonymous

Chapter Overview

Chapter 9 discusses the history of health care financing, budgetary leadership and management, budgets, cost containment, costing out nursing services, personal finances, and marketing.

Chapter Objectives

- Define capitation.
- Identify at least three prerequisites for budgeting.
- Compare at least four types of budgets.
- Differentiate at least three advantages and three disadvantages of budgeting.
- Select at least five strategies for cost containment.
- Explain fixed and variable costs as they relate to break-even points.
- Determine at least three factors to consider when costing out nursing services.
- Describe the four *P*'s of the marketing mix.
- Describe the Boston consulting group's grid of potential growth and profitability possibilities for identifying marketing strategies.
- Name the four stages in the life cycle of a product.
- Explain at least three ways to do pricing.
- Determine at least four promotion tools.

Online Resources

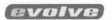

Critical thinking activities, worksheets, and case studies are available online at http://evolve.elsevier.com/Marriner/guide8e.

Major Concepts and Definitions

Accounting *a system for reporting business transactions and preparing financial statements*

Budget *a written plan for the allocation of resources and a control for ensuring that results comply with the plans*

Capitation *a fixed monthly fee for providing health maintenance services to enrollees*

Cost containment *holding back costs within fixed limits*

Economics *production, distribution, and consumption of wealth*

Costing out *calculating the cost of specific items*

Marketing *the business of buying and selling; the analysis, planning, implementation, and control of programs for exchanges of values with target markets to achieve organizational objectives*

Exchange *to give and receive resources*

Publics *distinct groups of people or organizations that have an actual or potential interest in or impact on an organization*

Market *a place where goods are bought and sold*

Image *sum of a person's beliefs, ideas, and impressions about an object or person*

Audit *to examine or correct financial accounts; identification, collection, and evaluation of information that needs examination to evaluate market relations*

Segmentation *subsets of the total market*

Marketing mix *product, price, place, and promotions*

Life cycle *introduction, growth, maturity, and market decline stages of a product*

Break-even calculations *computations to determine the point at which direct and indirect costs are equal to income*

Direct costs *specific costs of a program*

Indirect costs *generalized costs such as maintenance and administration allocated to the program*

Variable costs *costs that vary in direct proportion to volume*

Fixed costs *costs unrelated to volume*

Semifixed costs *costs that are fixed within a range of activity*

Semivariable costs *costs that are fixed at zero output and increase with volume*

HISTORY OF HEALTH CARE FINANCING

During the 1930s, most health care was privately financed. Insurance plans grew during the 1950s. During that time, cost-based pricing was used. The price of service was based on direct costs (such as salaries, benefits, supplies) and indirect costs or overhead costs (including services such as accounting, administration, housekeeping, medical records, depreciation, interest expenses, repayment of debt, return on investments, bad debts, other uncollectable accounts). The more treatments and services provided the more income to the health care providers. This retrospective approach increased hospital profits, increased health care costs, and in turn increased insurance rates.

Medicare was developed during the 1960s and brought average pricing to the health care market by establishing an average price that it would pay for services. That led to competition-based pricing, which forced providers to achieve the marketplace average or lose money.

Health costs have been rising because of the aging of the population and consequent increase in the number of individuals with chronic diseases and increased health care needs, the increased use of expensive technology, the availability of new and expensive treatment modalities, the rising cost of litigation, the increase in the number of uninsured people, and the increase in administrative costs. Previously, third-party payers paid hospitals for services. The employers paid the insurance premiums. The insurance companies paid the bills, and the customers felt little effect. During the 1980s, 1990s, and 2000s, insurance companies raised their premiums dramatically to meet the rising costs, which made it difficult for employers to pay the premiums. Consequently customers are required to pay larger portions of the costs as deductibles and are becoming increasingly aware of the high costs of health care and the need to be selective.

A *prospective reimbursement system* encourages the implementation of cost-effective health care services. The Tax Equity and Fiscal Responsibility Act of 1982 added case mix into Medicare reimbursement calculations through the definition of diagnosis-related groups (DRGs). A prospective payment system based on 467 DRG categories that provided pretreatment diagnosis billing categories for most U.S. hospitals reimbursed by Medicare was signed into law as HR 1900 (Public Law 98-21) by President Reagan. It used a prospective time frame rather than the traditional retrospective one. Reimbursement is based on case or costs related to the treatment of specific DRGs rather than on per diem costs or total hospital costs divided by patient-days. The payment unit is the diagnosis rather than the patient-day. Rates are determined from local, regional, and national rural and urban costs instead of the hospital's own costs. There are incentive payments when the length of stay is lower than average and disincentives when costs exceed the standard, so that hospitals profit from cost containment. Previously, hospitals were reimbursed for costs retrospectively and had little incentive to contain costs. The prospective payment system applies to all Medicare-participating hospitals

except long-term care, rehabilitation, children's, and psychiatric care hospitals. The results of the DRG-based system include a decrease in the number of patients in acute care settings because of early discharge, an increase in the acuteness of illness among hospitalized patients, an increase in the use of ambulatory and home care facilities, and a focus on cost-effectiveness.

Managed care became widespread during the 1980s. Coordination of high-cost health care services became a goal of health care insurance companies. Since 1988 there has been rapid growth in case management or utilization review organizations that monitor the delivery of care and are gatekeepers to providers of care. *Clinical pathways* use outcome criteria as indicators of quality. Cooperation among health care providers is necessary to achieve the expected outcomes in the most efficient manner. By the late 1990s, capitation and global payments were common.

Insurance companies have developed policies to control costs that direct beneficiaries away from providers that have charges above the marketplace average. By 2000, insurance companies were demanding discounted services. Insurance companies were contracting for discounts in or deductions from patient care charges that health care providers had to write off. The exclusive provider arrangement gives insurance coverage only for services rendered by a contracted professional or institution except when there is an emergency or when the insured individual is out of a given geographical area.

Health maintenance organizations (HMOs) provide comprehensive health care services to enrollees for a fixed periodic payment. *Capitation* is the fixed payment given to the provider per member per month for a specified amount of health care services. *Actuarial services* provide statistical analysis of demographic, financial, and utilization trends to predict health plan premiums or costs. The clients choose their physicians from a medical group roster. The primary care physician is a gatekeeper who assesses the patient and determines if referral to a specialist or hospitalization is necessary. The incentive is to keep patients healthy and to reduce physician, diagnostic, and hospital services. Under capitation, in which there is a fixed monthly fee no matter how much service is provided to the enrollee, the financial risk for provision of care is transferred from the payer to the health care delivery system. Visits to a physician and use of services are expenses, not revenue, to the provider. Hospitals have incentives to lower hospitalizations, decrease the length of stay, and minimize the variations in stay among patients with like diagnoses. Consequently, hospital utilization has dropped drastically, and hospitals have many empty beds. Hospitals have subcontracted some services, such as dialysis, to others for less cost. Because hospitals have large fixed costs in physical facilities, the trend of the 1980s and 1990s to give care outside the hospital may be reversed. Hospitals have become involved in delivery of services such as home health care and hospice care that previously were provided outside the hospital. Hospital administrators have become health care system managers.

Preferred provider organizations (PPOs) negotiate a special, usually reduced, rate for insurance plan beneficiaries, generally on a fee-for-service basis with incentives of lowered rates for consumers when they use the preferred providers. *Individual provider arrangements (IPAs)* allow health care providers to provide medical services in their offices for managed care or prepaid plans. This was one of the first alternative delivery prepaid plans with a set of benefits provided by a group of providers within a specific geographical area. During the 1940s, Kaiser Permanente became one of the first employers to provide such a plan.

Now managed competition exists among prepaid providers such as HMOs, PPOs, and IPAs and leads to early discharge of patients; early retirement of the better-paid senior nurses; narrow differentials in pay among nurses with associate, bachelor of science, and master of science degrees; slower wage growth rates; replacement of registered nurses (RNs) with less trained, more poorly paid, unlicensed personnel; increased use of advanced practice nurses as substitutes for physicians and psychologists; use of RNs

as utilization reviewers; and merging or resizing of agencies. In 2000, the federal government introduced ambulatory payment classifications as part of a new payment system for outpatient services, which changed the basis of payment for outpatient services from a flat fee for individual services to a fixed reimbursement for bundled services.

Supply and demand lead to demand-based pricing. Higher prices are paid for products or services that are in high demand. Reduced demand leads to lower prices. This makes entrepreneurial activities important both within the organization and to external markets. Entrepreneurs take risks for profits. Strategic planning is needed to determine which activities will be in the most demand and make the most profits. For example, a hospital may provide a food service instead of outsourcing that service and open the cafeteria to the public community for profit.

The providers played a major role in setting prices in the cost-based and charge-based systems. They assume increased financial risk in the flat-fee and capitated payment systems. Cost shifting by payers attempting to control their costs and by providers trying to pass on unpaid costs from one payer to other payers has caused a great increase in costs to the private sector. Consequently, employers and insurers have become increasingly involved in managing care.

Globalization has brought new challenges during the 2000s. Electronic communication facilitates instantaneous contact and worldwide collegial collaboration for solutions to biologic and technologic health care challenges. The Web allows the public to be aware of the latest diagnostic and treatment modalities and the "centers of excellence" at which those modalities are available. Assessable air transportation makes society highly and rapidly mobile. Consequently, diseases previously limited to remote locales can spread in epidemics and pandemics. The research and development for new drugs entails considerable cost and takes a prolonged time. The same is true for the development of diagnostic and technologic tools. While such work is being done, diseases can be spreading

RESEARCH Perspective 9-1

Data from Cowan MJ, Shapiro M, Hayes R, et al: The effect of a multidisciplinary hospitalist/physician and advanced practice nurse collaboration on hospital costs, *J Nurs Adm* 36(2):79-85, 2006.

Purpose: The purpose of this study was to compare nurse practitioner/physician management of hospital care, multidisciplinary team-based planning, expedited discharge, and assessment after discharge to usual management.

Methods: A comparative, two-group, quasiexperimental design was used and 1207 general medicine patients were enrolled. The experimental group included 581 patients and the control group included 626 patients. The control unit provided the usual care, whereas the experimental unit had three different components: an advanced

practice nurse who followed the patients during hospitalization and for 30 days after discharge, a hospitalist medical director and another hospitalist, and daily multidisciplinary rounds. Length of stays, hospital costs, mortality, and readmission 4 months after discharge were measured.

Results/conclusions: The average length of stay was significantly lower for patients in the experimental group than for those in the control group. The experimental treatment was more profitable for the hospital. There were no significant differences in mortality or readmissions.

in epidemic and pandemic magnitudes. The cost could be astronomical.

There is recognition that teams with diverse perspectives and experiences can achieve superior knowledge and process outcomes. The financial burden of epidemics and pandemics is a concern. The United States cannot be expected to underwrite the cost of epidemics and pandemics. It is important for the funding to be equitably shared by those at risk. The World Health Organization has been identified as a logical body to administer a program of that type. Its personnel could collect funds from numerous countries and facilitate the collaboration of researchers from around the world in the development of new diagnostic and technologic tools and drugs. The funds held by the World Health Organization could reimburse the cost of mobilizing research teams, human experts, and material supplies and technology when a global health care threat is identified by the World Health Organization, but the normal cost of research and development would be borne as the usual health care expense by each country. Multiple countries could then share the costs of prevention and treatment of epidemics and pandemics.

In the meantime, nurse managers and others need to prepare for large-scale infectious disease outbreaks. Clinical care protocols should

be developed, alternate space use designs should be planned, emergency staffing procedures should be developed, staff education with simulation drills should be conducted, and adequate disease testing equipment should be put in place. Although the preparedness is costly, it can be cheaper than failing to prepare (Institute for the Future, 2003; Nosek, 2004).

BUDGETARY LEADERSHIP AND MANAGEMENT

During the 1990s, 440 hospitals closed. Fifty-eight percent of the hospitals closed were in urban areas and 42% were located in rural areas (Office of Inspector General, 2001). This economic environment makes it increasingly important for nurses to understand economics and marketing, and to speak the related language.

Budgetary leaders inspire proactive fiscal planning, determine resource needs; guide the formulation of justification for resources; negotiate for needed resources; analyze expenses; anticipate, recognize, and creatively deal with budgetary problems; create a financially savvy work environment; involve group members in fiscal planning; and help groups find innovative ways to be more cost-effective (Table 9-1).

TABLE 9-1 Budgetary Leadership and Management

Leader	Manager
Inspires proactive instead of reactive fiscal planning	Coordinates fiscal planning to make it consistent with organizational goals and objectives
Determines resources and needs	
Guides formulation of justification for resources	Plans the budget
Negotiates for needed resources	Organizes the budget justification
Locates new sources of resources	Implements the budget process
Analyzes expenses	Determines resource requirements within constraints
Anticipates, recognizes, and creatively deals with budgetary problems	Coordinates expenses and budget control
Creates a financially savvy work environment	Documents needs to other administrative levels
Involves group members in fiscal planning	Organizes procurement of needed resources
Helps groups find innovative ways to be more cost-effective	Explains budgeting to others
	Evaluates technology

Modified from Huber D: *Leadership and nursing case management*, Philadelphia, 2006, Saunders; Marquis BL, Huston CJ: *Leadership roles and management functions in nursing: Theory and application*, ed 5, Philadelphia, 2006, Lippincott Williams & Wilkins.

The *fiscal manager* coordinates fiscal planning, plans the budget, organizes the justification, implements the budget process, determines resource requirements within the constraints, coordinates expenses and budget control, documents needs to other administrative levels, organizes needed resources, explains budgeting to others, and evaluates technology (Huber, 2006; Marquis & Huston, 2006).

BUDGETS

"Proportion your expenses to what you have, not what you expect."   —English proverb

A *budget* is a written plan for the allocation of resources and a control for ensuring that results comply with the plan. Results are expressed in quantitative terms. Although budgets are usually associated with financial statements, such as revenues and expenses, they also may be nonfinancial statements covering output, materials, and equipment. Budgets help coordinate the efforts of the agency by determining what resources will be used by whom, when, and for what purpose. They are frequently prepared for each organizational unit and for each function within the unit.

Planning is done for a specific period, usually a fiscal year, but may be performed for monthly, quarterly, or semiannual periods. The budgeting period is determined by the desired frequency of checks and should complete a normal cycle of activity. Setting budget periods that coincide with other control devices—such as managerial reports, balance sheets, and profit-and-loss statements—is helpful.

The extent to which accurate forecasts can be made must be considered. If the budget forecasts is forecasted too far in advance, its usefulness is diminished. On the other hand, factors such as seasonal fluctuations make it impossible to predict long-range needs from short budget periods. Managers therefore necessarily revise budgets as more information becomes available. Top management and the board of directors also may prepare long-term budgets of 3, 5, or more years, but these are not used as direct operating budgets (Huber, 2006; Yoder-Wise & Kowalski, 2006).

PREREQUISITES TO BUDGETING

Some conditions are necessary for the development and implementation of a budgetary program. First, a sound organizational structure with clear lines of authority and responsibility is needed. In such an organization, all employees know their responsibilities and the person to whom they are responsible; they have the authority to do what they are responsible for and are held accountable for their actions. Organization charts and job descriptions are available, and goals and objectives are set for areas of responsibilities. Budgets are then developed to conform to the pattern of authority and responsibility.

Nonmonetary statistical data—such as number of admissions, average length of stay, percentage of occupancy, and number of patient-days—are used for planning and control of the budgetary process. Someone must be responsible for collecting and reporting statistical data.

Charts of accounts are designed to be consistent with the organizational plan. Revenues and expenses are reported by responsibility areas, which supplies historical data that are valuable for planning and provides budgetary control for evaluation because performance can be compared with plans. Nurse managers focus their attention on the principle of management by exception by noting what is not going as planned so they can take necessary action.

Managerial support is essential for a budgetary program. Although budgeting is done at the departmental level, it must be valued by top administration. Managers must be willing to devote their time and energy to the budgeting process. They are most likely to do that when they are familiar, through budget education, with the principles of budgeting and its usefulness for planning and controlling.

Formal budgeting policies and procedures should be available in a budget manual, in which the objectives of the budgetary program are defined, authority and responsibility for budgeting are clarified, and instructions for budget development are discussed in detail. The manual should include samples of standardized forms, a calendar of the budgeting activities with the schedule for each stage of the program, and procedures for review, revision, and approval of budgets.

APPLIED ECONOMICS

Because decisions have become more complex and critical in the global economy, nurse leaders need to know more about economics than ever before. *Economic goods* are goods or services purchased by consumers from suppliers to provide a benefit to the consumer. Goods and services are acquired through an exchange, generally of money. *Wealth* is the value of the consumer's resources. *Income* is additional resources gained over time. Consumers do not have the wealth to buy everything they want, so they must make choices about what to purchase.

Utility is the benefit consumers get from the purchase of goods and services. It helps determine how much the consumer is willing to pay. *Marginal utility* is the additional utility gained by consuming one more unit. Marginal utility is not the same for all consumers or for all additional units. A person who likes chocolate is more willing to pay for a chocolate candy bar than a person who does not like chocolate but may not be willing to buy a second or third chocolate bar. People try to maximize their *total utility*. Total utility is maximized when a mix of goods is consumed so that the last unit has the same marginal utility per dollar spent as the first unit.

Supply and demand influence costs. *Supply* is the amount of goods or services that suppliers are willing to provide at a given price. *Demand* is the amount of goods or services consumers are willing to buy at that price. For an *equilibrium price*, the quantity offered and the quantity demanded are the same. As supply goes up and demand goes down, the price is likely to go down. As the supply goes down and the demand goes up, the price is likely to go up.

Elasticity of demand is the degree to which the demand for a good or service decreases in response to a price increase and increases in response to a price decrease. The demand for health care is generally inelastic. One is likely to have emergency surgery whether the price is up or down.

Economies of scale occur when the cost of providing goods or services falls as quantity increases and fixed costs are spread over the larger volume. Large volumes can eventually lead to decreasing returns to scale as more personnel and supplies are needed and costs consequently go up.

Incentives encourage action. Managers may use them to encourage good use of scarce resources.

Health insurance deductibles are incentives to encourage desirable behavior.

Market efficiency is the optimal allocation and use of goods and services resulting from supply and demand. Managers need to be attentive to having the goods and services desired available and not having an abundance of what is not wanted.

Redistribution of resources may be done to improve equality by moving resources to areas of high demand.

Market failure occurs when the free market does not operate efficiently and may result from lack of information, lack of direct patient payment, monopoly, government intervention and government-induced inefficiency, and other externalities (Finkler & McHugh, 2007; Samuelson, 2006).

ACCOUNTING

Accounting is a system that accumulates bookkeeping entries into summaries of the financial condition of an enterprise. The fundamental equation of accounting is as follows:

Assets = Liabilities + Fund balance

Assets are the valuable resources owned by the agency. *Liabilities* are what the agency owes. *Fund balance* is the agency's equity or undistributed profits. The *balance sheet* is a financial statement that shows the financial position of the agency at a specific time. The *income statement*, or statement of revenues and expenses, shows the financial results of the agency's activities for a specified period. *Depreciation* is the allocation of a portion of the cost of an asset with a multiyear life over the years the asset will be used. A *journal* is a book or computer file recording the financial events of the agency in chronologic order. *Ledgers* are sets of individual accounts to which information from the journal is transferred or posted so that the balance in any account can be determined and reported. *Fund accounting* is an optional accounting system used by not-for-profit agencies to establish a complete, distinct set of accounting records for separate accounts of agency assets.

These assets may be restricted and unrestricted funds set aside for specific purposes, such as endowments, renovations, or buildings (Finkler, 2004).

Several terms must be understood to interpret financial accounting reports. An *entity* is a definable organizational unit. The accountant considers only transactions between one entity and another. Transactions that occur within the entity or do not involve it are not considered. If each department is an entity, performance can be compared between departments. However, if the agency as a whole is the entity, the transfer of resources from one department to another is not taken into account. Accounts deal only with *transactions*, or definable changes in the financial situation of an entity: income, expenditure, depreciation. *Cost valuation* values goods at their cost minus any depreciation. *Double entry* compares the assets (what is owed to or owned by the entity) with the liabilities (what is owed by the entity to others). Accountants balance total assets with the total liabilities and net worth. The double entry makes it possible to know where the entity stands financially at any given time. *Accrual* allows one to determine the overall assets and liabilities by entering transactions on the accounting records at the time a commitment is made rather than waiting until it is billed or paid. *Matching* is the principle of matching revenues with expenses during a budget period.

There are several standard accounting practices. *Consistency* means that categories of transactions may not be changed during or between reporting periods without noting the changes and providing comparable figures. *Materiality* means that transactions can be combined for accounting purposes unless one transaction has a significant impact by itself. *Conservatism* is the act of understating revenue and overstating expenses to provide a margin of safety. Industry practices are specific to industries. Having special fund accounts designated by donors and establishing a separate account for charitable care provided are examples of industry practices (Young, 2004).

TYPES OF BUDGETS

Operating or Revenue-and-Expense Budgets

"To get money is difficult, to keep it more difficult, but to spend it wisely most difficult of all." —Anonymous

The *operating budget* provides an overview of an agency's functions by projecting the planned operations, usually for the upcoming year. The *operating table* shows an input-output analysis of expected revenues and expenses. Among the line items that nurse managers might include in their operating budgets are personnel salaries, employee benefits, insurance, medical-surgical supplies, office supplies, rent, heat, light, housekeeping, laundry service, drugs and pharmaceuticals, repairs and maintenance, depreciation, in-service education, travel to professional meetings, educational leaves, books, periodicals, subscriptions, dues and membership fees, legal fees, and recreation, such as Christmas parties and retirement teas.

Both controllable and noncontrollable expenses are projected. The manager determines the number of personnel needed and the level of skills required of each. Wage levels and quality of materials used are other controllable expenses. Indirect expenses, such as rent, lighting costs, and depreciation of equipment, are noncontrollable. The existence of noncontrollable expenses and the probability of rises in material prices or labor costs during the budgetary period demand that an operating budget include some cushion funds to provide for changes beyond the agency's control.

The operating budget deals primarily with salaries, supplies, and contractual services. Nonfinancial factors, such as time, materials, and space, can be translated into dollar values. Work hours, nurse-patient interaction hours, units of materials, equipment hours, and floor space also can be assigned dollar values (Huber, 2006; Marquis & Huston, 2006; Roussel, Swansburg, & Swansburg, 2006; Yoder-Wise, 2007; Yoder-Wise & Kowalski, 2006) (Table 9-2).

Personnel Budgets

Personnel budgets estimate the cost of direct labor necessary to meet the agency's objectives. They determine the recruitment, hiring, assignment, layoff, and discharge of personnel. The nurse manager decides on the type of nursing care necessary to meet the nursing needs of the estimated patient population. How many aides, orderlies, licensed practical nurses, and RNs are needed during what shifts, in what months, and in what areas? The current staffing patterns, number of unfilled positions, and last year's reports can provide a base for examination and proposals. Patient occupancy rates and the

TABLE 9-2 Operating Budget for a Medical Unit with Thirty Beds (December 2007)

Statistic	Actual	Budget	Variance
Patient-days	870	720	(150)
Full-time equivalents	79.2	71.4	(7.8)
Revenues			
Inpatient revenue	$1,287,000	$1,085,700	$201,300
Operating expenses			
Salaries, wages, benefits	$372,780	$246,450	($126,330)
Contract employees	3720	2000	(1720)
Overtime	7712	8640	928
Supplies	17,200	14,700	(2500)
Repairs	1000	1200	200
Travel	650	600	(50)
Continuing education	1750	2000	250
Total expenses	$404,812	$275,590	($129,222)

general complexity of patient cases affect staffing patterns; seasonal fluctuations must also be considered. Personnel budgets also are affected by personnel policies such as salary level for each position and number of days allowed for educational and personal leave. Overtime costs should be compared with the cost of creating new positions. Employee turnover, recruitment, and orientation costs must be taken into account (Finkler & McHugh, 2007; Marquis & Huston, 2006; Roussel, Swansburg, & Swansburg, 2006).

A *position* is a job for a person no matter how many hours worked. Personnel reports usually describe positions in terms of job categories and the number of hours regularly worked, such as full or part time. *Vacancy and turnover reports* use positions. However, *full-time equivalents (FTEs)* are more useful for payroll reports. An FTE is a conversion of hours to a standard base of one person working so many hours per day, so many days per week, and so many weeks per year (Table 9-3).

FTEs help in interpreting payroll reports, identifying trends, and comparing levels of utilization across time. Productive and nonproductive time should also be considered. *Productive worked time* includes straight time and overtime. *Nonproductive benefit time* includes holidays, vacation days, paid sick leave, and other paid nonworked time, such as continuing education hours. The most significant factor influencing paid FTEs is the fluctuation in nonproductive time. Variations in full-time and part-time staff or in professional versus nonprofessional personnel can be determined using FTEs (Finkler & McHugh, 2007; Huber, 2006; Roussel, Swansburg, & Swansburg, 2006; Sullivan & Decker, 2005).

Capital Expenditure Budgets

Capital expenditure budgets are related to long-range planning. *Capital expenditures* include expenditures on physical changes such as replacement or expansion of the plant, major equipment, and inventories. These items are usually major investments and reduce flexibility in budgeting because it takes a long time to recover the costs. For instance, a patient may be charged per

TABLE 9-3 Example of Full-Time Equivalent*

Time Frame	Total Hours	8-Hour Shifts
Per week	40	5
Per 2-week payroll period	80	10
Per 4-week payroll period	160	20
Per month	173.33	21.66
Per year	2080	260

*Full-time equivalent for person working 8 hours per day, 5 days per week, 52 weeks per year.

treatment or per day for the use of equipment, but it may take many months or even years to recover the cost of the equipment (Table 9-4).

The hospital administrator usually establishes the ceiling for capital expenses. For this budget the nurse manager must establish priorities if requests exceed available funds. When request forms for capital items are filled out, it is advisable to include names of manufacturers and suppliers, trade-in credits, and estimates of purchase, delivery, installation, and maintenance costs. Written justification for each item should be given.

Inventories are helpful in budgeting. If supplies are checked routinely, use and replacement figures are available for projection of future needs. Establishment of central supply services enhances budgetary control, and allotment of storage space facilitates inventory maintenance. Keeping stocked supply shelves on each unit with replacement service twice daily can provide a simplified recording system. Disposable equipment and supplies need careful evaluation to determine whether they are more economical than nondisposables (Huber, 2006; Marquis & Huston, 2006; Roussel, Swansburg, & Swansburg, 2006; Sullivan & Decker, 2005; Yoder-Wise, 2007). Capital expense replacements can also be projected (Grohar-Murray & DiCroce, 2003) (see Table 9-4).

Cash Budgets

Cash budgets are planned to make adequate funds available as needed and to use any extra funds profitably. They ensure that the agency has enough, but not too much, cash on hand during

TABLE 9-4 Capital Budget Request for Medical Unit Cost Center (Calendar Year 2007)

Type	Quantity	Description	Unit Cost	Extended Cost	Priority
Replacement	10	Intravenous pumps	$5000	$50,000	1
Replacement	10	Beds	$6000	$60,000	2

This is a 3-year replacement plan for 30 intravenous pumps and 30 hospital beds, 10 each budgeted per year over 3 years

the budgetary period. This is necessary because income does not always coincide with expenditures. The manager must anticipate fluctuations in resource needs caused by factors such as seasonal variations. If managers have insufficient cash on hand, they will not be able to purchase needed resources. At the other extreme, if too much cash is available, interest or other earnings that money could generate are lost. Budgeting of cash requirements may not significantly affect profits, but it does ensure a liquid position and is a sign of prudent management. Using a cash budget, the nurse manager estimates the amount of money to be collected from clients and other sources and allocates that cash to expenditures. If the budget is well planned, it will provide cash as needed and produce interest on excess funds (Yoder-Wise, 2007) (Box 9-1).

BOX 9-1 Types of Budgets

Operating budget (daily revenues and expenses to operate the health care institution)
  Revenues (income, return on investments and property)
  Expenses (costs)
    Personnel (employed people)
    Supplies (stock, materials—office supplies, pharmaceuticals, medical-surgical supplies)
    Other expenses (spending on items such as travel, training, dues, rentals, repairs, depreciation)
Capital expenditure budget (*capital* is often defined as something that costs more than $500 and is used more than once)
Cash budget (for money available for immediate use)

Flexible Budgets

Some costs are fixed and do not change with the volume of business. Other costs vary proportionately with changes in volume. Some variable expenses are unpredictable and can be determined only after change has begun—thus the need for *flexible budgets* to show the effects of changes in volume of business on expense items. Periodic budget reviews help managers compensate for changes. Relationships between the volume of business and variable costs may be predicted by a historical analysis of costs and development of standard costs (Roussel, Swansburg, & Swansburg, 2006).

Historical Approach to Budgeting

The historical approach is most effective for calculating the relationship between volume of business and variable costs when a company manufactures a few products or provides a few services and each product or service contributes a relatively stable percentage to the total sales volume. Using the historical approach, the nurse manager may observe that there are more fractures during skiing season. Consequently, more casting materials are used at that time, and there is a need for increased staffing on the orthopedic ward.

A supervising community health nurse in a small college town may note that there is less use of family planning services during the summer months and again during December when students leave for vacations. Consequently, there is less need for contraceptive devices and staffing during these months. There may be an increased demand for immunizations just before elementary schools open in the fall. By plotting on a graph the high and low volumes, the nurse manager can predict the expected costs for each level between the extreme volumes. This historical perspective helps determine the amount of supplies to stock and staffing patterns (Sullivan & Decker, 2005).

Standard Cost

Standard cost may be determined to predict what labor and supplies should cost. Multiplying the standard cost by the volume predicts the variable cost. Supervising community health nurses can predict the standard number of clinic visits and the number of birth control pills that will be required for each family planning client who has chosen birth control pills as a method of contraception. By multiplying the number of pills needed by each client by the number of clients using birth control pills, nurse managers can predict the inventory needed and the cost. They also can predict the number of clinic visits needed and plan staffing.

ZERO-BASED BUDGETING

Many budgeting procedures allocate funds to departments on the basis of their expenditures the previous year. Then the department managers decide how the funds will be used. This procedure usually allows for enrichment and enlargement of programs but seldom for decreases in or discontinuation of programs. Obsolescence is seldom examined, and this leads to increased costs.

With zero-based budgeting, no program is taken for granted. Each program or service must be justified each time funds are requested. Managers decide what will be done, what will not be done, and how much of an activity will be implemented. A decision package is prepared. The package includes a list of the activities that make up a program, the total cost, a description of what level of service can be performed at various levels of funding and the ramifications of including them in or excluding them from the budget. The manager may identify the activity, state the purpose, list related activities, outline alternative ways of performing activities, and give the cost of the resources needed.

After decision packages are developed, they are ranked in order of decreasing benefits to the agency. They can be divided into high-, medium-, and low-priority categories and reviewed in order of rank for funding. Resources are allocated based on the priority of the decision package. The cost of each package is added to the cost of approved packages until the agreed-on spending level is reached. Lower-ranked packages are then excluded.

A major advantage to zero-based budgeting is that it can develop managers' skills. It is likely the assumptions will be current and relevant. It forces managers to set priorities and justify resources. Unfortunately the process is time consuming, although some business may be very predictable over time. Instead of re-creating information, it may be more appropriate to give the attention to the areas that are difficult to budget (Huber, 2006; Nowicki, 2004; Roussel, Swansburg, & Swansburg, 2006).

PERIODIC BUDGETARY REVIEW

Managers should review the budget at periodic intervals, compare actual with projected performances, and make necessary changes. *Variance* is the difference between the budget and the actual results. It can be a positive profit or a negative loss. A *variance analysis* investigates the cause. If changes are too frequent or too great, the original budget becomes useless. One way to minimize variance between the annual budget and the revised budget is to anticipate factors such as increased labor costs and the inflationary cost of materials. When discrepancies are found between actual performance and the budget, management must determine the cause of variation to make appropriate adjustments for future plans. A variance may not be reason for changing the budget. It may be a symptom that alerts management to the need for further investigation and explanation. What may demand change is not the budget but the situation (Baker & Baker, 2003; Berkowitz, 2006).

Table 9-2 shows the variance in an annual budget. The variance analysis (Baker & Baker, 2003; Berkowitz, 2006; Sullivan & Decker, 2005) compares the actual results with the preestablished targets. In this case, one can see that the increase in patient-days has caused an increase in personnel expenses and supplies. Monthly variance analysis can help manage the budget. Causes or reasons for the variances are considered. There may be seasonal patterns or trends over time. When variance is greater than an established level, the manager may need to investigate the reasons and explain or justify the variance. The level may be a dollar amount or a percentage of the budgeted item. The variance percentage is calculated by dividing the dollar variance by the budgeted amount and multiplying by 100. For example:

$$\text{\$200 variance for repairs} \div$$
$$\text{\$1200 budgeted amount} =$$
$$0.16666$$

$0.16666 \times 100 = 16.6666\%$ under the budget for repairs

ADVANTAGES AND DISADVANTAGES

Advantages of Budgeting

Budgets plan for detailed program activities. They help fix accountability by assignment of responsibility and authority. They state goals for all units, offer a standard of performance, and stress the continuous nature of the planning and control process. Budgets encourage managers to make a careful analysis of operations and to base decisions on careful consideration. Consequently, hasty judgments are minimized. Weaknesses in the organization can be revealed and corrective measures taken. Staffing, equipment, and supply needs can be projected and waste minimized. Financial matters can be handled in an orderly fashion, and agency activities can be coordinated and balanced.

Disadvantages of Budgeting

Budgets convert all aspects of organizational performance into monetary values to provide a single comparable unit of measurement. Consequently, only those aspects that are easy to measure may be considered, and equally important factors, such as organizational development and research efforts, may be ignored. Symptoms may be treated as causes. Reasons for the symptoms should be explored; a decrease in revenue from the family planning clinic may be related to the way people are treated at the clinic, a new competitive service

in the neighborhood, or other factors. The budget may become an end in itself instead of the means to an end. Budgetary goals may supersede agency goals and gain autocratic control of the organization. There is a danger of overbudgeting so that the budget becomes cumbersome, meaningless, and expensive. Forecasting is required but uncertain, because budgetary control is subject to human judgment, interpretation, and evaluation. Skill and experience are required for successful budgetary control. Budget planning is time consuming and expensive.

BUDGETING PROCESS

Financial planning responsibilities must be identified before budget preparation is begun. The governing board, administrator, budget director, steering committee, and department heads are often involved in the budgetary process. The governing board is responsible for the general planning function. It selects the budget steering committee, determines the budgetary objectives, and reviews and approves the master budget. The administrator is responsible for the formulation and execution of the budget by correlating the governing board's goals with the guidelines for budget preparation and supervising the budget preparation. The budget director, who is responsible for the budgeting procedures and reporting, establishes a completion timetable, has forms prepared, and supervises data collection and budget preparation. The budget director serves as the chairperson of the steering committee, which approves the budget before it is submitted to the governing board. Department heads prepare and review goals and objectives and prepare the budgets for their departments.

The first step in the budget process is the establishment of operational goals and policies for the entire agency. The governing board should approve a long-range plan of 3 to 5 years that reflects the community's future health needs and the activities of other community health care providers. Because the situation changes over time, flexibility is built into the plan. Then operational goals must be translated into quantifiable management objectives for the organizational units. The department heads use the organizational goals as a framework for the development of departmental goals. A formal plan for budget preparation and review, including assignment of responsibilities and timetables, must be prepared. Historical, financial, and statistical data must be collected monthly so that seasonal fluctuations can be observed. Preparing and coordinating departmental budgets are important. During this phase, units of service, staffing patterns, salary and nonsalary expenses, and revenues are forecasted so that preliminary rate setting can be done. Next, departmental budgets are revised, and the master budget is prepared. At this point, operating, payroll, nonsalary, capital, and cash budgets can be incorporated into the master budget. Then the financial feasibility of the master budget is tested, and the final document is approved and distributed to all involved parties. During the budget period, there should be periodic performance reporting by responsibility centers (Huber, 2006; Yoder-Wise, 2007).

COST CONTAINMENT

The goal of cost containment is to keep costs within acceptable limits for volume, inflation, and other parameters. It involves cost awareness, monitoring, management, and incentives to prevent, reduce, and control costs.

Cost Awareness

Cost awareness focuses the employee's attention on costs. It increases organizational awareness of what costs are, what process is available for containing them, how they can be managed, and by whom. Delegating budget planning and control to the unit level increases awareness. Managers should be provided with a course on budgeting and should be oriented to the agency budgeting process before being assigned the responsibility of budgeting. They should have a budget manual that contains budget forms, a budget calendar, and budget periods.

Cost Fairs

Cost fairs in frequented areas, such as the cafeteria, increase awareness by displaying frequently disappearing items that are labeled with the cost per unit and by posting lists of estimated costs of inventory losses. Staff development programs, unit conferences, and poster contests help increase awareness. Tagging supply items with their costs and posting a computer printout of unit charges for supplies and services are revealing. Reviewing a patient's itemized bill during a conference can also be effective.

Cost Monitoring

Cost monitoring focuses on how much will be spent where, when, and why. It identifies, reports, and monitors costs. Staffing costs should be identified. Recruitment, turnover, absenteeism, and sick time are analyzed, and inventories are controlled. A central supply exchange chart prevents hoarding of supplies and allows identification of lost items.

Cost Management

Cost management focuses on what can be done by whom to contain costs. Programs, plans, objectives, and strategies are important. Responsibility and accountability for the control should be established. A committee can identify long- and short-range plans and strategies. A suggestion box can be used, as can contests for the idea that saves the most money.

Money has been saved by means such as forming a staff pool to maximize flexibility in staffing for census fluctuations, cross-training personnel, closing units for cleaning or remodeling and encouraging staff vacations when census is low, balancing the workload among shifts to minimize peaks and valleys in assigned tasks, reducing shift overlap, charting by exception, tape-recording shift reports, revising forms, improving drug ordering and delivery systems, controlling central supplies, not controlling oral analgesics, modifying food services, allowing volunteers to discharge and transport patients, reducing the amount of time nurses spend in nonnursing functions, and using guest relations personnel, a discharge holding area, outpatient clinics, progressive care, and ambulatory care.

Cost Incentives

Cost incentives motivate cost containment and reward desired behavior. Contests for the best money-saving ideas, perfect attendance, and nurse of the month help recognize personnel efforts.

Cost Avoidance

Cost avoidance means not buying supplies, technology, or services. Supply and equipment costs should be carefully analyzed. Costs and effectiveness of disposable versus reusable items are compared. The costs of receipt, storage, and delivery of disposables and labor and processing costs of reusable items are part of the analysis. The least expensive and most effective supplies, equipment, and services should be identified, and expensive and less effective items should be avoided.

Cost Reduction

Cost reduction means spending less for goods and services. The amount of reduction depends on the size of the agency, previous efficiency, the skill of managers, and the cooperation of employees. Safety programs that reduce the costs of workers' compensation and absenteeism programs that reduce sick time, absenteeism, and turnover reduce costs. Healthy living programs, such as exercise activities, stocking of heart-wise foods in the cafeteria, and smoking cessation classes, may help keep workers healthy and thus reduce sick time, absenteeism, and health care costs. Volume buying (getting a cheaper price because of the economies of scale), conservation of supplies, and careful handling of equipment to reduce cost of repairs help reduce costs. Costs can also be reduced through inventory control.

Inventory Control

The manager needs to determine the most economical level of inventory, because supplies represent a significant cost factor. The purchasing, order, storage, and costs of long and short stock must all be considered to determine the most economical level of inventory. The purchasing cost is the price paid per item. Cost may be related to the size of the order, with cost per item decreasing as the size of the order increases. The purchasing cost equals PD where P is the cost or price per unit and D is the number of units purchased.

The *order cost* is the cost of writing specifications, soliciting and analyzing bids, writing orders, receiving the supplies, accounting for the materials, and paying the bills. The order cost may be relatively large the first time an item is purchased or relatively small for routine purchasing processes. The order cost varies with the number of orders placed. The more orders per year, the greater the annual costs. Annual order cost equals $(D/Q)O$, where D is the number of units purchased, Q is the order size, and O is the average cost of placing a single order.

The *carrying cost* is the expense involved in holding inventories. It involves expenses such as storage, insurance, and security. To keep carrying costs down, small orders should be placed frequently; this approach is in direct conflict with keeping the purchasing and order costs low. Carrying cost equals the following:

$$HQ + \frac{IPQ}{2}$$

where H is the cost of storage per item and Q is the order size.

The opportunity cost element is as follows:

$$\frac{IPQ}{2}$$

where I represents the highest obtainable rate of return at the current interest rate, P is price per unit, and Q is the order size.

The *short* or *stock-out costs* involved in holding an insufficient amount of inventory must be considered. The manager considers the consequences of running out of stock. Not only is a sale lost, but also client satisfaction may suffer. Although this expense is difficult to measure, it is a real cost.

Total cost is expressed as follows:

$$TC = PD + \frac{DO}{Q} + \left\{\frac{HQ + IPQ}{2}\right\} + L + S$$

where

TC = Total cost

PD = Purchase cost

$\frac{DO}{Q}$ = Order cost

$HQ + \frac{IPQ}{2}$ = Carrying cost

L = Overstock cost

S = Stock-out cost

The economical order quantity is expressed as follows:

$$EOQ = \sqrt{\frac{2DP}{C}}$$

where

EOQ = Economical order quantity

D = Usage in units or demand

P = Order cost

C = Annual cost of carrying one unit in inventory

A large order size is merited when there is a large demand, high order cost, and low carrying cost. However, a small order size is desired when there is little demand for the item, the order cost is small, and the carrying cost is high.

A high inventory turnover is desired. Low inventory turnover may be caused by poor purchasing policies, overstocking, or a decrease in demand for the item. The inventory turnover can be calculated as follows:

$$\text{Inventory turnover} = \frac{\text{Total cost of supplies}}{\text{Inventories}}$$

To determine when to reorder, the manager must know the average daily usage and the lead time required to receive the supplies. The manager needs to keep on hand the average number of items used daily multiplied by the number of days it takes to receive the goods in order to not run out of stock.

Some managers use the ABC method for maintaining inventories. *A* refers to a small number of items that account for a large percentage of the budget and are carefully monitored; *B* refers to moderate-cost items that receive some monitoring; and *C* refers to a bulk of inexpensive, expendable items such as rubber bands that receive little monitoring (Roussel, Swansburg, & Swansburg, 2006).

Cost Control

Cost control is making effective use of available resources through careful forecasting, planning, budget preparing, reporting, and monitoring. Patient classification systems can be used to predict the appropriate staffing levels. Time management can help control costs. Making meetings worthwhile, reducing repetitious paperwork, improving communication systems, and streamlining the system help save time. Activities to promote retention of personnel, such as providing a good orientation program, ensuring careful placement and mentoring of new personnel, and helping people feel welcome and appreciated can reduce recruitment, orientation, and development expenses. Careful selection of supplies and equipment and in-service training to teach personnel how to use them can reduce frustration and damage. Proper charging of supplies and use of equipment through methods such as bar code scanning and issuance of charge slips could help the health care system recover millions of dollars lost because supplies were not charged to patients. Delegation of appropriate tasks to unlicensed personnel can save more expensive nurses' time for activities requiring more knowledge and skill. Teaching personnel how to delegate, supervise, and develop teams may help control costs in the long run.

Cost-Effectiveness and Cost-Benefit Analysis

Cost-effectiveness analysis is a method of economic evaluation that ranks programs by the cost of achieving the objective. Cost-effectiveness analysis compares costs and identifies the most beneficial outcomes for expenditures by specifying programs; identifying goals; analyzing alternatives; comparing costs per program, unit of service, and amount of service needed; assessing the effect of the outcome; and determining cost outcome and cost-effectiveness. Cost-effectiveness is measured in nonmonetary units, such as fewer readmissions to the hospital or fewer low-birthweight babies. *Cost-benefit analysis* is a procedure that determines the cost of installing and operating a program and converts that into a dollar amount. It also converts all benefits of the program into a dollar amount. A ratio of the two reflects the relationship of costs to benefits. Cost-benefit analysis is measured in monetary units, which facilitates reaching a conclusion regarding whether the program savings outweigh the costs. If the benefit/cost ratio is equal to or greater than 1, the investment is considered good. If the ratio is less than 1, it is not advisable to pursue the venture, because the number of dollars returned is less than the number invested. Such analysis often involves estimating the value of saving a life and adjusting the outcome for quality, which is measured as quality-adjusted life-years. Each increment of variable costs may not yield a comparable increment in work output. For example, adding one employee decreases the service volume for a time as the work increment of each employee decreases. Adding an employee may even cause a decrease in output for the group as communication problems and interpersonal conflict increase. *Break-even analysis* is used to calculate the break-even point for each program (Huber, 2006).

Break-Even Calculations

A *pro forma income statement* is a projection of the operations and activities of a business. The pro forma income and pro forma cash flow statements are used to develop the *pro forma balance sheet*. The pro forma balance sheet reflects the revenue to be generated and cost to be incurred over a period of time. It can be used to help calculate break-even points. *Full costs* equal all direct costs that can be traced to a source plus indirect costs such as those associated with maintenance,

administration, and the building that are allocated to that source. *Cost finding* is an attempt to determine the full cost and to allocate indirect costs. Indirect costs allocated may include housekeeping calculated by square feet, utilities by square feet, laboratory by number of tests, and dietary services by number of meals served.

The cost-volume-profit relationships can be visualized on a *break-even chart*. The manager considers variable, fixed, semifixed, and semivariable costs when doing a break-even analysis. *Variable costs* vary in direct proportion to volume (Figure 9-1). Two disposable syringes probably cost twice as much as one. *Fixed costs* are relatively fixed regardless of changes in volume (Figure 9-2). For example, a nurse receives a certain salary regardless of the number of injections the nurse gives. *Sunk costs* are fixed costs that cannot be recovered even if the service is not provided. *Semifixed costs* are fixed within a range of activity (Figure 9-3). One nurse can give just so many injections per shift, and beyond that a second nurse will need to be hired. *Semivariable costs* are fixed at zero output and increase with volume (Figure 9-4). The *break-even point* is depicted on a break-even chart where revenues equal expenditures (Figure 9-5). The formula for break-even analysis is as follows:

$$R = FC + VC + P$$

where

$$R = \text{Total revenue}$$
$$FC = \text{Fixed cost}$$
$$VC = \text{Variable cost}$$
$$P = \text{Profit}$$

Another break-even analysis equation is:

$$Q = \frac{FC}{P\text{-}VC}$$

where

$$Q = \text{Quantity}$$
$$FC = \text{Fixed cost}$$
$$VC = \text{Variable costs}$$
$$P = \text{Price}$$

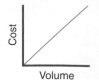

Figure 9-1 • Variable costs.

Figure 9-2 • Fixed costs.

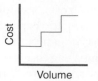

Figure 9-3 • Semifixed costs.

Direct costs are unique to the unit and can be identified with relative certainty. These costs, such as personnel time and supplies, would not occur if the unit were closed. *Indirect costs* or overhead costs are costs of shared resources, such as general administration, housekeeping, information systems, and maintenance, and are more difficult to calculate than are direct costs. *Average cost* is the full cost divided by the volume of service units. The average cost decreases as the volume of patients increases because the fixed costs are distributed over more patients. *Mixed costs* contain both the variable and fixed cost elements. *Marginal costs* are the extra costs created by providing care to one more service unit. It is the difference in the total costs before and after adding one more service unit. Decisions about changes should be made on the basis of marginal costs rather than average or full costs.

Cost estimation is the prediction of costs. It is a complicated process that involves dividing historical costs into fixed and variable components and adjusting historical costs for inflation to predict future costs. To adjust cost for inflation, the historical cost is multiplied by the current value of the appropriate price index divided by the value of that index when the cost was incurred. *Regression analysis* considers costs as the dependent variable and service units as the independent variable. The coefficient of the independent variable represents the variable costs, and the constant term of the regression represents fixed costs. *Contribution margin* is the price minus the variable costs per service unit and represents the additional financial benefit for each additional service unit (Finkler & McHugh, 2007; Gapenski, 2004; Huber, 2006; Roussel, Swansburg, & Swansburg, 2006)

Strategic Cost Decisions

"Not everything that counts can be counted and not everything that can be counted counts." —Albert Einstein

Adopting a strategic approach to cost containment involves taking a comprehensive view of the costs of the organization without being limited to direct, measurable costs. This approach uses a total cost perspective that includes a broad range of tangible and intangible operating and strategic costs. A cost audit is important in the creation of a cost-management strategy. The audit provides an assessment of the organization's cost position, compares it with that of competitors, and evaluates it for future profitability. This allows an assessment of the organization's current cost management processes.

Some accounting personnel may need to learn about the information needs of management. Defining what reports are required is important. In their cost containment efforts, managers and staff need to be supported with data that are focused rather than be overwhelmed with data that bury the critical information. Report formats should be clear and simple. Accountants' capabilities should be matched with the needs of management and staff.

Managers need to change their view of cost reductions from a negative exercise to something that can be creative and exciting. Then they should involve employees in this challenging and exciting process. Effective management

Figure 9-4 • Semivariable costs.

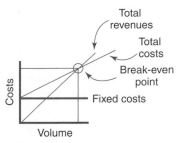

Figure 9-5 • Break-even costs.

communication is needed to increase employee awareness for and understanding of cost management. Having more employees involved in the task can create the greatest leverage. Brainstorming can be done with employees at all levels, who can then contribute to cost reduction. Short presentations about what actions are necessary and what employees can do, and rewards for results are key ingredients. Personal talks, videotaped presentations, newsletters, bulletin boards, staff meetings, and the grapevine can be used for communications. Meetings and discussions with employees can help alleviate fears and uncertainties about cost management.

Many ideas do not need simultaneous development and implementation. Factors such as what can be implemented quickly, cheaply, and with the greatest results should be considered. Short-term successes can be celebrated on the way to long-term improvements as management-employee attitudes and relationships change. Cost reduction successes should be rewarded. Recognition is a reward for most types of agency achievement. It can be formal, such as an employee-of-the-month program or public recognition in the form of a photograph and article in a newsletter or other media, or informal, such as a pat on the back or a simple "Thank you." Employees may quickly forget positive comments but remember any negative ones, so small token awards such as company pens or other items with the agency logo that may be handed out to customers can be used as a physical reminder of the manager's appreciation. Status rewards, such as employee of the month, can be used to create role models and heroes. Money can be awarded for proposing cost-reducing ideas, usually within a suggestion plan. An effective cost management strategy can take a long time to fully implement.

Persistence is a quality of good cost cutters. The long-run commitment to successful cost management strategies helps give the organization the competitive edge.

Cost cutting often involves workforce reduction. Increasing the number of cuts may become progressively less effective as muscle gets cut with fat. Attrition and early retirement are preferable to layoffs. Unfortunately, negative side effects can offset direct savings. High performers may become insecure and accept other positions, morale and productivity may drop, employees may stop suggesting ways to reduce costs, and absenteeism and grievances are likely to increase. Silent sabotage may occur in the form of increased employee theft; convening of the water cooler gang or gossiping about the company in a public place; employee huddling and chattering, which is gossip about what happened or might happen and causes hours of nonproductive time; stay-and-quit syndrome, in which employees lose their enthusiasm and refuse to go the extra mile; or work deviation, in which employees divert business by not providing good service. Restructuring work relationships, utilizing cross-skills, and gaining greater employee involvement may offer significant effects through increased productivity.

Across-the-board cuts may lead to customer complaints, inability to do the work, or lost time because of shortages of parts and lack of maintenance that consequently greatly increase costs. Focused cuts are more useful. Some managers concentrate on controlling direct expenditures and cut nickel-and-dime items such as free coffee. That can lead to greater losses because employees spend time complaining about the lost privilege instead of getting the work done.

Expenditures on "soft" items that lead indirectly to cost reductions are sometimes the first to be cut. Sometimes it is necessary to spend money to make or save money. Staff development, travel to gain new experiences, staff meetings held on company time, provision of seed money, and maintenance work can lead indirectly to cost savings.

Capital- or technology-intensive approaches may lead to cost reductions but may also result in higher overall costs, and implementation may be painful. Activity-based cost management should be used with caution, because a high percentage of the cost in health care organizations is indirect, and the indirect costs are not distributed evenly among units. Activity-based costing software packages convert financial information into a management tool by aligning costs with the various activities and by assigning costs directly to nursing practice. They can help differentiate value-added from non–value-added activities. Developing learning organizations, maximizing employee satisfaction, and simplifying and improving performance measures can be cost management strategies.

COSTING OUT NURSING SERVICES

The equation for the traditional model is the following:

$$NT \times (ANHS + BAI + ICA) = TNC \, per \, DRG$$

where

NT = Amount of nursing time per intensity level for a DRG

$ANHS$ = Average nursing hourly salary

BAI = Benefits across the institution

ICA = Indirect cost amount

TNC = Total nursing cost

The equation for the McCloskey model (Huber, 2006; McCloskey, 1989) is the following:

$$NT/NI \times (ANHS + BAI + EC + ICA) = TNC$$

where

NT = Amount of nursing time

NI = Nursing intervention (instead of intensity level for a DRG)

$ANHS$ = Average nursing hourly salary

BAI = Benefits across the institution

EC = Equipment cost (not in traditional model)

ICA = Indirect cost amount

TNC = Total nursing cost (instead of cost per DRG)

In general, the key problems related to costing out nursing are a lack of comparability of the data used, multiple definitions of costs, and neglect of variables that affect nursing care. We need a forum where administrators, researchers, educators, and staff can share ideas about cost-effectiveness. We need models to describe the relationships among cost, quality, and price of nursing functions. We need to continue to compare methods for costing out nursing care and to identify data sets needed to cost out nursing. Levels of care, expected outcomes, and cost of care can be related to pricing of nursing care. Nurses must be concerned about maintaining cost-effective, high-quality health care.

MARKETING

Marketing is the analysis, planning, implementation, and control of carefully formulated programs designed to bring about voluntary exchanges of values with target markets for the purpose of achieving organizational objectives. It relies heavily on designing the organization's offering in terms of the target markets' needs and desires and on using effective pricing, communication, and distribution to inform, motivate, and service the markets (Kotler & Keller, 2006).

Social Marketing

Social marketing is a fast-growing segment of nonprofit marketing in this age of rapid population growth and economic, social, and environmental problems. Firms should consider consumer short-run wants and long-run welfare and make decisions that are best for consumers and society in the long run. Social marketing applies generic marketing to change the social behavior of a target audience or the well-being of society in general. For example, health care agencies market antismoking campaigns, nutrition education, exercise programs, immunizations, cancer detection, healthy heart programs, safe sexual practices, and occupational safety. Marketing can be aimed at one-time or continuing behavior, high or low involvement, and individual or group behavior. Continuing high-involvement behavior of groups is the most difficult to change. Social marketing may try to create demand where none exists or influence negative demand, and may target relatively nonliterate audiences. It often deals with hard-to-research, sensitive issues or relatively invisible benefits while waiting for long-term change. If one is lucky, sustaining the new behavior becomes an issue. All companies have four basic social responsibilities: (1) economic—to be profitable; (2) legal—to obey the law and do what is legally correct; (3) ethical—to do what is right, just, and fair; and (4) philanthropical—to be a good citizen and contribute resources to improve the quality of life in the community (Andreasen & Kotler, 2002; Kotler & Armstrong, 2007; Pride & Ferrell, 2006; Yoder-Wise, 2007).

Trends in Marketing

Technology has caused changes in marketing. Before the Industrial Revolution peddlers carried products to the door. They took large pots and pans to communities with many children and smaller pots to retirement communities. Technology can now be used for a large-scale, individualized approach to large markets. The Industrial Revolution mass-produced products, created a faceless society, and led to marketing approaches that drew on economic sciences and consumer models that were based on rational behavior. Target groups were defined for marketing when people wanted the same things.

In cultures that value self-fulfillment and enjoyment of life more than being part of a group, consumption pressure aimed at the masses may not work. The new pattern finds people wanting

different things and showing less loyalty to brands. As people desire goods and services tailored to them, individual ordering emerges along with the mass markets. A modular product range can give customers broad choices while requiring the production of only a limited number of variants. There may be just a few colors, styles, and sizes, but that allows numerous possible combinations. These result in an abundance of diverse products that people can search out using the media to put together all kinds of options. A fast, interactive means of obtaining customized goods and services is thus created, and it is available 24 hours per day. Today's health care customers are educated, confident, assertive, and busy. They want convenience, mastery, quality, and lower costs.

People do not easily change their habits, so electronic media do not supersede everything but offer additional possibilities as people mail what they faxed or copy and distribute what they e-mailed. Agencies formerly used generic, thematic, one-sided bombardment advertising based on market research, generic models, and reported behaviors (which may not be actual behaviors) to manage target groups. Agencies are now more likely to engage in dialogue and to attend and react to actual behaviors by using media and marketing databases to manage personal client relationships (Table 9-5).

Leadership and Management of Strategic Planning for Marketing

Top-level administrators define the agency's mission, which is a statement of its purpose, and set goals and objectives, which will be detailed in each unit. An analysis of strengths, weaknesses, opportunities, and threats is desirable. Administrators also design the agency portfolio, which is the collection of products and services the agency provides. The marketing unit manager develops marketing plans from the strategic plan, implements the plan, evaluates the results, and takes necessary corrective action (Kotler & Armstrong, 2007; Pride & Ferrell, 2006) (Box 9-2). Market opportunities can be explored using a market expansion grid.

Agencies have the following market opportunities: (1) market penetration by using existing

TABLE 9-5 Trends in Marketing

From	To
Masses	Individual
Generic	Specific
Limited choice	Abundance
Print	Electronic
Passive	Interactive
Plenty of time	Fast, faster, fastest
9 AM–5 PM	24-hour service
Agency calls out to market	Agency listens and reacts
One-sided bombardment	Dialogue
Market research	Marketing databases
Generic models	Marketing databases
Generic, thematic advertising	Media
Reported behaviors	Actual behaviors
Management of target groups	Management of personal client relationships

products in existing markets, (2) market development by taking existing products into new markets, (3) product development by taking new products into existing markets, and (4) diversification by taking new products into new markets.

Marketing Concepts
Exchange

Marketing is based on resource dependency or *exchange*. Organizations offer satisfactions such as goods, services, or benefits to markets, which in return provide needed resources such as goods, services, time, money, or energy. Exchange involves four conditions: (1) there are at least two parties, (2) each party offers something that the other considers valuable, (3) each party is capable of communication and delivery, and (4) each party is free to accept or reject the offer (Pride & Ferrell, 2006).

Publics

A *public* is a group of people or organizations that has an actual or a potential interest or impact on a given agency. *Input publics* supply resources and constraints and consist of suppliers, donors, and regulatory publics. The agency's *internal publics* such as the board of directors, management, staff, and volunteers, then manage these inputs to accomplish the agency's mission. *Intermediary publics* are used to promote

and distribute goods and services to consumers. The *consuming publics* such as patients, clients, and students, consume the output of the organization. *Reciprocal publics* are interested in the agency, and the agency is interested in them. Patients are an example. *Sought publics* are desired by the agency but are not necessarily interested in the agency. For instance, wealthy people who are potential donors could be a sought public. *Unwelcome publics* are interested in the agency, but the agency is not interested in them. One unwelcome public consists of emergency department patients who come for nonemergency care. Publics are related to each other, as well as to the agency, and they influence each other's attitudes and behaviors. Publics are groups that have actual or potential interests in or impact on the agency.

Market

A *market* is a potential arena for the trading of resources. It is a group of people or organizations that have resources that they want to exchange, or might be willing to exchange, for distinct benefits. A market is composed of actual or potential buyers and is a place where people negotiate to transfer goods or services. The health care agency goes to the labor market to obtain employees, to the professional market to obtain physicians, and to the financial market to obtain capital.

Image

An *image* is the sum of impressions, beliefs, and ideas that people have of something. Publics with a positive image of an organization will be drawn to it, whereas those with a negative image will avoid or disparage it.

There are two opposite theories about image formation. *Object-determined theory* maintains that people perceive the reality of the object. They experience the object and process the sensory data in a similar way despite different backgrounds. Therefore when people see a building in a beautiful setting, they perceive it as a beautiful hospital. *Person-determined theory* maintains that people have different degrees of contact with an object; they selectively perceive different aspects of the object, and through individual ways of processing the sensory data, they experience selective distortion. Thus some people may perceive the hospital as beautiful and others may not.

Image is a function of deeds and communications. Good deeds about which others are not told and talk without action are not enough. A strong, favorable image develops from satisfied publics who tell others their opinions.

Buyer Decision Process

Both individuals and organizations follow similar processes when making buying decisions. First, the problem or need is identified. Second, specifications that must be met to solve the problem are identified. Then there is a search for products,

services, or ideas to meet the need. Alternatives are evaluated, a purchase decision is made, and then the product, service, or idea is reevaluated on performance (Kotler & Armstrong, 2005; Pride & Ferrell, 2006) (Figure 9-6).

Marketing Process

Marketing involves informing the market of services provided and fitting services to market needs. Different approaches to marketing have been developed. *Mass marketing* occurs when the seller mass-produces, distributes, and promotes one product or service to all customers. *Product-variety marketing* is carried out when the seller provides variety to customers by having two or more products with different features. In *target marketing* the seller identifies market segments, selects specific target markets, and then develops products or services and marketing mixes specific to each target market. The marketing process involves several steps as shown in Box 9-3.

Market Segmentation

An *audit* can be used to identify the bases for segmenting the market and to develop profiles of the segments. Marketing involves informing the market of services provided and fitting services to market needs. It is a complex process that generally includes the audit, market segmentation, marketing mix, implementation, and evaluation and control.

The *marketing audit* involves identification, collection, and evaluation of information that needs to be examined to evaluate market relations. Identification of the market and market segments is required. How large is the area to be served? Is it rural, urban, or both? How many potential customers are there? What are their ages, occupations, income levels, and interests? How many are aware of the organization's services? Are there seasonal differences? How satisfied are the clients with the services offered now?

The organization should be assessed. What is the mission of the organization? What are its philosophy, goals, objectives, and priorities?

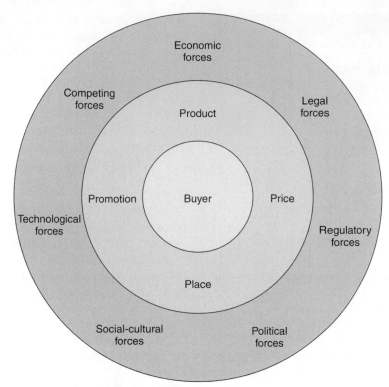

Figure 9-6 • Marketing environment model.

What are the services provided? What are the strengths and weaknesses? How do its services compare with those of others? What conditions of the industry affect the organization? What internal and external controls affect it?

As services are further analyzed, one should note distinctive superiorities. What services are heavily used? Why? What services are underused? Why? Are there voids? If so, can they be filled? How could needed materials, supplies, and personnel be obtained? Who pays for the services?

Who are the competitors? How many are there? Are their numbers increasing or decreasing? Who are the principal competitors? What areas do they serve? How do their size and strength compare? How do their charges compare?

What is the profile of present and future clients for the services? Are client profiles different for different services? What is the frequency of client usage of the services?

What are the perceptions of the nursing market? What are the internal perceptions of nurse recruitment? Focus groups can be formed to discuss reasons why nurses decided to work at the institution, the positive and negative aspects of the job, and ways working conditions can be improved. Interviews with directors of nursing education programs can be conducted to learn how the institution is perceived, where graduates of that school are going and why, and how personnel at the health care agency can influence those decisions.

What is the organization's pricing philosophy? How are prices determined? How do the staff, clients, and competitors view prices?

In what location is the service provided? How accessible is it to clients? How far will clients have to travel to obtain the service? Will personnel travel to provide a service? If so, how far will personnel travel? Will the agency charge for travel expenses?

BOX 9-3 Marketing Process

Defining problem and research questions
Designing the research project
  Reliability
  Validity
  Hypothesis
  Exploratory studies
  Descriptive studies
  Casual studies
Collecting data
  Primary data
  Secondary data
  Survey methods
  Interviews
    Mailings
    Telephone contact
    E-mail
    Personal interviews
    On-site computer
  Questionnaires
  Observations
Sampling
  Random
  Stratified
  Area
  Quota
Analyzing data
Interpreting and reporting findings

Data from Kotler P, Armstrong G: *Principles of marketing*, ed 12, Upper Saddle River, NJ, 2007, Prentice Hall.

What is the purpose of promotion? Is it reaching the intended publics? Is it effective? What media are being used? What media reach whom?

Many assessment tools can be used to collect data for the audit. Questionnaires administered by mail, telephone, or interview; in-depth interviews; and observations are common tools. A consumer panel can be used to discuss relevant issues. A mediator helps keep the discussions of a representative group of consumers on a specific topic in focus groups. Nominal groups aim at generating consensus about a particular issue. Records can be reviewed, and scientific research designs can be planned and implemented to collect data.

A sampling plan is important. Who will be surveyed? What will the sample size be? Large samples are more representative than small samples. How will the sample be chosen? A random sample is the most representative.

Statistical techniques, such as calculation of frequency distributions, means, and standard deviations, as well as regression analysis, correlation analysis, factor analysis, discriminate analysis, and cluster analysis, can be useful. Statistical techniques are technical; therefore statistical consultation is often advisable.

Profiles can be developed based on demographic, geographic, psychographic, and product-related variables. Demographic variables include age, gender, educational level, income, occupation, race, ethnicity, religion, family size, and family life cycle. Geographic variables include country; region; urban, suburban, or rural location; city size; county size; state size; climate; and market density. Psychographic variables include personality type, social class, lifestyle, benefits sought, readiness state (unaware, aware, informed, interested, desirous, intending to buy), rate of adoption (innovator, early adopter, early majority adopter, late majority adopter, laggard), user status (nonuser, ex-user, potential user, first-time user, regular user), user rate (light, medium, or heavy user), loyalty status (none, medium, strong, absolute), and attitude toward the product (enthusiastic, positive, indifferent, negative, hostile). Product-related variables include benefit expectations, price sensitivity, brand loyalty, and volume usage (Kotler & Armstrong, 2005; Pride & Ferrell, 2006).

Market Targeting

Targeting involves developing measures of segment attractiveness and selecting the target segment or segments to enter. *Segmentation* identifies subsets of the total market that have similar characteristics.

There are three major marketing strategies related to segments:

- Differentiated marketing aims directly and differentially at several specific segments.
- Concentrated marketing aims at a specific segment.
- *Undifferentiated marketing* ignores segments and deals with all as one market.

BOX 9-4 Marketing Mix
Product
Price
Place
Promotions

Data from Pride WM, Ferrell OC: *Marketing: Concepts and strategies*, Boston, 2006, Houghton Mifflin.

Market Positioning

The *product position* is the way customers describe the important attributes of the product or service. Leaders need to choose and implement a positioning strategy to obtain a competitive advantage, which often involves offering a greater value for a lower price or justifying a higher price by providing more benefits. The difference promoted should be important, superior, distinctive, affordable, and profitable. The difference should be communicated and made visible to the buyer.

Marketing Mix

A *marketing mix* is developed for each target segment. It involves the four *P*s: product, price, place, and promotions (Box 9-4). *Product* is something provided for consumption to satisfy a need or want. The inventory of services and analysis of costs, benefits, and target markets indicate which products are overused, underused, and cost-effective to provide and which are perceived as strong or weak. This information should be used to determine the appropriate product mix.

A *product line* is composed of similar services that are clustered to manage process, quality, costs, and marketing more efficiently. *Product-line analysis* is a method of analyzing products in terms of inputs and outputs and is built on total cost accounting principles. Because determination of actual cost per case is important, all costs for an admission are tracked. All hospital fixed overhead costs are allocated to patients and product lines. All costs from admission to discharge are determined and compared with the reimbursement per case. Length of stay by product line is important. When the patient's length

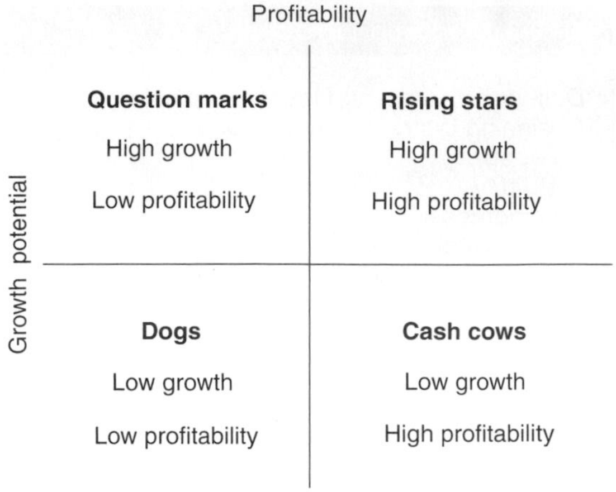

Figure 9-7 • Boston consulting firm's grid for classifying potential growth and profitability of products.

of stay is too long, the total cost may surpass the reimbursement per case even if the daily expense is reasonable.

Product-line analysis shows the relationship of inputs to outputs, gives profit and loss information for a product line, attaches all costs to a product line, increases cost awareness on the part of personnel, facilitates planning, promotes efficiency, encourages better review and control of resources, and promotes better decision making (Huber, 2006; Roussel, Swansburg, & Swansburg, 2006; Sullivan & Decker, 2005; Yoder-Wise & Kowalski, 2006).

A Boston consulting group developed a classification system for potential growth and profitability to identify marketing strategies for products (Figure 9-7). The group created a grid with growth potential indicated on the vertical axis and profitability along the horizontal axis. Low growth potential and profitability are represented at the lower left corner; the levels of these factors become higher toward the top and the right of the grid. Products with low profitability and low growth potential are labeled *dogs*. They drain the organization; the organization should divest itself of them if possible. Products in the upper left quadrant have low profitability and high growth potential. They are labeled *question marks*. Aggressive marketing to increase volume and therefore profitability is possible but risky. *Cash cows* with

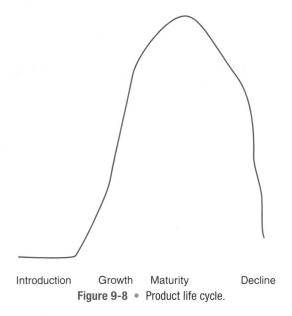

Introduction   Growth   Maturity   Decline
Figure 9-8 • Product life cycle.

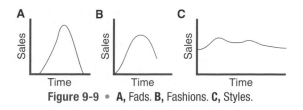

Figure 9-9 • **A,** Fads. **B,** Fashions. **C,** Styles.

high profitability but low growth potential, are in the lower right quadrant. Such products may be maintained so the profits can be used to finance other ventures or to cover other losses. In the upper right quadrant are the *rising stars* which have both high profitability and high growth potential. Promotional money should be put here to increase volume and profitability. After increasing growth, rising stars typically become cash cows.

Products have *life cycles*. The stages of the life cycle are as follows (Figure 9-8): The *introduction stage* is the beginning of a new product offering when the customer's response to the product and its growth potential are relatively unknown. The *growth stage* occurs when the number of customers and the size of the market increase. The *maturity stage* is the peak market level of the product. Competition enters the market to obtain a share. Marketing strategies during the maturity stage are designed to get and keep the agency's share of the market. The last stage is the *market decline stage,* when the market decreases because of the introduction of new ideas, products, technology, or changes in customer needs (Berkowitz, 2006).

Question marks occur during the introductory stage, when the future is risky but there is high growth potential. Rising stars form the growth stage, when profitability and growth potential are high. Cash cows are seen during the maturity stage, when there is high profitability but low growth potential. Dogs occur during the decline stage, with decreasing growth and profitability.

A *fad* is a fashion that peaks early and declines rapidly (Figure 9-9, *A*). A *fashion* is a currently popular style (Figure 9-9, *B*). *Style* is a basic mode of expression that is distinctive (Figure 9-9, *C*). For example, clothes may be casual or formal; art may be abstract or realistic. A style may last for decades, coming in and out of vogue with periods of renewed interest (Kotler & Armstrong, 2007).

Price is another major consideration. Because providers rather than patients usually determine the services used and health care bills are usually paid by third-party payers, nondollar costs such as time and convenience must be considered. Minimization of nondollar costs should benefit the health care agency and the consumer.

There are several pricing goals:
* *Profit-maximizing pricing* tries to set the maximum price that the demand for the product or service will bear.
* *Market-share pricing* sacrifices short-term profits for long-term market domination and attempts to identify the price that maximizes the agency's share of the market.
* *Market-skimming pricing* places a high price to ensure high profitability on a product or service when it is in high demand with no competition.
* *Current-revenue pricing* tries to maximize the current revenue.
* *Target-profit pricing* is designed to achieve a satisfactory profit.
* *Promotional, loss-leader pricing* sets the price lower than the cost or the competition's price

to introduce customers to the new product or service. Profits are regained when the customers purchase other products from the firm or organization.

- *Prestige pricing* sets unusually high prices to convey the image of quality or exclusivity.

Factors influencing pricing include the cost of the product, the demand for the product, and the competition for the product. When considering the cost of products or services in setting prices, one can use *mark-up pricing* by adding a certain percentage to the cost, *cost-plus pricing* by adding a fixed amount to the cost, and *target pricing* by setting the price so it yields a specific profit at a particular demand level. When considering the demand for the product or service, one can use *perceived-value pricing* by setting the price according to the customer's perception of the value of the product or service or *price-discrimination pricing* by varying the price from one customer or place to another. There might be a *sliding payment scale* according to the patient's income. One hospital in a corporation might charge more or less than others because of the clients' income in general or the facility's location in a rich or poor neighborhood. When considering competition, one can use *going-rate pricing*, which draws on the collective wisdom of the marketplace. In *sealed-bid pricing* the lowest bid gets the business.

Place involves the physical location, appearance of the location, its accessibility and availability, resource utilization, the expertise and courtesy of staff, referral mechanisms, and distribution. The goal is to provide the service to the consumer with efficient distribution and minimal inconvenience.

Marketing promotion informs potential consumers of the existence and availability of products and services and persuades them of the benefits of using these products and services. Tailoring services to consumer desires is important. Marketing promotion leads to awareness, understanding, interest, decision, utilization, satisfaction, reutilization, and recommendation.

Promotion tools include the following: (1) *advertising* which is any paid form of promotion; (2) *personal selling*, which is an oral presentation by a seller to a buyer; (3) *sales promotions*, which are short-term incentives for purchasing products or services; and (4) *publicity*, which is promotion that is not paid for by the agency. *Advertising* includes newspaper ads, magazine ads, journal ads, direct mail, fliers, billboard advertising, and ads in telephone directories and on radio and television. Printed materials can be used—for instance, calendars, matchbooks, pens, telephone stickers, newsletters, and booklets about topics such as diet, exercise, poison control, and first aid. Personal selling includes fund raising, lobbying, and sales calls such as presentations to community groups about health promotion, chemical dependency, weight control, exercise, birth control, and child care. Sales promotions include introductory offers, free samples, coupons, discounts, incentives, free lectures, and special credit cards. The best form of publicity is the word of mouth of satisfied customers or the grapevine. Other types are public service announcements, public relations campaigns, speakers' bureaus, interviews, health fairs, and screening programs.

Promotion has been revolutionized by technology. Personal computers and multimedia applications are readily available and make possible the use of graphics, moving pictures, and sound. *Multimedia notebooks* are portable compact computers that are so small they can be taken anywhere they are needed and used without a connecting lead. They are very convenient for traveling representatives. A *personal digital assistant (PDA)* is fitted with an optic device that allows one to write and draw on an electronic slate rather than type on a keyboard. *Television* facilitates visual communications. *Teletex* is a popular form of interactivity that allows choices to be made numerically by a standard remote control. People can get information about things such as the weather, traffic updates, airport arrivals, and stock indices. Then interests expressed by these choices can simultaneously become the focus of marketing via teletex. Travel arrangements can be booked when interest is expressed in a travel program. *Direct-response television* is interactive in that it uses a commercial to get customers to call a specific number. Most calls are made within

10 minutes of broadcast of the advertisement. Television *videotex* is an electronic information service that allows one to choose a teletex page from a menu. A telephone number must be dialed to get access to a specific page that lists a variety of services. *Near video on demand* allows customers to view films as they are repeated on a regular basis. The customer pays for what is viewed. The investment costs for near video on demand are considerably less than for *video on demand*, which is equivalent to having a video shop at home.

Computers can make databases easily accessible and retrievable. These databases can then be used to make marketing decisions. *Electronic bulletin boards* are computer network systems that link many computers by phone lines or satellite. They allow marketers to interact with data sources and clients almost instantaneously. Bulletin boards can permit customers to exchange ideas for problem solving, learn from each other, and give the agency new insights into marketing of products and services. The *Internet* is a collection of computers connected by phone lines that enables people to communicate around the world through e-mail, news groups, chat rooms, and more. It links companies with customers around the world by computer networks. Although the Internet has been in existence for a few decades, the *World Wide Web* was not developed until 1992. It organizes information available on the Internet into interconnected pages that may include text, graphics, sound, and video. Software packages that facilitate navigating the Web have made the Web a multimedia communication tool (Pride & Ferrell, 2006). Fax machines, sales-automation software, personal newspapers, video conferencing, cable television, and the Internet have revolutionized marketing.

Implementation

A marketing program can be implemented incrementally or as an entire package. Designing and implementing a marketing program are expensive projects and require personnel with expertise in marketing. Outside consultants can be hired when qualified people are not available within the organization. Dealing with local political conflicts, reaching communities that are out of touch with their own real demands, and sorting out real demands from surface expectations are challenging tasks.

Domestic marketing focuses on the market in the country of origin. Although there may not be an international marketing plan, sometimes international distributors or foreign companies purchase products or services, creating *limited exporting. International marketing* includes plans for marketing in one or more foreign countries. *Global marketing* involves strategies for marketing around the world.

Dealing with international and global markets is even more challenging than domestic

---

RESEARCH Perspective 9-2

Data from Findorff MJ, Wyman JF, Crogham CF, et al: Use of time studies for determining intervention costs, *Nurs Res* 54(4):280-284, 2005.

Purpose: The purpose of the investigation was to use time studies in calculating the program costs of personnel for use in future cost-effectiveness analysis of health interventions.

Methods: The time-study process was used to determine personnel costs in delivering an intervention. A step-by-step time study was conducted to illustrate how personnel costs associated with delivery of the intervention could be separated from those costs associated with implementation of research procedures in the determination of research costs.

Results/conclusions: The time study was able to provide an estimate of personnel time. The design of a time study should consider intervention components, staff involvement, and time for data collection.

marketing. Such markets have different political climates; different histories; cultural differences; different business customs; different laws, legal systems, and regulations; different technologic forces; different stages of economic development; different economic forces; and different local geography. Rather than dealing with one set of market conditions, marketers must address different conditions for each country and for each market within each country (Cateora & Graham, 2004; Pride & Ferrell, 2006).

Evaluation and Control

The last phase of the marketing process is *evaluation and control*. It involves identifying goals and objectives, measuring planned and actual results, determining reason for variance between planned and actual results, correcting action based on causal analysis, and revising goals. Evaluation can be performed more or less often—daily through weekly, monthly, yearly, or on a more extended basis—to determine whether implementation is accomplishing desired results.

Health Care Marketing and Ethics

Historically, many professionals argued that marketing of health care could sacrifice quality to achieve volume, could shift decision-making power to a public that is not qualified to make the decisions, would lower standards in the professions, could be harmful to professional image, and was thus unethical. Now many professional groups are marketing to increase awareness of services without sacrificing standards. Some say marketing has increased sensitivity to client needs. Others recommend marketing to recruit nurses. The American Marketing Association's Academy for Health Services Marketing has developed professional ethics for health care marketing. These include respecting the primacy of the client's welfare and confidentiality of the relationships with the client; providing communications to inform, not to deceive; being competitive and making fair comparisons; and being vigilant in the application of the standards. Marketing public relations has helped marketing campaigns be successful (Sullivan & Decker, 2005).

CHAPTER SUMMARY

Globalization gained attention during the 2000s in health care financing. There is recognition that worldwide teams with diverse perspectives and experiences can capture superior knowledge and process outcomes to develop new diagnostic and technologic tools and drugs, but there is also a concern about the financial burden of epidemics and pandemics that are occurring. Nursing leaders and managers need to know about economics, accounting, types of budgets, and cost containment because of the need for cost-effective, safe care. Nurses also need to know about marketing, particularly social marketing, and the marketing process.

CRITICAL THINKING ACTIVITY

Reflective Journal: Make observations in a clinical setting or reflect on past experiences. Answer the following questions: What are the sources of revenue for the agency? What is the unit charge for nursing services (e.g., hours of care, room rates)? What is the cost to a patient for 24 hours of care or cost per visit or other appropriate charge unit? Does the cost vary with the amount and type of care (e.g., care in an intensive care unit)? Do Medicare, Medicaid, and private insurance carriers reimburse the hospital at the same rate for the same care? What are the differences in reimbursement, and how is the deficit handled? Does the organization have a marketing plan? Who, if anyone, is responsible for the plan?

CASE STUDY

Services are changing from having physicians perform physical examinations to having nurse practitioners perform them. Consequently, there is reduced use of large gloves and increased use of smaller gloves. What factors should you consider when determining how many gloves to order and how often?

ONLINE RESOURCES

evolve Additional critical thinking activities, worksheets, and case studies are available online at http://evolve.elsevier.com/Marriner/guide8e.

REFERENCES

Andreasen A, Kotler P: *Strategic marketing for nonprofit organizations*, Upper Saddle River, NJ, 2002, Prentice Hall.

Baker JJ, Baker RW: *Health care finance: Basic tools for nonfinancial managers*, Sudbury, Md, 2003, Jones & Bartlett.

Berkowitz EN: *Essentials of health care marketing,* ed 2, Sudbury, Md, 2006, Jones & Bartlett.

Cateora PR, Graham JL: *International marketing,* ed 12, Boston, 2004, Irwin.

Cowan MJ, Shapiro M, Hayes R, et al: The effect of a multidisciplinary hospitalist/physician and advanced practice nurse collaboration on hospital costs, *J Nurs Adm* 36(2):79-85, 2006.

Findorff MJ, Wyman JF, Crogham CF, et al: Use of time studies for determining intervention costs, *Nurs Res* 54(4):280-284, 2005.

Finkler SA: *Financial management for public, health, and not-for-profit organizations,* ed 2, Upper Saddle River, NJ, 2004, Prentice Hall.

Finkler SA, McHugh M: *Budgeting concepts for nurse managers,* ed 4, Philadelphia, 2007, Saunders.

Gapenski LC: *Healthcare finance: an introduction to accounting and financial management*, Washington, DC, 2004, Aupha Press.

Grohar-Murray ME, DiCroce HR: *Leadership and management in nursing,* ed 3, Upper Saddle River, NJ, 2003, Prentice Hall.

Huber D: *Leadership and nursing care management,* ed 3, Philadelphia, 2006, Elsevier.

Institute for the Future: *Health and health care 2010: the forecast, the challenge,* ed 2, Boston, 2003, Jossey-Bass.

Kotler P, Armstrong G: *Principles of marketing,* ed 12, Upper Saddle River, NJ, 2007, Prentice Hall.

Kotler P, Keller KL: *Framework for marketing management,* ed 3, Upper Saddle River, NJ, 2006, Prentice Hall.

Marquis BL, Huston CJ: *Leadership roles and management functions in nursing: Theory and application,* ed 5, Philadelphia, 2006, Lippincott Williams & Wilkins.

McCloskey JC: Implications of costing out nursing for reimbursement, *Nurs Manage* 20(1):245-253, 1989.

Nosek LJ: Globalization's costs to healthcare: How can we pay the bill? *Nurs Adm Q* 28(2):116-128, 2004.

Nowicki M: *The financial management of hospitals and healthcare organizations,* ed 3, Chicago, 2004, Health Administration Press.

Office of Inspector General: *Hospital closures: 1990-1999*, Atlanta, December 2001, Office of Evaluation and Inspections.

Pride WM, Ferrell OC: *Marketing: concepts and strategies*, Boston, 2006, Houghton Mifflin.

Roussel L, Swansburg RC, Swansburg RJ: *Management and leadership for nurse administrators,* ed 4, Boston, 2006, Jones & Bartlett.

Samuelson WF: *Managerial economics,* ed 5, Hoboken, NJ, 2006, John Wiley & Sons.

Sullivan EJ, Decker PJ: *Effective leadership and management in nursing,* ed 6, Upper Saddle River, NJ, 2005, Pearson/Prentice Hall.

Yoder-Wise PS: *Leading and managing in nursing,* ed 4, St Louis, 2007, Mosby.

Yoder-Wise PS, Kowalski KE: *Beyond leading and managing: Nursing administration for the future*, St Louis, 2006, Mosby/Elsevier.

Young DW: *Management accounting in health care organizations*, Boston, 2004, Jossey-Bass.

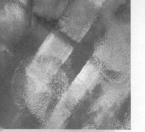

Organizational Concepts and Structures

10

"When you encounter difficulties and contradictions, do not try to break them, but bend with them with gentleness and time." —*Anonymous*

Chapter Overview

Chapter 10 outlines factors affecting organizational structures, explains organizational concepts, describes types of organizational structures including health care networks, and notes the effects of globalization.

Chapter Objectives

- Describe the relationships among span of management, flat or tall structures, and decentralization or centralization.
- Enumerate ways a manager can facilitate adjustments to mergers and acquisitions.
- Differentiate between line and staff authority.
- Identify at least three principles of organization.
- Describe disadvantages of the bureaucratic structure.
- Identify at least three adhocracy organizational models.
- Summarize the corporate model.
- Describe at least three factors affecting globalization.

Online Resources

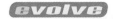

Critical thinking activities, worksheets, and case studies are available online at http://evolve.elsevier.com/Marriner/guide8e.

Major Concepts and Definitions

Organizational chart *a diagram that shows how the parts of an organization are linked*
Span of management *the number and diversity of people who report to a manager*
Centralize *to concentrate power or authority*
Decentralize *to distribute power and authority among more places*
Merger *the consolidation of two or more companies into one company*
Line authority *the formal chain of command*
Staff authority *advisory or service-oriented influence*
Organization *a consolidated group of elements; a systematized whole*
Structure *the way parts are arranged*
Hierarchy *a group of persons arranged by rank, grade, or class*
Bureaucracy *administration through departments and subdivisions managed by
    officials following an inflexible routine*
Adaptive *able to change to make suitable to new or changed circumstances*
Matrix *an organizational design that combines project management and
    bureaucratic structures*
Corporation *a legal entity governed by a board of directors or by shareholders*

FACTORS AFFECTING ORGANIZATIONAL STRUCTURES

*"Chaos results when the world changes faster
than people." —Anonymous*

Organizational structures are affected by the economic, political, social, regulatory, competitive, and technologic pressures in society and follow changes in vertical and horizontal integration, geographic dispersion, and unit volume. The structure delimits responsibilities, communication channels, and the decision-making environment. The organizational structure should facilitate implementation of the organization's vision, values, mission, philosophy, goals, objectives, strategies, policies, and procedures (Galbraith, 2002).

Organizational structures are moving away from simple, hierarchical structures with formal channels of communication, functional fiefdoms, and division of labor with simplification of work. Complex, flat organizations with cross-functional teams and free access to information are becoming more common.

Absence of boundaries empowers employees, and enrichment of work through performance of multiple tasks can increase creativity. Globalization is a reality. Focus has changed from product to customer centricity (Galbraith, 2005; Roussel, Swansburg, & Swansburg, 2006) (Table 10-1).

Responses to trends in health care include managed care; consolidations of health plans, hospitals, and physicians; physician and hospital integration; vertical integration with disease management; and horizontal integration for coordination of care. There has been an increase in primary care, outpatient services, self-care of chronic diseases, the uninsured population, and the use of Medicare by the aging population. New drugs, therapies, medical technology, and information systems are available; for example, electronic medical records and databases are increasingly being implemented in care. Telehealth has increased, as have e-mails between patients and their physicians. Costs are being shifted away from managed care organizations and insurance companies to physicians, hospitals, and the consumer (Coddington, Fischer, Moore, et al, 2000; Institute for the Future, 2000).

TABLE 10-1 Trends Affecting Organizational Structures

From	To
Hierarchical management structures	Flat organizations with cross-functional teams
Formal channels of communication	Free access to information
Functional fiefdoms	Absence of boundaries
Division of labor	Empowerment of employees
Division and simplification of work	Enrichment of work through performance of multiple tasks and expansion of knowledge
Simple	Complex

Leaders evaluate the organizational structure; model the use of decentralized power, responsibility, and accountability; encourage employees to follow the chain of communication; counsel employees who do not follow the chain of command; and help staff see how their roles fit into the structure. Leaders enable followers to function within the structure, encourage upward communication, facilitate the informal group, mold the organizational culture, support advisory personnel, and generate an empowering environment.

Managers develop the organizational chart, are knowledgeable about the structure, establish a chain of communication, and maintain and clarify the chains of communications. Managers monitor accountability, provide organizational charts, follow the chain of communication, use the informal organization, are knowledgeable about the culture, use advisory personnel, and evaluate the structure (Table 10-2).

ORGANIZATIONAL CHARTS

An organizational chart is a diagram that shows how the parts of an organization are linked. It depicts the formal organizational relationships, areas of responsibility, persons to whom one is accountable, and channels of communication. The informal organization is not usually depicted on an organizational chart. It is related to relationships that influence a great deal of what happens in organizations.

Managers should consider actual working relationships when drawing an organizational chart. The formal organization may not be functioning as outlined on an older chart. Rather, an alternate structure may have emerged that operates very effectively. It is essential, then, that the manager knows what is happening in actual practice. The process of drawing the chart demands a review of current practices, discovery of relationships not previously examined, and clarification of vague associations.

The organizational chart may be used for outlining administrative control, for making policy and planning (including organizational change), for evaluating strengths and weaknesses of the current structure, and for showing relationships with other departments and agencies. It can also be used to orient new personnel or to present the agency's structural design to others. The visual diagram of a chart is a more effective means of communicating the agency's organizational structure than is a written description.

Charts become outdated as changes are made. They usually do not diagram the informal structure which tends to have a great effect on the organization, the formal structure may be difficult to define, and duties and responsibilities may not be described. Charts may foster rigidity in relationships and communications. People may be sensitive about their relative status in the organization and may not want their positions revealed. It can be expensive to develop, disseminate, and store the charts. Vertical charts, depicting the chief executive at the top with formal lines of authority down the hierarchy, are most common, but other arrangements are used.

The informal structure could be superimposed on the formal structure or charted through the use of sociograms. Sociograms analyze data on the choice of, communication among, and

TABLE 10-2 Leadership and Management in Organizational Structure

Leader	Manager
Evaluates the organizational structure	Develops the organizational chart
Models use of decentralized process	Is knowledgeable about the structure
Models responsibility and accountability	Establishes a chain of communications
Encourages employees to follow the chain of communications	Maintains the chain of communications
Counsels employees who do not use the chain of communication	Clarifies the chain of communications
Enables followers to function within the structure	Monitors accountability
Helps staff to see how their roles fit into the structure	Provides organizational charts
Encourages upward communications	Follows the chain of communications
Facilitates the informal group	Uses the informal organization
Molds the organizational culture	Is knowledgeable about the culture
Supports advisory personnel	Uses advisory personnel
Generates an empowering environment	Evaluates the structures

Modified from Huber DL: *Leadership and nursing care management,* ed 3, Philadelphia, 2006, Elsevier; Marquis BL, Huston CJ: *Leadership roles and management functions in nursing,* ed 5, Philadelphia, 2006, Lippincott Williams & Wilkins.

interaction among members of a small group. Personnel may be asked with whom they prefer to work, or their interactions may be observed and charted. The person with the most relationships is often the leader. Members of the primary group are those most accepted by other group members. Managers should use this information to increase production because work groups based on sociograms are generally more productive than those designed arbitrarily. Sociograms usually do not become a part of formal documents but are very useful for enhancing team work.

Advantages of organizational charts are that they can contribute to sound organizational structures, map lines of decision-making authority, show formal lines of communication, help employees understand their assignments, especially in relation to others, and show how people fit into the organization (Box 10-1). Unfortunately, organizational charts can become obsolete quickly, usually show only formal relationships, usually do not show informal communications, may contribute to confusion about authority and status, and may show how things are supposed to be rather than how they are (Marquis & Huston, 2006).

Chain of Command

"A person remains wise as long as he seeks wisdom. The minute he thinks he has found it he becomes a fool." —Anonymous

The chain of command is the formal line of authority and communication. In hierarchies, authority and communication flow from the top down, and authority and responsibility are aligned. In newer organizational structures, the chain of command is flatter, with communications flowing in all directions, and authority and responsibility are delegated to the lowest operational level possible.

Centrality

Centrality refers to the location of a position in an organization where frequent communication occurs. It is determined by organizational distance. Employees with positions that are a short organizational distance from the center are able to receive more information than those more peripherally located. Middle managers tend to have a broad view of the organization because of the centrality of their positions—they receive upward, downward, and horizontal communications.

BOX 10-1 Advantages and Disadvantages of Organizational Charts

ADVANTAGES

Contributes to sound organizational structure
Maps lines of decision-making authority
Shows formal lines of communication
Shows how people fit into the organization
Helps employees understand their assignments

DISADVANTAGES

Becomes obsolete quickly
Shows only formal relationships
Does not show informal communications
May show how things are supposed to be rather than how they are
May help confuse authority and status

TABLE 10-3 Number of Staff Associates and Resulting Number of Potential Relationships

Number of Staff Associates	Number of Relationships
1	1
6	222
12	24,708
18	2,359,602

Unity of Command

Unity of command is represented by the vertical solid line between positions on an organizational chart. It indicates that one person has one boss. Unity of command is still supported in some structures, as in primary nursing. However, health care professionals are increasingly involved in matrix organizations, in which they answer to more than one person.

Authority, Responsibility, and Accountability

Authority is the official power to act. It is the power to direct the work of others.

Responsibility is a duty or an assignment. A person needs the authority necessary to accomplish the assignment.

Accountability is a moral responsibility. A manager may delegate responsibility but always remains accountable.

Span of Management

Initial work on span of management was quantitative and attempted to devise formulas for determining the most desirable number of people to report to a manager. General Hamilton, a British officer in World War I, concluded that managers at lower levels could direct more people than those at higher levels. He thought that

an effective span of control was three to six other people, especially at upper levels.

Hamilton's principle has been elaborated by A. V. Graicunas, a Lithuanian management consultant whose mathematical analysis of potential relationships illustrates the complex social processes between managers and their staff associates. Graicunas demonstrated that, as the number of staff associates responsible to a manager increases arithmetically, the number of potential interactions increases geometrically.

Graicunas's formula is as follows:

$$R = n\left(\frac{2^n}{2} + n - 1\right)$$

where R equals all types of relationships and n equals the number of subordinates (Table 10-3). Graicunas's formula illustrates how complex a situation can become as additional staff associates report to a manager. The larger the span of control, the more complicated the relationships become.

The optimal span of management depends on the time requirements for management. Managers' competence and qualifications and those of their staffs affect their time requirements. Some managers, because of their education and personal qualities, can work with more people than others. The better prepared staff members are for their jobs, the less time managers must devote to teaching, clarifying responsibilities, and correcting mistakes.

Much of a manager's time is spent explaining plans, giving instructions, and receiving information about problems and progress. Clear and concise communications transmit information quickly and accurately. Much communication can be written. However, some situations cannot be handled with planning documents, policy statements, written reports, memoranda, or other written communications; these require personal contact. Situations that can be handled by written communications may be better handled by personal contact. These might include delicate situations and instances in which attitudes are involved. Personal contacts require considerable time.

If plans are clear, staff associates will know what is expected of them without frequently checking with the manager. If staff associates do their own planning, they will need more supervision. However, establishment of clear policies to guide their planning will reduce demands on the manager. Clear and complete policy statements can also simplify managers' decision making and allow expansion of their span of management. Deciding every problem individually requires more time than making policy decisions that anticipate problems.

The demands on the staff vary according to the complexity of functions. Standardization reduces time requirements because people know what is expected. Routine work requires less time than innovative work. One can expect that as the degree of difficulty of performing a task satisfactorily increases, so does the demand on the manager. As the variability of functions increases, more time must be spent by the manager because more factors and interrelationships must be considered. Interdependent functions require more management time than independent functions because of the increased need for coordination. The greater the geographic separation of personnel reporting to the manager, the more limited the span of control. The greater the nonmanagerial responsibilities, the less time the manager has for management. Managers in organizations with flat structures have a broader range of management than those in organizations with tall structures, and lower-level managers have a broader range than top management (Huber, 2006; Marquis & Huston, 2006; Sullivan & Decker, 2005).

Levels of Management

Top-level managers generally make decisions with the help of few guidelines or structures, coordinate internal and external influences, and view the organization as a whole. These managers include the chief executive officer, the organization's highest-ranking individual, and the top-level nurse manager. The titles vary but include chief nurse executive, president, vice-president, and director. Middle-level managers conduct day-to-day operations with some involvement in long-term planning and policy making. Their titles also vary but include unit manager, head nurse, and patient care coordinator. First-level managers are concerned with a specific unit's work flow. They deal with immediate day-to-day operations problems. Their titles vary and include case manager, nurse practice coordinator, primary care nurse, team leader, and charge nurse (Marquis & Huston, 2006). The trend is to expand the span of top-level management to multiple organizations and to global relationships, the span of middle-level managers to multiple units, and the span of lower-level managers to cases across agencies.

Flat Versus Tall Structures

The flat structure is developed along horizontal dimensions according to the number of organizational functions that are identified separately. There are few levels of management. The tall structure is developed along vertical dimensions by the use of a scalar process that is the direct line of command from top to bottom that defines relationships among levels in an organization. The scalar process expands vertically by dividing labor further, which necessitates more personnel and accomplishes the work through increased delegation. Because there are advantages and disadvantages to both the flat and tall structures, it is best to maintain a reasonable balance of dimensions. Changes within the organization bring imbalance over time, so the organizational structure should be reviewed periodically.

The flat structure shortens the administrative distance between top and bottom levels in the organization, thereby minimizing distortions because lines of communication are shorter. Communications are direct, simple, fast, and clearly apparent to employees. Another advantage of the flat structure is that large groups have a greater variety of skills available and are capable of solving a greater variety of problems. This structure is believed to contribute to high employee morale and to help develop capable, self-confident staff. It lends itself to a democratic approach and general management, which are preferred by many people. This minimal social stratification is consistent with an egalitarian political and social philosophy, which is currently popular.

A flat structure may be impractical in large organizations, however. Large groups have more difficulty reaching a consensus and require more coordination. The flat structure places tremendous pressure on each manager because of the large amount of authority and responsibility and high penalties for failures. Overburdened managers may not have the time to select, evaluate, and teach subordinates or the energy to think and plan. They may have difficulty making and communicating decisions (Yoder-Wise, 2007).

Tall structures lend themselves to authoritarianism, which is most effective in situations requiring rapid changes and precise coordination.

In a tall structure, messages from managers are given more attention than those from peers and consequently pass through levels quickly. The narrow range of management allows staff to evaluate decisions frequently. With small groups, decision making taking less time and there is more opportunity for members to participate and to understand the goals. Such interaction facilitates group cohesiveness.

Multiple management levels are expensive because of the large number of executives needed. Each additional level makes communication more cumbersome. The more levels through which communications passes, the greater the distortion. Therefore a tall structure reduces the understanding between higher and lower levels and increases impersonality (Sullivan & Decker, 2005) .

Decentralization Versus Centralization

With centralization, decisions are made at the top levels. With decentralization, decision making is diffused throughout the organization. It is relative, for the degree of decentralization is greater when more important decisions affecting more functions are made at lower levels with less supervision. Several factors must be considered

 RESEARCH Perspective 10-1

Data from Adams CE, Michel Y, DeFrates D, et al: Effect of locale on health status and direct care time of rural versus urban home health patients, *J Nurs Adm* 31(5):244-251, 2001.

Purpose: The purpose of this study was to determine whether health status differed between rural and urban home health patients and whether locale was a significant predictor of time spent in home direct care.

Methods: The investigation was a secondary analysis that compared outcomes and resource utilization in home health patients. Data were collected retrospectively in four Medicare-certified home health agencies on a convenience sample of 2788 patient episodes of care. Patient health status was measured using items from the Outcome Assessment and Information Set. Direct care time was the time clinicians spent in the home and was obtained from itinerary records.

Results/conclusions: Significantly more urban than rural patients were female. Urban patients were significantly older by an average of 2 years. Significantly more urban than rural patients had been discharged from an inpatient care facility within the previous 14 days, had a good rehabilitation prognosis, and had a good overall prognosis. When the home health care episode ended, significantly more urban than rural patients remained in the home. On average, rural patients received more registered nurse direct care time than urban patients. Total direct care time was increased by an average of 150 minutes for patients living in rural locations. Urban patients were healthier than rural patients.

when determining the optimal degree of decentralization for an organization. People in top management need to have a positive attitude toward decentralization, and they need competent personnel to whom they can delegate authority. The latter need access to the information necessary for decision making.

The number of people who need to interact to solve a problem should be considered. In general, the larger the organization, the greater the number of complex decisions that must be made and that can overburden top management and delay decision making. With smaller, decentralized units the number of decisions made by each manager is reduced and the time available to devote to each problem is increased. Agencies tend to be more centralized during their early, formative years. If the agency gradually expands from within, it is more likely to remain centralized. An organization that grows rapidly through acquisitions is more likely to be decentralized. Thus decentralization is more common in organizations with geographic dispersion of operations. Some functions lend themselves more readily to decentralization than do others. Production, marketing, personnel, and some purchasing may be readily decentralized. In contrast, finances, accounting, data processing of statistics, and purchase of capital equipment are likely to remain centralized.

The advantages of decentralization seem to outweigh the disadvantages. Decentralization increases morale and promotes interpersonal relationships. When people have a voice in governance, they feel more important and are more willing to contribute. This increased motivation provides a feeling of individuality and freedom that in turn encourages creativity and commits the individual to making the system successful. Decentralization fosters informality and democracy in management and brings decision making closer to the action. Thus decisions may be more effective, because the people who know the situation and have to implement the decisions are the ones who make them. Because managers do not have to wait for the approval of their superiors, flexibility is increased, and

reaction time is decreased. Fewer people have to exchange information; hence, communications are swift and effective. Coordination improves, especially coordination among services, coordination of production with sales, and coordination of costs with income. Products or operations that are minor in terms of the total production receive more adequate attention. Plans can be tried on an experimental basis in one unit, modified, and proven before being used in other units. Risks of losses of personnel or facilities are dispersed.

Decentralization helps determine accountability. It makes weak management visible because divisions are semiindependent and often competitive. Operating on the premise that people learn by doing, decentralization develops managers by allowing them to manage. A management pool can be developed, which eases the problem of succession. There is usually less conflict between top management and divisions. Decentralization releases top managers from the burden of daily administration, freeing them for long-range planning, goal and policy development, and systems integration.

Nevertheless, several problems can also result from decentralization. An organization may not be large enough to merit decentralization, or it may be difficult to divide the organization into self-contained operating units. Top administrators may not desire decentralization. They may feel it would decrease their status, or they may question the abilities of the people to whom they would delegate accountability. They may feel that most people prefer to be dependent on others and do not want decision-making responsibility. An increased awareness of division consciousness and a decrease in company consciousness may develop. Divisions may become so individualized and competitive that they sacrifice the overall objectives for short-range profitability and work against the best interests of the whole organization. Because of conflicts among divisions, it may be difficult to obtain a majority vote, and compromises may result. If the majority vote is delayed, it may come too late to be effective.

Decentralization involves increased costs. It requires more managers and larger staffs. Managers may be underused. Divisions may not adequately use the specialists housed at headquarters. Functions are likely to be duplicated between divisions and headquarters. Because decentralization develops managers, there are novice managers in the system that will make mistakes. Division managers may not inform top management of their problems. There are difficulties with control and nonuniform policies. Some restrictions on autonomy remain. Even with decentralization, people in top management remain responsible for establishing long-range objectives and goals, setting broad policies, selecting key executives, and approving major capital expenditures, even when recommendations are made by committees (Huber, 2006; Roussel, Swansburg, & Swansburg, 2006).

Departmentalization

Departmentalization results from limitations on the effective span of management, division of work, and need for cooperation. Its primary purpose is to subdivide the organizational structure so that managers can specialize within limited ranges of activity. Organization of the agency influences group behavior and the effectiveness of the group. The objectives of the agency can be met most easily if the group is properly organized. Two common types of departmentalization are input and output. The input, or process, orientation includes function, time, and simple numbers as bases for departmentalization, whereas the output, or goal, orientation includes product, territory, and client divisions.

Input

The input, or process-oriented, structure emphasizes specialization of skills. It reinforces professional skills by uniting people with similar expertise in the same department. For example, the focus may be on cardiac nursing, respiratory nursing, or transplant nursing, depending on the departmentalization. It is possible for professionals to advance within their field of expertise instead of advancing through the administrative hierarchy. Unfortunately, the process-oriented structure emphasizes professional skills over organizational goals. Conflicts increase as communication and cooperation decrease. Input organization provides less favorable training for general administrators than does a goal-oriented structure.

In departmentalization by function, activities are grouped according to similarity of skills or a set of tasks necessary to accomplish a goal. Logical, simple, and commonly used, this method of departmentalization facilitates specialization that contributes to economical operations. It groups functions that can be performed by the same specialists with the same type of equipment and facilities. Less demand for one product may be counteracted by a greater demand for another product. Consequently, staff, equipment, and facilities will have optimal utilization. The combination of administrative activities also is economical. One manager is responsible for all related activities; therefore coordination is improved because it is more easily achieved. The agency benefits from having a few people with outstanding abilities, for only top management is able to coordinate the major functions. For example, the hospital may be organized by medical, surgical, and pediatric units.

Functional departmentalization also has its disadvantages. As the size of the agency increases, centralization may become excessive, which makes effective control more difficult. The necessary additional organizational levels may slow communications and delay decision making. It becomes more difficult to measure performance. Functional departmentalization does not provide good training for general managers. They become experts in their particular function, have little opportunity to learn about other functions, and may emphasize their previous function while deemphasizing other functions when they become general managers.

Time factors are another basis for organization. Acute care services require coverage 24 hours per day, 7 days per week, whereas preventive services may require coverage for only 8 to 12 hours per day for 5 or 6 days per week at the most.

Output

The output, or goal, structure emphasizes service to the client. It collects all the work for a project under one manager and reduces dependence on other units for needed resources. This allows considerable autonomy, and the client, workers, and goals are readily identified. Systems and procedures are highly standardized. Family planning, pregnancy counseling, and school health are examples of services available from some health departments.

Unfortunately, these units may stress their own goals while deemphasizing agency goals. Duplication of equipment and services may occur. Equipment may not be fully utilized, or smaller-scale equipment may be less effective.

A product or group of closely related products may be the basis of organization for autonomous departments. Emphasis is on the product instead of the process. Improvement, expansion, and diversification of the product are possible because one manager is responsible for all activities affecting that specific product. Organization on the basis of products has become increasingly popular. It is common for schools of nursing to organize according to the "products" turned out—medical, surgical, obstetric, pediatric, psychiatric, geriatric, and community health nurses.

Departmentalization by territories is particularly useful for physically dispersed activities when branches provide similar services at each location. This method serves the local clients with greatest efficiency. Managers consider local circumstances that might be overlooked by a central manager. Departmentalization by territories uses local people who are familiar with local conditions. It reduces delivery time and may reduce transportation costs for raw materials and finished products. It is particularly useful for production and sales and when perishability is a problem. However, financial management works best if centralized.

Departmentalization by client makes sense when service is important and the welfare of the client is of primary interest. For example, a health center may have obstetric, pediatric, and adolescent clinics. Clinics may be open nights and weekends for working people. Schools of nursing may offer night classes for working students. This allows better use of facilities and is more satisfactory to the client. However, pressure for special consideration and treatment of specific groups may exist, and coordination problems may increase (Galbraith, 2002; Galbraith, Downey, & Kates, 2002; Roussel, Swansburg, & Swansburg, 2006).

Clusters

Clusters are two or three clinically similar units that share resources such as staff, equipment, and educational materials. Clustering fosters collaboration and consultation among nurses, decreases the isolation of decentralization, and enhances professional marketability by expanding knowledge and skills.

Units forming cluster work groups should develop written agreements describing how the cluster will work, emphasize sharing of resources, and arrange for personnel to meet each other through in-services and social events. New staff should know that clustering is an expectation and should be oriented to the cluster units. Staff should be oriented to cluster units before being shared and during nonstressful times. Cross-training facilitates cost-effectiveness, safety, and satisfaction in provision of nursing services. Nurses are prepared to work in two or more units as needed.

Line-Staff Relationships
Line Authority

Line organization is the oldest type of structure. It is a chain of command or a manager-staff or leader-follower relationship. The manager delegates authority to staff. This progression is the basis for the term *line authority*. The command relationship is a direct line between manager and staff and is depicted by a solid line on organizational charts. The line positions are related to the direct achievement of organizational objectives. This arrangement fosters quick decision making, because managers are given complete charge of their areas and at most would need to consult only with their immediate managers. Buck passing is reduced, and authority relationships are clearly understood. The manager has the right to give orders, demand accountability, and discipline violators (Figure 10-1).

Staff Authority

Staff support line-authority relationships and are advisory or service oriented. Staff authority is depicted by a dashed line on the organizational chart. Staff handle details, locate required data, and offer counsel on managerial problems. Staff functions through influence, for they do not have authority to accept, use, modify, or reject plans. They make the line more effective, but organizations can function without staff authority.

The two major categories of staff are personal and specialist. Personal staff includes the assistant and general staff. Specialist staff is composed of advisory, service, control, and functional personnel.

Assistant Staff

A personal staff member may be called an *assistant*, a *staff assistant*, or an *administrative assistant* and is responsible to one line manager. The assistant's chief purpose is to extend the line manager's capacity for completing a large amount of work by doing the more routine tasks that the manager would otherwise have to perform. The duties vary widely from one manager to another but might include activities such as mail answering, data collection for decision making, consolidation of information from various reports, preparation of documents, development of budgets, interpretation of plans to others, and substitution for the manager at various meetings and functions.

Personal staff members have no specific functions. Their duties vary with the assignments. They do not act on their own behalf but rather as personal representatives of a manager. The only specific authority they have comes from a manager on a limited basis, usually for a specific job over a brief time span. With delegated authority, the personal staff member can give instructions in the manager's name and

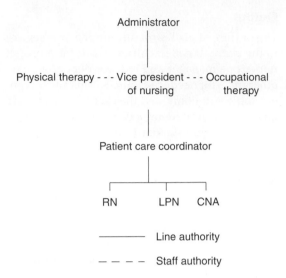

Figure 10-1 • Line-staff relationships.

make decisions that affect the organization. It is important for assistants and the people with whom they work to know the extent of their influence. Misuses of and misunderstanding about the assistant are all too common. Some feel that the assistant is unnecessary and that the duties should be delegated to other line managers. When the assistant takes over tasks that belong to others misunderstanding and poor cooperation result. Some assistants give the impression that they are the manager instead of just acting for one.

General Staff

The general staff is composed of top administrators. The top administrator makes the decision after receiving input from key people who together have the necessary expertise to make sound decisions for the agency. This is a coordinated group performing to maximize results. They serve in an advisory capacity by collecting and sharing information and are functional through their supervisory activities. The military has used this concept extensively, but it is relatively uncommon in business. Rotating general staff members to various areas and levels within the organization fosters an understanding of line problems.

Advisory Staff

Advisory staff counsel line managers. They study problems, collect and analyze data, offer alternatives, and prepare plans. Their work may be accepted, rejected, or modified by the line manager. Although ideas are heard, they are not always implemented. This puts staff on the defensive, because they must sell their ideas. It is important that they counsel rather than suggest or confirm just what the line manager wants. The chances that an idea will be approved are increased when staff has discussed proposed recommendations with line managers who will be affected by the decision and have received their approval before presenting the plan to the top administrator. Careful evaluation of the plan is important. The better prepared the advice, the more likely the staff will be heard and their suggestions implemented. If they work in seclusion, secretly preparing reports without listening to or discussing the reports with line managers, they are likely to get a suspicious and negative reception from others.

Service Staff

Service staff is not advisory. They perform a centralized service that has been separated from the line to prevent duplication and to allow more economical performance and good control. Such staff includes dietary and laundry services in a hospital. Line managers rely on service staff to get the job done. They do not do it themselves.

Control Staff

Control staff also do not advise. They control by restraining line authority. They have direct or indirect control over certain line performance. They control directly by acting as an agent for a line manager or indirectly through evaluation of procedural compliance and interpretation of policies and reports. Quality control personnel and affirmative action officers are members of the control staff.

Functional Staff

Functional authority exists when a specialist is given decision-making authority for specific activities outside the formal chain of command. This authority may be delegated to line, staff, or service managers and may be exercised over line, staff, and service personnel. Functional staff has limited line authority with power to determine standards in their areas of specialization and to enforce them. This authority is usually of an impersonal nature in the form of schedules, inspection reports, and written orders. It breaks the scalar chain and violates the principle that personnel should only be accountable to one superior. Although it is implemented in the interest of convenience and efficiency, its use should be restricted because it can damage line authority, destroy departmentalization, and create confusion.

Line-Staff Conflict

Conflict is likely to arise in any situation in which two or more people must interact to get results. Line-staff conflicts occur when there is a lack of understanding of the roles and functions of others and when their lines of responsibility, accountability, and authority are not clear. Line and staff have different responsibilities and goals. Line is generalized, whereas staff is specialized. Line managers are likely to be pragmatists who have received their positions because they provided competent service. They may not have much formal education but pride themselves on common sense. Staff managers probably consider themselves experts by virtue of their extensive formal education or experience in their areas of competence or both. In addition to their differences in responsibilities and backgrounds, they also have different loyalties. Line managers identify with their work group; staff managers are inclined to be loyal to their professional colleagues and the company as a whole.

Improving Line-Staff Relationships

Certain conditions can be created to foster the integration of line-staff efforts. It is helpful if both line managers and staff members have participated in determining objectives and plans and their method of implementation. Participation increases everyone's awareness of the overall goals to be accomplished. Each should be briefed on the roles and functions of other team members.

The lines of responsibility, accountability, and authority should be clearly established and publicized. A team-effort atmosphere is more likely to prevail in structures that allow line and staff members to interact with open communications and that have a problem-solving focus.

ORGANIZATIONAL STRUCTURE

Organizational Redesign, Restructuring, and Reengineering

So that market position can be maintained by reducing the cost of health care, jobs are being redesigned, organizations are being restructured, and systems are being reengineered. Redesign focuses on individual jobs in one setting, although it may be occurring in several areas simultaneously or consecutively. Inefficient distribution of activities, excess specialization, role overlap, and waste are examined so that the job can be redesigned to encompass appropriate tasks and require appropriate qualifications in order to be efficient and effective. Such redesign is also intended to facilitate motivation, higher-quality work, greater job satisfaction, less absenteeism, and lower turnover. Unfortunately downsizing and restructuring efforts such as differentiation of practice and shared governance can lead to resistance, job dissatisfaction, and decreased motivation initially. People may not desire growth or changes in their jobs. Some fear the increased productivity and sense job insecurity. There may not be clarity about what is to be accomplished. Consequently, restructuring organizations and reengineering systems are important (Hall, 2006).

Restructuring and reengineering deal with the entire organization's structure to improve its functioning and productivity. Restructuring changes the structure of the organization. It naturally follows organizational affiliations, mergers, consolidations, and integrations. Downsizing or right sizing by cutting the number of positions is also restructuring that requires redesign.

Reengineering examines the process of health care delivery to improve it. Although it is collaborative, patient centered, and data driven, it usually involves the entire organization and makes changes that affect the organization and its members. It is complex and often radical. Common practices have been path development, coordination among departments, case management, implementation of patient-focused care, and development of multiskilled workers.

The role of the nurse manager throughout redesigning, restructuring, and reengineering includes team building, coaching, mentoring, initiating change, reducing costs, and improving quality of care (Sullivan & Decker, 2005). Substantial increases in spending related to use of agency nurses, overtime, orientation, and ongoing educational expenses have been noted after restructuring (Hall, 2006).

 RESEARCH Perspective 10-2

Data from Milisen K, Abraham I, Siebens K, et al: Work environment and workforce: A cross-sectional questionnaire survey of hospital nurses in Belgium, *Int J Nurs Stud* 43(6):745-754, 2006.

Purpose: The purpose of this study was to investigate Belgian hospital nurses' perceptions of work environment and workforce issues, quality of care, job satisfaction, and professional decision making.

Methods: All 13,958 eligible nurses in the 22 hospitals selected were surveyed using the BELIMAGE questionnaire; 9638 questionnaires were useable for statistical analysis.

Results/conclusions: Concerns about the quality of leadership and management, insufficient staff, time demands, and stressful work environment were experienced as obstacle to providing good nursing care. Four out of ten nurses would not choose nursing as a career again, and 54.3% had contemplated leaving the profession. To deal effectively with professional and workforce issues in nursing, investments need to focus on redesigning the work environment to support nurses in providing comprehensive professional care.

Formal

Although planning is the key to effective management, the organizational structure furnishes the formal framework within which the management process takes place. The organizational structure should provide an effective work system, a network of communications, and identity to individuals and the organization and should consequently foster job satisfaction. Agencies contain both informal and formal structures.

Informal

The informal organization comprises personal and social relationships that do not appear on the organizational chart. This might include a group that usually takes breaks together, works together on a particular unit, or takes a class together. Informal organization is based on personal relationships rather than on respect for positional authority. It helps members meet personal objectives and provides social satisfaction. People who have little formal status may gain recognition through the informal structure. Informal authority is not commanded through organizational assignment. It comes from the follower's natural respect for a colleague's knowledge and abilities.

Informal structure provides social control of behavior. The control can be either internal or external. If pressure is intended to make a member conform to group expectations, it is internal. Kidding a member about her dirty shoelaces is an example. On the other hand, an attempt to control the behavior of someone outside the social group, such as the manager, is external control.

The informal structure also has its own channels of communication, which may disseminate information more broadly and rapidly than the formal communication system. Unfortunately, this grapevine may circulate rumors whose content is not authentic. The best way to correct an invalid rumor is for managers to provide accurate information. It is better that they not state that they are correcting the rumor, for in doing so they may strengthen it, and the facts they give may then be seen primarily as a subterfuge to refute the rumor.

The informal organizational structure is important to management. The manager should be aware of its existence, study its operating techniques, prevent antagonism, and use it to meet the agency's objectives.

Principles of Organization

Certain principles of organization help maximize the efficiency of the bureaucratic structure. The organization should have clear lines of authority running from the highest executive to the employee who has the least responsibility and no authority over others. There should be unity of command, with each person having only one boss. All employees should know to whom they report and who reports to them. The authority and responsibility of every individual should be clearly defined in writing. This reduces role ambiguity. Employees should know what is expected of them and what their limitations are. This prevents gaps among responsibilities, avoids overlapping of authority, and helps determine the proper point for decision making. Although many people do not think it is necessary to have their responsibilities in writing, it can be revealing to ask them to write what they believe their functions are and to note the duplicated efforts and jurisdictional disputes. When someone leaves an agency, it is not uncommon for no one to know exactly what that person did. Under such circumstances it can be difficult to justify replacement and to offer a meaningful orientation to a new employee.

A clear definition of roles is necessary for effective delegation, but it does not guarantee it. Role clarity allows employees to know what is expected of them, to whom they report, and to whom they should go for help. In contrast, role ambiguity leads to anxiety, frustration, dissatisfaction, negative attitudes, and decreased productivity. Job descriptions increase productivity and satisfaction; however, they should not be so exact that innovation is discouraged.

Ordinarily increased delegation and general rather than close supervision increase performance effectiveness, production, and employee satisfaction. The employee should be given formal authority commensurate with the responsibility delegated. It is not uncommon for managers to delegate authority and then undermine it by making decisions that were supposedly delegated. For example, if patient care coordinators are responsible for the quality of care given on their units, they should not have to accept members on their team who have been hired by the director without consulting them. In turn, patient care coordinators should not tell patients that they can have a bath at a certain time without consulting the person assigned to give that bath. Preferably the patient assistant and the patient will determine when various routines can be performed in accordance with the physician's orders and the manager's rationale.

The delegation of responsibility should be accompanied by accountability. The most effective control systems are probably those that provide feedback directly to the accountable person; this seems to increase motivation and provide direction. When feedback from a manager is given as performance evaluation rather than as guidance, it tends to be nonfunctional and only infrequently contributes to improvement of performance. The delegation of functions along with accompanying responsibility and accountability is particularly difficult for managers because they remain responsible for the actions of their staff members. They are as responsible as their staff members for their members' performance. Consequently, the span-of-control principle becomes important.

Three types of categorization are commonly used to define span of control: (1) function or process, (2) product or service, and (3) region. Function is associated with specialization. Specialization may apply both to individuals and to departments or divisions. For example, one nurse may pass medications and give treatments, another may just start intravenous lines, and patient assistants may give the baths and change linens. There may be a surgical nursing division with departments for specific types of surgery. It is preferable that if a person is accountable for carrying out more than one type of responsibility, the responsibilities be similar. Efficiency is maximized if employees perform predominantly the tasks they do best and in which their proficiency will consequently continue to increase; they may, however, become bored. It is not uncommon to find individuals within an organization who are assigned several unrelated tasks. Although that may be feasible for some people in given situations, it is not considered good organization, and their replacements are not likely to be successful. It is more viable to hire personnel to fill the organizational structure than to change the structure to fit personnel.

Having individuals consistently perform the same or similar tasks and having divisions with specific functions can help expand the range of control. Similarly, having departments that provide specific services, such as cardiac intensive care, or produce certain products can influence the structure. Organization by geographic location becomes increasingly viable when operations are scattered. Many agencies use a combination of these methods. For instance, a school of nursing may be organized according to campuses (regional division); according to undergraduate, graduate, and continuing education (product division); or according to inpatient, outpatient, medical-surgical, maternal-child, or some other service division; or it may assign individual faculty members to teach according to specialization (functional division).

The organizational structure should be flexible enough to permit expansion and contraction in response to changing conditions, without disruption of the basic design. It should also be kept as simple as possible, because additional levels of authority complicate communications and excessive use of committees may impede progress (Galbraith, 2002).

The formal organizational structure is defined by executive decision determined by planning. It can be diagrammed to show the positions in the organization and the relationships among them. It describes positions, task responsibilities, and relationships. The two basic forms of formal organizational structure are the hierarchical or bureaucratic model and the adaptive or organic model (adhocracy).

Bureaucratic Structure

A hierarchy or bureaucracy is an organizational structure designed to facilitate large-scale administration through coordination of the work of many personnel. It is associated with subdivision, specialization, the need for technical qualifications, rules and standards, impersonality, and technical efficiency. Figure 10-2 illustrates a typical bureaucratic hierarchy in which the managers are responsible to the vice president or director of nursing. The vice president or director, in turn, must answer to the hospital administrator, who is accountable to the board of directors. Managers also have authority over their staff associates, who are accountable to their managers (Sullivan & Decker, 2005).

Dual Management

A dual management approach separates technical and administrative responsibilities. It has one hierarchy in which technical professionals make technical decisions and control technical matters and another hierarchy in which management makes decisions about issues such as personnel and budget. This dual hierarchy gives equal status to managers and technical professionals. It provides a set of titles and job descriptions for each hierarchy.

Advantages of the Bureaucratic Structure

Bureaucracy is suited for work requiring large numbers of moderately educated people who perform routine tasks. Orientation is easy, because workers carry out few procedures within a narrowly circumscribed job description. Orders can be transmitted quickly.

Disadvantages of the Bureaucratic Structure

There are disadvantages to the bureaucratic model. It may be detrimental to healthy personality patterns by predisposing people to an authoritarian leadership style, increasing insistence on the right of authority and status, and fostering a pathologic need for control. If managers do trust the technical competence of their staff associates, they may feel insecure and fear those associates. Autocratic behavior may become a defense mechanism, so that managers use power and fear to control staff members and enforce norms through arbitrary or rigid rules. The use of reward and punishment to produce desired behavior may alienate personnel. Self-serving behavior patterns may develop because of competition to advance individual interests. Aloofness can result from the specialization, which leads to impersonality. Personnel

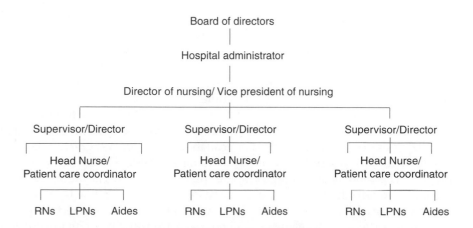

Figure 10-2 • Bureaucratic hierarchy.

may develop a ritualistic attachment to routine, experience monotony and alienation, become attached to subgoals, and show resistance to change.

Line and Staff Structure

A line-staff organization develops when a simple line structure is altered to provide support to line authorities. The line functions are command and control. The staff functions are separate from those of the chain of command, involve specialization, and support line authorities (see Figure 10-1). The advantage of line-staff structures is that the executive can delegate tasks that the executive does not have the skill or time to do. Disadvantages are that executives may get the credit for staff recommendations; staff may increase their influence by usurping the authority of the executive by making decisions without consulting the executive; and the executive may ignore the staff's recommendations.

Adhocracy Models of Organizational Structure

Adhocracies or organic models are organizational frameworks that are free form, open, flexible, and more fluid than older bureaucratic models. Boundaries separating internal and external relationships are easily penetrated. Temporary affiliations such as consultantships are formed.

The underlying assumptions, aims, and structures of adaptive frameworks differ from those of the bureaucratic model. They have resulted from behavioral research to facilitate job satisfaction and creativity as well as efficiency. They give greater recognition to the informal structure and encourage the group to improve its own norms. Adaptive models recognize realities and are designed to meet them. They are less likely to use organizational charts, because the relationships are flexible. Job descriptions are also less meaningful. The models are ambiguous, and consequently organizations following these models must be staffed by independent, self-reliant people who have a high tolerance for ambiguity. Such models lend themselves to participative management. Motivation is derived from system needs, task-related factors, and peer pressure rather than from supervision. Rewards are based on individual and group results rather than subjective evaluations from managers. The term *adhocracy* comes from "ad hoc committee." Adhocracies are loosely structured project organizations (Marquis & Huston, 2006).

Task Force

Task forces are sometimes used for special projects. The task force has a mission, a leader, and a projected completion date for its work. To be most successful, the project should be short range. There must be a pool from which to select talent, and task force members should be readily reabsorbed by the organization. Personnel are relieved of their usual tasks and given a temporary assignment, usually to investigate, analyze, research, and plan. They are less often used to make decisions and take actions. Establishment of a task force allows personnel with special qualifications to combine their expertise and concentrate on a project in a manner that would not be possible while they were performing their usual duties. Structural flexibility is accomplished by adding members when their potential contribution is high and removing them when their specific talents are no longer required. The task force can be an efficient problem-solving method and can offer training opportunities for managers. It can unleash creative energies and introduce innovations.

On the other hand, the task force can be disruptive to the organization. Key personnel may be away from their jobs for unknown lengths of time. As members experience different qualities of supervision in moving from one team to another, they may become more critical of the less capable manager. Assignment to a task force may make employees consider themselves better than their peers. They may feel independent and detached from their usual work groups. It is not uncommon for personnel to be promoted and removed from their original departments after the task force has completed its responsibilities.

Reabsorbing the task force member back into the organization is sometimes difficult, and that realization is almost certain to increase the employee's anxiety; in other cases what began as a short-range, problem-solving task force may become an unwanted permanent arrangement (Huber, 2006; Roussel, Swansburg, & Swansburg, 2006).

Project Management

The project organizational design is used for large, long-range projects in which a number of project groups are created and managed throughout the various phases of their existence. This method is useful for one-time projects when the task is unfamiliar and complex; when considerable planning, coordination, high-risk research, and development are involved; and when there is a long lead time between planning and production.

There are several types of project units. The general, or functional, management type is the most common. Project activities are carried out within functional groups that are managed by department heads. The general manager coordinates the activities. With this type of arrangement there is no strong central project authority, and consequently decisions are likely to be made to the advantage of the strongest functional group rather than in the best interests of the project. Lead time and decision-making time are increased because the coordination and approval of all functional groups are required.

Aggregate project management has appointed managers who have their own staffs and full authority over their projects. Those project managers manage from a pool of funding and other resources that they do not have to share with other projects or functional managers. All people involved in a project report directly to the manager, which gives the manager a high degree of control over each project. This allows rapid reaction time and reduces lead time. Project management is highly regarded by outside sources. The people involved tend to be loyal to the project because it is their only job at the time.

There are disadvantages to aggregate management. In this management method, production elements are not shared with other projects. Consequently there is duplication of functional activities among projects, and managers cannot keep all production elements in use at all times. There is also a lack of career continuity. Anxiety may increase as the time nears for completion of a project, because project personnel do not know where they will be assigned next. It is difficult to balance workloads as projects begin and reach completion. Aggregate management is not often used.

Project management offers several advantages. It visualizes projects and focuses on results. It provides control over the project, shorter development time, improved quality, and lower program costs. This yields higher profit margins and positive customer relations. Project management facilitates coordination among functional areas and good mission orientation for people working on the project. It can help elevate morale and develop managers.

Project management also has numerous disadvantages. It requires changes in patterns of interaction and disrupts the established hierarchical arrangements, span of management, unity of control, resource allocation, departmentalization, priorities, and incentives. Work groups are disrupted, and interfunctional groups develop. Duplication is common. Interdepartmental consensus is used and tends to increase fears of invasion from other departments.

Project managers tend to depend on functional managers for resources. This dependence can create a conflict over those resources. Hence the project may deplete the functional department of premium professional talent, and the competition for talent may disrupt the stability of the organization and interfere with long-range interests by disrupting traditional business. Some professionals complain that higher-level ego needs are not met. Project personnel are more likely to be anxious about the loss of their jobs, frustrated by make-work assignments between projects, and confused by a lack of role definition. They are concerned about setbacks in their careers and upset by the apparent lack of concern about their personal development. Conflicts of allegiance result and undermine loyalty to the organization. Shifting of personnel can disrupt their training. What is learned may not be transferred from one project to another. Long-range planning suffers when people are more concerned with their temporary projects (Huber, 2006; Roussel, Swansburg, & Swansburg, 2006).

Matrix

Matrix organizational designs try to combine the advantages of project and functional (bureaucratic) structures. The functional line organization provides support for the project line organization. In a functional organization the functional manager has the authority to determine and rate goals, select personnel, determine pay and promotions, make personnel assignments, and evaluate personnel and the project. Managers are responsible to their superiors but work independently. In a matrix organization the functional manager shares those responsibilities with the project manager, because management by project objectives is important to the matrix organization. The project manager uses people assigned to functional areas to complete the project while they are still assigned to the functional area. Thus the worker has two bosses, and conflicts can arise between project and functional managers (Yoder-Wise, 2007). Initially, the functional manager may experience a sense of loss in status, authority, and control. Therefore it is important for managers to be able to persuade others by using their personal qualities and knowledge of the program. The functional and project managers need each other's cooperation for approvals and sign-offs. The intent in the matrix organization is to have the decision making as far down in the organizational structure as possible. This encourages group consensus. Most decisions are made at the middle management level, which frees top administration for long-range planning. Matrix organizations are more decentralized with fewer levels of decision making and have less rigid adherence to formal rules than line-staff or functionalized structures (Figure 10-3).

The matrix organization increases the amount of contact among individuals, and its complexity makes conflict inevitable. Increased communication is essential. Recognizing and dealing with differences are necessary because collaborative behavior is required. Team building between departments is encouraged, and consultants are used as connections between parts. Managers need human relations training. Provision of organizational charts showing task responsibilities and levels of responsibility may reduce conflict.

A matrix organization fosters flexibility in dealing with change and uncertainty. It enables managers to balance conflicting objectives by maximizing technical excellence through efficient use of resources. Because decision making is moved down in the organization, opportunities are provided for personal development and motivation. Commitment is improved, and top management is freed for long-range planning.

Because people are more familiar with bureaucratic structures, there is considerable need to orient personnel to the matrix structure and philosophy. Rigid lines of authority, inflexible boundaries separating jobs and divisions, unambiguous resource allocation to divisions, and specific loyalties that exist in bureaucracies are not appropriate in dynamic organizations with overlapping and sometimes contradictory interests and goals. Because of the multiple and often ambiguous roles, however, some personnel may get frustrated and feel insecure. Matrix structures are increasingly common in health care systems. Because of their generalized education and time spent with patients, nurses are well qualified to coordinate the clinical and nonclinical care of patients. That may involve integrating care from nutritionists, occupational therapists, pharmacists, physicians, physiotherapists, and social workers (Galbraith, Downey, & Kates, 2002; Huber, 2006; Marquis & Huston 2006; Roussel, Swansburg, & Swansburg, 2006; Westphal, 2005) (Box 10-2).

Collegial Management

Collegial management restricts monocratic authority by maintaining a division and balance of power among the top management group

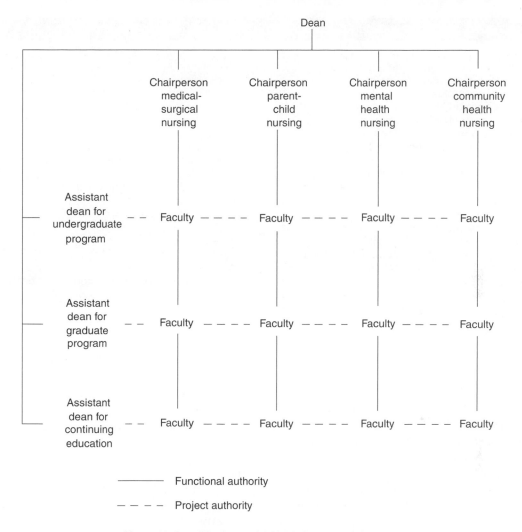

Figure 10-3 • Adaptive model. Matrix for a school of nursing.

through collective responsibility. It is most commonly used in Germany and Holland but is also employed in Austria, Switzerland, and France. Consequently, it is often referred to as *European-style management*. The directors usually represent functional areas of the organization. They may or may not have a chairperson. If so, the chairperson may be the first among equals and merely speak for the directors, may coordinate the work of the others, or may be recognized as the general manager or chief executive. The directors may have vice directors.

The decision-making process varies from one country to another, but in every case it is the board that makes policy decisions. Essentially, the directors need to persuade each other. Although chairpersons may not have strong decision-making powers, they do have strong veto powers.

Collegial management has several strengths. It limits autocratic leadership, breeds democratic management, and ensures representation of each functional area. Because of their collective responsibility, directors are better informed

BOX 10-2 Advantages and Disadvantages of the Matrix Organizational Structure

ADVANTAGES

Manages dual demands
Is good for complex work
Focuses on products and functions
Is good for uncertain environments
Is good for nonroutine technologies
Involves high interdependence between
    functions
Provides collaborative management
Allows flexible, efficient use of scarce resources
Is adaptive
Is innovative
Allows decisions to be made close to operations
Provides fluidity
Encourages improved interpersonal skills and
    conflict management, which leads to
    achievement and job satisfaction

DISADVANTAGES

Involves dual authority (one line, one project)
Is complicated
May be viewed as confusing
Has a complex structure
Needs well-educated personnel
Involves complex communications
Requires advanced interpersonal relationship
    skills
Requires group and teamwork skills
Generates role conflicts
Leads to role ambiguity
Requires frequent meetings
Is time consuming
Requires special learning in conflict
    management
Can lead to stress in interpersonal relationships

Data from Grohar-Murray ME, DiCroce HR: *Leadership and management in nursing,* ed 3, Stamford, CT, 2003, Appleton & Lange; Sullivan EJ, Decker PJ: *Effective leadership and management in nursing,* Upper Saddle River, NJ, 2005, Prentice Hall.

about the functional areas that are not their own; this broadens the approach to problem solving. Collegial management prevents precipitous decisions, encourages long-range planning, and fosters objective appraisal of functions. Camaraderie is possible.

Collegial management also has limitations. The need for consensus can slow decision making. Consensus based on compromise may be an inferior solution. Logrolling results when directors give reciprocal support to programs that are not viable. Collegial management requires considerable expensive executive time to deal with what may be relatively minor matters or what may be others' functional affairs; this results in a diffusion of responsibility. The management process may even cease at times, especially when policies and programs are to be determined. Differences of opinions may smolder and lead to rudeness and cold wars. Communications are more likely to be vertical than horizontal; coordination is thus a problem. The encouragement of group action may stifle a strong creative director. Because of the inherent problems in collegial

management, some organizations are moving toward committee management with an executive to coordinate policy.

Shared Governance

Shared governance was one of the more radical changes during the 1980s. It was an accountability-based governance system for professionals that empowered individuals within the decision-making system and increased nurses' authority and control over their nursing practice. Group professional communications took on an egalitarian structure when joint practice committees were developed to assume power and accountability for decision making. A typical model of shared governance is a committee structure in which representative staff nurses belong to nursing committees that are assigned specific management or clinical functions. The committees are typically composed of a staff nurse or administrative chair appointed by an administrator and representatives of staff and administration. The nursing committee chairs and nursing administrators comprise the nursing council or cabinet that makes the final decisions on recommendations from the committees. Schryer (2004) found that overdelegating to novice nurses did not create an environment that fostered success. Resistance came from nurse managers who were reluctant to change their roles from those of autocratic decision makers to coaches, consultants, teachers, collaborators, and facilitators of shared decision making. The turnover rate increased after implementation of shared governance committees.

Participatory Management

Participatory management is the foundation for shared governance. However, it allows participation only in decision making in which someone else has the power to make the final choice. In this model, staff nurse representatives are members of forums or committees that deal with designated issues. Managers are also members. Recommendations go to an executive committee, which has staff representation as well as manager membership. The nurse executive retains the decision-making authority and may or may not agree with committee recommendations.

Self-Governance

Self-governance goes beyond participatory management and shared governance to structures that allow nursing staff to govern themselves. These professional practice models place autonomy, authority, and control of services to clients with the professionals providing the care. Staff nurse representatives are members of councils with authority for specified functions. The council chairs comprise the management committee charged with making the final operational decisions for the organization. Bylaws are developed to specify the authority, responsibility, communication channels, and coordination of the self-governance structure. The councils have the authority to make decisions and are responsible for the results. It is important to clarify what decisions councils will make, what shared decisions will be made by staff and managers, and what decisions will be the responsibility of administration. Councils typically have functional accountability for practice, nursing professional development, peer behavior, and governance with a coordinating council.

Systems Design Approach

Systems design is an adaptive organizational model. It has been facilitated by the use of computers. The systems approach can be applied to bureaucracies that are considered closed systems or to adaptive models viewed as open systems. The design develops from the flow of work and information. It considers relationships, time, and decision points.

Mixed Model

A mixed model may be the most viable. Bureaucratic design can work very well for routine functions. Adaptive designs may be more useful for research and development. However, the success of any organizational design depends largely on the managers' skills and the staffs' adaptability.

Corporate Model

A corporation is any group of people who act as one body. Corporations are required to register their articles of incorporation, which specify the purposes and functions of the organization. Corporations may be private or public and proprietary (for profit) or not for profit. A public corporation is subject to government regulations, may issue and trade stock, and is expected to return a profit to the owners of the stock. Most individual investor-owned hospitals are operated for a profit but are privately owned, not public, corporations. However, many hospital management firms are publicly held corporations that manage both for-profit and not-for-profit hospitals. Most private corporations are smaller than public corporations.

Corporate growth leads to mergers, buyouts, and other business transactions to increase the value of the business. Large multihospital corporations have emerged in the health care arena. Nurses have opportunities for leadership and management positions in the corporations and may operate their own corporations.

The physician's share of the health care dollar has increased in the newer delivery systems as the hospital's share has decreased and services have moved out of the hospital. Services still tend to be illness based, medically dominated, interventional, and expensive. Decentralization through the use of holding companies with multiple subcorporate entities that provide a range of services is the trend. This has created a need to restructure nursing. There is also a trend toward emphasis on disease prevention and globalization of health care.

For nursing service to be a corporate entity it must be able to sustain its own activities without dependence on other units. Nursing practice must be clearly defined and its contribution to profitability clearly identified. The holding company's mission and purposes must be reflected in the philosophy, purpose, and objectives of the nursing service corporate entity. The relationship to the marketplace and plans to meet market demands should be outlined. Remuneration of nurses should reflect the value of their work in the marketplace.

As nursing becomes increasingly decentralized and incorporated, it also becomes increasingly important to create a network instead of preserving a pyramid. A coordinating council may centralize the activities of individual councils for practice, education, research, and quality assurance. This provides an opportunity for the chairpersons of the individual councils to meet together to discuss issues, coordinate the work of the councils, and make decisions that affect the entire corporate nursing entity.

The corporate nursing staff should meet at least once per year to (1) review, revise as necessary, and approve the nursing staff bylaws; (2) review, discuss, and revise as appropriate the nursing organization's long- and short-range planning process, goals, and objectives; (3) debate issues of concern and vote on them as appropriate; (4) review, discuss, and approve the coordinating council's activities; (5) provide opportunities for informal networking; and (6) provide education sessions.

Interorganizational Relationships

Health care organizations have been forming relationships with one another to survive the increased competition for resources. Horizontal integration occurs when the organizations provide the same or similar services, such as dietary and laundry services. One provides dietary services to the other, whereas that other provides the laundry services for both organizations. Vertical integration is an arrangement among dissimilar but related organizations to provide a continuum of services. It could include an affiliation of a health maintenance organization with a pharmacy, hospital, home care agency, and long-term care facility. Vertical integration can improve coordination of services, quality, efficiency, and cost-effectiveness (Sullivan & Decker, 2005). Brown, Alikhan, and Seeman (2006) used a survey to identify system priorities shared by hospitals in the Ontario hospitals system.

Continuum of Multiorganizational Arrangements

Rakich, Longest, and Darr (2001) describe a continuum of multiorganizational arrangements:
1. Informal affiliations are joint undertakings without written agreements.
2. Formal affiliations occur when two or more organizations formalize the undertaking of limited activities.
3. Shared or cooperative services have a common management; for example, joint purchasing or shared laundry facilities for two or more organizations.
4. Consortia and alliances are limited voluntary associations for specific purposes, such as management information systems and labor relations.
5. Management contracts occur when one organization supplies the senior management for the other.
6. Umbrella organizations are new corporations that span but do not replace the existing organizations.
7. Mergers occur when one organization maintains its name and identity, and another is dissolved and absorbed into it.

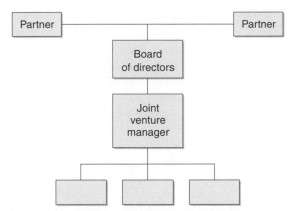

Figure 10-4 • Merger collaborative organizational structure. (Modified from Nadler DA, Gerstein MS, Shaw RB, et al: *Organizational architecture: Designs for changing organizations*, San Francisco, 1992, Jossey-Bass, p 94.)

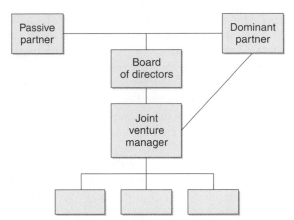

Figure 10-5 • Acquisition instrumental organizational structure. (Modified from Nadler DA, Gerstein MS, Shaw RB, et al: *Organizational architecture: Designs for changing organizations*, San Francisco, 1992, Jossey-Bass, p 96.)

8. Consolidation occurs when two or more organizations dissolve and are unified into a new legal organization. Management contracts, umbrella corporations, mergers, and consolidations are multiorganizational systems.

Mergers

Mergers occur when one organization purchases another of approximately the same size. There are some multiinstitutional relationships for sharing assets such as a central laundry service, a purchasing department, or a home health agency. However, mergers usually restructure the relationship of one health care organization with another. Acquisitions occur when one organization is considerably larger than the other. Both mergers and acquisitions are used to acquire complementary services or products that are connected by common clients and technologies. By increasing the size of the organization, they increase organizational power and leverage through expansion of product or service offerings, market access, distribution networks, and capital access; promotion of economies of scale; enhancement of diversification, name, and reputation; and expansion of access to technology, people, and management resources. They gain financial benefits by eliminating employees who have responsibilities that overlap both entities. However,

this makes employees nervous, strains organizational cultures, and often brings out the worst of behaviors. Nurse managers need to resolve their own negative feelings and help employees understand and adjust to the changes (Figures 10-4 and 10-5).

It is appropriate for the nurse manager to assess attitudes toward the merger through a questionnaire, personal interviews, or focus groups. Only personnel who are supportive of the merger should be assigned to leadership positions to accommodate it. Managers need to keep staff informed about the changes. Maintaining open communications can help minimize pluralistic views about the merger. Staff may need assistance in understanding the new organizational culture, and managers can help them recognize the unique qualities of the merging agency. Managers should periodically assess how personnel are responding to the merger, identify problems, and engage in problem solving (Roussel, Swansburg, & Swansburg, 2006).

Health Care Networks

Health maintenance organizations (HMOs) are associations of health care professionals and facilities that provide a health care package for a fixed sum of money paid in advance for a specific period of time. The HMO contracts with health care professionals and facilities to provide care. The members can seek care outside the network at their own additional expense. The plan will not cover expenses for care outside the plan that is not preapproved. Primary care physicians usually see the client first and decide if a specialist is needed. Specialists may have contracts with the plan, but the plan may or may not allow members to make appointments with them directly. Consequently, patients are not guaranteed the right to see a specialist for consultation or care unless the primary care physician gatekeeper approves.

Preferred provider organizations (PPOs) are groups of health care professionals and hospitals that contract with an employer, insurance company, or other third-party payer to provide health care to a group. The services are not fixed or prepaid, and more customer choice is allowed than with an HMO. Consequently, PPOs are more expensive, and customers pay an even greater percentage of fees for services rendered by providers outside the PPO. Individual practice associations provide insurance coverage, set health care services rates, and bill a fee for services.

Physician-hospital organizations (PHOs) allow a hospital and the medical staff to have joint managed care contracts. They vary in terms of administration, credentialing, governance, managed care contracting, and structure. The impetus for their creation usually comes from the hospital, which incorporates a not-for-profit organization with a hospital and a physician board. Management skills and infrastructure are critical to the survival of PHOs, which will have to develop networks to provide a broader spectrum of services to remain competitive. An external focus and customer orientation are important to success. Care management, risk management, information management, and relationship management are all important components of PHOs to help them provide cost-effective care in a timely manner. Management service organizations provide medical practice management, physician recruitment, information systems, billing and collection systems, quality monitoring, and other services.

DISEASE MANAGEMENT

Disease management is a population-based health strategy that has an intense focus on a given disease or health condition and provides care to groups needing specialized health services. Disease management programs were developed largely as managed care health plans. Disease management programs may be offered by health plans or can be developed in an organization or obtained by contract from another organization. They primarily focus on chronic diseases because chronic diseases place a large burden on society through lost productivity and increased health care costs. The prevalence of chronic diseases increases as people get older, but they are increasingly appearing in younger people.

Disease management models can span the continuum of care starting with risk identification. Primary prevention and lifestyle and behavioral changes can be taught at this level. There is a need for care coordination for people identified to be at risk and a need for case management for the approximately 20% of the population needing integrated economic and care management. Disease management empowers individuals, along with their physicians and other care providers, to manage chronic diseases and conditions such as asthma, congestive heart failure, diabetes, and obesity to prevent complications through adherence to medication regimens, regular monitoring of vital signs, and consumption of a healthful diet, regular exercise, and adoption of other healthy lifestyle choices (Huber, 2006).

DEMAND MANAGEMENT

The third-party payer system that arose from an incentive in the tax code made employer-provided health care dominant and has increased reimbursement through Medicaid. Consumers are frustrated by limited provider choices determined by a bureaucracy, insurance paperwork, interference with medical care, and a lack of attention to health promotion and personal responsibility for the consequences of one's own health choices (Gingrich, Pavey, & Woodbury, 2006).

Herzlinger (2004) believes that the system would be improved by discontinuing the current third-party payment system and letting consumer demand determine the health care market. She maintains that money not spent on insurance could be used for health expenses or for a medical savings account. She wants health care to function as a business market and believes that competitive forces can increase productivity and innovation. She envisions specialized clinics that cater to individuals with specific diseases like asthma and diabetes.

Burns (2006) has declared that biotechnology, information technology, genomics and proteomics, medical devices, and pharmaceuticals supply the majority of innovative products used by physicians and health care facilities, and these products are increasingly demanded by consumers. They are also responsible for a disproportionate amount of health care costs. He recommends convergence among these sectors to add value.

Porter (2006) wants to create results-value–based competition. He argues that we have been cost shifting and restricting services, which has resulted in high costs, poor quality, inefficiency, and consumer dissatisfaction rather than creating value for clients. There has been a zero-sum situation among health plans, networks, and hospitals rather than the addition of value related to diagnosis, treatment, and prevention. He wants positive-sum competition.

Quality is more efficient, effective, and economical. Better providers generally add value for less cost because there are more accurate diagnoses, fewer treatment errors, fewer complications, faster recovery, less invasive treatments, and minimization of the need for more treatment. Better health is less expensive than illness. If providers competed on value added, they could magnify each other's gains.

Demand management focuses on customer expectations. Demand forecasting assesses trends and anticipates shifts in demand. That helps improve revenue and decrease inventory carrying costs. Research methods are used to acquire, process, and apply information on customer desires and preferences (Shillito, 2001).

Technology can be used to identify the mass market, the target market, the customer, and even to do one-on-one marketing (Sharp, 2003). Spector (2001) describes the lessons learned from Nordstrom, the number one customer service company, about providing customers with choices, creating an inviting place, hiring nice people, selling the relationship, empowering employees to take ownership, being innovative, promoting competition, and committing 100% to customer service. Timm (2001) explains the importance of one-to-one customer contact in the future and the need to exceed customer expectations. This requires dealing with customer turn-offs and dissatisfactions, encouraging positive attitudes, and using behaviors that win customer loyalty, such as friendly written messages and telephone, e-mail, and website techniques. Leaders need to be aware of generational differences.

By the early 2000s, private case management companies had become common. Directories, buying guides, market research data, statistical reports, databases, and mailing lists for managed care and health care organizations were available. Case managers had access to over 100,000 providers of home care, rehabilitation, long-term care, addiction care, behavioral and psychiatric care, and clinical specialty care. The position of clinical nurse leader, a new role for masters-prepared nurses to serve as lateral integrators of care, was gaining popularity. Clinical nurse leaders serve as patient advocates throughout the many components of the health care continuum and as information managers for the many disciplines involved in patient care (Wiggins, 2006).

CONTINUUM OF CARE

Historically the United States has had a two-tiered system for delivering health care: inpatient hospitalization and outpatient treatment. Treatment was often costly. The increasing need for cost containment and the development of flexible benefit programs led to creation of a continuum of care. This allowed payers to ensure that patients could be directed to the most cost-efficient and clinically appropriate services. Expansion of services covered by benefit plans lowered costs, and those additional services enhanced patient treatment and improved patient outcomes. Common treatment settings on a continuum of care include, but are not limited to, the following (Huber, 2006):

- Prevention and early intervention services provide screening in primary care offices and nonclinical settings such as schools and workplaces.
- Outpatient offices or clinics are facilities where patients may be seen by one or more clinicians and may be treated individually or as part of a family or group.
- Employee-assistance programs are worksite programs that help in identifying and resolving personal concerns associated with job performance that interferes with productivity.
- Intensive outpatient programs provide individual or group treatment to patients at least three times a week.
- Intensive case management coordinates the financial, legal, and medical services the patient needs to live successfully at home.
- Home-based treatment involves the provision of intensive therapy to a patient or family by a person or team who makes visits to the home.
- Family support services are services to support and train families in caring for a person at home.
- Partial hospitalization of daily or weekly treatment services are structured programs to which an individual, group, or family goes during the day only. The individuals return home at night.
- Therapeutic foster homes are foster homes in which the foster parents provide a therapeutic environment and supervised care.
- Group homes are residential homes that provide a therapeutic family-type environment. They may serve as a step-down from a more intensive level of care.
- Rehabilitation services address functional problems and deficits that interfere with a person's ability to live in the community. They may provide evaluation, treatment, consultation,

educational or vocational placement, family or caregiver support, and training.

- Residential treatment centers are facilities in which intensive and comprehensive treatment is provided by a multidisciplinary team 24 hours a day on a long-term basis.
- Assisted living facilities are for people who cannot live independently. Food preparation, laundry services, cleaning, and so on, may be provided.
- Respite care is care provided to give the usual caregivers some temporary relief, either with prior planning or on an emergency basis.
- Hospice care may be provided at home or in an inpatient setting once the patient has agreed to receive palliative care only.
- Crisis residential programs provide short-term crisis intervention, usually for fewer than 15 days, and individualized treatment with 24-hour supervision.
- Personal emergency response systems are electronic communication systems that can summon emergency assistance 24 hours a day. They automatically dial for help after activation of a remote button typically worn around the neck.
- Emergency or crisis services provide emergency care and include emergency departments and mobile crisis teams.
- Acute inpatient hospital-based treatment is medically directed interdisciplinary treatment, including 24-hour professional nursing care.
- Hospital treatment provides comprehensive treatment based on the patient's needs.
- Consumer programs provide support and structure through social centers, clubhouses, day programs, drop-in centers, and self-help groups like Alcoholics Anonymous or Narcotics Anonymous.

INTEGRATED HEALTH CARE SYSTEMS

The objective of integrated health care systems is to keep people healthy and treat them in the lowest-cost setting possible, which makes primary

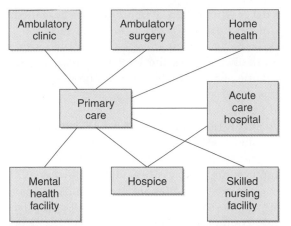

Figure 10-6 • Integrated health care system. (Modified from Grohar-Murray ME, DiCroce HR: *Leadership and management in nursing,* Stamford, CT, 1997, Appleton & Lange, p 144.)

<table>
<tr><td colspan="2">**BOX 10-3** Degrees of Integration of Organizations</td></tr>
<tr><td colspan="2">**NONE**
Separate holdings
Loosely coupled</td></tr>
<tr><td colspan="2">**MODERATE**
Coupled
Operationally integrated</td></tr>
<tr><td colspan="2">**COMPLETE**
Consolidated</td></tr>
</table>

care and managed care pivotal (Figure 10-6). Efforts are aimed at improving health care outcomes at reduced cost while ensuring patient satisfaction. This requires inventing and managing new health care systems. There is a trend toward a reduction in the number of managers and the levels of management, retention and training of workers with multiple skills, data-based decision making, and continuous quality improvement. Hospitals are joining together and linking health promotion programs, clinics, ambulatory care, acute care, home care, and long-term care into integrated health care (Grohar-Murray & DiCroce, 2003). A moderate rate of integration seems desirable. When the parent organization in an acquisition moves in quickly and tries to integrate in a fast and intense way by imposing its own policies and procedures, the management of the acquired agency often leaves, followed by the technical staff; therefore the parent organization loses the leverage that was to be gained from the acquisition. If the integration occurs too slowly, people experience a high level of stress because they do not know what is going to happen to them. This brings out undesirable behaviors, and the best people may accept positions elsewhere.

When there is no integration, the parent organization may adopt a hands-off approach and let the acquiree operate its separate holdings. Except possibly for submitting to limited financial controls and reviews of productivity at the board level, the acquiree remains autonomous. In coupled integrations, some of the activities or functions of the acquired agency are integrated with those of the parent organization, whereas others are left independent and separate. In loosely coupled acquisitions, a minimum of activities are integrated. Most are left separate and independent. The acquiree functions largely as an independent entity. In moderately coupled integrations the degree of integration is greater. Operationally integrated organizations still can be identified as separate entities, but the key procedures and operations are tightly linked to those of the parent organization. With complete integration, the organizations are consolidated or merged into one (Box 10-3). There are phases to the integration of health care systems, including assessment, planning and design, implementation, and development.

Assessment Phase

During the assessment phase the organization should assess its strategic plan, its ability to handle the operating requirements for a joint venture, and its readiness to manage change. Is the joint venture an appropriate strategic action to address the problem, or are there less complicated alternatives? Is the problem temporary, not meriting a joint venture, or is it a long-term problem that could best be addressed by integration?

All partners should agree on the long-term goals and their compatibility with individual organizational goals. Convergent objectives are those the organizations share and are probably the primary reason the joint venture is being considered. Compatible objectives are those held by each organization that are unique to it but are compatible with shared objectives. Objectives in potential conflict require the most careful assessment. These may involve differences in management style, strategies, or other factors that present a potential threat to the viability of the venture. It is better to articulate the potential problems and address them before the joint venture is undertaken than to be surprised by them later.

The internal operating and management requirements for the joint venture should be carefully considered. Partners will need to be cooperative and flexible while sharing responsibilities. It can be difficult for some managers to give up power and control. People are likely to resist change. Having a specific plan for the implementation of the change can help in managing the change. Is the organization ready to manage change? Is there a deliberate plan of action to minimize disruption during the implementation of change? Is there understanding of the relationship of this venture to the strategic plan? Is there an understanding of the opportunities being sought? Does the other organization provide the resources, skills, or other attributes that are needed? Is the other organization financially sound, trustworthy, and respected? Are the management styles and cultures compatible? Are the people cooperative, flexible, skilled in conflict resolution, and experienced in joint ventures? Are people willing to make a commitment, learn, and make comparable contributions? Do people understand the joint venture's business?

Planning and Design Phase

After agreeing to integrate, partners need to plan and design the joint venture. The main work in the second phase is to plan the structure, staffing, management style, and support systems. How involved will each partner be in the operations? Who will make what decisions? Who will report

what to whom? How will the venture be staffed? How will the organizations relate to each other? Chances for success increase when one partner primarily manages the joint venture. The joint venture general manager needs autonomy to act quickly to achieve the responsiveness required to be successful. When both partners are heavily involved in the operations, it slows down decision making. They need compatible styles and orientations, common understanding of the joint venture's necessities, and skills at conflict management and human relationships. Achieving the necessary relationships takes considerable commitment, time, and effort. Managers need to be able to handle much ambiguity and uncertainty. A participative style in which input is solicited from all partners tends to produce more commitment to plans than an autocratic style. The venture manager should be positioned as the leader for the venture and as the person who is in control. The venture manager and staff need to establish an independent identity and allegiance to the venture. People from both partner organizations may staff the venture in a collaborative structure. In general, however, staff should not be employed from the passive partner organization, because that can create allegiance problems and managerial interference by the passive partner. Staff should be qualified to perform the required tasks, should be viewed as competent, and should be respected. A compensatory reward system should be established that is consistent with the performance criteria and expectations of the venture.

Implementation Phase

The implementation phase focuses on successful startup and execution of the venture. It deals with the organization's culture and major organizational change, which typically involves issues of power, anxiety, and control. During change, individuals and groups often compete for power. Change threatens the balance of formal and informal power. As uncertainty increases, so does the political behavior of people who want to protect their positions and gain power. Competition for control emerges. If the venture is expected to be successful, managers may compete for positions and promise appointments to their staff based on networks rather than job requirements. If failure is anticipated, managers may protect themselves, thus withholding commitment, energy, and resources from the venture and contributing to a self-fulfilling prophecy of failure. During organizational change, people are usually concerned about what will happen to them, become anxious, and experience stress. The redistribution of people, material, tasks, and systems during the change usually results in some loss of managerial control and a deterioration of performance. Managers can help shape the political dynamics associated with change by supporting the change and by getting the support of key power groups. Providing anchors to anxious people can help stabilize the organization. Managers should give assurances about what is not going to change, warn people in advance of what changes will occur, explain the need for the change, and send consistent messages.

Development Phase

Next, attention must be given to the development of the people in the venture. It is important that they feel identity with the venture and independence from the partner organizations. The venture should be seen as distinct from the partner organizations. Building allegiance to the venture and severing formal ties to the partner organizations are necessary. People must not think they can just return to the parent organization if the going gets rough. They need commitment to the venture. The strategic plan can help people assess where they fit into future options.

People need to be trained to deal with the characteristics of future organizations. Organizations can be expected to be networks that cooperate with each other to survive in a competitive market. Organizational forms will be fluid and transitory with fuzzy boundaries. Social and technical systems will be used to create high-performance work systems. Teams will be the norm at all levels and will have relative autonomy. Norms and values will dominate

over rules and direct supervision and will facilitate the cohesion necessary to achieve coordination and direction. There will be an emphasis on system-level learning and preparation of people to understand the broad strategic issues and the specific tasks required to accomplish the strategic plan. Pareto's law states that in most situations about 20% of the causative factors account for about 80% of the effects; it advises us to pay attention to the 20% of the factors that truly matter in shaping the future and to focus on the 20% of personnel who will make 80% of what happens happen.

"Worse than a quitter is a person who is afraid to begin."   —Anonymous

GLOBALIZATION

Globalization and its implications for health have been receiving increasing attention in medicine and public health. The worldwide spread of disease; the speed of change; and the number, ease, and complexity of connections are leading to globalization. The rapid movement of capital, goods and services, drug-resistant infectious diseases, contaminated foodstuffs, legal or banned toxic substances, and terrorism are a threat to the health of all countries (Pappas, Hyder, & Akhter, 2003). The World Health Organization reported that the following conditions contributed to about one third of deaths worldwide in 2003: underweight and malnutrition in children; adverse consequences of unsafe sex; high blood pressure and cholesterol level; tobacco and alcohol consumption; unsafe water, sanitary conditions, and hygienic conditions; indoor smoke; iron deficiency; and obesity. The World Health Organization identified the following as priorities for attention in 2004 and 2005: cancer, cardiovascular disease, diabetes, food safety, healthful environment, health systems, HIV/AIDS, malaria, maternal health, mental health, safety of the blood supply, tobacco use, and tuberculosis (Dickenson-Hazard, 2004). Infectious diseases pose the risk of epidemics and pandemics. Electronic communications facilitate worldwide collegial collaboration in finding solutions to biologic and technologic health care challenges, but there is a need to mobilize research efforts, human experts, and material supplies and technology. The World Health Organization could play a major role in meeting the challenges of globalization (see Chapter 9).

The unprecedented interconnectedness of health care around the world through computers, telecommunications, and rapid air transportation is creating a new era in health care, and these new global systems should draw on nursing leadership talents (Nash & Gremillion, 2004). The centrality of nurses in global health care provides an opportunity to create new knowledge through health care research (Schultz, 2004). The ability to conduct global nursing dialogues helps cultivate new ideas and foster synergy (Rantz, Zazworsky, Zerull, et al, 2004). Nursing leaders and managers need to be aware of real and potential areas of conflict of interest and be prepared to prevent and deal with such conflicts (Willers, 2004). Nurses of many cultures need to work together, but nurses have much in common despite cultural differences (Thompson, 2004). Case management and clinical paths provide groundwork for the management of outcomes in global patient care (Bower, 2004). Information technology is the foundation of global health care and the marketing of it (Simpson, 2004). Globalization is a challenge and opportunity for nursing leaders and managers.

CHAPTER SUMMARY

Restructuring and integration are occurring in response to a rapidly changing health care environment. This makes it important for nurse leaders and managers to understand the factors affecting organizational structures, organizational concepts, and the advantages and disadvantages of various types of organizational structure. Nurses need to know how to work across the entire continuum of care in integrated health care systems and beyond.

CRITICAL THINKING ACTIVITY

Reflective Journal: Make observations in a clinical setting or reflect on past experiences. Answer the following questions: What is the organizational structure of the facility? How does the structure support the organizational purposes? Where is the top nursing position in the organization? Compare the nursing position with those of medicine and other powerful departments. Outline the similarities and differences in the management responsibilities of lower-level, middle-level, and top-level nursing managers in the agency.

CASE STUDY

Develop an organizational chart for General Hospital. Identify a possible restructuring of units to maximize hospital profits by serving the changing needs of the community. Consider changing General Hospital's underused medical-surgical units to accommodate the increasing demand for geriatric, home health, and ambulatory care services. Develop a new organizational chart, noting span of management, flat or tall structure, decentralization or centralization, and line authority. List the advantages and disadvantages of the new organization and discuss them with your classmates.

ONLINE RESOURCES

evolve Additional critical thinking activities, worksheets, and case studies are available online at http://evolve.elsevier.com/Marriner/guide8e.

REFERENCES

Adams CE, Michel Y, DeFrates D, et al: The effect of locale on health status and direct care time of rural versus urban home patient, *J Nurs Adm* 35(1): 244-251, 2001.

Bower KA: Patient care management as a global nursing concern, *Nurs Adm Q* 28(1):39-43, 2004.

Brown AD, Alikhan LM, Seeman NL: Crossing the strategic synapse: Aligning hospital strategy with shared system priorities in Ontario, Canada, *Health Care Manage Rev* 31(1):34-44, 2006.

Burns LR: *The business of healthcare innovation*, Cambridge, UK, 2006, Cambridge University Press.

Coddington DC, Fischer EA, Moore KD, et al: *Beyond managed care: how consumers and technology are changing the future of health care*, San Francisco, 2000, Jossey-Bass.

Dickenson-Hazard N: Global health issues and challenges, *J Nurs Scholarsh* 36(1):6-10, 2004.

Galbraith JR: *Designing organizations: An executive guide to strategy, structure, and process revised*, San Francisco, 2002, Jossey-Bass.

Galbraith JR: *Designing the customer centric organization: A guide to strategy, structure, and process*, San Francisco, 2005, Jossey-Bass.

Galbraith JR, Downey D, Kates A: *Designing dynamic organizations*, New York, 2002, American Management Association.

Gingrich N, Pavey D, Woodbury A: *Saving lives and saving money*, Washington, DC, 2006, Alexis de Tocqueville Institution.

Grohar-Murray ME, DiCroce HR: *Leadership and management in nursing,* ed 3, Stamford, CT, 2003, Appleton & Lange.

Hall LM: Examining the human capital costs of nursing following restructuring, *J Nurs Adm* 36(5):231, 2006.

Herzlinger RE: *Consumer-driven health care: Implications for providers, payers, and policy-makers*, San Francisco, 2004, Jossey-Bass.

Huber DL: *Leadership and nursing care management,* ed 3, Philadelphia, 2006, Elsevier.

Institute for the Future: *Health and health care 2010*, San Francisco, 2000, Jossey-Bass.

Marquis BL, Huston CJ: *Leadership roles and management functions in nursing: Theory and application,* ed 5, Philadelphia, 2006, Lippincott Williams & Wilkins.

Milisen K, Abraham I, Siebens K, et al: Work environment and workforce problems: A cross-sectional questionnaire survey of hospital nurses in Belgium, *Int J Nurs Stud* 43(6):745-754, 2006.

Nash MG, Gremillion C: Globalization impacts the healthcare organization of the 21st century: demanding new ways to market product lines successfully, *Nurs Adm Q* 28(2):86-92, 2004.

Pappas G, Hyder AA, Akhter M: Globalization: Toward a new framework for public Health, *Soc Theory Health* 1(2):91-100, 2003.

Porter ME: *Redefining health care: Creating value-based competition on results*, Boston, 2006, Harvard Business School Press.

Rakich JS, Longest BB, Darr K: *Managing health services organizations,* ed 3, Baltimore, 2001, Health Professions Press.

Rantz M, Zazworsky D, Zerull LM, et al: The power of dialogue with the global nursing exchange, *Nurs Adm Q* 28(1):19-26, 2004.

Roussel L, Swansburg RC, Swansburg RJ: *Management and leadership for nurse administrators*, Boston, 2006, Jones & Bartlett.

Schryer N: Implementing organizational redesign to support practice: the Tulane model, *J Nurs Adm* 34(9):400-406, 2004.

Schultz AA: Role of research in reconstructing global healthcare for the 21st century, *Nurs Adm Q* 28(2):133-135, 2004.

Sharp DE: *Customer relationship management systems handbook*, Boca Raton, Fl, 2003, Auerbach Publications.

Shillito ML: *Acquiring, processing, and deploying the voice of the customer*, Boca Raton, Fl, 2001, St. Lucie Press.

Simpson RL: Global informing: impact and implications of technology in a global marketplace, *Nurs Adm Q* 28(2):144-150, 2004.

Spector R: *Lessons from the Nordstrom way: How companies are emulating the #1 customer service company*, New York, 2001, John Wiley & Sons.

Sullivan EJ, Decker PJ: *Effective leadership and management in nursing*, Upper Saddle River, NJ, 2005, Prentice Hall.

Thompson PA: Leadership from an international perspective, *Nurs Adm Q* 28(3):191-199, 2004.

Timm PR: *Customer service: career success through customer satisfaction*, Upper Saddle River, NJ, 2001, Prentice Hall.

Westphal J: Resilient organizations: Matrix model and service line management, *J Nurs Adm* 35(9):414-419, 2005.

Wiggins MS: The partnership care delivery model, *J Nurs Adm* 36(7-8):341-345, 2006.

Willers L: Global nursing management: Avoiding conflicts of interest, *Nurs Adm Q* 28(1):44-51, 2004.

Yoder-Wise PS: *Leading and managing in nursing,* ed 4, St Louis, 2007, Mosby.

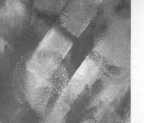

Organizational Culture, Change, and Innovation

"We cannot direct the wind, but we can adjust our sails." —Anonymous

Chapter Overview

Chapter 11 explains individual and organizational culture, diversity, process of change, cultural change, behavioral aspects of organizational change, resistance to change, oscillation, strategies for change, and innovation.

Chapter Objectives

- Describe the interrelationship of values, attitudes, perception, personality, and roles.
- Identify four factors in organizational culture.
- Explain how managers can use heroes.
- Describe a cultural network.
- Identify at least two rituals.
- Define three strategies for effecting change.
- Define at least three types of change.
- Describe the five tracks that must be carefully planned to facilitate complex organizational change according to Kilmann.
- Discuss what occurs in the three developmental stages of an organization.
- Compare creativity and innovation.

Online Resources

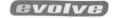
 Critical thinking activities, worksheets, and case studies are available online at http://evolve.elsevier.com/Marriner/guide8e.

Major Concepts and Definitions

Values *basic convictions and beliefs about what is desirable or important*
Attitudes *mental states of readiness*
Perceptions *awareness of the environment gained through the senses*
Personality *a relatively stable set of characteristics and temperament*
Roles *expected behaviors in given situations*
Myers-Briggs Type Indicator *a tool for self-examination of one's strengths and weaknesses and how one differs from others*
Assumptions *suppositions, presumptions, things that are taken for granted*
Symbols *objects or acts that represent other things*
Language *choice of words and sounds used to express thoughts and feelings*
Behaviors *actions or mannerisms*
Organizational culture *customary way of thinking and behaving that is shared by members of an organization*
Hero *a person honored for outstanding qualities*
Cultural network *primary informal means of communication in an organization*
Rituals *customary observance or practice*
Change *to become different*
Change agent *one who helps bring about change*
Organizational development *stages of birth, youth, and maturity of organizations*
Innovation *the use of change to introduce a new product or service*

CULTURE OF INDIVIDUALS

The culture of an individual includes the individual's values, attitudes, perceptions, interpersonal needs, roles, and cognitive styles. Managers need to be aware of these factors when planning change. It is also helpful to understand collective and expert culture. The collective culture is highly affiliative staff that can embrace the mission, values, and vision statements of the organization. However, the expert culture such as doctors does not feel that one needs mission or value statements. Expert cultures are motivated by feelings of accomplishment and power instead of affiliation. The experts have had to compete to get good grades, get into the best schools, and get the best jobs. Success has been obtained by outperforming the competition rather than through teamwork. Achievement, intense focus, stamina, quick decision making, and personal accountability have been reinforced for experts. Teamwork, consensus building, interdependency,

and following orders are not a part of the expert culture. Understanding the expert culture can help one understand physicians and other expert health care professionals (Atchinson & Bujak, 2001). There is a trend toward interdisciplinary education of professionals with some focus on working as teams.

Values

Values represent basic convictions about what is right, good, or desirable; as a result, they help an individual decide which mode of conduct is preferable to others. Value systems express an individual's values in order of their relative importance and provide the foundation for attitudes, perceptions, personality, and roles. These values cloud objectivity and rationality by influencing interpretations of what is right and wrong and implying that certain behaviors or outcomes are preferred over others. They are relatively stable and enduring and generally influence decisions and behaviors (Sullivan & Decker, 2005).

Attitudes

"Some people grin and bear it. Others smile and change it." —Anonymous

Attitudes are mental states of readiness that are organized through experience and exert specific influences on a person's response to the people, objects, and situations to which they are related. Attitudes, like values, are learned from parents, teachers, and peers, but attitudes are less stable than values. They influence decisions and behavior and are close to the core of personality.

In the late 1950s, Leon Festinger proposed the theory of cognitive dissonance to explain the link between attitudes and behavior. *Cognitive dissonance* means a perceived inconsistency or incompatibility between attitudes and behavior. Festinger maintained that this inconsistency is uncomfortable and that people will try to reduce the dissonance and consequently the discomfort. People seek a stable state with a minimum of dissonance. For example, if people think they are being paid more than they are worth, they are likely to work harder, whereas if they think they are underpaid, they may slow down and do less (Festinger, 1957).

Tolerance of ambiguity and perceived locus of control influence people's attitudes toward change. Environments are increasingly chaotic, complex, temporary, and overloaded with information. The ability to process information is affected by one's attitude toward change. *Tolerance of ambiguity* refers to the degree to which a person is threatened by unpredictability or has difficulty coping with complex situations. People who have a tolerance for ambiguity and complexity are more adaptive. Tolerance of ambiguity involves at least three factors: tolerance of novelty, tolerance of complexity, and tolerance of insolubility. *Tolerance of novelty* is tolerance of new and unfamiliar information and situations. *Tolerance of complexity* is tolerance of situations that involve multiple unrelated things. *Tolerance of insolubility* is tolerance for situations that are difficult to solve because of unavailability of information and lack of identification of alternative solutions.

The perceived locus of control can be internal or external. Perceiving an *internal locus of control* means that the person feels responsible for the success or failure of a situation. Perceiving an *external locus of control* means that the person feels that someone or something else has caused the results. A person who perceives the locus of control to be internal is more adaptable than one who perceives the locus of control to be external.

"A wise man changes his mind, a fool never." —Anonymous

Perceptions

Perception is a psychological process that makes sense out of what the individual sees, hears, smells, tastes, or feels. The individual's previous experiences and personal value system affect perception; thus people may perceive the same situation differently. There are also differences in people's ability to process data, to remember facts, and to explore alternatives. Perception involves receiving, organizing, and interpreting stimuli. These perceptions then influence behavior and form attitudes. People select various cues that influence their perceptions and consequently often misperceive another person, group, or object.

Selective perception means that people select information that supports their viewpoints. Knowing oneself increases the accuracy of one's perception of others. People tend to identify their own characteristics in others. Consequently, people who accept themselves are more likely to view others favorably.

A *stereotype* is a judgment made about people on the basis of their gender, ethnic background, or other group characteristic that can contribute to selective perception. A *self-fulfilling prophecy* occurs when people expect certain behavior, use selective perception to see this behavior, and treat others as if they behaved in this way. For example, if a nurse manager thinks members of certain ethnic groups are lazy and irresponsible, the manager may not assign them challenging tasks. That could lead to boredom and demotivation, which reinforce the stereotype and thus create a self-fulfilling prophecy.

Interpersonal Needs

Interpersonal orientations are not actual behaviors but rather are the tendencies to behave in certain ways. They are influenced by one's basic needs with regard to relationships with others. People need people and tend to seek compatible relationships with others in social situations. There are at least three basic needs: inclusion, control, and affection. Inclusion involves introversion, extroversion, joining and including others, and the desire to be included by others. Control relates to the need to balance influence and power in relationships. People differ in their need to control others or be controlled by others. People also have a need for affection, which is the need for intimacy and the desire for close personal relationships with others.

Personality

Personality is a relatively stable set of characteristics, temperaments, and tendencies that is significantly molded by inheritance as well as by social, cultural, and environmental factors.

Cognitive Styles and the Myers-Briggs Type Indicator

People gather and process information differently. The Myers-Briggs Type Indicator is an evaluation tool based on a model of cognitive styles which holds that people gather information through sensing and intuiting and process or evaluate the information through thinking and feeling. Sensing focuses on detail or specific attributes rather than on the relationships among factors. Intuiting emphasizes commonalities and generalizations in relationships among factors. Thinking systematically evaluates information, whereas feeling gives an internal sense of what to do.

The Myers-Briggs Type Indicator is a useful method for performing self-examination to understand one's strengths and weaknesses and the ways in which one differs from others. Isabel Briggs-Myers (1995) has identified four dimensions of psychological type: (1) attitude toward life, (2) perceptual function, (3) judgment function, and (4) orientation to the outer world. Each of the four dimensions has two categories, so that 16 different types are possible, as shown in Table 11-1.

Introverts like to work alone, think before they act, do not like interruptions, like quiet for concentration, may work on a project for a long time, are interested in ideas, are careful with details, may have difficulty remembering names and faces, and may have trouble communicating. *Extroverts* like to be around people, communicate freely, may act without thinking, like variety and action, and may become impatient with slow jobs. *Sensing* types tend to be good at detail work, are not usually inspired, rarely make errors of fact, are patient with routine details, enjoy using skills they know, like established ways of doing things, and work steadily step by step to an end. *Intuiting* types like solving new problems, enjoy learning new skills, follow their inspirations, and work in bursts of energy to reach conclusions quickly. *Thinking types* value logic, organize ideas into logical sequences, tend to be brief and businesslike, and may seem impersonal. *Feeling types* value sentiment, tend to be friendly and agreeable, may undervalue thinking, and are likely to ramble. They are usually stronger in social skills than in executive ability. *Judging types* like to plan their work and follow the plan, make decisions quickly, and get things done. *Perceiving types* are curious, may start too many projects, and may have trouble finishing them or coming to a conclusion.

Leaders should know their own styles and those of the people with whom they work. When leaders are aware of their own limitations, they can consult opposite types to compensate. By knowing their associates' strengths and weaknesses, they can maximize the strengths, minimize the weaknesses, and develop strong teams (Barr & Barr, 1989; Briggs-Myers, 1995).

TABLE 11-1 Myers-Briggs Type Indicator

Dimensions	Contrasting Categories	
Attitudes toward life	Introversion	Extroversion
Perception	Sensing	Intuiting
Judgment	Thinking	Feeling
Orientation to outer world	Judging	Perceiving

RESEARCH Perspective 11-1

Data from Dunham-Taylor J: Nurse executive transformational leadership found in participative organizations, *J Nurs Adm* 30(5):241-250, 2000.

Purpose: This study explored transformational leadership, stage of power, and organizational climate.

Methods: Three hundred ninety-six randomly selected hospital nurse executives and the 1115 staff members reporting to them rated the nurse executives' leadership style, staff extra effort, staff satisfaction, and work group effectiveness using Bass and Avolio's Multifactor Leadership Questionnaire. The executives' bosses (360 subjects) rated executive work group effectiveness. Executives completed Hagberg's Personal Power Profile and ranked their organizational climate using Likert's Profile of Organizational Characteristics.

Results/conclusions: Nurse executives used transformational leadership fairly often, had staff who were fairly satisfied, were very effective according to their bosses, were most likely at stage 3 (power by achievement) or stage 4 (power by reflection), and rated their hospital as a Likert system 3 (consultative organization). Staff satisfaction and work group effectiveness decreased when nurse executives were more transactional (focused on management tasks and trade-offs to meet goals). Transformational leadership (influenced changes in perception) scores tended to be higher for nurse executives who had higher educational degrees and were in more participative organizations.

Roles

Role theory is a collection of concepts, definitions, and hypotheses that predict how actors will perform in certain roles and under what circumstances given behaviors can be expected. Roles are acts or behaviors expected of a person who occupies a given social position. Positions are locations in social systems, such as nurse or teacher. People who occupy a position collectively share common behaviors. Specific behaviors associated with positions constitute roles. Positions and roles have counterparts or counterroles, such as nurse-client, teacher-student, or leader-follower.

Positions may be ascribed or achieved. A person has little or no control over ascribed positions such as age, gender, or birth order in the family. Some degree of control is possible for achieved positions, such as marital status, occupation, and social status.

Role structure involves individuals, behaviors, and positions. The individual (or actor, ego, referent, or self) has a set of attributes that can be described from a variety of viewpoints. An interactionist would look at the interaction of roles, the psychiatrist at personality, and the structuralist at position tasks. Behaviors are actions taken by the role enactor. These acts are learned and influenced by norms. They are often voluntary and goal directed. *Prescription* refers to what should be done by a person in a certain position. Positions often require specific skills, intelligence, or temperament and may be held based on one's age, gender, and education. Positions often imply titles, such as nurse or teacher. People in positions are exchangeable, but the positions are not.

Role socialization is a process of acquiring specific roles and involves role expectations, role learning, and role enactment. *Role expectations* are beliefs held by others about the specific behaviors inherent in specific positions; they may be general or specific, formal or informal, and extensive or narrow in scope. Some expectations are very clear, whereas others are not. General expectations allow more latitude in the implementation of the role than do specific ones. For example, nurses should be kind and gentle in general. More specifically, nurses use two-way communications skills. Some formal expectations are written, such as codes of ethics and behavioral objectives, whereas informal expectations are communicated indirectly. Expectations related to age and gender are extensive in scope in that they transcend other roles. Expectations that apply in only a few positions are narrow in scope. Thus, only nurses working in cardiac intensive care units are expected to read and interpret electrocardiograms, and only nurse managers are expected to write budgets.

Role learning involves locating oneself accurately in the social structure. It begins at infancy and early childhood as one prepares eventually to assume adult responsibilities. It involves the development of basic skills such as language, interpersonal competence, and role taking. *Role taking* is the ability of the person to act out perceptions of how she or he and others would behave in certain positions. Playing nurse is an example of role taking.

Role enactment refers to behaviors and is related to the number of positions one holds, the intensity of involvement in those positions, and their preemptiveness. One holds multiple positions at any one time, a situation that sometimes causes conflict and difficulty with role enactment. One may not have enough time to implement each role effectively, and there can be conflicts between various role expectations. A professional nurse who takes a course will have less time for child care. *Intensity of involvement* is the degree of effort exerted to enact a role. It may vary from noninvolvement to engrossing involvement. For example, a nurse may merely pay for membership in an organization or may become an officer and serve on several committees. *Preemptiveness* is the amount of time a person spends enacting one role compared with others.

Role stress or role dissonance is the difference between role enactment and role expectations. The greater the difference, the greater the stress. *Role ambiguity* results from a lack of clear role expectations. *Role shock* arises from discrepancies between anticipated and encountered roles. *Role conflict* is a consequence of contradictory or mutually exclusive roles.

DIVERSITY

"It's OK to be different." —Anonymous

Diversity is a state of being different and having variety. There is strength in diversity. At the center of diversity is the individual's personality. Other internal factors include age, gender, race, ethnicity, physical ability, and sexual orientation. External factors include education, work experience, income, religion, marital status, parental status, personal habits, recreational habits, geographical location or living environment, and appearance. Organizational factors include work content field; functional level classification or job roles; division, department, or work environment; seniority; management status; work location; and union affiliation.

Respect for diversity comes through finding and acknowledging that good comes from these differences. Culture is an accumulation of attitudes, beliefs, concepts of the universe, experiences, hierarchies, meanings, notions of time, possessions, religion, roles, spatial relations, and values. It is a system of knowledge and a way of life shared by a large group of people. It is cultivated behavior.

Multiculturalism refers to the maintenance of several different cultures simultaneously. It usually applies to distinct cultures of immigrant groups in developed countries rather than to indigenous peoples. This contrasts with *monoculturalism,* which is a prescribed cultural homogeneity. *Cross-culturalism* refers to mediating between cultures. *Transculturalism* means bridging significant differences in cultural practices (Grunitzky, 2004).

Cultural differences are common in several areas, including the following:

Values and norms. People in the United States may value individual orientation, independence, and direct confrontation of conflict, whereas other cultures may prefer a group orientation, conformity, and harmony.

Beliefs and attitudes. People in the United States may believe in egalitarianism, gender equity, and individual control over one's own destiny, and may challenge authority, whereas those in other cultures may tolerate a more hierarchical structure, respect authority, accept different roles for men and women, and think individuals should accept their destinies.

Mental processes and learning style. People in the United States may have a linear, logical, and sequential mode of thinking with a problem-solving approach, whereas those in other cultures may have a lateral, holistic, simultaneous style and greater acceptance of life's difficulties.

Sense of self and space. The culture in the United States may be informal and use handshakes, whereas other cultures may be more formal and use hugs and bows, as well as handshakes.

Relationships with family and friends. People in the United States may focus on the nuclear family, value youth, and emphasize responsibility for self, whereas those in other cultures may focus on the extended family, respect age, and feel loyalty and responsibility to the family.

Time and time consciousness. People in the United States may value promptness and be linear and exact with regard to time consciousness, whereas those in other cultures may use time to enjoy relationships and may be elastic and relatively less time conscious.

Communication and language. People in the United States may use explicit, direct communications with an emphasis on the content, whereas those in other cultures such as Asians and Native Americans may use implicit, indirect communications that emphasize the meaning of the context of words.

Food and eating habits. People in the United States may view eating as a necessity and consume fast food, whereas those in other cultures may view dining as a religious and social experience.

Dress and appearance. People in the United States may dress for success and accept a wide range of dress codes, whereas those in other cultures may see dress as a sign of position and prestige. They may follow religious rules for dress.

Work habits and practices. People in the United States may emphasize tasks, intrinsically value work, and reward workers based on individual achievement, whereas those in other cultures may put an emphasis on relationships, believe that work is a necessity of life, and reward seniority and relationships.

A culture of poverty has been said to exist. Members of racial or ethnic minorities are at higher risk for lower socioeconomic status, less health insurance, and diseases. Opportunities for education, occupations, income, and home ownership have been fewer for those in minority groups. School systems and recreation facilities are often poorer in the inner city and rural areas than in the suburbs. Lack of financial support, less education, and less insurance lead to poor decisions such as going to the emergency department for treatment of nonemergency conditions.

Non-Hispanic whites and Asians have a higher median income than African-Americans, Hispanics, and Native Americans. They also tend to be better educated. Hispanics and Mexican-Americans have a higher rate of noninsurance. They are less likely to engage in preventive measures because they are more interested in the present than in the future.

The economic and social conditions contribute to the increasing level of violence. Unemployment is associated with violence because people have time on their hands and may feel frustrated, guilty, and inadequate. Public places such as businesses, churches, playgrounds, restaurants, and schools have become places where random acts of violence occur. Homicide is a leading cause of death among African-American men. Women, children, and the elderly are groups that are vulnerable to violence. People living in poverty are at higher risk for many diseases. Social, economic, and health problems influence health care and the cultures of health care organizations (Cherry & Jacob, 2002).

Cultural imposition occurs when one culture forces its values and beliefs onto another culture or subculture. *Cultural imperialism* is a situation in which one country has control over other countries onto which it imposes its own culture; it is often characterized by struggles over the control of raw materials and world markets. *Ethnocentrism* is the belief that one's own race, culture, or values are superior to those of others. It is the lowest level of intercultural sensitivity. There are several stages in the development of intercultural sensitivity. (1) Denial of differences is the inability to recognize cultural differences. Isolation in homogeneous groups does not allow people to notice and interpret cultural differences. (2) Separation allows for some awareness of cultural differences but often yields undifferentiated broad categories such as "Asian" or "black." These are only broad categories for different cultures, based on ignorance, that have a relatively benign effect. (3) Defense against difference is the recognition of cultural differences accompanied by a negative evaluation of variations from the dominant culture. The greater the variation, the more negative the evaluation. This may be characterized by the dualistic thinking of "us" versus "them" accompanied by overt negative stereotyping and attempts to convert to the dominant culture. (4) Minimization of difference is the recognition and acceptance of superficial cultural differences, such as eating customs. The assumption is that all human beings are essentially the same. There is an emphasis on the similarity of people and basic values. (5) Acceptance of difference is recognition and appreciation of cultural differences in both behaviors and values. It emphasizes acquisition of knowledge about cultures, including an increased awareness of one's own culture. (6) Adaptation to difference includes a shifting of the frame of reference to understand and be understood across cultural boundaries, empathy, and communication skills that enable intercultural communication. One is able to consciously shift perspective into an alternative cultural worldview and act in culturally appropriate ways. (7) Integration of difference is the internalization of bicultural frames of reference. It is the acceptance of an identity that is not based entirely in one culture (Gardenswartz & Rowe, 2003).

MANAGEMENT OF CULTURAL DIVERSITY

The leader or manager needs to help staff deal with cultural diversity through awareness building, discrimination control, and prejudice reduction. First-line managers need knowledge about common beliefs and practices of the diverse cultures. The organizational mission and goal statements should address diversity. People who want to deal with diversity issues should be supported and open communications should be encouraged. Development and implementation of a culture audit, including the use of focus groups, interviews, and questionnaires, can help describe the culture. Homogeneous groups who are provided with a safe problem-solving environment can make recommendations for resolving difficulties. Long-term contact among culturally and ethnically diverse people can increase awareness. Working with diverse groups may require more time and effort because of the conflict management that is needed before a mature group emerges. The importance of cultural diversity should be apparent in organizational philosophy and goals. Orientation programs, seminars, role playing, skill building, and workshops can be used to facilitate intercultural sensitivity. Informal networks for coaching, tutoring, mentoring, and role modeling can help people develop intercultural skills. Leaders should be role models for integration of differences. Diversity accountability should be visible in hiring, promotion, and staff support actions. Leaders and managers must be compliant with federal, state, and local regulations. Translation services should be available as necessary. People should be aware that foreign or minority staff may not consider themselves of lesser status than the majority and that some of the majority may have felt they were part of an oppressed group at some time. People with different lifestyles should not be treated as if they need interventions, because they may be happy with their choices. Emotional outbursts may not be anger but may be a communication style. Managers should take time to get to know the staff and help give them a sense of dignity and value. Managers should recognize and value diversity and provide incentives to staff for integrating cultural values into their practice (Green-Hermandez, Quinn, Denman-Vitale, et al, 2004; Raso, 2006; Scalzi, 2006).

All managers should participate in discrimination control. Discrimination is the mistreatment of people based on factors irrelevant to the quality of their work, such as race, gender, age, or handicap. Active recruitment, selection, retention, and promotion of women and minorities; monitoring of their progress; establishment of affirmative action committees to monitor the fairness of policies and their implementation; and creation of advisory groups representing minorities can help control discrimination. Managers and staff can attend in-service sessions about the appropriate actions to take when they are aware of discriminatory behavior. Open discussions between representatives of conflicting groups may help minimize discrimination and should focus on the strengths each group brings to the situation to help in reaching organizational goals. Clearly written policies and provision of equal support and career development resources to all employees can help reduce the risk of reverse discrimination, which occurs when a person of a particular ethnic group is chosen over someone else who has better credentials. People need to be aware that physical features do not always denote a specific race or ethnic group. Jamaicans and Puerto Ricans are not African blacks, and Hispanics may have Asian features. Managers should implement standards of performance and ensure fairness.

Prejudice reduction is more difficult than awareness building or discrimination control. Prejudice is an internal, abstract perception. Organizations can attempt to control the manifestations of prejudice. People who observe and report prejudice can help reduce it. Discouraging racial and gender-related comments usually decreases the number of such comments made.

ORGANIZATIONAL CULTURE

Organizational culture is the customary way of thinking and behaving that is shared by all members of the organization and must be learned and adopted by newcomers before they can be accepted into the agency. Culture is learned, shared, and transmitted. It is a combination of assumptions, values, symbols, language, and behaviors that manifest the organization's norms and values. Objective aspects of the organizational culture are those that exist outside the minds of the members of the organization and include artifacts such as pictures of leaders, monuments, stories, ceremonies, and rituals. Subjective aspects are related to assumptions and mindsets, and include such things as shared assumptions, values, meanings, and understanding of how things will be done.

Values are the basic beliefs of the organization. Agencies with strong cultures have a complex system of values that are discussed openly by managers and are accepted by members. These values establish the standards for achievement in the organization. They are the essence of the organization's philosophy. They provide a sense of direction, guide daily behavior, serve as an informal control system, and help in setting priorities and planning strategies.

Heroes personify the values of the organizational culture. They show that success is attainable, set a standard for performance, preserve what is special in the organization, motivate employees, serve as role models, and symbolize the organization to the outside world (Shani & Lau, 2000).

The *cultural network* is the primary informal means of communication within the organization that carries the corporate values and heroic mythology. Managers should use this network to understand what is going on and to get things done (Deal & Kennedy, 2000)

Artifacts, or articles made by human work, include a range of verbal and physical symbols, such as stories, myths, verbal or visual forms of humor, rituals, ceremonies, analogies, metaphors, pictures, logos, office décor, and dress. *Gestures*

RESEARCH Perspective 11-2

Data from King T, Byers JF: A review of organizational culture instruments for nurse executives, *J Nurs Adm* 37(1): 21-31, 2007.

Purpose: The purpose was to review instruments that measure organizational culture.

Methods: A search of over 100,000 articles about organizational culture, quality improvement, patient safety, and organizational effectiveness was performed using the key term *organizational effectiveness,* and 3824 articles dealing with this topic were identified. Those articles were then reviewed to identify the instruments used to assess organizational culture in the work environment.

Results/conclusions: Eight instruments met the inclusion criteria: the instrument developed by the Agency for Healthcare Research and Quality, the Hospital Survey on Patient Safety Culture, the Nursing Unit Cultural Assessment Tool, the Organizational Beliefs Questionnaire, the Organizational Culture Inventory, the Organizational Culture Profile, the Organizational Description Questionnaire, and the Quality Improvement Implementation Survey. It is important to understand the health care organizational culture to plan, implement, and evaluate infrastructure change through the use of evidence-based leadership to develop cultures that promote safe, effective, high-quality patient care.

are a nonverbal form of communication. *Gossip* is talk or rumors about others. *Jargon* is specialized vocabulary or idioms specific to a way of work. A *joke* is a funny anecdote. *Slang* is a specialized vocabulary of idioms outside the standard language. A *signal* is given by a gesture. A *slogan* is a catchword or motto. Stories may describe conflicts, heroes, or traditions. *Legend* is the story of a saint or some wonderful event. *Myths* are fictitious traditional stories with a historical basis used to explain something. A *saga* is a long story of adventure or heroic deeds. *Songs* are poetry or verse that is sung. Verbal forms of humor could be jokes, whereas visual forms could be cartoons posted on bulletin boards.

Rituals are the day-to-day routines that show employees how they are to behave. Policies and procedures clarify routines. Inductions, promotions, planning retreats, and retirements are rituals that reinforce the values of the organizational culture. *Ceremonies* are extravagant rituals that give visible evidence of the agency's values. Ceremonies keep the values, beliefs, and heroes visible.

Analogies speak to similarities between things that are otherwise unlike or that bear a partial resemblance. For example, the organization may be said to be like a battlefield. *Metaphors* are figures of speech in which one thing is likened to another and is spoken of as if it were the other thing. Organizations can be described using many types of metaphors: (1) anthropologic (a family, Big Daddy, the Prodigal Son), (2) mechanistic (an assembly line, a factory, a well-oiled machine), (3) television (sitcom, soap opera), (4) military (battles, battle zone, captain, enemies, troops), (5) sports (quarterback, stars, teams), and (6) animal (chicken, sly fox) (Roussel, Swansburg, & Swansburg, 2006; Shani & Lau, 2000; Sullivan & Decker, 2005). Morgan (2006) uses machine, organismic, brain, cultural, political, and psychic prison metaphors to describe organizations.

Types of Culture

Schneider (1998) has identified four core cultures with a leadership and management focus: (1) control, (2) collaborative, (3) competence, and (4) cultivation: The *control culture* is authoritative, cautious, conservative, definitive; the leader is firm, impersonal, tough minded, realistic, systematic, task driven, objective, and prescriptive. The *collaborative culture* is adaptive, collegial, democratic, first among equals, informal, participative, personal, relational, supportive, and trusting; the leader functions as a coach, integrator, team builder, and trust builder. The *competence culture* is assertive, challenging, persuasive, efficient, emotionless, formal, impersonal, intense, objective, rational, and task driven; the leader is an assertive, visionary standard setter who recruits the most competent people and then stretches them. The *cultivation culture* is attentive, emotional, enabling, humanistic, nurturing, people driven, personal, promotive, and relaxed; the leader is a catalyst, cultivator, empowerer, inspirer, promoter, and steward (Schneider, 1998).

Cooke and Rousseau (1987) have identified three culture types: (1) positive, (2) passive-defensive, and (3) aggressive-defensive. In a *positive culture* members are proactive and interactive to meet their satisfaction needs. That culture is based on humanism, affiliation norms, achievement, and self-actualization. In passive-defensive and aggressive-defensive cultures people protect their security and status in reactive, guarded ways. *Passive-defensive* culture is based on conventional, approval, dependent, and avoidance norms. *Aggressive-defensive* culture is based on power, oppositional, competitive, and perfectionistic norms. Leaders need to diffuse negativism in oppositional norms and act as role models for desirable behaviors, encouraging a cultural transition to more positive norms.

Integrated or Differentiated Frames of Reference

Organizations may be integrated or differentiated. Organizations may have action, content, and symbolic consistency. *Action consistency* occurs when content themes are consistent with the formal and informal practices and the artifacts of the organization. *Content consistency* is congruence among content themes. *Symbolic consistency* is congruence among artifacts and informal and formal practices. *Integration* means that an organization has a single culture with a high level of consistency and consensus. Highly integrated cultures can be repressive and nonadaptive. *Differentiation* recognizes and allows for variation of cultures within the organization, such as subcultures (Sullivan & Decker, 2005).

Subcultures/Microsystems

Subcultures/microsystems have the same elements that cultures have, including distinct patterns of shared ideologies and sets of cultural forms. They are collective, dynamic, emotionally charged, historically based, and inherently symbolic. The degree of distinctiveness of subcultures varies. Some resemble the dominant culture in which they are embedded, and others deviate greatly from it. The more unique the subculture, the more it encourages members to weaken their commitment to the dominant culture and violate significant aspects of it. Organizations are usually multicultural; that is, they have multiple subcultures within them. Frequency of interactions provides the basis for subcultures. Long periods of close association are necessary for subcultures to develop distinctive ideologies. It is shared experiences which stimulate that collective sense making. Shared personal characteristics, such as age, education, ethnicity, occupational training, and social class, also facilitate sense making because people do not need to displace their old beliefs and values very much when they find a common ground with each other. Cohesion is also important to subcultures and is facilitated by small group size; agreement on group goals; existence of tasks requiring interdependence; similarity of member characteristics, such as interests and values; physical isolation from others; threats from the outside; and performance success, failure, or crisis. When groups are cohesive, the members are attracted to each other, spend time together, and consequently influence each other. Subcultures tend to form strong norms that govern the behavior of members. The occupational cultures of professionals are created and maintained through rituals, rules, and specialized language. These subcultures or microsystems are important for the development and deployment of the macrosystem's strategic plan (Kosnik & Espinosa, 2003; Schein, 2004).

Social cohesiveness is not the same as a subculture. When neighbors respond to a natural disaster, they have social cohesiveness for a while; but when the circumstances that brought them together end, so do the mutual influence and strong emotional bonds. Subcultures are more enduring than social cohesiveness. People's occupations are the most pervasive source of subcultures in an organization. An occupation consists of a set of tasks, and members of the occupation claim exclusive rights to perform and control those tasks. Members of the occupation identify themselves with other members of that occupation and come to share beliefs, norms, and values in a variety of ways. Language, myths, rituals, songs, and taboos help members vent their emotions and learn ways to frame their activities so they are not overwhelmed. Members then form favorable self-images and social identities from their work that become part of their presentation of self. Members of occupations may live near one another, spend time together, encourage their children to enter the same profession, and link families through marriage. The subculture then becomes prone to ethnocentrism.

Countercultures

Countercultures develop to oppose the dominant culture. Mergers, rebellious innovators, chronically discontented employees, and those engaging in illegal or other deviant behaviors encourage the formation of countercultures.

Leaders help shape the culture by identifying and projecting a vision, demonstrating a philosophy, modeling values, setting policies, creating systems, and supporting a reward system. Leaders must ensure congruity between strategic plans and decision-making processes. They need to identify the actual norms, establish desired norms, identify and close culture gaps, and sustain culture changes. Leaders help others understand and make sense of events and cope with change, instability, and unexpected events. Leaders need to help members of the organization adapt to the dynamic life cycle of the organization. Open and collaborative interaction among leaders and followers is important (Ashkanasy, Wilderom, & Peterson, 2004).

CHANGE

"If you're not confused, you're not paying attention." —Tom Peters

Forces That Influence Change

There are internal and external forces that influence change. Internal forces originate from operations inside the organization, which may result from external changes, and include change in priorities, need for increased productivity, need for cost containment, staffing pattern changes, shifts in philosophy, work process changes, and need for quality of work life. External forces include health care economics, technology, restructuring, diversity, and changing demographics.

Lack of financial resources and adequate technology can slow change, but attitudes and behaviors are even more significant barriers to change. Change can be slowed by inflexible policies and procedures; satisfaction with the status quo; dysfunctional teamwork and work overload even before the change process is initiated; lack of confidence in the leaders; lack of vision; concern about the effect on oneself; and territoriality.

It is helpful if people want a change and believe that change will make things better. Motivated workers who are adaptable, creative, willing to try new innovations, and have the necessary skills or are willing to learn them can facilitate change. Stability of the progressive workforce, commitment of the workforce, and patience are necessary to adapt to the paradigm shifts effecting change (McConnell, 2006; Zohar, 1997) (Table 11-2). Leaders are visionary role models who focus on the future. Managers process the changes and understand the future directions (Huber, 2006; Marquis & Huston, 2006) (Table 11-3).

Strategies for Effecting Change

Whether working with individuals, groups, or systems, the nurse manager is sure to be involved in the management of change. Several strategies for managing change have been identified and can be useful for nurses.

Empirical-Rational Strategies

Empirical-rational strategies are based on the assumption that people are rational and behave according to rational self-interest. It follows then that people should be willing to adopt a change

TABLE 11-2 Trends: Paradigm Shifts Effecting Change

From	To
Automatism	Holism
Fragmentation	Integration
Emphasis on separate parts	Emphasis on relationships
Determinate	Indeterminate
Control	Trust
Certainty/predictability	Uncertainty/ambiguity/rapid change
Reductive	Emergent
Isolated/controlled	Contextual/self-organizing
Parts defining the whole	Whole being greater than the sum of the parts
Top-down management	Bottom-up leadership
Hierarchy	Nonhierarchical networks
Reactive	Imaginative/experimental
Power from top	Power from interacting centers
Competition	Cooperation
Single viewpoint	Many viewpoints
Knowing	Discovering
Quality of work	Quality of life

Data from Zohar D: *Rewiring the corporate brain: Using the new science to rethink how we structure and lead organizations*, San Francisco, 1997, Berrett-Koehler.

TABLE 11-3 Leadership and Management for Change

Leader	Manager
Is visionary in identifying needed change	Assesses the driving and restraining forces
Is a role model and change agent	Identifies and implements strategies
Is sensitive to timing of initiatives	Seeks subordinates' input
Is creative in identifying solutions	Supports and rewards individual efforts
Focuses on the future	Understands future directions

Data from Huber LL: Change and innovation. In Huber LL, editor: *Leadership and nursing care management*, ed 3, Philadelphia, Elsevier, 2006; Marquis BL, Huston CJ: *Leadership roles and management functions in nursing: Theory and application*, ed 5, Philadelphia, 2006, Lippincott Williams & Wilkins.

if it is justified and if they are shown how they can benefit from the change.

Nurse managers who use empirical-rational strategies are likely to want the appropriate persons for specific positions. Desirous of having people perform jobs for which they are well qualified, nurse managers give considerable attention to recruitment and selection of personnel. Staff development through independent study, in-service education, continuing education, and formal degree programs is encouraged. Systems analysis, operations research, and implementation of research findings are consistent with the empirical-rational philosophy, as is long-range futuristic planning.

Normative-Reeducative Strategies

Normative-reeducative strategies are based on the assumption that people act according to their commitment to sociocultural norms.

The intelligence and rationality of people are not denied, but attitudes and values are also considered. The manager pays attention to changes in values, attitudes, skills, and relationships in addition to providing information.

Believing that the basic unit of the social organization is the individual, the nursing manager fosters the development of staff members through means such as personal counseling, training groups, small groups, and experiential learning because people need to participate in their own reeducation. Organizational development programs are promoted, and it is typical to collect data about the organization, give data feedback and analysis to appropriate people, plan ways to improve the system, and train managers and internal change agents. The relationships between internal change agents and other personnel can be a major tool in reeducating others.

Power-Coercive Strategies

Power-coercive strategies seek to obtain the compliance of less powerful people with the leadership, plans, and directions of more powerful individuals. These strategies do not deny the intelligence and rationality of people or the importance of their values and attitudes, but rather they acknowledge the need to use sources of power to bring about change. The use of strikes, sit-ins, negotiations, conflict confrontation, and administrative decisions and rulings are power-coercive strategies (Bennis, Benne, & Chin, 1985).

Types of Change

The variables of mutual goal setting, the power ratio between the change agent and the client system, and the deliberativeness of change are differentiating factors in the change process. In *coercive change* there is nonmutual goal setting, an imbalanced power ratio, and one-sided deliberativeness. In *emulative change*, transition is fostered by promoting identification with and imitation of power figures. *Indoctrination* uses mutual goal setting, has an imbalanced power ratio, and is deliberative. Subordinates are instructed in the beliefs of the power sources. *Interactional change* involves mutual goal setting and fairly equal power, but no deliberativeness. Parties may be unconsciously committed to changing one another. *Natural change* occurs through accidents and acts of God. It involves no goal setting or deliberativeness. *Social change* is directly related to interactional change. In this case, an individual conforms to the needs of a social group. When there is greater deliberativeness on the power side, change becomes

indoctrination. *Technocratic change* involves collecting and interpreting data to bring about change. A technocrat merely reports the findings of the analysis to bring about the change.

Process of Change

Several theorists have identified phases or levels of change (Table 11-4).

Lewin: Phases of Change

Lewin's framework specifies three phases of change: (1) unfreezing, (2) moving, and (3) refreezing (Lewin, 1947, 1951) (Figure 11-1). *Unfreezing* is the development through problem awareness of a need for change. Even if a problem has been identified, people must believe there can be an improvement before they are willing to change. Coercion and the induction of guilt and anxiety have been used to accomplish unfreezing. Removal of people from the source of their old attitudes to a new environment, punishment and humiliation for undesirable attitudes, and rewards for desirable attitudes have been used to effect change.

Stress may cause dissatisfaction with the status quo and become a motivating factor for change. Points of stress and strain should be assessed. Change may begin at a point of stress

TABLE 11-4 Comparison of Selected Planned Change Theories

Lewin	Lippitt	Havelock	Rogers
1. Unfreezing	1. Diagnosing the problem 2. Assessing the motivation and capacity for change 3. Assessing the change agent's motivation and resources	1. Building a relationship 2. Diagnosing the problem 3. Acquiring the relevant resources	1. Awareness 2. Interest 3. Evaluation
2. Moving	4. Selecting a progressive change objective 5. Choosing the appropriate role for the change agent	4. Choosing the solution 5. Gaining acceptance	4. Trial
3. Refreezing	6. Maintaining change 7. Terminating the helping relationship	6. Stabilizing and undergoing self-renewal	5. Adoption

Data from Bennis, Benne, & Chin, 1985; Havelock,1973; Lippitt, Watson, & Westley, 1958; Rogers, 2003; Roussel, Swansburg, & Swansburg, 2006; and Yoder-Wise, 2006.

but ordinarily should not be started at the point of greatest stress. It is most appropriate for it to start with a policymaking body that considers both formal and informal structures. The effectiveness of the change may depend on the amount of involvement of all personnel in fact finding and problem solving.

Moving is working toward change by identifying the problem or the need for change, exploring the alternatives, defining goals and objectives, planning how to accomplish the goals, and implementing the plan for change. *Refreezing* is the integration of the change into one's personality and the consequent stabilization of change. Frequently personnel or the system return to old behaviors after change efforts cease. Leaders' attention to accomplishing related changes in neighboring systems, providing momentum to perpetuate the change, and making structural alterations that support the procedural changes help to stabilize the change (Ashkanasy, Wilderom, & Peterson, 2004). First-level managers can apply Lewin's ideas on planned change to nursing care. The unfreezing phase is assessment, problem identification, creation of a felt need, and problem solving to make a plan of care. Moving is implementing the plan and considering alternate plans. Refreezing is evaluation and reaffirmation of the plan. Nursing managers can use Lewin's force-field analysis to help plan change.

Lewin's force-field analysis provides a framework for problem solving and planned change. The status quo is maintained when driving forces equal the restraining forces (Figure 11-2), and change will occur when the relative strength of opposing forces changes. Consequently, when planning change, the manager should identify the restraining and driving forces and assess their strengths.

Driving forces may include pressure from the manager, desire to please the manager, perception that the change will improve one's self-image, and belief that the change will improve the situation. *Restraining forces* include conformity to norms, morals, and ethics; desire for security; perception of economic threat or threat to one's prestige and homeostasis; and regulatory mechanisms for keeping the situation fairly constant.

Once the driving and restraining forces have been identified, the manager determines their relative strengths. Which are the major factors advancing or resisting change? Which are important or moderately important? Which have little effect for or against change? These might be listed in columns under "driving" and "restraining" and then ranked (Box 11-1).

To help visualize these forces, the manager can draw a diagram as shown in Figure 11-3, write in key words to identify the forces, and draw arrows toward the status quo line to represent the strength of the forces. The longer the line, the stronger the force.

Next, the manager plans strategies for reducing the restraining forces and strengthening the driving forces. Managers may conduct some experiential learning exercises to facilitate the change of group norms, explain each person's role in the change with emphasis on security, and provide some status symbols to reduce the threat to people's prestige. They should also help workers

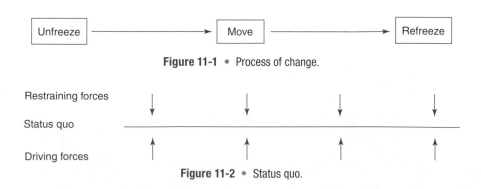

Figure 11-1 • Process of change.

Figure 11-2 • Status quo.

identify how the change will improve their situation. Steps should be taken to improve self-images. For instance, people may be taught new tasks to prepare for the change, to reduce the threat to their prestige and their fear of making fools of themselves when doing something new, and to improve their self-images. If managers perceive that the workers want to please them, they may inform the workers that they desire the change and provide positive reinforcement for accomplishing it. Keeping the goals in mind, the manager should assess the results of implementing the strategies and revise plans as necessary. Top-level leaders and managers can use Lewin's force-field analysis to plan for organizational changes, whereas first-level managers can use it to help plan changes to promote health, prevent disease, improve care for chronic diseases, and facilitate recovery from acute illness (Yoder-Wise, 2006).

Havelock: Phases of Change

Havelock (1973) modified Lewin's phases into six phases: (1) building a relationship, (2) diagnosing the problem, (3) acquiring the relevant resources, (4) choosing the solution, (5) gaining acceptance, and (6) stabilizing and undergoing self-renewal.

Lippitt: Planned Change

Lippitt, Watson, and Westley (1958) added to Lewin's work and identified seven phases of planned change. As noted earlier, planned change involves mutual goal setting, an equal power ratio, and deliberativeness. First, the client must feel a need for change. The manager, as the change agent, can stimulate an awareness of the need for change, help the client become aware of the problems, and indicate that a more desirable state of affairs is possible. The change agent assesses the client's motivation and capacity for change and the change agent's motivation and resources. Thus unfreezing occurs.

Next, a helping relationship must be established and the moving process begun. Managers, as change agents, must identify with clients' problems while remaining neutral so that they can remain objective. The change agent needs to be viewed as an understandable and approachable expert. The success or failure of most planned action will depend largely on the quality and workability of the relationship between the change agent and the client. The problem must be identified and clarified. Collection and analysis of data can facilitate this process. Alternative possibilities for change should be examined. Goals and objectives are planned. The client's emotional and material resources are examined. Strategies for change are determined. The success of planned change is evaluated by the outcomes. It is the active work of modification that completes the moving process.

The refreezing process occurs during the sixth phase—generalization and stabilization. All too often clients slip back into their old ways after change efforts cease. The spread of change to neighboring systems and to subparts of the same system aids the stabilization process. Change momentum, positive evaluation of the change, receipt of rewards for the change, and accomplishment of related procedural and structural changes increase the stabilization. The helping relationship ends, or a different type of continuing relationship is established. Dependency is the major factor determining when the relationship will end (Lippitt, Watson, & Westley, 1958; Lippitt, 1973).

Kilmann: Organizational Planned Change

Kilmann (1991) has identified five stages of organizational planned change: (1) initiate the integrated program for cultural change, (2) diagnose the problems, (3) schedule the tracks, (4) implement the tracks, and (5) evaluate the results (Box 11-2).

The five tracks are as follows: (1) culture, (2) management skills, (3) team building, (4) strategy structure, and (5) reward system (Box 11-3). They require implementation in that order to be most successful. The culture track helps explain organizational differences in decision making and actions, much as personality explains differences in individuals. The culture track reveals the norms of the organization. It exposes the old culture and helps create a new culture. Without an adaptive culture it can be impossible to make improvements, so the cultural barriers must be removed before proceeding to another track.

First, one needs to clarify the actual norms. For instance, one could ask members to list current dos and don'ts. The members can then list what they want the norms to be and identify the culture gaps. Culture gaps are often related to the following: (1) task support—norms related to helping others, sharing information, and showing concern for efficiency; (2) task innovation—norms related to performing new activities, trying different approaches, and being creative; (3) social relationship—norms about mixing business with pleasure and socializing with co-workers; and (4) personal freedom—norms for pleasing oneself, using self-expression, and exercising discretion. Culture gaps are generally largest at lower levels in the organization.

Closing the culture gaps then becomes an issue. If the managers and staff decide that changes should occur, those changes can be more easily made. Adaptive cultures have internal control. Control is a social reality but not necessarily an objective one. To establish desired norms, members can be asked to list norms they think would lead to organizational success. Then work groups need to develop a sanctioning system to monitor and enforce the new norms. Work groups should decide what will be done if a member violates a new norm or performs the desired behavior. The open sanctioning system is probably more equitable than the old unconscious sanctions.

BOX 11-1 Driving and Restraining Forces

DRIVING FORCES

Rank	Factor
1	Pressure from manager
4	Desire to please manager
2	Desire to improve self-image
2	Desire to improve situation

RESTRAINING FORCES

Rank	Factor
4	Conformity
4	Security
2	Economic threat
3	Threat to prestige

SCALE

1 = little strength
2 = moderate strength
3 = important strength
4 = major strength

Data from Lewin K: Defining the "field at a given time," *Psychological Review* 50: 292-310, 1943. Republished in *Resolving social conflicts & field theory in social science*, Washington, DC, 1997, American Psychological Association.

BOX 11-2 Five Stages of Organizational Planned Change

Initiate the integrated program of cultural change.
Diagnose the problems.
Schedule the tracks.
Implement the tracks.
Evaluate the results.

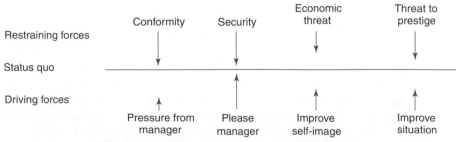

Figure 11-3 • Strength of driving and restraining forces.

Now it becomes important to sustain the cultural change. If the new culture is not supported by the remaining four tracks, it is likely that the culture will revert to the dysfunctional ways. The management skills and team-building tracks develop leadership to support the adaptive culture. The strategy structure track will document the new systems, and the reward system track will support the new norms.

In the management skills track, managers are taught the five steps of problem management: (1) sensing problems, (2) defining problems, (3) deriving solutions, (4) implementing solutions, and (5) evaluating outcomes. Next, managers examine their personality types. Because one's personality type determines how one will assimilate information and make decisions, managers should be aware of their own styles and the styles of associates so they can compensate for their natural inclinations and acknowledged limitations and develop strong work teams.

Managers also need to learn assumptional analysis: how to uncover assumptions, classify them by amount of certainty and importance, and synthesize assumptions. Outdated assumptions can lead to the wrong strategy structure and reward systems. In a climate of trust and openness, associates should be able to examine previously unstated assumptions so they are not held back by faulty assumptions.

The team-building track activates the new culture and skills throughout the entire organization. Team building involves the following: (1) reuniting the work group, (2) identifying work group problems, (3) identifying solutions and developing action plans, (4) implementing the plans, and (5) evaluating and monitoring the outcomes. Interteam building is also included in this track. Everyone in the organization needs to learn how to cope with difficult people, understand his or her own personality style, and appreciate the styles of others.

In the strategy structure track, strategy sets the direction and structure organizes the goals, tasks, people, and other resources to accomplish the plans. This involves operationalizing strategy, designing subunits, and implementing structure. The reward system track ensures that associates are rewarded for doing the right things for the right reasons.

Kotter: Process for Leading Change

Kotter (1996) outlines an eight-stage process for leading change as follows: (1) establish a sense of urgency, (2) create and guide teams, (3) develop a vision and strategy, (4) communicate the change vision, (5) empower employees for broad-based action, (6) generate short-term wins, (7) consolidate gains and produce more change, and (8) anchor new approaches in the culture. He discusses how failure to do these things is a reason that transformation efforts fail (Box 11-4).

Smith: Levels of Change

Smith (2002) identified the following seven levels of change: (1) being effective—doing the right things; (2) being efficient—doing things right; (3) improving—doing the right things better; (4) cutting—doing away with things; (5) copying—doing things other people are doing; (6) being different—doing things no one else is doing; (7) doing the impossible—doing things that can't be done.

Innovation

To change is to be different, to alter, or to replace with something else. To create is to produce, and creativity is imaginative and original. Innovation is the introduction of something new. Creativity is the mental work behind developing something new, whereas innovation is the result of creativity and is the introduction of what was created. A nurse can create a product or service (creativity), then put it into

---

BOX 11-4 Kotter's Eight-Stage Change Process

Establishing a sense of urgency
Creating and guiding teams
Developing a vision and strategy
Communicating the change vision
Empowering employees for broad-based action
Generating short-term wins
Consolidating gains and producing more change
Anchoring new approaches in the culture

---

use (innovation), and consequently, change something (Huber, 2006; Roussel, Swansburg, & Swansburg, 2006).

Rogers: Stages of the Innovation Process

Rogers (1983, 2003) developed a model of the stages in the innovation-decision process: (1) knowledge, (2) persuasion, (3) decision, (4) implementation, and (5) confirmation. The *awareness knowledge* stage involves information seeking and processing to determine the advantages and disadvantages of an innovation. Innovation requires more information collection than complex activities. *How-to knowledge* is the information necessary to implement the innovation properly. The "earlier knowers" tend to have more formal education, higher socioeconomic status, more exposure to interpersonal channels, more change agent contact, and more social participation than the "late knowers."

The *persuasion stage* is a feeling phase in which people form a favorable or unfavorable attitude toward the innovation. People want to know how easily the innovation can be implemented and what the advantages and disadvantages are for the individual. A preventive innovation is an idea aimed at preventing an unwanted occurrence in the future. The rate of adoption of preventive innovations is slower than that of nonpreventive innovations.

The *decision stage* is when people engage in activities to decide whether to adopt or reject an innovation. An adoption is a decision to implement the innovation. A rejection is a decision not to implement the innovation. Active rejection occurs after one has considered adoption, but in passive rejection one does not even think about adoption.

In the *implementation stage*, the innovation is put to use. This stage is easier for early adapters and more difficult when working with a group of people. The adoption may involve reinvention by copying or imitating something that has worked somewhere else, or an innovation can be modified before adoption and implementation. What works in one situation may not work in another, but an innovation may stimulate ideas that can work. After the new idea is institutionalized, the innovation loses its distinction as a new idea.

In the *confirmation stage*, people seek reinforcement for the decision made. They try to avoid dissonance, which is an internal disequilibrium between what is expected and what exists. The felt need to know stimulates the knowledge stage. When people know about an innovation and have a favorable attitude toward it, people experience dissonance between what they know and what they are doing. That facilitates the decision and implementation stages. If, after adoption, people decide that they should not have implemented the new idea, they may discontinue the innovation to decrease the dissonance. They may discontinue the innovation to replace it with a better idea or process, or they may discontinue it because of disenchantment with its performance. Later adopters are more likely to discontinue innovations than are early adopters. Sometimes adopting an innovation means discarding previously adopted ideas (Festinger, 1957; Rogers, 2003).

Rogers (2003) identified five categories of adopters: (1) innovators, (2) early adopters, (3) early majority, (4) late majority, and (5) laggards. In the 1983 edition of his book, he also listed another category, rejectors.

Innovators are venturesome, daring, and risk taking. They are enthusiastic people who thrive on change. The innovator may not be very well respected by peers. Innovators play a key role in the diffusion of innovations by being gatekeepers and introducing new ideas from the outside into the system.

Early adopters are usually more popular with peers than are innovators. They are open and receptive to new ideas. Peers tend to check with early adopters for advice and information about the innovation before deciding to adopt it.

The *early majority* are often the opinion leaders in an organization and adopt new ideas shortly before their average peers. They make up about one third of the members in the network. They may consider a new idea for some time before deciding to adopt it.

The *late majority* are skeptical and cautious about new ideas. They do not adopt an idea before most of their peers do and adopt it only after most of the uncertainty has been resolved.

The *laggards* are the last people in the social system to adopt a new idea. They tend to associate with other people who have traditional values and think more of the past than the future.

The *rejectors* were identified in Rogers's 1983 book as opposing change and encouraging others to reject change too. They interfere with the success of the change process (Huber, 2006; Marquis & Huston, 2006).

Rogers (2003) also identified several factors that help explain different rates of adoption: (1) relative advantage, (2) compatibility, (3) complexity, (4) trialability, and (5) observability.

Relative advantage is the degree to which the change is considered better than the idea that it supersedes. The perceived advantage is more influential than the real advantage. People want to know, "What's in it for me?"

Compatibility is the degree to which the innovation is compatible with values, past experiences, and needs. If there are negative perceptions of a past experience, an attitude of "here we go again" can interfere with successful adoption.

Complexity is the perceived difficulty in understanding and using the innovation.

Trialability is the degree to which people have the opportunity to test out the innovation on a small scale. Phasing in an innovation may be more acceptable to people than implementing it all at once. This allows tweaking of the new change. Anthony, Eyring, and Gibson (2006) indicated that most new strategies will encounter a problem in some fundamental way. It is important to have a rigorous and quick way to isolate the problem by running experiments and adapting.

Observability is the degree to which the results of the innovation are visible to others. People will probably be more willing to adopt an innovation when they can see desirable benefits (Geibert, 2006; Huber, 2006). Geibert (2006) has used diffusion-of-innovation concepts to enhance implementation of an electronic health record system to support evidence-based practice.

Kanter (2006) has identified the classic traps for innovation. These include hurdles that are too high, a scope that is too narrow, controls that are too tight, connections that are too loose, separations that are too sharp, leadership that is too weak, and communications that are too poor. She recommends that managers widen the search and broaden the scope because sometimes small bits of tinkering can become big innovations. Flexibility should be added to planning and control systems so that innovations can occur outside the normal planning cycles. A reserve pool of special funds should be available to take advantage of unexpected opportunities. Kanter recommends facilitating close connections between innovators and the mainstream staff. Leaders should encourage mutual respect by convening discussions to lessen tensions and antagonism. She warns not to give the innovators big perks because others may then sabotage the innovator's efforts. Kanter encourages the selection of leaders with good communication skills who will surround the innovators with a supportive culture for collaboration.

Hamel (2006) noted that managerial work for innovation includes setting goals and laying out plans, motivating and aligning effort, coordinating and controlling activities, accumulating and allocating resources, acquiring and applying knowledge, building and nurturing relationships, identifying and developing talent, and understanding and balancing the demands of outside constituencies.

Herzlinger (2006) has identified three kinds of innovations that she thinks could make health care cheaper and better. They are to change the ways consumers buy their health care, develop technology, and develop business models for the horizontal and vertical integration of health care organizations. She acknowledges that forces such as accountability, customer reactions, funding, actions of industry players, and public policy can help or hinder efforts for innovation.

ORGANIZATIONAL DEVELOPMENT

Organizations progress through three developmental stages: (1) birth, (2) youth, and (3) maturity (Box 11-5). The creation of a new organization and its survival as a viable system are primary concerns during the birth stage. Gaining stability and developing a reputation and pride are the focuses of the youth stage. The maturity stage involves achieving both uniqueness and adaptability and contributing to society.

As organizations are born and grow, they pass through increasingly complex stages. They must develop internally and generate new control processes to cope with the amount of turbulence and complexity in the environment. At each stage the environment can become more unknown, unsettled, and difficult. A crisis develops during each stage. Changes in organizational and decision-making structures are needed to adapt to this new complexity. The new organization copes by developing job descriptions, programs, policies, and procedures. However, as the organization grows and becomes more complex, these policies do not cover the exceptions. As a result, the organization develops a set of hierarchical positions to make judgments about the exceptions to the existing job descriptions and policies. As the organization becomes larger and more complex, the managers in the hierarchy become overloaded. They do not have time to deal with all the exceptions and cannot make sense out of the situation.

BOX 11-5 Developmental Stages of an Organization

Birth: Creation and survival as a viable system
Youth: Stability, reputation, pride
Maturity: Uniqueness, adaptability, contribution to society

Consequently, in the third stage, accomplishing orderliness by developing broader goals is required. However, as the organization becomes increasingly complex, conflicts arise among factions, and the organization regresses to hierarchical structure again.

A decentralized system of departments reduces the interconnections among divisions and reduces the number of communications necessary to make decisions; however, as the evolutionary cycle continues, conflict develops among decentralized departments.

In the last stage, a vertical information system is developed so that standardized accounting and statistical reporting data from each department are consolidated at the top, and then resources are allocated among departments. Because all the complex information in turbulent systems cannot be reduced to numbers, human contacts made among department members become a major coping mechanism. Liaisons, teams, committees, task forces, and integrator roles are used. A learning organization is important to respond to needed changes and to survive (Schein, 2004; Senge, 2006).

BEHAVIORAL ASPECTS OF ORGANIZATIONAL CHANGE

In an adaptive culture, members of an organization support each other's efforts to identify and solve problems. The members believe they can manage the problems, have confidence and enthusiasm, and are receptive to change. In a dysfunctional culture, members continue behaviors that have worked in the past but are no longer effective. A cultural rut develops when members do not adapt to change and continue to function out of habit even when success is not forthcoming. Culture shock occurs when the members realize that the organization is out of touch with its setting, mission, and assumptions.

Many people are unaware of the factors that initiate change or influence its direction. Even when they are known, some forces are beyond their control. Some factors that effect change in an agency stem from society, such as new knowledge and technology, new social requirements, changing client needs and demands, and increased competition. Even when these are known in advance and anticipated, they cannot be controlled by an agency.

The efficiency of an organizational structure is hard to measure, and the factors contributing to success or failure may be impossible to isolate. Organizational structure may not be the problem. A few ineffective people can disrupt an otherwise sound structure, and good people can make a bad structure work. High labor costs, inadequate equipment, ineffective advertising, changing client needs, and increased competition may contribute to inadequate profits.

Some symptoms reflect inefficiencies within the organization and indicate a need for change. If slow and erroneous decision making is a problem, one may question the qualifications of the person making decisions, the level at which responsibility is placed, and the accessibility of the necessary information. Poor communications, a dearth of innovation, and failure in functional areas are other symptoms indicating a need for change. Diagnosis of the problem is extremely important for planned change. Minor adjustments rather than major reorganizations may correct some problems. However, even a small change in one part of an organization can cause a chain reaction throughout the agency. This domino effect creates problems with coordination and control and brings about a need for comprehensive planning.

Change disrupts equilibrium. Equilibrium can be maintained only when opposing forces are equal. Production may be maintained when the forces fostering production, such as pressure of the manager to produce, desire for favorable attention from the nursing manager to further one's own gain, and desire to earn more through an incentive plan, equal the forces limiting production, such as the informal group's standard against rate busting (doing more work than the average), resistance to training, and the feeling that the job and product are not important. However, when the forces in one direction or the other change in relation to one another, a new grouping forms and change is inevitable.

Changes involve (1) endings, (2) transitions, and (3) beginnings. People grieve when they lose something, when they are threatened with the loss of something, and when they never had and never will have something. With change, people go through the grieving process, which Kübler-Ross (1997) has identified as progressing through the stages of denial, anger, bargaining, depression, and then acceptance. Three phases of loss and mourning are (1) protest, (2) despair, and (3) reorganization. If people do not work through acceptance and reorganization, they may show disengagement (withdrawal), disidentification (sadness and worry), disorientation (confusion), or disenchantment (anger). Disengaged workers may quit and leave or quit and stay, or retire in place. They tend not to ask questions, not to seek information, not to discuss, and to fulfill only the basic requirements, and they may be hard to find. People experiencing disidentification have lost their self-identities and are vulnerable, like a lobster that has cast off its shell so it can grow. They may sulk, reminisce, dwell on the past, continue to do the old job, and resist performing new tasks. People experiencing disorientation have lost sight of where they fit into the organization. They do not know the priorities, do the wrong things, get very detail oriented, and get others to ask questions. Disenchanted people know that what is gone is gone and may become angry and negative. They may talk in a raised voice or refuse to talk, show self-pity, walk out, engage in sabotage, and back stab. Disenchantment can lead to personal problems, destructive behavior, and slow death of the organization (Finkelman, 2006; Marquis & Huston, 2006).

Resistance to Change

Caution should be used when making organizational changes. Changes are disturbing to those affected, and resistance often develops. Giving the structure a chance to work may be better than changing it. Although changing the organizational structure may appear easy on paper, it is quite complicated in reality. It affects the attitudes and effectiveness of personnel whose prestige and status are threatened. Resistance to change is a common phenomenon, whether the change is initiated by positive stimuli, such as growth or promotion of an employee, or negative forces, such as poor management. Personnel develop vested interests, preferences, habits, and rigidities that attract them to the existing structure. People tend to consider the effects of the change on their personal lives, status, and future more than on the welfare of the agency. Change introduces the risk of error, fear of failure when trying something new, resistance to admission of weakness, fear of losing a current satisfaction, or a fatalistic expectation based on previous unsuccessful attempts to change. Change is most threatening in the presence of insecurity. Even logical, necessary changes produce resistance.

Causes of resistance to change include the following: threatened self-interest; embarrassment; insecurity; habits; complacency; inaccurate perceptions; perceived loss of power, rewards, or relationships; objective disagreement; psychological reactions; low tolerance for change; opposition of the change to current trends; and previous system stability for a long time (Grohar-Murray & DiCroce, 2003).

Harper (2001) identified seven types of individuals representing different levels of commitment to change: (1) covert resisters—people who resist the change behind the scenes; (2) overt resisters—those who openly resist the change; (3) skeptics—people who need to be convinced of the need for the change; (4) observers—those who watch and withhold judgment about the need for or merit of the change; (5) participants—people who accept the change and go through the necessary actions; (6) committed—those who embrace the change; (7) champions—those who are the initiators of the change (Box 11-6).

BOX 11-6 Seven Levels of Commitment

Covert resistance
Overt resistance
Skepticism
Observation
Participation
Commitment
Championing

Changes in personnel are normal, but they are accelerated during organizational changes. Unless managers are to become obsolete, they must change with the times. Some quickly increase their managerial knowledge and skills. Unfortunately, others are inflexible, overly conservative, and negative. Executive obsolescence is increasingly common with the rapid changes in society. Managers who previously performed competently may be overwhelmed with increasingly complex duties, or they may have been promoted during an emergency to a position for which they were inadequately prepared. Staff must also keep increasing their knowledge and skills.

What can a person do about an unqualified incumbent? In developing a strategy, one should consider the ramifications of a given action on the individual and on the group. The strategy should depend on the particular circumstances. An incompetent staff member may be counseled toward satisfactory performance. Weaknesses should be identified and means to overcome them defined. On-the-job training, in-service education, college courses, and independent study may be explored. A contract may be written between the employer and the incompetent subordinate, specifying what skills are to be developed to what level of achievement and in what time frame.

Incompetent executives may be transferred to positions for which they are more qualified. They may be moved from line to staff authority. The change is most attractive when the advisory staff position is at a higher organizational level than the present line position, carries prestige, and maintains the current salary. Executives may be told there is a problem in the new area that they are to solve. This method fosters high morale and loyalty. It removes an incompetent individual from line authority when damage could be done but uses the executive's knowledge and skills to solve specific problems. This is an expensive method, however.

Termination of employment is the most extreme way to handle incompetence. It is either direct or indirect. In the direct method, employees are informed that their work does not meet the minimal criteria and they are expected to leave the agency. The indirect method may involve giving incompetent employees nothing to do, withholding information from them, leaving their names off memoranda, excluding them from conferences, and generally making them so miserable they will voluntarily resign.

New managers may be hired, particularly when new positions become available during reorganization. They often bring new ideas, objectivity, and enthusiasm to the job. Recruitment is important for development of an executive pool. The best managers do not need to hunt for jobs. The jobs hunt for them. The agency should let its need be known and seek good managers aggressively. Similar agencies may be a resource for managers with new ideas and different approaches. Graduates may be recruited from university programs. Recruiting through advertisements in professional journals and through employment agencies is useful for locating potential managers and well-qualified staff.

Promotions within the agency provide incentives and supply the executive pool. However, some personnel may not be interested in managerial work, and competent, satisfied employees may lack managerial potential.

Oscillation

Fritz (1996, 1999) explained that organizations either oscillate or advance. If they oscillate, success is neutralized. If they advance, success is possible. Successes breed further success, but with oscillation, success is short term. Because oscillation occurs over a long period and the organization is moving in the desired direction some of that time, oscillation can be hard to observe.

A conflict of interest causes oscillation between tension and resolution. For example, there is tension in a desire for change, which leads to a resolution through change effort; but that creates tension in a desire for continuity, which leads to change avoidance. That further leads to tension in a desire for change, which leads to change effort, which then causes tension in a desire for continuity, which in turn leads to change avoidance. Organizations often oscillate between centralized and decentralized decision making, expansion and limitation, growth and stability, investment and cost cutting, and long-term and short-term benefits (Figure 11-4).

Problem-solving approaches identify a problem and take action to solve the problem, which

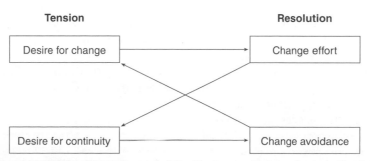

Figure 11-4 • Oscillation. (Modified from Fritz R: *Corporate tides: The inescapable laws of organizational structure*, San Francisco, 1996, Berrett-Koehler.)

lessens the intensity of the problem; this in turn leads to less action and then to reintensification of the problem. That is oscillation, because as problems are solved, the motivation for change is reduced. Problem solving focuses on how to eliminate an unwanted situation instead of envisioning the desired situation. Successful organizations often use a continuous quality improvement approach within structural tension. Personnel are clear about the desired outcomes and work on improving processes. Then success is measured against standards that reflect improvement toward the vision.

Organizations advance when there is structural tension that requires structural understanding, leadership, and organizational learning. If the structure remains unchanged, behavior will revert to previous organizational behavior. A change in structure facilitates change in organizational behavior. The structural change is hierarchical because the organization's purpose gives direction to the strategies that are steps to move the organization from the current state to the desired vision. Progression creates a cycle that leads to results that are evaluated. That leads to adjustments and refinements, which in turn lead to new actions or continuous quality improvement and increased capacity over time because structural tension is continually renewed. Organizations without vision cannot create structural tension and will oscillate instead of advancing. Values that dominate in an organization will displace competing lesser values and thus reduce oscillation. Leadership is a critical factor in clarifying the vision. Leaders need to be clear about both the vision and the present reality to create the necessary structural tension. They make decisions about competing interests based on values. When leadership is weak, workers support their own interests; this leads to conflicts and oscillation. Leaders need to create fair situations and reward people based on their merits and the accomplishments of the team. Organizations renew themselves by learning, which is best motivated when it serves a desired outcome. Training that is directly related to the organization's vision and values is a powerful instrument for change toward expanding capacity.

Gradual changes made in progressive phases are usually less disturbing than radical, sweeping, unpredicted changes. Changes in the structure resulting from sharply defined events that have already been planned—such as changes in size, scope, or objectives—are easier to execute than shifts in personnel, which involve infinitely complex human relations. Careful planning, appropriate timing of communications, adequate feedback, and employee confidence in management can reduce resistance to change.

Informing personnel of the reasons for change can further reduce resistance, especially when the advantages of the change are stressed. Personnel can be involved by requesting their input, including feelings, suggestions, and talents. Their negative as well as positive feelings should be respected. Communicating honestly about the changes, giving specific feedback, asking what assistance is needed to help them cope, and recognizing their contributions to the implementation of the changes can further minimize resistance.

> *"There comes a moment when you have to stop revving up the car and shove it into gear."* —David Mahoney

Types of Organizational Change

Organizational structure usually grows vertically, then horizontally, and from a functional type to a divisional type. Initially there is vertical growth, but as the amount of work and its complexity increase, horizontal growth occurs. Usually organizations develop from a functional structure, which is departmentalized by major functions, into one with divisions by product or territory. There is now rapid horizontal globalization in health care.

Nursing Leaders and Managers Planning for Change

> *"… the very speed of change introduces a new element into management…to make more and more decisions at a faster and faster pace."* —Alvin Toffler

Decisions made without knowledge of the culture could have unanticipated and undesirable consequences, so plans for change begin with an evaluation of the existing organization. The Competing Values Framework of Cameron and Quinn (2006) can be used to identify the values orientation that characterizes organizations and creates the market, adhocracy, clan, and hierarchy cultures. An organizational audit provides a detailed analysis of the organization, reveals the extent to which goals are accomplished, and examines the use of personnel and the growth of individuals. An organizational audit is performed by collecting and reviewing all available written material about the organization, including the statement of the mission or purpose, information on the scope of the agency, goals and objectives, organizational chart, job descriptions, annual reports, performance appraisals, and qualifications needed and not needed by personnel in their present positions. The planner notes whether the reviewed materials are consistent, looks for gaps and overlapping of functioning, and determines if all activities contribute to the major goals of the agency. The Organizational Culture Assessment Instrument can be used to diagnose organizational culture, which is the primary source of resistance to change.

Departmentalization, span of management, and balance and emphasis are analyzed. Authority relationships are studied. Leadership patterns, delegation, decentralization, use of committees, and provision of controls are considered. The Management Skills Assessment Instrument can be used to identify key competencies that leaders and managers need to develop to encourage organizational change (Cameron & Quinn, 2006; Schein, 2004). The agency may be compared with what is considered an ideal agency or with competitors to identify areas of need and to propose recommended changes. Personnel may be surveyed to identify areas needing improvement. The quantitative approach may be used when ratios are appropriate, such as in figuring the range of management. Then various organizational patterns are designed, and position breakdown using existing personnel is

developed. Personnel who are needed but not presently available and people who are available but are not qualified or needed are identified.

A job description and requirements must be compiled for each position. Each person's qualifications can then be compared with the job requirements. Notations are made of job requirements for which skills are not possessed. Those qualities that can be developed on the job within reasonable time limits should be separated from required skills that cannot be acquired. Unused abilities should be compared with the requirements of other jobs for which the individual may be better qualified.

> *"If everything seems under control, you're just not going fast enough."*   —Mario Andretti

CHAPTER SUMMARY

As a change agent, the manager assesses the culture, identifies the problem and the need for innovations, assesses the staff's motivations and capacities for change, determines alternatives, explores ramifications of those alternatives, reviews resources, determines appropriate helping roles, establishes and maintains a helping relationship, recognizes the phases of the change process and helps the staff through them, and chooses and implements techniques for planned change as identified by Lippitt, Watson, and Westley (1958). The nursing manager facilitates planned change by being a catalyst, solution giver, process helper, and resource linker (Havelock, 1973).

CRITICAL THINKING ACTIVITY

Reflective Journal: Make observations in a clinical setting or reflect on past experiences. Answer the following questions: Is the organization going through changes? If so, what are some of them? How are people responding?

CASE STUDY Primary nursing with all nursing care given by registered nurses (RNs) has been practiced for the past several years on the unit for which you are the patient care coordinator. In an effort to cut costs, the hospital is going to hire technicians to work with RNs and implement a "partners in practice" model. What will you do as patient care coordinator to help change the organizational culture?

ONLINE RESOURCES

evolve Additional critical thinking activities, worksheets, and case studies are available online at http://evolve.elsevier.com/Marriner/guide8e.

REFERENCES

Anthony SD, Eyring M, Gibson L: Mapping your innovation strategy, *Harv Bus Rev* 64(9):148-149, 2006.

Ashkanasy NM, Wilderom CPM, Peterson MF, editors: *Handbook of organizational culture and climate*, Thousand Oaks, CA, 2004, Sage Publications.

Atchinson TA, Bujak JS: *Leading transformational change: The physician-executive partnership*, Chicago, 2001, Health Administration Press.

Barr L, Barr N: *The leadership equation: Leadership, management and the Myers-Briggs*, Austin, Tex, 1989, Eakin Press.

Bennis WG, Benne KD, Chin R: *The planning of change*, ed 4, Fort Worth, TX, 1985, Holt, Rinehart and Winston.

Briggs-Myers I: *Gifts differing: Understanding personality type*, Palo Alto, CA, 1995, Holt, Rinehart and Winston.

Cameron KS, Quinn RE: *Diagnosing and changing organizational culture: Based on the competing values framework*, San Francisco, 2006, Jossey-Bass.

Cherry BC, Jacob SR: *Contemporary nursing issues, trends, and management*, ed 2, St Louis, 2002, Mosby.

Cooke R, Rousseau D: Behavioral norms and expectations: A quantitative approach to the assessment of organizational culture, *Group Organ Stud* 13:245-273, 1987.

Deal TE, Kennedy AA: *Corporate cultures: The rites and rituals of corporate life*, Cambridge, MA, 2000, Persens Publishing.

Dunham-Taylor J: Nurse executive transformational leadership found in participative organizations, *J Nurs Adm* 30(5):241-250, 2000.

Festinger L: *A theory of cognitive dissonance*, Stanford, Calif, 1957, Stanford University Press.

Finkelman AW: *Leadership and management in nursing*, Upper Saddle River, NJ, 2006, Pearson/Prentice Hall.

Fritz R: *Corporate tides: The inescapable laws of organizational structure*, San Francisco, 1996, Berrett-Koehler.

Fritz R: *The path of least resistance for managers: Designing organizations to succeed*, San Francisco, 1999, Berrett-Koehler.

Gardenswartz L, Rowe A: *Diverse teams at work: Capitalizing on the power of diversity*, Alexandria, Va, 2003, Society for Human Resource Management.

Geibert RC: Using diffusion innovation concepts to enhance implementation of an electronic health record to support evidence-based practice, *Nurs Adm Q* 30(3):203-210, 2006.

Green-Hermandez C, Quinn AA, Denman-Vitale S, et al: Making nursing care culturally competent, *Holist Nurs Pract* 18(4):215-219, 2004.

Grohar-Murray ME, DiCroce HR: *Leadership and management in nursing*, Stamford, CT, 2003, Appleton & Lange.

Grunitzky C, editor: *Transculturalism: How the world is coming together*, Nashville, TN, 2004, True Agency.

Hamel G: The why, what, and how of management innovation, *Harv Bus Rev* 84(2):72-84, 2006.

Harper SC: *The forward-focused organization: Visionary thinking and breakthrough leadership to create your company's future*, New York, 2001, American Management Association.

Havelock RG: *The change agent's guide to innovation in education*, Englewood Cliffs, NJ, 1973, Educational Technology Publications.

Herzlinger RE: Why innovation in health care is so hard, *Harv Bus Rev* 84(5):58-66, 2006.

Huber DL: Change and innovation. In Huber DL, editor: *Leadership and nursing care management*, ed 3, Philadelphia, 2006, Elsevier, pp 805-826.

Kanter RM: Innovation: The classic traps, *Harv Bus Rev* 84(11):72-83, 2006.

Kilmann RH: *Managing beyond the quick fix*, San Francisco, 1991, Jossey-Bass.

King T, Byers J: A review of organizational culture instruments for nurse executives, *J Nurs Adm* 37(1):21-31, 2007.

Kosnik LK, Espinosa JA: Microsystems in health care: Part 7. The microsystem as a platform for merging strategic planning and operations, *Jt Comm J Qual Saf* 29(9):452-459, 2003.

Kotter JP: *Leading change*, Boston, 1996, Harvard Business School Press.

Kübler-Ross E: *On death and dying*, New York, 1997, Simon & Schuster.

Lewin K: Frontiers in group dynamics: Concept method and reality in social science, social equilibria and social change, *Hum Relat* 1(1):5-41, 1947.

Lewin K: *Field theory in social sciences*, New York, 1951, Harper & Row.

Lippitt G: *Visualizing change: Model building and the change process*, La Jolla, CA, 1973, University Associates.

Lippitt R, Watson J, Westley B: *The dynamics of planned change*, New York, 1958, Harcourt, Brace & World.

Marquis BL, Huston CJ: *Leadership roles and management functions in nursing: Theory and application*, ed 5, Philadelphia, 2006, Lippincott Williams & Wilkins.

McConnell CR: *Umiker's management skills for the new health care supervisor*, ed 4, Boston, 2006, Jones & Bartlett.

Morgan G: *Images of organizations*, ed 2, Thousand Oaks, CA, 2006, Sage Publications.

Raso R: Cultural competence: Integral in diverse populations, *Nurs Manage* 37(7):56, 2006.

Rogers EM: *Diffusion of innovations*, ed 3, New York, 1983, Free Press.

Rogers EM: *Diffusion of innovations*, ed 5, New York, 2003, Free Press.

Roussel L, Swansburg RC, Swansburg RC: *Management and leadership for nurse administrators*, ed 4, Boston, 2006, Jones & Bartlett.

Scalzi C: Barriers and enablers to changing organizational culture in nursing homes, *J Nurs Adm* 36(5):230, 2006.

Schein EH: *Organizational culture and leadership*, San Francisco, 2004, Jossey-Bass.

Schneider W: Why good management ideas fail— understanding your corporate culture, 1998 (website): www.parshift.com/Speakers/Speak016.htm. Accessed February 10, 2007.

Senge PM: *The fifth discipline*, New York, 2006, Doubleday.

Shani AB, Lau JB: *Behavior in organizations: An experiential approach*, Boston, 2000, Irwin/McGraw-Hill.

Smith R: *The seven levels of change: Create, innovate and motivate with the secrets of the world's largest corporations*, ed 2, Arlington, TX, 2002, Summit Publishing Group.

Sullivan EJ, Decker PJ: *Effective leadership and management in nursing*, Upper Saddle River, NJ, 2005, Prentice Hall.

Yoder-Wise PS: *Leading and managing in nursing*, ed 4, St Louis, 2006, Elsevier.

Zohar D: *Rewiring the corporate brain: Using the new science to rethink how we structure and lead organizations*, San Francisco, 1997, Berrett-Koehler.

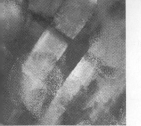

Selection and Development of Personnel

12

Chapter Overview

Chapter 12 discusses leadership and management in relation to recruitment and development of personnel, screening of staff, equal opportunity and affirmative action, Americans with Disabilities Act, multicultural workforce, cultural diversity, sexual preference and gender, generational differences, job descriptions, job analysis, orientation, staff development, career planning, career mapping, group process, and team development.

Chapter Objectives

- Identify three activities related to selection of personnel.
- Define affirmative action.
- Discuss at least four cultural phenomena and their influence on the interviewing process.
- Describe features of job descriptions.
- Differentiate the advantages and disadvantages of career ladders.
- Discuss the importance of orientation.
- List at least six ways to accomplish staff development.
- Describe career mapping as a part of career development.
- Diagram four stages of group, or team, process and the major activity in each stage.
- Compare groups and teams.

Online Resources

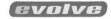 Critical thinking activities, worksheets, and case studies are available online at http://evolve.elsevier.com/Marriner/guide8e.

Major Concepts and Definitions

Personnel *individuals employed in an agency or department*

Recruitment *the process of enlisting personnel for employment*

Retention *capacity to retain employees once they are hired*

Affirmative action *actions taken to remedy past discriminatory practices*

Cultural diversity *variations among cultures in communication style, sense of personal space, social organization, sense of time, environmental control, and biologic characteristics*

Orientation *familiarization with and adaptation to an environment*

Job analysis *the study of a position to determine what knowledge, skills, aptitudes, and personal characteristics are needed to carry out certain responsibilities*

Job evaluation *the process of measuring the remunerative worth of a job in relationship to that of other positions*

Job design *specification of what the job requires, job methods, and the relationship among the organizational, social, and personal needs of the worker*

Job rotation *a horizontal job enlargement technique*

Job enrichment *a vertical approach to job design that uses more of the abilities and skills of personnel*

Job descriptions *specifications that are the requirements for given jobs*

Career ladder *vertical clinical or management advancement*

Staff development *education of employees*

Preceptor *a teacher or instructor*

Mentor *a wise and faithful counselor*

Career mapping *a strategic plan for one's career*

Group process *how the group functions*

CAREER PLANNING FOR JOB CANDIDATES

What job applicants do to choose a field of nursing and what they do to apply for a job are used by leaders and managers to select and develop personnel. Managers use the application form, resume, and interview to make hiring decisions.

Choosing a Field of Nursing

There are many opportunities in nursing for the new or experienced nurse. From the 1930s until the 1990s about 70% of nursing was done in hospitals. Hospital nurses can do medical, surgical, obstetric, pediatric, and psychiatric nursing or nursing in subspecialties, such as intensive cardiac care. Community health nursing, home care, hospice care, managed care, industrial nursing,

school nursing, work in a physician's office or clinic, rehabilitation nursing, long-term care, and health promotion are other opportunities. The federal government offers additional options, such as a career in the U.S. Army, Navy, or Air Force and work in the nursing service of the U.S. Department of Veterans Affairs or the Indian Health Service. Teaching, consulting, conducting research, serving as a staff member of a professional organization, and being an independent nurse practitioner are among the numerous possibilities.

To set short-term and long-range goals, one considers the importance of salary, fringe benefits, retirement plans, work hours, and opportunities for advancement. Climate and geographic location are also considerations. Fulfilling short-term goals can help position one for accomplishing long-range goals. For example, it is advisable to get some clinical experience before applying for teaching or consultation positions. Trends should be taken into consideration in setting long-term goals. The population is growing older and acquiring chronic diseases; health care reform is focusing on access to safe, high-quality, economical care. Care is moving from the hospital to the community. Ambulatory care and home care are increasing, and health promotion is being encouraged.

Searching and Applying for Job Openings

After deciding what type of nursing one wants to do and the geographic area where one wants to practice, one needs to locate job openings. Professional journals advertise positions, and college placement services and employment agencies maintain job listings. Recruiters are often at professional meetings. One can ask friends, acquaintances, and relatives if they know of openings. The Web can be searched, and employers can be contacted directly.

Application Form

The institutions of choice must be contacted to obtain an application form to start the hiring process. The application should be an attractive, typed document to give a good first impression. In many cases a form can be found online.

Résumé

A résumé is a summary of information about one's education, employment, and professional and personal history. It is typically a prerequisite for an interview because the employer uses the résumé to determine which candidates will be interviewed. Consequently, the résumé should be carefully developed and updated periodically.

Résumés should be printed on high-quality 8½- by 11-inch typing paper using a laser printer; they should never be handwritten. The contents should be well arranged, with major and minor headings to facilitate reading. The content should be concise yet complete, but not crowded. Résumés should contain the following information:

Identification: Full name, address, and telephone number should appear at the beginning of the résumé.

Job objective: Including or excluding a job objective is controversial. Some say it limits the scope of employment, whereas others argue that the personnel manager should know what position the nurse is seeking. Preparing separate résumés for each job that customize the job objective and accent the characteristics qualifying the nurse for a particular job is appropriate.

Education: The names and locations of schools attended, dates of attendance, and diplomas or degrees conferred should be listed in reverse chronologic order. Continuing education, such as workshops, in-service education, and home study courses, indicates an interest in self-improvement and is appropriate to list. If the grade point average is high, it is appropriate to cite it.

Work experience: Previous employment should be indicated in reverse chronologic order by listing the name and location of each agency, dates of employment, position title, and responsibilities. New graduates can list their student clinical experiences. It is appropriate to give a reason for leaving a position.

Military service: If the applicant has served in the armed forces, a summary of the military record should be included. Branch of service, years in the service, rank achieved, awards and distinctions, special assignments, skills, and knowledge acquired are some of the items appropriate to include.

Affiliations: Memberships, offices held, and committee activities in professional organizations, learned societies, and civic and social groups may be listed. Religious and political affiliations should be included with discretion.

Honors and awards: Scholarships, honors, and awards may be cited by stating the honor, the organization that conferred it, the location, and the date.

References: If references are available, the résumé should state that they will be provided on request. The applicant should always check the willingness of people who might serve as references. Because almost anyone could write a letter, it is appropriate to ask, "Do you think you know my work well enough to write me a good recommendation letter?" That gives the reference writer an opportunity to decline to write a letter if the person is not comfortable doing so. The applicant may also compile a file of letters of reference by asking teachers, supervisors, or peers to write letters of reference addressed "to whom it may concern" at the time of job termination. This is an opportune moment to make such a request because the nurse's performance is vivid in the reviewer's mind. It may prevent the reviewer from having to write more than one letter when copies are acceptable, and the applicant does not have to be concerned about locating the person later. Compiling such a letter file allows the applicant to send the most informative and appropriate letters of reference. It may be helpful to get several original copies of each letter so that letters with the original signature can be submitted. Otherwise, the original letters are kept and the appropriate photocopies are sent with the résumé.

Cover letter: The résumé should be accompanied by a cover letter stating the applicant's interest in working for the specific agency, the special qualifications and interests the applicant brings, the applicant's availability, and how the applicant can be reached. It may be possible to submit the résumé and cover letter online.

Interview

An interview allows the employer to determine if the applicant meets the requirements for the position being sought, and it allows the applicant to obtain information about the agency. First impressions are important. The interviewer will quickly assess the applicant's manners and appearance. The applicant may be questioned about dependability, responsibility, and ability to work with others. The compatibility of the applicant's goals with available opportunities may be explored.

Background Check

Initial registered nurse (RN) licensure requires fingerprinting and background check. Federal regulations require background checks for some health care providers.

Preemployment Physical

A preemployment physical may be required, and drug and alcohol screening may be included.

Job Procurement

A nurse is likely to apply for more than one job at a time. Once a position has been accepted, the other agencies should be informed of the decision in a friendly and professional way because the nurse may apply to those agencies again in the future.

LEADER AND MANAGER RESPONSIBILITY FOR RECRUITMENT AND RETENTION OF PERSONNEL

Leaders predict and plan for the future. They serve as role models, promote the image of the organization, identify and recruit well-qualified people, and assign the new personnel so as to achieve success for them and the organization. Leaders model continued professional development, encourage career planning and development of all employees, and support employees' personal career decisions. They encourage mentorships, coach employees, assess the learning deficits of staff, and plan strategies to minimize the deficits.

Managers share responsibility for recruitment and retention of well-qualified people. They help establish criteria for selection of personnel and structure interviews to increase the validity and reliability of recruitment. They apply their knowledge of legal requirements for hiring and make placement decisions based on employee strengths and the organization's needs. Managers monitor orientation, in-service, and continuing education; disseminate career information; and post job openings.

They select preceptors for staff, encourage role modeling and mentoring, evaluate staff development needs, and help formulate staff development policies (Marquis & Huston, 2006; Workman, 2006) (Box 12-1).

BOX 12-1 Leadership and Management for Recruitment and Retention

LEADER

Predicts the future

Plans for the future

Role models for recruitment

Uses interview process to promote image of the organization

Identifies and recruits well-qualified people

Assigns new personnel so as to promote success

Serves as role model for continued professional development

Encourages career planning and development for all employees

Supports employees' personal career decisions

Encourages mentorships

Coaches employees

Assesses the learning deficits of staff

Plans strategies to minimize the deficit

MANAGER

Shares responsibility for recruitment and retention of staff

Structures interview process

Increases validity and reliability of recruitment process

Helps establish criteria for selection

Applies knowledge of legal requirements for hiring

Makes placement decisions based on employee strengths and organizational needs

Monitors orientation, in-service, and continuing education

Disseminates career information

Posts job openings

Selects preceptors for staff

Encourages role modeling and mentorships

Evaluates staff developmental needs

Helps formulate staff development policies

Modified from Workman LL: Staff recruitment and retention. In Huber DL, editor: *Leadership and nursing care management*, ed 3, Philadelphia, 2006, Elsevier; Marquis BL, Huston CJ: *Leadership roles and management functions in nursing: Theory and application*, Philadelphia, 2006, Lippincott Williams & Wilkins.

RECRUITMENT EFFORT

"Cast a wide net and carefully sift through what you catch in it." —Linda S. Goldzimer

The acquisition of qualified people by any agency is critical for the establishment, maintenance, and growth of the organization. Therefore active recruitment is important, and the attraction of qualified applicants is the first step in selection of personnel. Methods for active recruitment include employee recommendations and word of mouth; attractive, informative websites; advertisements in local newspapers, nursing organization bulletins, and nursing journals; recruitment literature, such as fliers and newsletters; direct mail; computerized databases; posters; career days and job fairs; partnerships with schools of nursing; contacts with schools' graduating classes; placement services; open houses; organizational presence at nursing conventions; and provision of frequent, low-cost, credit-carrying continuing education courses for outsiders as well as employees (Box 12-2).

Word of mouth can be very effective, but it can also lead to the hiring of friends and relatives of the current workforce; this practice may foster nepotism and violate equal opportunity employment requirements. The use of advertisements in professional journals, in newspapers, and on radio and television; employment

---

BOX 12-2 Recruitment Methods

Employee recommendations

Word of mouth

Advertisements

Fliers

Newsletters

Bulletins

Posters

Career days

Job fairs

Placement services

Open houses

Nursing conventions

agencies; partnerships with schools of nursing; and contacts with schools' graduating classes offers the prospective employer a broader field for selection and more opportunities to hire from minority groups. Hiring minority group members to meet public policy goals may require active recruitment (McConnell, 2006).

Each institution should have someone who is responsible for recruitment. Recruiters should know nursing qualifications and the needs of the institution. They should be able to represent the institution with candor and enthusiasm. It is important that the recruiter relate well to people. Referrals from employees should be sought and in-house applicants encouraged; however, favoritism should not be shown. To aid in the selection of the best candidate for the job, an adequate budget should be provided to place the necessary advertisements; these advertisements should depict an institution that cares about employees and patients. That image should also be reflected at open houses, during conventions, and at high school and college career days. Printed recruitment materials should state that the institution complies with the employment practices of equal employment opportunity/affirmative action/ Title VI/Title IX/Section 504/Americans with Disabilities Act/Age Discrimination in Employment Act. The image portrayed on the Internet may have even more influence on the public and RNs (Kasoff, 2006).

The content of advertising is more important than the form. The recruiter should determine the needs and desires of potential applicants and demonstrate how the institution will meet those needs. Recruiters need to be attentive to the generational differences among mature veterans, baby boomers, and X and Y generations. Applicants are likely to be interested in the opportunity to give high-quality care, possibilities for advancement, opportunity for self-fulfillment, adequate income, good fringe benefits, adequate support systems, fellowship with colleagues, intellectual stimulation, educational opportunities, opportunity to be a leader, and, for some, child or elder care facilities. New graduates are likely to be interested in thorough orientation, in-service

education, staff development, and intern programs. Some nurses will be interested in tuition reimbursement and release time to work on educational degrees. Single people will be more interested in health benefits than married people whose spouses have family coverage. Older nurses will be increasingly interested in retirement plans. Refresher courses, chartered buses for people who live in suburban areas, child and elder care programs, part-time work, and flexible personnel policies may appeal to inactive nurses.

Mature nurses born from 1922 to 1945 are likely to hold the traditional values of adherence to rules, conformity, dedication, duty before pleasure, hard work, honor, respect for authority, and sacrifice. The baby boomers born between 1946 and 1964 may be taking care of children and aging parents; may value personal gratification and growth, health, and wellness; and may look forward to retirement. They may need an organization that allows flexibility to deal with their responsibilities to both children and parents and are likely to want money for security. Generation X members born between 1965 and 1980 are likely to consider family and leisure higher priorities than work. They may value balance, diversity, global thinking, informality, and self-reliance. They may also like flexibility to balance work and family, adequate income, and use of technology. Generation Y individuals born between 1980 and 2000 are the youngest group of employees and are likely to value achievement, civic duty, diversity, morality, and sociability. The nurse recruiter needs to assess nurses' interests and show how the institution can address their concerns (Hart, 2006).

The recruiter should respond to inquiries immediately. There should be daily phone coverage and 24-hour call-back response time. Postcards or letters for applications and résumés should be acknowledged. Packages of recruitment materials can be mailed to interested persons. Out-of-town or out-of-state applicants should be assisted with information about the community and housing. Applicants should know whom to contact and have access to toll-free telephone numbers, a specific mailing address, fax number, e-mail address, and websites with feedback buttons. Travel reimbursement for an interview with paid room and meals is attractive (Roussel, Swansburg, & Swansburg, 2006).

Records of inquiries noting the origin (how the job applicant learned of the opening) and disposition (hired or not and length of tenure) should be compiled and evaluated. The most productive recruitment method should be maximized. Recruitment is everyone's job. Current employees should understand that what they say to others at church or the grocery store affects recruitment and should preferably be positive. Some institutions have an RN recruitment and retention committee to advise about recruiting and retraining staff (Kelly, 2006; Thorgrimson & Robinson, 2005).

The major sources of personnel are persons seeking their first jobs, dissatisfied employees, and unemployed individuals. These classifications are important, because the categories indicate types of information the nursing manager should obtain, and they influence the selection process. Recent graduates or nurses who have not practiced since graduation may have a limited idea of job opportunities. Their choice of a first job may be strongly influenced by their education, achievement level, geographic preference, salary, mate's occupation, and peer pressure. They are likely to take several jobs before settling down. This variety of jobs, along with growing family responsibilities and maturity, helps develop the nurse's capabilities.

Dissatisfied employees are often not actively seeking other employment but are likely to be receptive to news of openings and job offers. If the nursing manager attributes the dissatisfaction to the misuse of the person's talents and abilities, the nursing manager may explore how to employ that person more effectively within his or her own agency. Job dissatisfaction is not uncommon, because every job has disadvantages. Agencies that require special job skills should expect applications from nurses who are looking for a better job with fewer disadvantages.

Hiring an unemployed worker who has been released from a previous job because of an infraction or a quarrel with the previous employer demands careful assessment. The nursing manager may wish to hire nurses who were fired because they refused to falsify records or perform a task for which they were not adequately prepared. The nursing manager would not want to hire a nurse who was fired because of high absenteeism and irresponsibility, unless the nurse could adequately explain the situation and assure the nursing manager that the problem has been resolved. For instance, the prospective employee might have been caring for a dying child at that time or undergoing a marital crisis that has since ended in divorce.

International recruitment of foreign-educated nurses requires attention to governmental and institutional requirements (Lee & Mills, 2005). Foreign nurses may need extra orientation and mentoring to learn a new culture. Although Filipino nurses may have studied the same curriculum, have used the same textbooks, and speak English, they have probably not had the opportunity to do stethoscope assessments, start intravenous lines, or insert nasogastric tubes or urinary retention catheters. In the Philippines, family members tend to basic personal care such as feeding and bathing the patients. Nurses usually do what the doctors order and tend to one or two patients. Therefore, Filipino nurses may need to be encouraged to express their views and participate in decision making. They may need coaching about how to manage time to care for multiple patients and may need to gradually add more patients to their assignments. Not only do they need to learn a new job, they may need to learn how to use the bus system and find grocery stores, especially ones that sell foods common to the Philippines. They may need help learning how to do the cooking and laundry, and so on. Helping new foreign staff form strong bonds with other nurses from their country is helpful (Kinderman, 2006).

If nurse applicants have been laid off from previous jobs because of slack times or budget cuts, the nursing manager should consider the chances of the nurses' returning to their old jobs when the slack time has ended. Seniority and other vested interests may influence nurses' desires to return to their previous positions.

Because of the costs of recruiting, selecting, and training employees, the decreased quality of care while new workers are being oriented, and the emotional drain of turnover on continuing employees, serious attention should be given to retention efforts. Exit interviews, particularly anonymous questionnaires, can help identify the reasons people resign. Posttermination questionnaires mailed to the homes of former employees 1 or 2 months after their resignation may obtain more accurate information than does the exit interview. After a period of time has elapsed, a person may be less emotional and more objective with some distance from the job and may feel more anonymous with less fear of retaliation. In addition, attitude surveys can be administered to current employees to identify sources of dissatisfaction and concern. Focus groups can be used to identify and solve problems. Once stressors are identified, strategies to reduce them can be planned. It is important to meet personnel's psychosocial needs for advancement, responsibility, achievement, and recognition. Nurses want input into decision making and control over their own lives. Savings from decreased turnover can eventually exceed the cost of higher direct care nurse staffing. A return-on-investment approach can help justify recruitment expenses (Baggot, Dawson, Valdes, et al, 2005).

Screening of Potential Staff

"Hire people with the desired values. You can teach them skills later." —Anonymous

Investment in well-qualified nurses can produce a high rate of return; and errors, whether they be failing to hire a promising nurse or hiring someone who falls short of the organization's expectations, can be expensive mistakes. In general there are three underlying philosophies in the screening process:

1. The manager should screen out applicants who do not fit the agency's image. Although this practice is common among some corporations, it is not a standard procedure for selecting health care personnel.
2. The manager should try to fit the job to a promising applicant. Examples include creating part time positions, split-shift hours, and opportunities for handicapped people.
3. Usually the manager should try to fit the applicant to the job. This philosophy assumes that both the person and the position are unique.

The essential and desirable qualities for an applicant can be identified. Each of the search and screening committee members can list what she or he thinks are essential and desirable qualities for an applicant for a specific job; the committee members can then discuss the qualities and come to consensus. Next, a qualification assessment form can be developed that lists the essential and desirable qualities; has columns labeled "yes," "?," and "no" for indicating whether the applicant has each quality or not; and includes a column for comments.

Application Forms and Résumés

Once the applicants have been found, they should be asked to submit biographic data. The application form is a quick way to collect demographic information. For the manager, personal history data—educational background, work experience, and other pertinent information—can be used to do the following:

- Determine whether the applicant meets minimal hiring requirements, such as minimal educational level or minimal job experience
- Collect background data useful in planning the selection interview
- Obtain names of references who may be contacted for additional information about the applicant's work experience and general character
- Collect information for personnel administration, such as Social Security number.

Letters of Reference

Letters of recommendation may be requested from references listed on the application form, previous employers, or both. However, these letters may be inaccurate and misleading, because the people writing them may not have had sufficient exposure to the applicant to become familiar with the applicant's capabilities, or they may not even have known the applicant. Because of the rapid turnover of nursing personnel, it is possible that few current staff members worked with the previous employee, and the current manager, who joined the agency after the applicant had resigned, may have to write the letter of reference based on an inadequate personnel file. The applicant may not know the current whereabouts of previous managers. To prevent these problems, employees could ask that a letter of reference be sent to a placement bureau at the time of termination, but this measure does not necessarily solve the problem. They have no assurance that the letter writers can express themselves well or are even willing to be accurate.

Because a new employer may sue if the newly hired employee does not measure up to the qualities described in the letter of recommendation, letters now tend to be brief, stating only verifiable information such as length of employment, job description, and responsibilities. However, a "to whom it may concern" letter is not considered legally binding and may include more information about the former employee's characteristics (Luthy & Feathers, 2007).

The right to privacy prevents unwanted disclosure of personal information to the public or a third party, including age, disability, marital status, medical information, national origin, race, religion, or sex. Defamation common law principles prevent impugning reputation, saying something that is not true, or saying something that causes damage to the person. However, negative employment references may not be legally actionable if they are based on an evaluation of a person's ability and work, are made by a person who has knowledge of the person's ability and work, limit information to job specifics, satisfy legitimate business needs, are not done in malice, and have their accuracy verified prior to disclosure. Letters of reference should be used cautiously. Most emphasis should be placed on characteristics consistently cited and on the general tone of the letters.

Interview

> "It's a heck of a lot easier to hire the right people to begin with than to try to fix them later." —Brad Smat

After the initial screening, the most qualified applicants should be given a preemployment interview to predict their success in the job. Information obtained from the application form and letters of reference should be taken into consideration in conducting the interview. The purposes of the interview are to obtain information, to give information, and to determine if the applicant meets the requirements for the position. The interviewer judges the applicant's dependability, willingness to assume responsibility for the job, willingness and ability to work with others, interest in the job, and adaptability; the consistency of the applicant's goals with available opportunities; and the conformity of the applicant's manners and appearance to job requirements. The interviewer answers questions, explains policies and procedures, and helps acquaint the applicant with the position. Finally, the interviewer must predict whether the applicant's overall performance will be satisfactory. The value of the interview is determined by the interviewer's ability to evaluate applicants and to predict accurately their future success.

The interview has definite purposes, and social chitchat should be avoided, although a brief warm-up period may help put the interviewee at ease. One of the main purposes is to learn about the prospective employee. Therefore it behooves the interviewer to concentrate on listening as well as to provide necessary information and answer questions from the applicant. Managers should avoid giving clues about what pleases or displeases them, should not be argumentative, and should try to avoid making a premature judgment. They should also beware of the halo effect, that is, judgment based on appearances. Although individuals wear clothing that reflects their personalities, they are likely to select clothes for the interview that project the image they wish to convey.

It is advisable to train managers in the art of interviewing. Training might include methods of establishing rapport with an interviewee, interviewing techniques, therapeutic communication, and ways of predicting applicant job performance. It is helpful to construct an interview recording form designed for the needs of the agency or for a specific position. Use of the job description to define and specify job dimensions on the form increases interviewer reliability. A personal profile of what characteristics the person hired should have, including education, experience, abilities, aptitudes, and interests, is helpful. Standardization of the interview promotes nondiscriminatory hiring practices and is particularly important when more than one person does the interviewing.

The heading of the interview form contains the date, name of the applicant, position desired, and interviewer's name. The body of the form lists traits required for the position. This allows the interviewer to assess applicants more systematically. One area might be work history. Does the applicant's work history indicate that the applicant has the ability to learn and understand the requirements of the job for which he or she is applying? More specifically, is there any evidence of lack of ability? Has the applicant had past experience in performing the same or similar tasks? Is the person familiar with the equipment and procedures? Has the applicant had special project or task force assignments? Has he or she shown job progression? Education is another area to be evaluated. Has the applicant had adequate formal education? Is there evidence of on-the-job training? Has the applicant participated in continuing education or in self-initiated skill development by reading books and journals and watching related television specials? Is the applicant active in professional organizations?

Certainly the applicant's dependability demands assessment. Is it likely that the applicant will have a good attendance record and maintain good work habits? Or is there evidence of poor work habits or work performance? What do past attendance and safety records indicate? Of equal concern is the applicant's sense of responsibility. Will the applicant seek assistance when needed and take the initiative when appropriate to get the job done? Will the applicant see jobs through to the end? Is there evidence of past independent thought and action, or does the applicant tend to blame others for problems? Finally, is the applicant capable of assuming leadership when required?

Job interest, poise, manners, appearance, and aspirations are other areas to investigate. Is the applicant cooperative and able to get along with others and work well as a team member, or does the person prefer to work alone? Is there evidence of success or friction with managers, peers, and staff associates? Is the applicant open to criticism, or does he or she react excessively? Is the applicant involved in the community? Has the person been open and candid during the interview?

The interviewer greets the applicant, introduces herself or himself to the applicant, and makes brief comments about the agency and the position available. The interviewer confirms the position for which the person is applying and explains the plan for the interview. Information on the application is discussed, and clarification is sought if necessary. The applicant's qualifications are discussed, preferably using the structured interview format. If the applicant appears qualified, the agency and position can be discussed in more detail, and subsequent hiring procedures can be explained before the interview is terminated.

During the interview the interviewer explains the purpose and plan of the interview. This helps create a positive climate. The interviewer learns the most by listening rather than talking and can encourage the job candidate to talk freely by asking open-ended questions. These are nondirective questions that help reveal feelings and attitudes. Examples of nondirective questions are the following: What qualifies you for this job? What aspects of your last job appealed to you? How were your relations with your peers?

Closed-ended questions are directive and can often be answered with "yes" or "no." They solicit less information than open-ended questions but are appropriate for obtaining objective and factual information. The following are examples of closed-ended questions: Who was your last employer? How long did you work for that agency? Did you get along with your co-workers? Do you think you are qualified for this job?

The funnel technique incorporates both open-ended and closed-ended questions. When using the funnel technique, the interviewer starts with an open-ended question, such as, "What subjects did you like most in school?" This produces objective information and sets a nonthreatening tone. The scope of the discussion is then funneled by asking a self-appraisal question, such as, "Why do you think you liked those courses in particular?" This elicits subjective information. The interviewer closes the discussion of a particular subject by asking direct questions to clarify the self-appraisal. A direct question might be, "What classes did you take for your nursing electives?"

A grid of topics to explore and use of the funnel technique can help the interviewer sequence questions in a logical order and decide what kind of questions to ask. Initially it may be helpful to fill in the topics and potential questions.

The questions may be modified during the interview (Table 12-1).

After information is obtained from the candidate, it is appropriate for the interviewer to share information about the job, policies, the agency, and the procedure for informing the interviewee of the hiring decision. The applicant is given an opportunity to ask questions. The interviewer closes the interview by telling the applicant when and how she or he can expect to learn of the decision. For example, the interviewer can say, "I will be interviewing a few more applicants this week. You can expect to hear from me by the first of next week" or "You should receive a letter regarding our decision within 2 weeks."

The facts collected during the interview are used as the basis for assumptions or inferences. They should be checked throughout the interview as new information is collected. It is possible to make both positive and negative assumptions from the same information. For example, if an applicant did not work for 3 months between jobs, the negative assumption could be that the person was escaping, undirected, or lazy. A positive inference could be that the applicant was clarifying goals and fulfilling personal objectives. Inferences are often more reflective of the person making them than of the applicant, which makes it particularly important to test interpretations.

TABLE 12-1 Topics and Questions to be Explored during an Employment Interview

Topics to Explore	Open-Ended Questions	Self-Appraisal Questions	Direct Questions
Education	Why did you choose to go to that school?	What courses were most useful to you, and how where they useful?	What courses did you take as electives?
Prior employment	Where have you worked?	What did you like best about your last job? What did you like least about your last job?	How long did you work there? What was your title? In what service areas did you work?
Life experiences	What life experiences have you had that help qualify you for this job?	How will raising your own children help you in this job?	How long have you spoken Spanish? How frequently do you use sign language?
Professional goals	What are your professional goals?	How do you plan to accomplish your goals?	What do you plan to be doing 5 years from now?

Women, men, minority applicants, and persons with disabilities should be treated in the same professional manner. The same general questions and the same standards should be required for all applicants. The interviewer should follow a structured interview plan to help achieve fairness in interviewing and should treat all applicants with fairness, equality, and consistency.

Interviewers can talk about applicants' qualifications, abilities, experiences, education, and interests; the duties and responsibilities of the job; where the job is located; travel, equipment, and facilities available; and the organization's missions, programs, and achievements. These topics are acceptable, but there are questions the interviewer may not ask (see Legal Interviewing Questions).

Discriminatory behavior is improper even when it is not intended, and appearance is as important as reality. Questions not related to the job have been used in a discriminatory way and should be avoided. Because improper significance might be given to questions regarding marriage plans or family matters, the interviewer should not inquire about marital status or non-marital arrangements; the occupation or earnings of the significant other; the feelings of the significant other about the applicant's work life, travel arrangements, or possible relocation; medical history concerning pregnancy or any questions relating to pregnancy; or the presence of children, the number of children, and their ages. The interviewer should use either first or last names for all candidates and persons involved in the recruitment. A photograph may not be required before employment. When discussing the location of employment, the interviewer should mention special features such as lakes, parks, and urban areas; sports, cultural, and other recreational features; and renting and buying options.

Interviews do have limitations. Their reliability and validity are questionable. Intra-rater reliability (reliability of repeated interviews by the same person) is higher than inter-rater reliability (reliability of repeated interviews by different people). Intra-rater and inter-rater reliability are lower with unstructured interviews than with structured interviews. Even if the interview process has reliability, interview ratings may not be a valid predictor of job performance. Validity tends to increase when a team approach is used. Interviewers seem to be influenced more by unfavorable than by favorable information. Attitudes and biases of interviewers affect how applicants are rated. Fortunately, there are interventions to reduce subjectivity. Conducting multiple interviews using a team approach with a structured interview format for each job classification reduce biases. Training people how to carry out interviews is helpful. The scenario method can be used to check the problem-solving ability of applicants (Anderson, Smit-Voskuijl, Voskuijl, et al, 2006; Marquis & Huston, 2006; Sullivan & Decker, 2005).

Legal Interviewing Questions

When interviewing applicants for positions, the interviewer should remember that some employment inquiries are acceptable, whereas others are not (Table 12-2). The purpose of the question determines its propriety. Appropriate inquiries have a direct relationship to the applicant's capacity to do the job. Inappropriate questions may elicit answers that will limit the person's opportunities because of ancestry, race, color, age, religion, gender, marital or parental status, or handicap. Some information needed for payroll or personnel purposes—such as age, proof of citizenship, and number of dependents—can be obtained after the person has been hired. Questions about the applicant's religious preferences, gender, marital status, credit rating, number and ages of dependents, or marital and family plans are not appropriate. Although the interviewer may ask about academic and professional education and schools attended, the interviewer may not ask about the racial or religious affiliation of the schools or the date of the schooling.

Applicants with disabilities should also be asked questions relevant to the job. Whether the individual needs any reasonable accommodations or assistance during the hiring or interviewing process and whether the individual is able to perform essential job functions with or without

TABLE 12-2 Legal Interviewing Guidelines

Subject	May Ask	May Not Ask
Age	Nothing	Any question to determine age
Arrest record	Nothing	Any questions to determine arrests
Availability for Saturday, Sunday, or holiday work	Whether the applicant can meet the work schedule	Any question about religious observance
Availability for weekend work or travel	Whether the applicant can meet the work requirements	Any question unrelated to work requirements
Citizenship	Whether the applicant is legally able to work	Any questions to identify country of origin
Convictions	Whether the applicant has pled guilty to, has pled "no contest" to, or has been convicted of anything other than a misdemeanor or summary offense	Whether the applicant has pled guilty to, pled "no contest" to, or been convicted of a crime
Disability	Whether the applicant, with or without reasonable accommodations, is able to perform the functions of the job	Whether the applicant has ever been disabled, suffered from a work-related injury, received workers' compensation, had a major illness, or missed work because of illness, or has any physical defects that interfere with some work or the duties of the position for which the person is applying
Education	Questions about vocational, academic, or professional education and schools attended	Any question designed to determine protected status
Family status	Whether the applicant can attend orientation and meet the requirements of the job	Whether the applicant is married, single, or divorced; ages of children or parents; plans to have children; spouse's job; family responsibilities
Languages	What foreign languages are read, spoken, or written and degree of acquired fluency	How or where the skill was acquired
National origin	Nothing	Any questions about lineage, ancestry, national origin, descent, or place of birth
Organizations	Questions about memberships in professional organizations related to the job	Any questions about membership that would indicate race, creed, gender, national origin, religion, or an affiliation with a labor organization
Pregnancy	Questions about the applicant's anticipated duration of time on the job or ability to meet orientation or attendance requirements	Any questions designed to learn about current, past, or future pregnancies
Relatives	What are the names of the applicant's relatives employed with the agency or a competitor	What are the names and addresses of relatives other than those employed by the agency or a competitor
Religion	Nothing	Any questions about religious denominations, church, pastor, or religious holidays observed
Gender	Nothing	Any questions about gender

reasonable accommodations may be discussed. The interviewer should avoid discussions of past or present serious illnesses or physical or mental conditions; the nature or severity of an apparent disability; problems an individual may have had because of a disability; and the reason the person became disabled.

Questions that would identify the person as being over 40 years of age or general questions about disabilities are not acceptable. Applicants may be asked to prove they are over 18 years of age and are able to perform job-related functions. The interviewer can ask for an address and length of residence in a city or state but not for rental or home ownership information. The name and address of a person to contact in case of an emergency may be solicited, but not the name and address of a relative. Inquiries about relatives who work in the agency or the name and address of parents if the applicant is a minor are acceptable.

Questions about the ability to read, write, or speak a language are acceptable, but questions about the applicant's primary language or the way the applicant acquired the ability to use a language are unacceptable. The applicant's legal right to remain in the United States can be questioned, but questions about the naturalization of parents or spouse are unacceptable. The applicant may be asked to list membership in clubs, organizations, societies, and associations, except those that would indicate the national origin, race, color, or religion of the applicant. Requests for all memberships are not appropriate. General questions about military service are inappropriate.

Because people are presumed innocent until proven guilty, records of arrests without convictions are meaningless. The interviewer may inquire about an applicant's conviction record for jobs for which that is relevant.

When interviewing minority candidates, the interviewer should not pretend interest in, or knowledge of, an ethnic culture or use ethnic vernacular or a foreign language the interviewer does not speak well. It is inappropriate for the interviewer to talk about his or her minority friends or to expect the candidate to know all other minority members. Lack of eye contact should not be judged negatively, because some cultures interpret direct eye contact as disrespectful. The interviewer should be aware that body language and tone of voice give messages that provoke confidence or mistrust and suggest support or indifference.

The interviewer should avoid references to the applicant's personal happiness and should not suggest an interest in hiring a woman, member of a minority group, or person with a disability to improve the affirmative action or equal opportunity profile. Applicants should be considered for a position based on qualifications.

The manager should be aware that some minority applicants may not have well-defined aspirations and career goals because their opportunities may have been limited and they may feel they have little control over their careers. Minority applicants often have frequently changed jobs in search of better pay. Therefore steady work and work progression histories may be of little use in evaluating minority applicants who have had limited opportunities (Cahn, 2002; Cox, 2001; Sullivan & Decker, 2005).

Testing

Personality and interest testing is sometimes performed, but this must be done by a trained psychologist. Ability tests are rarely used when hiring nurses. However, in-basket exercises, problem analysis, mock selection interviews, oral presentations, and debates have been used to select management personnel. Testing is useful for selecting clerical help. Tests can measure the knowledge and skills possessed and estimate the rate at which the applicant can acquire the knowledge and skills required for the position. These tests measure clerical and mechanical aptitudes, general intelligence, and mental, perceptual, and psychomotor abilities (Guion & Highhouse, 2006).

Background Checks

Nurses and recruiters need to be familiar with the laws about background checks. Federal regulations require background checks for some health care providers, and many agencies have started requiring them even if not required by law.

RESEARCH Perspective 12-1

Data from Krugman M, Smith K, Goode CJ: A clinical advancement program: Evaluating 10 years of progressive change, *J Nurs Adm* 30(5):215-225, 2000.

Purpose: The purpose of this study was to report the evolution of a clinical advancement program, UEXCEL, at the University of Colorado Hospital and the outcomes associated with evaluation over time.

Methods: Structure and progression of program development and change were outlined. Evaluation data were collected using a 23-item clinical ladder satisfaction scale developed by Strzelecki. Data were collected in 1993, 1994, 1996, and 1998 using standard survey methods. Trends in the University of Colorado Hospital data across units and time periods were determined and were compared with those in other institutional evaluation data sets.

Results/conclusions: Improvement in nurse satisfaction with the UEXCEL program was steady and incremental. Satisfaction improved after each program revision. A significant demographic trend was the correlation between higher level of education among registered nurses and program satisfaction. The authors concluded that successful clinical advancement programs need to balance professional dimensions and requirements for a clinical ladder with significant human resource rewards to create a model that motivates nurses to advance in their professional development, contribute to improved patient care outcomes, and commit to advancing the profession.

Of particular interest are patient or child abuse, neglect, and rape.

Preemployment Physicals

Preemployment physicals including drug and alcohol screening may be performed. However, they must meet the requirements of the federal Drug-Free Workplace Act of 1988, and candidates cannot be discriminated against because of disability.

Job Descriptions

Job descriptions are important to have available for the recruitment and hiring of staff. It is very important to match the employee to the job description for which the person is being hired. Job descriptions generally contain specifications that describe the requirements for the job, major duties and responsibilities, and organizational relationships of a given position. The title of the job indicates the major responsibilities and sets that job apart from others. The job description is a summary of primary duties in a complete but not detailed fashion. Job relationships and professional affiliations may be cited. Education, experience, and worker traits such as aptitudes,

interests, and temperament may be included. The physical demands and working conditions of the job may be mentioned. Job descriptions should be up to date, accurate, and realistic in terms of the resources available. The use of standard forms for all jobs within a category facilitate comparison.

Job descriptions should arrange duties in a logical order, state them separately and concisely, and use verbs to describe the action. They should be specific rather than vague and should avoid generalizations by using quantitative words whenever possible. To indicate frequency, the descriptions can note that an activity is performed daily, periodically, or occasionally when the percentage of total time spent on the specific activity cannot be determined.

Job descriptions are useful for recruitment, placement, and transfer decisions. They can also be used to guide and evaluate personnel. Job descriptions help prevent conflict, frustration, and overlapping of duties (Box 12-3).

Job Analysis

Job descriptions are derived from job analysis and are affected by job evaluation and design (Sullivan & Decker, 2005).

BOX 12-3 Sample Job Descriptions

VICE PRESIDENT FOR NURSING

Description of Work

General statement of duties: Performs administrative work in planning, coordinating, and directing the nursing service.

Supervision received: Works under general direction of the hospital administrator.

Supervision exercised: Supervises assigned personnel as a significant part of the duties.

Examples of Duties

(Any one position *may not* include all of the duties listed, nor do the listed examples include all tasks that may be performed by individuals in positions of this class.)

Directs and administers the nursing service, including inpatient and ambulatory care; develops and implements policies and patient care standards for all nursing service areas.

Participates in the planning and development of hospital policies and practices; works closely with administrative and medical personnel in coordinating nursing service functions with those of all other hospital departments and services.

Develops and implements staffing and ratio patterns to meet patient care and medical service needs; directs the broad planning of in-service training and orientation programs for nursing staff; directs research activities for continuing education and coordinates the clinical experience of nursing students.

Develops nursing service philosophies and goals in accordance with hospital policies; encourages and provides channels for staff participation in achieving these goals; interprets nursing service objectives to administrative and medical staff.

Serves on various hospital and community committees for the coordination of nursing services with other patient care and educational services; participates in professional organizational activities and represents the hospital in working with various service agencies and volunteer groups.

Directs the preparation of budgets for nursing service staffing, equipment, and supplies; develops systems and standards for patient care records and reports.

Directs the recruitment, selection, transfer, and promotion of nursing personnel and the maintenance of personnel records.

Performs related work as required.

Qualifications for Appointment

Knowledge, skills, and abilities: Extensive knowledge of professional nursing theory and practice. Extensive knowledge of modern principles and practices of hospital operation and nursing administration. Ability to plan, organize, and direct large-scale and comprehensive nursing activities. Ability to supervise, educate, and motivate employees. Ability to communicate effectively orally and in writing. Ability to establish and maintain effective working relationships with administrative and medical personnel, employees, the public, and other agencies.

Education: Minimum of graduation from a 4-year college with attainment of a master's degree in nursing and major course work in nursing administration or education. Related doctoral degree is desirable.

Experience: Five years of professional nursing experience including 3 years in an administrative capacity.

Necessary special requirement: Possession of a license to practice as a registered nurse as issued by the state board of nursing.

CLINICAL SPECIALIST I

Description of Work

General statement of duties: Performs advanced professional nursing work in a recognized medical specialty field.

Supervision received: Works under the general supervision of an administrative supervisor.

Supervision exercised: Supervises personnel as assigned or provides full supervision incidental to the other duties.

Continued

BOX 12-3 Sample Job Descriptions—cont'd

Examples of Duties

(Any one position may not include all of the duties listed, nor do the listed examples include all tasks that may be performed by individuals in positions of this class.)

Performs advanced professional nursing work in specialized medical fields such as mental health, respiratory care, and other recognized medical specialties in accordance with standard nursing procedures and medical direction.

Interviews patients to obtain general background information and identify problems; evaluates patients' behavior and assesses immediate and long-range needs; schedules and conducts individual and group psychotherapy sessions.

Participates as a member of a professional medical, psychiatric, or social public health team in evaluating, developing, and implementing health care plans.

Makes rounds with physician to review condition of patients; develops nursing care plans; participates in the care of the critically ill.

Participates in the orientation and in-service training of professional nursing personnel in teaching new, advanced, or complicated methods and procedures; interprets nursing services to patients and hospital personnel.

Performs related work as required.

Qualifications for Appointment

Knowledge, skills, and abilities: Thorough knowledge of professional nursing theory and practice. Thorough knowledge of modern nursing care principles and practices in a recognized medical specialty. Ability to motivate and train employees. Ability to communicate effectively orally and in writing. Ability to establish and maintain effective working relationships with patients, employees, the public, and other agencies.

Education: Attainment of a master's degree in nursing.

Experience: Two years of experience in an appropriate nursing clinical specialty.

Necessary special requirement: Possession of a license to practice as a registered nurse as issued by the state board of nursing.

Job Design

Job design specifies the job content (what the job requires), job methods (how to do it), and the relationship among the organizational, social, and personal needs of the worker. It involves observation, recording, and analysis of current jobs to make work more efficient and to provide incentives for the workers, thereby reducing costs and improving job satisfaction.

Job Simplification

Another technique, job simplification, removes the more difficult parts of a job so that the worker can do more of what remains. For example, a nurse can be hired to start all intravenous lines. The treatment nurse, team leader, and primary nurse then do not have to start any intravenous lines and therefore can give other medications and treatments to more patients. Work simplification, however, tends to lead to boredom.

Job Rotation

Job rotation is another horizontal job-enlargement technique. Nurses may rotate shifts and assignments among different units and different patients on the units. This practice complicates continuity of care, however, and often leads to additional frustration. Community health nurses may be rotated through clinic assignments. For instance, a nurse may work well-baby clinics one month; family planning clinics the next; and immunization, tuberculosis, or venereal disease clinics at other times. Again, this can disrupt continuity of care.

Job Enrichment

Job enrichment is a vertical approach to job design that uses a fuller range of the abilities and skills of personnel. When planning job enrichment, one should consider skill variety—the number of different talents and skills needed to do a job; task identity—the degree to which one can do a job from beginning to end with a visible outcome; task significance—the degree to which the job has an impact on others; autonomy—the degree of independence and discretion the job holder has to plan and implement the job; and feedback—the degree to which the job holder receives clear feedback about the effectiveness of his or her performance. These core job dimensions contribute to the psychological states that affect work outcomes. Skill variety, task identity, and task significance contribute to the experience of the meaningfulness of work. The job holder may experience responsibility for outcomes through autonomy and knowledge of the results through feedback. This should contribute to motivation, high-quality work performance, and satisfaction, which in turn help reduce absenteeism and turnover.

For example, community health nurses may have a specific set of clinics at which they work in addition to their family caseload. Continuity is preserved because nurses are always at the assigned clinics. They need to develop their expertise, knowledge, and skill in all the relevant clinical areas. In the past hospital units have switched from functional or team nursing to primary nursing so nurses could give total patient care and could assume additional responsibility and accountability.

Personnel may also be assigned more tasks. For instance, staff nurses can teach patient care assistants to do additional treatments. This may relieve some monotony from job simplification, but many workers are already very busy, and the new tasks may prove to be no more meaningful than the others.

Job enrichment is intended to increase motivation and productivity while reducing absenteeism and turnover. It can, however, increase anxiety, conflict, and feelings of exploitation. Skill levels of personnel limit the amount of job enrichment possible. Managers may not be willing to trust workers, and some workers may not be willing or able to do more work.

Job Evaluation

Job evaluation is a process of measuring the remunerative worth of a job in relation to that of other positions, both internal and external to the organization. On the assumption that workers will be more satisfied if they perceive pay rates to be consistent, the objective of evaluation is to compare jobs and establish a consistent pay base, so that employees in responsible positions receive more pay than those with less demanding jobs. A point system, ranking of jobs, job grading, and job-to-job comparisons are used. Consideration is given to education, mental and manual skills, responsibility for resources (personnel, materials, finances), mental and physical effort, and working conditions, such as exposure to dangerous or disagreeable elements. Under the point system the nurse manager assigns numerical values to specific qualifications (Box 12-4). Once point values have been assigned to various job factors, they can be added to determine a grade. The grades for various jobs can be ranked, and job-to-job comparisons can provide a basis for determining pay.

Job evaluation is a systematic rather than a scientific process, and its high reliability does not ensure validity. The management values used to choose and weigh factors may not be consistent with the values of other personnel, or the selected values may differ among work groups. Although relative pay rates can be determined by job evaluation, the absolute levels are often negotiated by the individual or by unions.

The number of grievances related to pay rates commonly increases after the introduction of job evaluation because personnel now have an objective basis for a grievance. Before job evaluation, employees had little concrete data on which to base grievances. They complained that they were not getting paid enough; management insisted that they were. After job evaluation, employees have criteria to use in filing grievances.

The transition period is especially troublesome. Problems related to adjusting the worker's present pay to the new pay structure may interfere

BOX 12-4 Job Evaluation

QUALIFICATIONS	POINTS
Education	
Less than a high school diploma	10
High school diploma	20
High school diploma plus a special training course	30
Associate degree or 3 years in a work-study program and passage of accrediting examinations	40
Baccalaureate degree and passage of accrediting examinations	50
Master's degree in area of specialty needed for the position	60
Doctoral degree in area of specialty appropriate for the position	70

Mental Skills

Work is simple and repetitive and is performed according to instructions.	10
Work involves a variety of duties that are performed according to procedures but requires alertness to identify needed changes.	20
Work involves a variety of complicated duties and some independent actions in adapting procedures to specific situations.	30
Work involves planning, organization, implementing, and evaluating actions related to patient care.	40
Work involves development of policies and procedures, organizations of functions, development of staffing patterns, and budget preparation.	50

Manual Skills

Work involves the normal manual skills, such as lifting, pushing, folding, writing, filing.	10
Work involves above-normal manual skills, such as accurate measurement, administration of medications and treatments, manipulation of instruments, typing, bookkeeping.	40
Work involves considerable manual skill, such as administration of complex treatments and manipulation of complex equipment.	50

RESPONSIBILITY FOR RESOURCES

Personnel

Supervises no one	10
Supervises fewer than 10 people	20
Directs up to 25 people	30
Directs up to 50 people	40
Directs up to 100 people	50
Directs more than 100 people	60

Finances

No responsibility for budget	10
Responsible for budget up to $10,000	20
Responsible for budget up to $25,000	30
Responsible for budget up to $100,000	40
Responsible for budget over $100,000	50

LEVEL OF EFFORT

Mental

Requires little thinking or judgment	10
Requires some alertness while performing repetitious tasks according to directions	20
Requires mental effort for problem solving	30
Requires considerable mental effort for decision making and problem solving	40
Requires continuous mental effort for dealing with the most difficult situations	50

Physical

Light work requiring little physical effort, usually seated	10
Light physical effort, use of light materials, frequently seated	20

BOX 12-4 Job Evaluation—cont'd

Sustained physical effort, seldom seated, continuous activity	30
Considerable physical effort, continuous activity, lifting	40
Working Conditions	
Good working conditions—light, ventilation, freedom from disagreeable elements such as dirt, heat, wetness, odors, noise	10
Average working conditions with occasional exposure to disagreeable elements and danger	20
Fair working conditions with frequent exposure to disagreeable elements and danger	30
Poor working conditions with continuous exposure to disagreeable elements and danger	40

---

with traditional lines of promotion. Adjusting a worker's pay upward to the new rate is acceptable to employees, but some may then file grievances to recover back pay. Granting back pay, however, could undermine the agency's budget. Therefore management may decide that payment will be retroactive only to a specified date. The case of an employee who has previously been overcompensated is a more difficult situation. To prevent dissatisfaction, personnel can be assured that no one's pay will be reduced as a result of the new pay schedule. However, it is possible to deny any pay increase to the individual who was overcompensated until others' salaries have been raised and all have been realigned to the new pay schedule. That can be demoralizing to the overpaid individual, of course, but the previous situation was demoralizing to other employees. More acceptable options may be to promote the individual to a job commensurate with the pay or to give the overpaid employee additional responsibilities in the present position to make the current job commensurate with the salary. After the individual vacates the position, the salary for the job can be realigned to a lower level in keeping with the pay schedule (Roussel, Swansburg, & Swansburg, 2006).

EQUAL OPPORTUNITY AND AFFIRMATIVE ACTION

The employer is subject to a number of legal requirements that have been legislated to provide equal opportunity and affirmative action in the workplace. Nurse leaders and managers need to be familiar with the current laws. Requirements

for providing equal opportunity are contained in Title VI and Title VII of the Civil Rights Act of 1964, Title IX of the Education Amendments of 1972, the Equal Pay Act of 1963, and the Age Discrimination in Employment Act of 1967. Affirmative action requirements are contained in Executive Order 11246, Section 503 of the Rehabilitation Act of 1973, and Section 402 of the Vietnam Era Veterans' Readjustment Assistance Act of 1974.

The Equal Pay Act of 1963 as amended by the Education Amendments of 1972 makes it illegal to pay lower wages to employees of one gender when the jobs men and women perform are of equal responsibility and accountability, are performed under similar working conditions, and require equal mental and physical effort and equal skill, experience, training, education, and ability (Guido, 2007).

Title VI and Title VII of the Civil Rights Act of 1964, as amended by the Equal Employment Opportunity Act of 1972, prohibit discrimination in any term, condition, or privilege of employment because of race, color, religion, gender, or national origin. Title IX of the Education Amendments of 1972 prohibits discrimination on the basis of gender in any educational program or activity receiving federal financial assistance. Prohibition of sexual discrimination applies to both males and females. A male successfully sued a skilled nursing facility for refusing to hire him in *Little Forest Medical Center of Akron v Ohio Civil Rights Commission* (1993). Discrimination is not an issue when bona fide occupational qualifications are considered. For example, if an employee must be able to lift 150 lb, any man or woman who could lift 150 lb would be a viable applicant (O'Keefe, 2001).

The Age Discrimination in Employment Act of 1967 makes discrimination against older male and female employees by employers of 20 or more persons, employment agencies, and unions illegal. A 1986 amendment prohibits discrimination against persons older than 40 years. A 1978 amendment prohibited mandatory retirement under the age of 70 years, but a 1987 amendment removed even that restriction except in certain job categories. Some possible exceptions include cases of poor performance evaluations and limited occupational qualifications, such as lack of physical endurance. *Goodhouse v Magnolia Hospital* (1996) involved a 53-year-old nurse who was terminated after 23 years of employment when there was a reduction in force. She applied for another position that was available in the facility but was not hired. She sued claiming age discrimination. She was awarded $100,000, and the hospital was ordered to reinstate her. At that time, average dollar amounts of settlements were higher in age discrimination cases than in cases involving disability, race, or gender discrimination. Age-based harassment, such as making age-related comments, is also a violation of employee rights. In *Madel v PCI Marketing, Inc.* (1997), the employer was held liable for using the word *old* with lewd language and for referring to the sleeping quarters as the "geriatric wing" (Grohar-Murray & DiCroce, 2003; Guido, 2007; O'Keefe, 2001; Sullivan & Decker, 2005).

Executive Order 11246 (as amended Executive Order EO 11375) prohibits all government contracting agencies from discriminating against any employee or applicant for employment and requires that contractors take affirmative action to ensure that applicants are hired and that employees are treated during employment without regard to their race, color, religion, gender, or national origin.

Sections 503 and 504 of the Rehabilitation Act of 1973 prohibit discrimination because of handicap in employment and in programs and activities receiving federal funds. Section 503, in addition, requires contractors to take affirmative action to employ and advance in employment qualified handicapped individuals.

The Pregnancy Discrimination Act of 1978 prohibits sexual discrimination against women who are or could become pregnant. An employer may not refuse to hire a woman because of pregnancy if she is able to perform the major aspects of a job, and she must be allowed to work as long as she is able to do her job. It also protects the woman's fetus. However, the act does not mandate that pregnant women receive preferential treatment. A suit was brought on behalf of a pregnant nurse who was fired because she refused to care for a patient with acquired immunodeficiency syndrome in *Armstrong v Flowers Hospital, Inc.* (1994). The Supreme Court ruled that policies that are written for fetal protection violate Title VII of the Civil Rights Act of 1964 in the case *UAW v Johnson Controls, Inc.* (1991). Consequently employers can inform a job applicant or employee of risks, but the woman must be allowed to decide whether or not she accepts a job assignment. Disability benefits and sick leave for women unable to work because of pregnancy-related reasons are to be granted on the same basis as for employees unable to work for other medical reasons (Grohar-Murray & DiCroce, 2003; O'Keefe, 2001).

Section 402 of the Vietnam Era Veterans' Readjustment Assistance Act of 1974 requires contractors to take affirmative action to employ and advance in employment qualified disabled veterans and veterans of the Vietnam era.

Executive Order 11246 addresses affirmative action and requires employers to make extra efforts to recruit, employ, and promote qualified members of formerly excluded groups. It is based on the premise that unless action is taken to overcome systematic exclusion and discrimination based on national origin, race, color, gender, or religion, employment practices will perpetuate the status quo indefinitely. In addition to the elimination of all existing discriminatory practices, affirmative action requires actions beyond neutral nondiscrimination.

In 1980, the Equal Employment Opportunity Commission established guidelines establishing that sexual harassment in the workplace violates Title VII of the Civil Rights Act and making employers liable for an act of sexual harassment committed by an employee even if the employer had no prior knowledge of the reported sexual harassment. The guidelines define sexual harassment as including conditions in which (1) submission to sexual advances is explicitly or implicitly a condition of an individual's employment, (2) submission to or rejection of sexual advances is used as a basis for employment decisions, and (3) the sexual advances interfere with work performance or create an intimidating, hostile, or offensive work environment. The victim does not have to be of the opposite gender of the harasser, but can be anyone affected by the offensive behavior. Examples of actions creating a hostile working environment are asking questions or making comments about one's sexual life; sending e-mails of a sexual nature; using computer screen savers that are sexually explicit and in view of others; making offensive comments of a sexual nature; repeating gossip, jokes, or stories with sexual content; displaying cartoons, drawings, graphics, photographs, or posters of a sexual nature; making obscene gestures; whistling; and touching the body (Grohar-Murray & DiCroce, 2003; O'Keefe, 2001; Sullivan & Decker, 2005).

The Immigration Reform and Control Act of 1986 mandates that employers verify the identity of employees and sanctions employers that knowingly hire an unauthorized alien (Grohar-Murray & DiCroce, 2003).

Three categories of individuals with disabilities are protected by the Americans with Disabilities Act (ADA, 1990): (1) individuals who have a physical or mental impairment that substantially limits one or more major life activities, (2) individuals who have a record or history of a physical or mental impairment that substantially limits one or more major life activities, and (3) individuals who are regarded as having such an impairment whether they have the impairment or not. Disability in a major life activity includes difficulty in caring for oneself, walking, breathing, hearing, seeing, speaking, or learning. The act specifically excludes the following from the definition of disability: drug and alcohol abuse, homosexuality or bisexuality, transvestism, transsexualism, pedophilia, exhibitionism, voyeurism, gender identity disorders, other sexual identity disorders, compulsive gambling, kleptomania, pyromania, and psychoactive substance use disorders.

The requirement that the individual be able to perform "essential" functions ensures that a person with a disability will not be considered unqualified because of inability to perform marginal or incidental job functions. If the person is qualified to perform essential job functions except for limitations caused by a disability, the employer must consider whether the individual could perform these functions with a reasonable accommodation. A written job description prepared in advance of advertising or interviewing applicants for a job could be considered as evidence in determining the essential functions of the job (US Equal Employment Opportunity Commission, 2002).

Many people who have learning disabilities work. Leaders and managers should develop personnel policies that clarify that the institution will comply with federal and state Equal Employment Opportunity and ADA regulations. It is appropriate to hire an administrator to oversee disability issues and to provide training to that person regarding legal obligations and institutional grievance policies. Staff should also be educated about the policies, and copies of the policies should be readily available to all. People who have attention-deficit/hyperactivity disorder are likely to be forgetful, have a short attention span, be hyperactive, and be inattentive to detail. They may need flexible work hours, opportunities to take frequent short breaks to get focused, written instead of verbal directions, and regular feedback. Dyslexia is another common learning disability. This disorder makes it difficult for the person to accurately recognize, read, and write words. People with dyslexia do better with verbal instructions. Web adaptation software for dyslexic individuals may magnify text, increase the spacing between letters and words, sharpen images, and allow different-colored text and background. Other low-cost electronic aids include graphic organizers for creating and writing documents, screen reading and voice-recognition software, and talking calculators. Because people have different auditory, tactile, and visual learning styles, it is good to have manuals on tape and digital recordings; computers with text-reading programs and voice dictation; and handouts with illustrations and paraphrased instructions (NetDoctor, 2007).

Physical impairments include but are not limited to orthopedic, visual, speech and hearing impairments, cerebral palsy, epilepsy, muscular dystrophy, multiple sclerosis, cancer, diabetes, tuberculosis, infection with human immunodeficiency virus (HIV), drug addiction, and alcoholism.

Mental impairments include but are not limited to mental retardation, organic brain syndrome, emotional or mental illness, and specific learning disabilities.

Temporary conditions may be considered a disability depending on the duration and the extent to which one or more major life activities are limited. Qualified individuals with a disability must meet the essential eligibility requirements of the agency, with or without (1) reasonable modification to the agency's rules, policies, or practices; (2) removal of architectural, communication, or transportation barriers; or (3) provisions of auxiliary aids or services.

People who pose a direct threat to the health or safety of others are not qualified for protection under the ADA. Such a determination may not be based on generalizations or stereotypes but must be based on an individualized assessment that relies on current medical evidence or the best available objective evidence to assess (1) the nature, duration, and severity of the risk; (2) the probability that the potential injury will actually occur; and (3) the possibility of mitigating or eliminating the risk by reasonable modification of policies, practices, or procedures. Modifications that fundamentally alter the nature of the program, service, or activities are not required.

An agency should have procedures by which people who identify potential difficulties in meeting essential performance standards can receive appropriate assistance and guidance. When a person believes that he or she cannot meet one or more of the standards without accommodations or modifications, the agency must determine on an individual basis whether or not the necessary accommodations or modifications can be made. Reasonable accommodations are defined by the ADA to include (1) making existing facilities readily accessible to and usable by individuals with disabilities, and (2) restructuring the job; instituting part-time or modified work schedules; acquiring or modifying equipment or devices; making appropriate adjustments or modifications to examinations, training materials, or policies; providing qualified readers or interpreters; and making other similar accommodations for individuals with disabilities. Each agency should rely on its legal resources to make informed decisions.

The ADA mandates that people with disabilities not be disqualified from employment just because of an easily accommodated disability, but it does not mandate that people with disabilities be hired before fully qualified people without disabilities. In the case of *Zamudio v Patia* (1997), the court required the employer to inform Ms. Zamudio when a position became available for which the reasonable accommodations she required could be carried out but did not require the employer to hire her before better-qualified people or people with more seniority. Nor does the court require job restructuring when the person needing accommodation qualifies for other jobs that do not need accommodation, such as in the case of *Mauro v Borgess Medical Center* (1995). The Michigan court denied an operating surgical technician accommodation to continue working in the operating room. Mauro tested positive for HIV and consequently was moved to an equivalent position that did not require patient contact.

The ADA also recognizes essential job functions that a person must be able to perform to be qualified for a given position. The court found that the ability to restrain patients is an essential job function for a psychiatric nurse in the case of *Jones v Kerrville State Hospital* (1998). Ability to work rotating shifts was considered an essential job function in the case of *Laurin v Providence Hospital and Massachusetts Nurses Association* (1998).

Numerous lawsuits have been filed under the ADA. Some other relevant cases are the following: *Howard v North Mississippi Medical Center* (1996) found that migraine headaches and latex allergies are not disabilities; *Jessie v Carter Health Care Center, Inc.* (1996) found that pregnancy is not a disability; *Webb v Mercy Hospital* (1996) found that erratic behavior does not give notice to the employer that the individual has mental impairment; *Thompson v Holy Family Hospital* (1997) found that a nurse with a lifting disability is not qualified for protection under the ADA; *Wilking v County of Ramsey* (1997) found that a nurse taking medications for depression is not disabled; and *Cody v Cigna Healthcare of St. Louis, Inc.* (1998) found that depression and anxiety are not disabling conditions (Grohar-Murray & DiCroce, 2003; Guido, 2007; O'Keefe, 2001; Sullivan & Decker, 2005).

The Family and Medical Leave Act of 1993 provides job security during unpaid leave while a male or female employee is caring for a new infant of the employee or a new foster or adopted child; is caring for a spouse, child, or parent who has a serious health problem; or is personally seriously ill. The act helps in balancing the demands of work and home for single parents who are employed full time and for two-parent households in which both parents work full time, which puts job security and parenting at odds. Aging parents are also putting increasing demands on working children. To be eligible for the benefits of the Family and Medical Leave Act, the employee must have worked at least 12 months and at least 1250 hours during the previous 12 months. The employee is eligible for 12 weeks of unpaid leave in a 12-month period. The employer may require the employee to use all or part of any paid vacation, personal leave, or sick leave as part of the 12-week family leave. The employee's job and benefits are protected during the leave, and on return, the employee is to be given the original job or an equivalent job with equivalent pay (Guido, 2007; O'Keefe, 2001).

Equal employment opportunity policy concerns implementation of employment practices that do not discriminate against or impair employment opportunities of protected groups. Affirmative action differs from equal employment opportunity in that it enhances employment of protected groups. A major portion of an affirmative action program must recognize and remove barriers and establish affirmative measures to remedy past discriminatory practices. Such measures include providing additional aid to prepare disadvantaged people for jobs. It is noteworthy that Supreme Court rulings state that such measures are not restricted to workers who have individually been victims of discrimination.

Development of an affirmative action program includes the addition of affirmative action intent to the agency's philosophy; creation of affirmative action policies and procedures; appointment of a manager responsible for the program; inclusion of affirmative action responsibilities in appropriate job descriptions; and publication of the affirmative action commitment internally to all employees and externally to sources for recruitment, to minority and women's organizations, to organizations of handicapped individuals, to appropriate veterans' service organizations, to community agencies, and to the community in general.

The affirmative action policy is disseminated internally by including it in the policy manual, annual reports, and other media, such as the agency newsletter. It can also be posted on bulletin boards. Nondiscrimination clauses are included in union agreements. Articles about the affirmative action program, its progress, and the activities of disadvantaged workers are published in agency publications. When employees are pictured in handbooks or advertising brochures, minority and nonminority men and women should be included.

Top administration should discuss the intent of the policy and individuals' responsibilities for its implementation with management personnel. Special meetings should be scheduled with all employees, and the policy should be discussed in orientation and management training classes.

A workforce analysis of job classifications by departments is the first step toward identifying where members of minority groups, women, and men are currently employed and discovering areas of concentration and underuse. The availability of minority individuals, women, and handicapped persons with the requisite skills is considered when determining whether there is underuse: How many minority members, women, and handicapped persons are in the geographic area from which the institution recruits? What percentage of the total workforce in the area are members of minority groups, women, and handicapped persons? How many are unemployed? How many can be recruited from the local community or the nation? Are there training programs available to prepare minority members, women, and handicapped people with skills the agency can use? Can the agency prepare minority individuals, women, and handicapped personnel? An agency may be able to prepare nurses' aides or assistants but may need to rely on other institutions to prepare licensed practical nurses or vocational nurses and RNs. Are there disadvantaged people already employed by the agency who are transferable or promotable? Programs to correct underuse must be developed when there are fewer minority members, women, and handicapped persons in a job classification than would be expected by their availability.

Once management has completed its use and availability analysis, it establishes goals and timetables to improve use. To correct identifiable deficiencies, management needs goals that are measurable and attainable. Goals for minority group members and women are presented separately. These goals and the timetables for completion, along with supportive data and analysis, are major parts of the written affirmative action program.

Next, programs to achieve these goals must be developed and implemented. This phase begins with a review of the employment process to identify barriers. Recruitment procedures and the selection process—including job requirements, job descriptions, application forms, testing, and interviewing—are examined. The upward mobility system, including training, assignments, job progressions, seniority, transfers, promotions, and disciplinary action policies, is reviewed. Wage and salary structure, benefits, conditions of employment, and union contracts are also studied. Appropriate changes are made, and an internal audit and reporting system to monitor and evaluate the affirmative action program is implemented. Records of referrals, placements, transfers, promotions, and terminations should be maintained for 3 years. Formal reports regarding attainment of goals and timetables are prepared on a regular basis. The manager of the affirmative action program reviews the reports with other managers, advises top administration of the program's effectiveness, and submits recommendations for improvement of unsatisfactory performance.

Compliance status is not judged solely by whether goals have been met by the time set for achieving them. The program's content and the efforts made toward realization of the goals are factors that are considered in determining its effectiveness. It is important to keep in mind that goals are not inflexible quotas that must be met but are targets that are reasonably attainable through good faith efforts. Goals therefore should be realistic, measurable, and achievable by the time established (Doverspike, Taylor, & Arthur, 2000).

MULTICULTURAL WORKFORCE

Multiculturalism is working together toward a cohesive society while understanding, respecting, and protecting cultural differences. Diversity comes in many forms: race, ethnicity, culture, age, gender, sexual preference, educational level, income level, physical attributes, skills, learning styles, mental abilities, and parental status.

Prejudice is an unreasonable bias that is formed before facts are known. It is an opinion or judgment that is often unfavorable. It may be suspicion, intolerance, or even hatred of others who are different from the opinion holder. It may result in judgments or actions that are harmful to another. To stop and overcome prejudice and to be open minded, do the following: Try to get to know people who are different from you. Eat at foreign restaurants. See some foreign films. Check the library for books, films, and videotapes about other countries and cultures. Participate in diversity training. Attend a college course on diversity. Learn a new language. Participate in community work with organizations serving people who are culturally different. Travel to other countries. Write to a pen pal and exchange information about each other's lives. Invite someone to your home. See the person, not the label. Even if you have had a bad experience with someone from a certain group, give everyone a chance. Do not judge everyone in a group as the same. Recognize feelings of prejudice and deal with them (Cox, 2001).

Discrimination is the act of treating someone unfairly because of differences. Such behavior may be based on stereotypes. Stereotypes are fixed patterns that make people view everyone in a group as alike instead of as individuals.

Ethnocentrism is a tendency to view other groups or cultures in terms of one's own. It is a belief in the inherent superiority of one's own group or culture that is often accompanied by a feeling of contempt for other groups and cultures. The creation and maintenance of a diversity-friendly multicultural workplace requires recruitment of individuals from diverse groups, implementation of policies and procedures that support diversity, and intolerance of "isms" (Cox, 2001).

CULTURAL DIVERSITY

Understanding cultural variables can help leaders and managers recruit, retain, direct, and evaluate personnel. People bring with them assumptions, attitudes, and behaviors related to their cultural heritage. The recognition of and respect for cultural differences help foster positive relationships. Leaders and managers need to have an awareness of how their own cultural background affects their performance (see Table 5-2 regarding Title VII of the Civil Rights Act of 1964, which prohibits employers from engaging in conduct that creates a hostile environment for individuals of any given race, religion, gender, or national origin).

Individuals within any given cultural group vary widely, but the majority of individuals in such a group generally share common norms and traits. Communication is an important aspect of one's culture. Communication includes both spoken and nonverbal expression. Misunderstandings can result from silence, words used, tone of voice, voice pitch, and body movements. What a person says and does can be interpreted in a variety of ways. Unless the person's cultural heritage is understood, an interpretation could be wrong.

Someone speaking loudly with animation might be misinterpreted as being aggressive, pushy, or rude. Someone speaking in a soft, low voice may be viewed as passive, afraid, or shy.

The context of speech refers to the use of emotion in communications. Mexican-Americans, Irish-Americans, and Italian-Americans often use emotions, whereas African-Americans, German-Americans, and Jewish people rarely do. Kinesics is the use of gestures, stances, and eye movements when communicating. Alaskan Eskimos blink to indicate agreement. Irish- and Italian-Americans use gestures, stances, and eye movements to emphasize points. Persons in certain socioeconomic groups in India are supposed to avoid eye contact with persons in lower or higher socioeconomic groups and persons of the opposite gender.

Dialect and language styles often differ among cultural groups. Some cultures convey feelings and emotions through touch. Others find touch intrusive or consider it to have sexual connotations.

There are four zones of interpersonal space: (1) intimate, (2) personal, (3) social consultative, and (4) public. Each zone is associated with distinctive distance and intimacy techniques for verbal and nonverbal communication. The intimate zone is 0 to 18 inches and is reserved for those with close personal relationships; entering this zone is considered taboo in some cultures.

Personal space, 18 inches to 4 feet, is the area in which touching by family and friends and those in some counseling interactions is permitted. The social consultative zone, 4 to 12 feet, is for casual social interactions. The public zone, beyond 12 feet, is beyond the sphere of personal involvement, and verbal communication in this zone is usually formal. The preferred distance between people in the United States is 2 to 3 feet. In general, Asians usually do not mind closer distances, whereas African-Americans tend to not want their personal space invaded.

Leaders and managers need to be aware of these differences in space as well as other cultural differences that can impact recruitment and retainment of personnel. See Chapters 1 and 2 for more information on cultural differences.

People tend to be past, present, or future oriented. People who value the past maintain tradition and are not likely to set goals for the future. People who focus on the present tend to be unappreciative of the past and do not plan for the future. People with a future orientation plan and organize for the future.

People in the United States tend to be individualistic and desire to control their own lives. Chinese-, Mexican-, Vietnamese-, and Puerto Rican–Americans tend to consider the family as the most important social organization. Some cultural groups, such as Italians and Appalachian people, extend their families beyond blood lines.

Environmental control relates to the ability to control nature and direct the environment. Some groups believe they can control nature; others feel controlled by it. Still others, such as many Native American nations, believe humans should attempt to live in harmony with nature.

There are also biologic variations among cultures. Features, skin color, body size, and enzyme differences are related to cultural heritage. Understanding cultural variables can help leaders and managers recruit, retain, direct, and evaluate personnel. Understanding cultural variables can help one understand oneself better, as well.

African-American households are often headed by a single female parent. Large extended family networks usually are important, the elderly are respected, and church affiliation and religious beliefs are sources of strength. African-Americans are likely comfortable with close personal space when interacting with family and friends. They may have a past, present, or future orientation depending on their socioeconomic background. Relationships are important, so an individual may be late to an appointment because a relationship was considered more important than getting to an appointment on time. African-Americans are at higher risk for cancer, diabetes mellitus, heart disease, hypertension, lactose intolerance, and sickle cell anemia than whites. It is important to clarify the meaning of verbal and nonverbal communications, build a relationship on trust, and involve family members. African-Americans may want to use herbs, laying on of hands, and prayer for healing.

Asian-Americans usually respect the past but also pay attention to the present and future. They may have a preference for formal personal space except among close friends and family. Touching someone's head is disrespectful, because the head is considered sacred. Touching members of the opposite sex is not acceptable, and Asians usually do not touch each other during conversations. Large extended family networks are common, and family units are structured and hierarchical. Members value tradition, loyalty, and education. A healthy body is viewed as a gift from ancestors, and health is considered a state of physical and spiritual harmony. Illness is believed to be an imbalance between yin (positive energy) and yang (negative energy). Yin foods are cold and are eaten for hot illnesses. Yang foods are hot and are eaten for cold illnesses. Asian-Americans are at high risk for cancer, heart disease, hypertension, lactose intolerance, and hereditary anemia. Others interacting with them should avoid physical closeness, touching, eye contact, and hand gesturing. It is preferable to have same-sex caregivers. Flexibility and family involvement can be encouraged. Acupuncture, herbs, incense, consumption of appropriate hot or cold foods to restore balance, massage, and prayers may be used as alternative modes of healing.

Hispanic-Americans tend to have a present time orientation. They are comfortable with close contact, are tactile, and value the physical presence of others. The needs of the family have priority over individual needs. Men tend to be the ones who work for pay, whereas the women are caretakers and homemakers. They may consider health a reward from God and illness a punishment. They view health as a balance between hot and cold and wet and dry. Hispanic-Americans are at risk for diabetes mellitus, heart disease, hypertension, lactose intolerance, and parasites. Health workers should be polite, protect modesty and privacy, offer to call clergy for patients, ask if it is all right to touch a child before examining the child, and be flexible with time issues. Hispanic-Americans may use consultation with lay healers, herbs, consumption of hot or cold foods to restore balance, prayers, and religious medals as alternative modes of healing.

Native Americans tend to be oriented to the present and to personal space. Members just lightly touch another person's hand as a greeting. Massage may be used for a newborn to promote bonding between the mother and infant. Some tribes prohibit touching of a dead body. Members are usually family oriented. The basic family unit is the extended family. Elders are honored, and grandparents may be the head of the household. Sacred myths and legends supply spiritual guidance, and religion and healing practices are integrated. Health is considered a state of harmony among the person, family, and environment. Illness is considered a disequilibrium between the person and environment that is caused by supernatural forces. Natural and religious folk medicine may be used along with traditional health care. Native Americans are at risk for alcohol abuse, arthritis, diabetes mellitus, gallbladder disease, heart disease, injury, lactose intolerance, and tuberculosis. Members are reluctant to undergo screening for illness because of the perceived power of language, and it is not acceptable to talk about cancer. Health care providers should clarify communications, modify their own body language, and understand that lack of eye contact is respectful. Herbs, consultation with traditional healers, and restoration of balance between the person and nature may be alternative modes of health care (Silvestri, 2005).

Alaskan Natives have strong family ties and value spirituality. Women may neglect their own health to take care of their families. There is often a subsistence lifestyle.

Many Puerto Rican–Americans live in northeast urban areas like New York and Philadelphia. They have strong family ties and many single-parent, female-headed households. Lifestyles differ, but core values and religion are similar across geographic regions.

Most Cuban-Americans are political exiles seeking to escape from an oppressive government regime. They tend to have take-charge attitudes and may engage in self-care. They seem to have fatalistic attitudes about cancer (Huber, 2006).

SEXUAL PREFERENCE AND GENDER

Sexuality characteristics involving sexual orientation relate to the gender identification of the individual, not to human sexuality. Nursing leaders and managers need to be familiar with the laws regulating recruitment and retention of individuals with different sexual orientations (see Table 5-1 regarding Title VII of the Civil Rights Law of 1964, which prohibits employers from engaging in conduct that creates a hostile environment for individuals of any race, religion, gender, or national origin). *Transgendered* is an umbrella term used to refer to transsexuals, intersexuals, cross-dressers, transgenderists, and others. The gender identity of transsexuals does not match their biologic gender. Biologic males may identify with females and biologic females with males. Such individuals are often motivated to change their anatomy to more closely match their gender identity. Transgenderists are similar to transsexuals but choose to not have genital surgery. Cross-dressers' gender expression is sometimes different from their biologic gender. Intersexuals are not typically male or female. Gay men are biologic males who identify as men and are attracted to other men. Gay men who dress in women's clothing are called *drag queens*. There are also female-to-male transsexuals, and it is more common for women to wear men's clothing than for men to wear women's clothing. Lesbians are biologic females who identify as females and are attracted to other women.

Individuals go through three phases of "coming out." First is comparison, in which people compare what they hear, see, and feel with what they observe in other people, and start to reassess their own sexuality. Second is support and change from tolerance to acceptance to support. Third is incorporation or integration and a sense of pride. Gay individuals typically have more in common with "straight" people than they have differences from them.

Organizations also have three phases of coming out. The first phase is acknowledgment that gay people exist in the workplace. Second is accommodation by actions such as offering partner benefits to same-gender and unmarried opposite-gender couples and substituting the word *partner* for *spouse* in organizational policies. Third is incorporation, in which sexual orientation is viewed as a fact of life. At this stage the organization implements nondiscrimination policies, applies change-agent methodologies, and provides educational programs, brown bag meetings, mentoring, coming-out coaches, referral services, community outreach initiatives, assistance in dealing with spirituality and religion issues, a hot line to report harassment and discrimination, awards for promoting a safer work environment, and encouragement of gay employees to bring their partners to events. Organization leaders should be clear and articulate about the mission, vision, values, and philosophy of the organization (Winfeld & Spielman, 2001).

GENERATIONAL DIFFERENCES

People born from around 1925 to 1945 are known as traditionalists and as the silent generation (Table 12-3). Nursing leaders and managers need to be familiar with the laws regulating recruitment and retention of such employees (see Table 5-1 on the Age Discrimination in Employment Act). The career goal of individuals of this generation is to build a legacy, and they are rewarded by the satisfaction of a job well done. They consider no news as good news and learn the hard way. They view retirement as a reward. They value honesty, integrity, family, and work and are loyal, hard workers. They may have live unbalanced lives because they were consumed by work. They often lack formal education. They are motivated by the message, "Do it!" This group tends to welcome retirement after long years of hard labor. They see retirement as a time for leisure and a chance to do things they did not have the time or money to do before. Social Security has helped make that possible. Unfortunately, some early retirees have reported that their standard of living has declined since retirement, and some are not confident that they will have enough money

to remain comfortable for the rest of their lives (Goldberg, 2000; Lancaster & Stillman, 2002; Zemke, Raines, & Filipczak, 2000).

People born from about 1946 to 1964 are known as the baby boomers. They want to build a stellar career and are rewarded by things such as money, title, recognition, and a corner office. They invented the 60-hour work week believing that hard work and loyalty would pay off. Feedback once per year with lots of documentation suits them. Managers are afraid that if one trains them too much, they will leave the organization. Baby boomers want to find meaning for themselves in their work and view retirement as a time to retool. They tend to value optimism, team orientation, personal gratification, health and wellness, and personal growth. Their service orientation, drive, and ability to be good team players are assets, whereas their lack of budget-mindedness, discomfort with conflict, conformity, sensitivity to feedback, and self-centeredness are considered liabilities. They are motivated by messages such as, "We need you," "You are important," "I approve of you," "You are valued." They have a spending style of "buy now and pay later with plastic." As they near retirement, they need more opportunities that will challenge them because many are likely to work until about age 70. Many retirees would prefer to work at least part-time. Although they have worked excessive hours during the past few decades, many would like a slower pace now. They are willing students if treated respectfully. Adult education programs have increased significantly. Older workers are as productive as younger ones and have fewer on-the-job accidents. With the shortage of nurses and the cost of recruiting, hiring, and developing new employees, it is appropriate to encourage the most experienced nurses, even those with the highest pay, to continue to work. A phased-out retirement with a gradual reduction in the number of days worked or perhaps the number of hours worked per day has possibilities. Besides full-time permanent work, one can consider options such as part-time permanent work, full-time or part-time temporary work, contract work, consultation, telecommuting from

TABLE 12-3 Generational Differences

Years	1925-1945	1946-1964	1965-1980	1981-1984
Title	Traditionalists, matures, veterans, seniors, silent generation	Baby boomers	Generation X, baby busters, postboomers	Generation Y, nexters, millennial generation, Internet generation
Career goals	Build a legacy	Build a stellar career	Build a portable career	Build parallel careers
Rewards	Satisfaction of a job well done	Money, title, recognition, corner office	Freedom	Meaningful work
Feedback	No news is good news	Once per year with lots of documentation	Frequent feedback	Feedback when desired
Training	Learn the hard way	Train them too much and they will leave	The more they learn, the more they stay	Continuous learning is the way of life
Balance	Support for shifting the balance	Balance others, find meaning for self	Balance now, not at age 65 years	Give flexibility to balance own activities
Retirement	Reward	Retool	Renew	Recycle
Core values	Honesty, integrity, work, family	Optimism, team orientation, personal gratification, health and wellness, personal growth	Diversity, global thinking, balance, technoliteracy, self-reliance, informality	Optimism, civic duty, confidence, achievement, sociability, morality, diversity
Assets	Loyal, hard working	Service oriented, driven, good team players	Adaptable, technoliterate, independent, creative	Act collectively, multitaskers, technically savvy, tenacious
Liabilities	Has unbalanced life, consumed by work, lacks formal education	Not budget minded, uncomfortable with conflict, reluctant to go against peers, sensitive to feedback, self-centered	Impatient, has poor people skills, inexperienced, cynical	Needs supervision and structure, inexperienced
Defining events	Depression, World War II, Korean War, New Deal, radio, silver screen, rise of labor unions	Assassinations, Vietnam War, civil rights, cold war, women's liberation, space race, Woodstock, love-ins, laugh-ins	Watergate, Challenger disaster, fall of Berlin Wall, Persian Gulf War, computers, birth control pills, less parental supervision (latchkey kids), single-parent homes	Schoolyard violence, Oklahoma City bombing, terrorism, multiculturalism, crack cocaine, AIDS epidemic, computers, television talk shows
Heroes	Charles Lindbergh, Amelia Earhart, Joe Louis, Babe Ruth	Gandhi, Martin Luther King, John Kennedy, John Glenn	None	Princess Diana, Mother Teresa, Bill Gates, Tiger Woods, Christopher Reeve

Continued

TABLE 12-3 Generational Differences—cont'd

Years	1925-1945	1946-1964	1965-1980	1981-1984
Cultural memorabilia	Radio shows, Saturday afternoon matinees, cowboy and Indian movies, serial movies, swimming hole, work	Ed Sullivan Show, fallout shelters, Slinkies, TV dinners, poodle skirts, pop beads, hula hoops, peace sign	Platform shoes, pet rocks, Cabbage Patch dolls, *ET, The Brady Bunch, Dynasty, The Simpsons*	American Girl dolls, Barney, Beanie Babies, Teenage Mutant Ninja Turtles, virtual pets, Oprah, Rosie, the Spice Girls, the X Games
Messages that motivate	"Do it or else I will use the switch", "I want you to … ," "Do it"	"We need you," "You are important," "I approve of you," "you are valued"	"We don't have many rules," "Do it your way," "We have the latest technology"	"You can be a hero here," "You can help turn this company around," "You will work with creative people"
Spending style	Cautious, conservative, spends on necessities	Buy now, pay later, pay with plastic	Cautious, conservative	Spend parents' money as fast as possible

AIDS, Acquired immunodeficiency syndrome.

Modified from Lancaster LC, Stillman D: *When generations collide*, New York, 2002, HarperCollins; and Zemke R, Raines C, Filipczak B: *Generations at work: Managing the clash of veterans, boomers, Xers, and nexters in your workplace*, New York, 2000, American Management Association.

home, and on-call work. Intelligence is believed to remain constant until at least age 70 years (Goldberg, 2000; Karp, Fuller, & Sirias, 2002; Lancaster & Stillman, 2002; Raines & Hunt, 2000; Zemke, Raines, & Filipczak, 2000).

Members of Generation X were born from around 1965 to 1980. They want to build a portable career, are rewarded by freedom, and like frequent feedback. The more they learn in an organization, the more likely they are to stay. They want balance in their lives now. They see retirement as a period of renewal. Their core values include diversity, global thinking, balance, technoliteracy, self-reliance, and informality. Their assets are adaptability, technoliteracy, independence, and creativity, whereas impatience, poor people skills, inexperience, and a cynical nature are viewed as liabilities. They are motivated by statements such as, "We don't have many rules," "Do it your way," and "We have the latest technology." The Generation Xers are self-reliant, are seeking a sense of family, and

want a balance between work and family. They like informality, approach authority casually, and have a nontraditional orientation to time and space. They may do well with management by objectives rather than a requirement to be in a specific place at a specific time. They want a fun, relaxed workplace. They want ideas to be evaluated on their merit, not on the basis of years of experience. They appreciate hands-off supervision. They do not read as much as the mature generation but use computers more and like their freedom. Thus a variety of learning materials, such as books, computer programs, CD-ROMs, audio and video materials, and face-to-face instruction, should be made available but not mandatory. Managers should be available to answer their questions when they come to the manager. They should be encouraged to think about what they have learned on a regular basis. It is good to give them mentors and lots of positive constructive feedback. Development is important to Generation Xers, so managers should let them know that this is part of the job. An employee assistance program, particularly for low-wage workers, that covers transportation, child care, language skills, financial literacy, transition to home ownership skills, and completion of paperwork for food stamps and immigration matters can help employee retention. Employees may appreciate not only child care but also convenient postage, banking, dry cleaning, and shoe repair services, and the possibility of picking up a carry-out dinner on their way home from work. Their spending habits tend to be cautious and conservative. Many are struggling to make ends meet. They are the first generation that probably will not be able to have a better lifestyle than their parents did. They will probably lose money in Social Security. They are willing to work hard but want fair pay for the hours worked and want a life beyond work (Karp, Fuller, & Sirias, 2002; Lancaster & Stillman, 2002; Raines & Hunt, 2000; Tulgan, 2000; Zemke, Raines, & Filipczak, 2000).

People born from around 1981 to 1994 may be called Generation Y or the Internet generation. They are interested in building parallel careers. They are rewarded by meaningful work and like feedback when they ask for it. They view continuous learning as a way of life and want to be given flexibility so they can balance their own activities. They see retirement as a time to recycle. Their core values include optimism, civic duty, confidence, achievement, sociability, morality, and diversity. Their assets include collective action, multitasking, technologic savvy, and tenacity, whereas their need for supervision and structure and their inexperience are seen as liabilities. They are motivated by the following messages: "You can be a hero here," "You can help turn this company around," and "You will work with creative people here." The majority of the Generation Yers were planned children, and many appreciate being wanted. Like their grandparents, they have a more strict moral code, and consequently rates of teenage pregnancy, teen abortions, drug use, drunk driving, and high school dropout are down. Unlike their parents, they expect to work more than 40 hours

per week to achieve their goals. They have an optimistic, can-do spirit. They will need plenty of orientation to the job. The long-term goals of the organization should be made clear to them. Managers should learn the goals of these personnel and try to integrate these goals with the organizational goals. This generation engages in "gender bending" as men do more of the household tasks and women assume more traditional male tasks. Generation Y has a new confidence, is the most education-minded generation in history, is leading a wave of volunteerism, and is paving the way to a more open, tolerant society. Generation Yers are comfortably self-reliant, want technology and other things right now, and desire opportunities. There is a greater generation gap than that between other generations. Their spending style is to spend their parents' money as fast as they can (Bennis, Spreitzer, & Cummings, 2001; Bennis & Thomas, 2002; Lancaster & Stillman, 2002; Raines, 2003; Raines & Hunt, 2000; Tulgan & Martin, 2001, Zemke, Raines, & Filipczak, 2000).

Tulgan and Martin (2001) have identified 14 things that Generation Yers expect their superiors to do:

1. Provide challenging work that really matters.
2. Balance clearly delegated assignments with freedom and flexibility.
3. Offer increasing responsibility as a reward for accomplishments.
4. Spend time getting to know staff members and their capabilities.
5. Provide ongoing training and learning opportunities.
6. Establish mentoring relationships.
7. Create a comfortable, low-stress environment.
8. Allow some flexibility in scheduling.
9. Focus on work but be personable and have a sense of humor.
10. Balance the roles of boss and team player.
11. Treat Generation Yers as colleagues, not as interns or "teenagers."
12. Be respectful and call forth respect in return.
13. Consistently provide constructive feedback.
14. Reward Generation Yers when they've done a good job.

ORIENTATION

Orientation is critically important for job satisfaction and retention for both new and experienced nurses and other personnel of any age who are starting a new job. Induction is the first 2 or 3 days of orientation. It can be carried out by personnel department employees for all new hires. It includes describing to new employees the history of the organization and its vision, purpose, and structure and informing them about working hours, holidays, vacation time, sick time, paydays, performance standards and evaluation, labor contracts, grievance procedures, parking facilities, eating facilities, health services, and educational opportunities. That is more information than new employees can remember. It is advisable to provide the information in a handbook and to reference the handbook during the induction. Both new employees and experienced nurses in new positions need orientation. The manager introduces the nurse to the new job, agency policies, facilities, and co-workers. Orientation is important, and the manager who does not take the time to assist a new employee is making a serious mistake.

Communicating what the regulations are and exactly what is expected of the nurse diminishes uncertainty, relieves anxiety, and prevents unnecessary misunderstandings. The employee's feeling of security usually increases when someone is considerate enough to help the employee adjust to a new situation. The manner in which nurses are treated during their first day at a new job may be critical to their future job satisfaction and performance.

Because of the potential for information overload, induction and further orientation should be conducted over time. A checklist for orientation that indicates the content, time frame, and person who is responsible for teaching the information can be helpful (Box 12-5). It is appropriate to use an orientation schedule (Box 12-6).

Orientation to the institution typically includes a tour of the facilities; a description of the organizational structure; a discussion of different departmental functions; a presentation of the organization's philosophy, goals, and standards; an interpretation of administrative policies and procedures; and possibly an explanation of the relationships of the organization with the community. Next, nurses will need an orientation to the nursing service, including interdepartmental relationships, departmental organization, administrative controls, philosophy, goals, policies, procedures, and job descriptions.

After the general orientation, new nurses may be assigned to an experienced nurse for orientation to their specific jobs. New nurses will need a tour of the unit so that they know the location of supplies, equipment, and policy and procedure books. Information about how the unit is run, specific methods of practice, and communication systems is important. Introductions to other personnel can help the new person feel welcome.

Frequent visits to see that the nurse is comfortable and that the orientation is progressing satisfactorily are helpful. Documentation of the orientation process is useful. The documentation may be a simple checklist that itemizes information such as the organizational structure, specific policies, fire and disaster plans, tour of the facilities, and procedures, with space for a signature. It can be retained in the personnel file.

Nurse internship programs are common to assist newly graduated nurses in making the adjustment from the student role to a staff nurse position. The instructor and head nurse usually work together to identify teaching-learning needs, plan rotation schedules, and evaluate the intern's performance. Classes are held on a regular basis for orientation, role adjustment, problem solving, and information about pathophysiology. There is a concentration on the mastery of technical skills. Some programs also present leadership instruction. The use of nurse internship programs helps new graduates build self-confidence, lowers frustration levels, increases nursing care planning, improves patient care, increases job satisfaction, and reduces turnover.

In-service education helps keep employees' skills and knowledge up to date. It usually involves the use of new equipment, new patient

BOX 12-5 Sample Orientation Checklist

INFORMATION/ACTIVITY	TIME FRAME	PERSON/DEPARTMENT RESPONSIBLE
History of organization	Day 1	Personnel department
Vision, purpose of organization	Day 1	Personnel department
Structure of organization	Day 1	Personnel department
Payroll information	Day 1	Personnel department
Tour of facilities	Day 1	Staff development department
Introduction to unit heads and purpose of departments	Day 1	Staff development department
Employee and organizational responsibilities, rules of conduct	Day 1	Personnel department
Fire and safety video	Day 1	Staff development department
Personnel policies	Day 2	Personnel department
Tour of unit	Day 2	Preceptor
Introductions to unit personnel	Day 2	Preceptor
Work schedules, staffing, scheduling policies	Day 2	Preceptor
Cardiopulmonary resuscitation recertification	Day 2	Staff development department
Universal precautions update	Day 2	Staff development department
Workload assignments	Day 3	Preceptor
Introduction to charting	Day 3	Preceptor
Reporting of accidents	Day 3	Preceptor
Use of services such as nutrition, occupational therapy, physical therapy, pharmacy, radiology, clinical laboratory	Day 3	Preceptor
Job description	Day 3	Preceptor
Standards of performance	Day 3	Preceptor
Staff development	Day 3	Preceptor
Employee appraisal system	Day 3	Preceptor
Promotion and transfer policies	Day 3	Preceptor
Work with preceptor while assuming more responsibility	Week 2	Preceptor

care procedures, and new services. The Joint Commission requires that nursing in-service sessions be offered on a continuing basis and that employee attendance be documented.

Near the end of the probationary period, it is advisable to have a systematic evaluation. The nurse should know what characteristics will be evaluated. Two independent judgments, such as those of the manager and a head nurse, may be secured and used to check the reliability of the evaluation. The results of the evaluation are indicative of the success of the selection process.

Orientation alone does not socialize people to the organization. Socialization is the sharing of attitudes and values through role modeling, myths, and legends. It is less structured than orientation. All employees need socialization. Instilling a clear understanding of the value system throughout the organization is the socialization process for creating team spirit that is found in excellent organizations. It is correlated with lower levels of dissatisfaction, absenteeism, and attrition (Marquis & Huston, 2006; Sullivan & Decker, 2005).

CAREER MAPPING

"If a man proceeds confidently in the direction of his dreams and endeavors to live the life he has imagined, he will meet with success unexpected in common hours." —Henry David Thoreau

BOX 12-6 Sample Orientation Schedule

DAY 1

8:00-10:00 AM   Welcome by personnel department
Delivery of employee handbook; overview of organizational history, vision, purpose, and structure; payroll information

10:00-10:15 AM   Provision of bread, coffee, and fruit
10:15-11:30 AM   Tour of facilities by staff development department
11:30 AM-12:00 PM   Introduction of unit heads and purpose of units by staff development personnel
12:00 PM-1:00 PM   Lunch with unit heads
1:00-2:15 PM   Information on employee and organizational responsibilities, rules of conduct by personnel department
2:15-2:30 PM   Break, refreshments
2:30-4:00 PM   Presentation of fire and safety video by staff development department

DAY 2

8:00-10:00 AM   Explanation of personnel policies by personnel department
10:00-10:30 AM   Arrival on unit, break with preceptor
10:30 AM-12:00 PM   Tour of unit with preceptor
12:00-1:00 PM   Introduction to unit personnel
1:00-3:30 PM   Cardiopulmonary resuscitation recertification by staff development department
3:30-4:00 PM   Universal precautions update by staff department

DAY 3

Work all day with preceptor on unit and shift
Receipt of workload assignment
Introduction to charting
Explanation of accident reporting
Guidelines for use of services such as nutrition, physical therapy, occupational therapy, pharmacy, radiology, clinical laboratory

DAY 4

Work all day with preceptor on unit and shift
Provision of job description
Clarification of standards of performance

DAY 5

Work all day with preceptor on unit and shift
Explanation of staff development practices
Description of employee appraisal system
Clarification of promotion and transfer policies

WEEK 2

Work with preceptor on unit and shift, gradual assumption of more responsibilities to full workload by day 5 of week 2

Career mapping is the development of a strategic plan for one's career. It provides a direction for formal education, experience, continuing education, professional associations, and networking. Nurses need to assess their own values and define success for themselves. Job security, sense of accomplishment, and opportunities for professional advancement are often considered important. Other issues to consider are work hours, salary, fringe benefits, retirement plans, organizational and geographic climate, and location.

Nurses also need to assess their skills. What do they do well, do poorly, want to do, not want to do, or have the potential to develop? Once they have (1) assessed interests and skills, they

RESEARCH Perspective 12-2

Data from Laborde SA, Lee JA: Skills needed for promotion in the nursing profession. *J Nurs Adm* 30(9):432-439, 2000.

Purpose: The purpose of this research was to identify the relative importance of interpersonal skills and technical skills for promotion within the nursing profession and to examine the difference between the perceived and actual importance of these skills.

Methods: A stratified random sample of 219 nurse administrators at a large southeastern United States hospital rated hypothetical candidates for managerial positions based on mailed scenarios. Respondents were assigned to upper, middle, or lower management based on the following categorization: top managers are those responsible for the operations of multiple services; middle managers are those responsible for coordinating nursing units; and first-line managers are those responsible for the production of nursing services. The beta weights of the regression equation were used to test the hypotheses. A chi-square analysis of interpersonal skills did not find a statistically significant relationship between position and number of skills used.

Results/conclusions: A larger number of technical skills were found to influence promotion to first-line management positions than to middle management positions. Interpersonal skills seemed important for promotion to all levels of management. Significant differences were found between decision makers' perceptions of a skill's importance and the skill's actual importance to promotion decisions.

should (2) determine goals, (3) develop a map, and (4) pursue strategies to maintain the map. It is appropriate to make a list of interests and skills and to establish 1-, 5-, and 10-year plans. The time frame can be illustrated in a career map with a 10-year time period across the top of the paper. Then years of specific experience can be written in under "Dates" and types of education can be entered under "Experiences." The individual might focus on continuing education classes for a time or work on an advanced degree during certain periods.

Ongoing maintenance of the map will reflect advancement efforts: writing, personal presentations, networking, and professional development. The curriculum vitae and the résumé are used interchangeably to present the individual in writing. A curriculum vitae is a listing of educational, professional, and scholarly accomplishments and is most commonly used in academic settings. A résumé is a concise history of education and experiences in a few pages. The vitae should have an attractive format and contain information such as professional goal, education, work experience, professional memberships, continuing education, research, publications, and presentations. If there have been no accomplishments in a category to date it is best to omit that category from the vitae. Résumés are updated periodically, especially when the individual is applying for a job. It is helpful to keep information files listing continuing education, organizational memberships, offices, committees, research, publications, and presentations so that accurate information is available for updating the résumé. A cover letter should accompany a résumé to introduce the sender and explain the purpose for sending the résumé, such as interest in a different position or application for an award.

The applicant must appear in person for an interview. One-on-one interviews are common. The applicant is typically asked the following questions: What are your goals? What are your strengths and weaknesses? Why do you want to work here? What do you have to offer this agency? In serial interviews the applicant sees one person after another. Looking attractive, having a positive attitude, remaining consistent, and treating each interviewer as if that person alone will make the decision are appropriate. Serial interviews become increasingly common as a person applies for jobs higher in the hierarchy. The interviewers are interested in the interrelationship with their specific areas of responsibility. The applicant's communication skills are tested during group interviews, when several people interview the applicant at once. Stress interviews are sometimes used to test an applicant's reactions to stress. They may leave a very negative feeling about the job; the applicant should try to remember that such a test is not a personal attack.

It is helpful to network with colleagues inside and outside the organization. Nurses should identify individuals who have influence over their career, who can serve as mentors, who can provide career guidance, and who can serve as references. They should join professional organizations to meet colleagues with similar interests. They should volunteer for committee work. They should attend conventions and meetings. Business cards should be made and exchanged with colleagues. They should keep in touch with colleagues, ask for what they need, give feedback, and follow up with contacts.

Careers typically progress through the stages of exploration, early career trial and establishment, middle career growth and maintenance, and later career plateau and decline. The exploration stage includes identifying the right career and getting the appropriate education. The early career involves getting the first job, adjusting to a daily work routine, choosing a specialty, receiving transfers and promotions, and broadening the perspective of the organization and profession. During the middle career people establish their professional identities, choose among alternative career paths, and take on more responsibility. In the later career people train others, shape the future of the organization, plan for retirement, deal with a reduced workload and less power, and may help prepare their replacement through succession planning.

Exploration typically occurs during ages 15 to 22 years, early career during ages 22 to 38 years, middle career from 38 to 55 years, and later career from 55 to 70 years. However, some women raise a family before they start the exploration stage, and many interrupt their careers to raise a family. It is more common for women than for men to have discontinuous careers because of family responsibilities. People may change careers during their lifetimes too.

The individual progresses in professional development by systematically reviewing professional journals, collecting and filing articles and materials topically, developing a professional library, attending continuing education offerings, achieving professional certification, chairing a committee to develop leadership skills, presenting an in-service session, and fostering a support group.

Career Ladders and Performance Management Plans

"There are two educations, one should teach us how to make a living and the other how to live." —John Adams

Zimmer (1972) designed a clinical ladder to create a work environment that would nurture and challenge professional growth and recognize clinical excellence to meet the professional's needs for growth and recognition and the institution's requirement for a stable, experienced nursing staff. It was a ladder for clinical advancement with rungs for vertical advancement that provided recognition for nurses who chose to stay at the bedside. Clinical ladders evolved into career ladders and proliferated during the 1970s and early 1980s. Career programs varied from simple two-level clinical ladders to multitrack and multilevel systems that include provisions for evaluation. The concept has declined and reemerged.

Advantages of career ladders include potential to increase positive self-image, increase motivation, improve personal and professional satisfaction, provide opportunity for professional growth, provide a system of rewards for accomplishments, encourage development of peer review, improve recruitment and retention, and improve cost-effectiveness through lower attrition rate and retention of experienced nurses. A five-hospital system evaluation of a clinical ladder program provided information related to costs, financial impact, and benefits that help justify the salary increments for ladder programs (Drenkard & Swartwout, 2005). The satisfaction, nurse retention, and cost savings caused by reduced turnover justify the cost of the salary increments for the ladder programs. Lack of recognition for work performance has been one of the biggest barriers to staff satisfaction and consequently contributes to turnover. In the early 2000s, it was estimated that it cost $42,000 to replace a medical-surgical nurse and $64,000 to replace a specialty RN because of the cost to recruit, hire, and orient to higher skill level requirements (Drenkard & Swartwout, 2005). The clinical ladder programs recognize, reward, and retain professional nurses who choose to remain in direct clinical practice.

Potential problems with career ladders include the difficulty of designing them and their potential negative psychological effect. A newly hired experienced nurse may enter the career ladder at the same level as an inexperienced, newly graduated nurse. There may be fewer monetary differences between clinical levels than between administrative levels. Competency is difficult to define, and nurses on tracks may be evaluated by administrators instead of peers (Zimmer, 1972).

During the 1990s, career management plans based on management by objectives emerged. These plans can involve identifying the vision, mission, strategies, and core competencies needed to accomplish the strategies that are consistent with the values of the organization. Forms can be developed to help identify and track the desired outcomes or objectives, desired behaviors, information sources such as reports, self-assessment and feedback from others, actual behavior, and degree of achievement when the actual behavior is compared with the desired behavior. Then a developmental plan can be prepared by identifying the behavior to be enhanced, describing developmental activities, and specifying what is to be done by whom by when. An interim review

and coaching log can be maintained. There can be an end-of-cycle review noting employee's and manager's comments with the dated signature of each.

DEVELOPMENT OF PERSONNEL AND SUCCESSION PLANNING

"Cultivation to the mind is as necessary as food to the body." —Anonymous

Career planning focuses on what is best for individuals within the organization. Succession planning focuses on what is best for the organization and involves organizational assessments, action plans, and mechanisms to identify employees with leadership potential (Bonczek & Woodard, 2006). Key components of succession planning include development of an organizational plan with targeted roles and skills needed through out the agency and personalized plans for the development of targeted individuals and groups (Redman, 2006). The goal goes beyond just replacing people. It is continuity to ensure strategic and operational effectiveness. Once the target role has been identified, finding the right person is important. Getting affirmation from the person's boss and assessment of interest and agreement from the individual is critical. After these approvals are obtained, it is appropriate to have the person work with a formal or informal coach or preceptor with appropriate resources allocated for the leadership development (Bennis, 2006; Beyers, 2006; Blouin, McDonagh, Neistadt, et al, 2006).

Coaches need to be sensitive to the generational cultural differences. As noted earlier, there are four generations currently working. These are the veterans, baby boomers, Generation X, and Generation Y. The veterans may be willing to be coached if they understand the need for change and respect the leader. The baby boomers generally like coaching to help meet their goals and provide lifelong learning. Generation Xers may view the coach as a surrogate parent to help them assimilate into the workplace culture while bypassing the politics. Generation Y people are generally happy to be coached (Cadmus, 2006).

Personnel must be developed at all levels in an organization. In fact, the Veterans Health Administration facility has a three facility-level succession plan and individual development programs in place (Goudreau & Hardy, 2006). There is also an electronic database of nurse leaders ready for leadership assignments (Weiss & Drake, 2007) Nurse researchers also need mentoring (Lynn, 2006). Walrath and Theodoropoulos (2004) reported three initiatives implemented at Virginia Hospital Center. The accelerated patient care assistant program provided 96 hours of classes and 80 hours of clinical experience in 6 weeks. Individuals received tuition and their salary during the class and clinical experiences. In return, they were to remain employed with the hospital for at least 6 months. The workforce enhancement program offered employees an opportunity to participate in a certificate-granting program or to earn credits toward an associate degree. The general education requirements could be completed in 1 year at the hospital site. A student nurse mentorship program was used to recruit and retain graduate nurses. The program did decrease the turnover among mentorship participants (Nelson, Godfrey, & Purdy, 2004).

Graduate nurses experience stress in transitioning from student to practicing professional nurse. Research results indicated that nurses did not feel confident, comfortable, or skilled for the first year after being hired, which indicates that extended orientation and support programs are necessary to facilitate successful entry into practice (Casey, Fink, Krugman, et al, 2004). Personnel at the University of Michigan Health System developed "preceptor action days" that included coaching, education, and skill training in how to be a preceptor for more than 400 RN preceptors. The program contributed to a 68% decrease in RN vacancy rate over a 2-year period. Satisfaction with preceptors increased over that time (Baggot, Hensinger, Parry, et al, 2005).

McNally and Lukens (2006) used an internal and external coach partnerships to provide individual and group coaching to 64 clinical leaders at Multicare Health System. The external coaches were perceived to be more objective and a source of broader experiences. They had exposure to many experiences by serving multiple clients, and coaching was often their only job. The disadvantages of external coaches were that they are difficult to locate and they require work and time up front to learn the nuances of the given organization. Internal coaches know the culture and policies of the organization and already have a credible reputation. Unfortunately, coaching may simply be added to other responsibilities, which leaves less time and energy for coaching as well as the other responsibilities. A combination of both internal and external coaches was considered the best solution. Developmental strategies such as application of a variety of management and leadership tools, clarification of roles, dialogue, feedback, on-the-job-training, teaching, and referral to other departmental resources were used. Topics included building accountability, developing one's career, making decisions, determining vision, discerning authority, promoting personal well-being, modeling values, providing a leadership presence, and running effective meetings. Similar projects had considerably increased productivity.

There have been several attempts to make it easier for employees to obtain nursing education. Hackensack University Medical Center used a trilevel system that (1) provided a financial support base, (2) established partnerships with academic institutions, and (3) provided incentives to encourage nurses to pursue certifications and advanced degrees. Salaries were differentiated by educational level (Cheung & Aiken, 2006).

Taking the classroom to the nurses was one technique used in education and practice partnerships. North Shore–Long Island Jewish Health System partnered with educational institutions to offer RN to bachelor of science in nursing (BSN) and master's programs for nurses on site. Assessment indicated that the practical barriers to obtaining a baccalaureate degree faced by RNs were too high. These barriers included program focus on the traditional post–high school graduate without work or family obligations, interference of class times with work schedules, time-consuming commutes, and financial obligations. St. Mary Medical Center administration did a similar approach and arranged for academic programs to be offered on site so that students could complete an accelerated RN to BSN program in 18 months (Cheung & Aiken, 2006).

Premier Health Partners needed educational programs to graduate more nurses in less time. Selected employees attended a 15-month long program in return for a 3-year work commitment. Computer-assisted classrooms were developed to facilitate educational programs (Cheung & Aiken, 2006).

The Children's Hospital of Philadelphia provided clinical scholarships to staff to complete an on-site BSN program in 18 to 24 months. Classes met weekly. On-site certification courses were also offered two to three times a year. A Future Nurses Club had RNs inviting employees from nonnursing areas to meet monthly. Registered nurses served as preceptors to introduce the employees to various clinical and professional aspects of patient care so people could make informed career decisions (Cheung & Aiken, 2006).

At the Mayo Clinic in Phoenix, baccalaureate- and master's-prepared staff nurses could be offered the opportunity to be chosen as adjunct faculty for Arizona State University. The university provided the resources to prepare the RNs for their new role. The Mayo Clinic provided classroom and clinical space where their own staff would teach 20 nursing students pursuing a baccalaureate degree. The hope was that the graduates would join the Mayo staff and that the staff would be enriched from the teaching experience (Cheung & Aiken, 2006).

The University of Pittsburgh Medical Center developed a Health Care Leadership Academy for nurses with high potential (Wolf, Bradle, & Nelson, 2005). Many schools of nursing have started clinical nurse leadership programs, and nurses in practice and in education are partnering to develop the future nursing administration curricula (Harris, Huber, Jones, et al, 2006).

Staff development goes beyond orientation. It is a continuing liberal education of the whole person to develop the individual's potential fully. It promotes aesthetic sensibilities as well as providing technical and professional training and may include orientation, preceptorships, mentorships, skill checklists, internships, in-service education, continuing education, courses, conferences, seminars, journal or book clubs, programmed learning, computer modules, independent study, formal education, refresher courses, and career development.

Nurse managers play an important role in the support of staff development and have a responsibility to review the goals of the staff development program and to provide a budget for development activities. They can engage in coaching by sharing ideas and telling stories about what it takes to succeed. They invest in relationships and plan stretch goals collaboratively with staff. They participate in needs identification and analyze how education effects change in nursing services. They then develop doable projects and actions to deal with the identified needs, delegate tasks to people according to their interests and talents, and provide feedback (Hargrove, 2000).

In addition, they must be careful to differentiate staff development needs from administrative needs. If staff nurses know how to do a procedure properly but do not do it because the necessary supplies and equipment are not available to them, the need is administrative rather than educational. Nursing managers are legally liable for the quality of nursing services. Their ability to document staff development provides strong supportive evidence for them. Employee receptiveness to staff development efforts depends largely on the reward system developed. Positive reinforcement through recognition, such as oral praise on the unit or acknowledgment of accomplishments in a newsletter, is useful. Staff development can also be linked to retention, pay raises, advancement to other positions, or termination. The novice-to-expert theory can be used to guide staff development (Benner, 1984; Hargrove, 2000; Jacobs & Osman-Gani, 2006; Wilson, 2005).

Preceptorship

*"To encourage others is to strengthen
the team." —Anonymous*

Preceptorships may be used to help recruit, retain, orient, and develop staff. They may be used before students graduate to orient them to the agency and to recruit them for hire. If students have worked at an agency before graduation and are familiar with it, they can make more sound decisions about where to work, are not as likely to be unprepared for the work situation, and consequently are likely to be retained longer. The preceptorship also gives agency personnel an opportunity to evaluate students and determine if they are suitable candidates for employment.

During the preceptorship, faculty members facilitate, monitor, and evaluate student learning. Faculty members direct students to resources, offer suggestions regarding patient care problems, and lead discussions at conferences. Faculty members are responsible for student learning and encourage students to apply class content.

The preceptor is responsible for the quality of patient care and facilitates the student's learning. Preceptors are liaisons between students and the agency. They help students learn skills and learn how to organize their work. They provide real-life experiences for students before graduation to help reduce the difficulties of transition from school to work.

The professional nurturance of a preceptorship can be likened to the "good old boy" network or to godparents who look after godchildren. The preceptorship allows students to use and augment their knowledge and skills so they can assume increasing responsibilities. They gain experience with a variety of patients and different levels of staff. They have opportunities to discuss and adjust to professional-bureaucratic conflicts. Preceptorships are a potential recruitment tool for the agency and can increase the job satisfaction of nurses. Preceptors may even learn from the students and are likely to find the preceptor role challenging and stimulating.

There are also disadvantages to preceptorships. They add to staff nurses' responsibilities and require time. Sometimes busy nurses have little time to spend with students. It becomes difficult for faculty members to evaluate students because they have little direct observation of the students' work. The use of preceptors requires considerable planning and coordination. Role descriptions should clarify who chooses learning experiences for the student, who supervises the student, and who evaluates the student. Practical tools for evaluating the student, preceptor, and faculty should be developed and used. Educational and service administrative support is needed.

The faculty member serves as a preceptor of preceptors. Holding a workshop to prepare preceptors is desirable. It is appropriate to discuss and clarify role descriptions, skill inventory lists for students, and guidelines for preceptor evaluation of students. Information about teaching methods, counseling, and evaluation is useful. Finding a time and place for the workshop and getting release time for the preceptors may create problems. Awarding continuing education credits for the workshop and preceptor experience may be considered as a way to reward preceptors.

The preceptor model can also be used by the staff development department for nurses after a graduate has been hired. The staff development faculty may present formal content in orientation and development programs that is reinforced by preceptors on the units. Preceptors can also be used for succession planning as nurses progress through their careers. Recruitment and retention of well-qualified nurses provides a return on investment that can be used to justify the costs of recruitment and retention efforts (Baggot, Dawson, Valdes, et al, 2005; Baggot, Hensinger, Parry, et al, 2005).

Mentorship

*"I hear and I forget. I see and I remember.
I do and I understand." —Confucius*

Preceptors are role models who may become mentors. Mentors give their time, energy, and material support to teach, guide, assist, counsel, and inspire other nurses. It is a nurturing relationship that cannot be forced. Close, trusted counselors, usually in their forties or fifties, acquaint younger nurses, usually in their twenties or thirties, with the values, customs, and resources of the profession. The mentor is a confidant who personalizes role modeling and serves as a sounding board for decisions. The mentor is a resource person who supports the development of the younger person through influence and promotion.

There are phases to the mentoring process (Box 12-7). At first, during the invitational stage, mentors must be willing to use their time and energy to nurture someone who is goal directed, willing to learn, and respectfully trusting of the mentor. The younger professionals have a career goal, a vision of what they want to become; the mentors are people who have reached that goal and are willing to share the secrets of their success. Then there is a period of questioning, when the younger person has self-doubt and fears of being unable to meet the goals. The mentor helps clarify those goals and provide guidance. Next, mentors share information about power and politics, tell how they became successful, and serve as a sounding board. The transitional phase is the final phase, in which mentors help students

---

BOX 12-7 Phases of the Mentoring Process

INVITATIONAL

Mentor uses time and energy to nurture a younger professional who is goal directed, willing to learn, and respectfully trusting of mentor.

QUESTIONING

Mentored individual experiences self-doubt and questions goals. Mentor helps clarify goals and provides guidance.

TRANSITIONAL

Mentor helps younger professional personalize learning and become aware of own strengths and uniqueness. Mentored individual is now prepared to be a mentor.

---

personalize learning and become aware of their own strengths and uniqueness. Younger nurses are then prepared to be mentors and to tell others how they became what they are.

Mentorship should provide an opportunity to share information, review work, provide feedback, explore issues, plan strategies, and solve problems. It helps socialize novices into professional norms, values, and standards. Career advancement and success are promoted, which increases self-confidence, self-esteem, and personal satisfaction.

GROUP PROCESS

"Two heads are better than one." —Old adage

Group process is critical for group and team development. How the group functions, communicates, and sets and achieves objectives is related to group dynamics. Both task-oriented behavior and maintenance-oriented behavior are necessary for adequate group development. Teams function at a higher level of cooperative productivity than groups, but they need to go through the group development process to become proficient.

People who assume group task roles coordinate and facilitate the group's efforts to identify the problem, explore alternative options, identify the ramifications of the options, choose the most viable option, and implement and evaluate the plan. There are numerous group task roles, and any member of the group may fulfill a number of these roles at different times (Box 12-8).

Initiators-contributors propose new ideas or different ways of approaching a problem. Their task is to identify the problem, clarify the objectives, offer solutions, suggest agenda items, and set time limits. Information seekers search for factual information about the problem, whereas opinion seekers clarify values pertinent to the problem and its solutions. Unlike information seekers, information givers identify facts, share experiences, and make generalizations.

BOX 12-8 Group Process Roles

GROUP TASK ROLES	GROUP MAINTENANCE ROLES	DYSFUNCTIONAL ROLES
Initiator-contributor	Gatekeeper	Aggressor
Information seeker	Encourager	Dominator
Opinion seeker	Harmonizer	Recognition seeker
Information giver	Compromiser	Special-interest pleader
Opinion giver	Follower	Blocker
Elaborator	Group observer	Self-confessor
Coordinator	Standard setter	Help seeker
Orienter		Playboy
Critic		
Energizer		
Procedural technician		
Recorder		

Opinion givers state their beliefs and what they think the group should value. Their focus is on values rather than on facts. Elaborators develop suggestions, illustrate points, and predict outcomes. Coordinators clarify relationships. Orienters summarize the discussion, activities, and points of departure to provide perspective on the group's progress toward its goal. Critics may measure the group's achievement against a set of standards and evaluate the problem, content, and process. Energizers stimulate the group to increase the quantity and quality of their work. Procedural technicians facilitate group action by arranging the room for the meeting, distributing the materials, working the audiovisual equipment, and generally functioning as the "go-for"—the person who obtains for what is needed. Recorders keep an account of the discussion, suggestions, and decisions.

The roles of group building and group maintenance focus on how people treat each other while accomplishing a task. Gatekeepers regulate communication and take actions to ensure that everyone has an opportunity to be heard. Encouragers radiate warmth and approval. They offer commendation and praise and indicate acceptance and understanding of others' ideas and values. Harmonizers create and maintain group cohesion, relieving tension through their sense of humor and helping others reconcile their disagreements. Compromisers promote group process by yielding status, admitting mistakes, modifying their ideas for the sake of group cohesiveness, maintaining self-control for group harmony, or generally making compromises to keep the group action oriented. Followers, acting as a passive audience, go along with the group. Group observers keep records of the group process and give interpretations for evaluation of the proceedings. The quality of the group process is compared with standards by the standard setters.

Some members of the group may try to satisfy their individual needs irrespective of the group tasks or maintenance roles. For example, aggressors meet their needs at the expense of others by disapproving of others and deflating their status. Dominators assert authority or superiority by using flattery, interrupting others, and giving directions authoritatively. Recognition seekers call attention to themselves by boasting and acting in unusual ways. Special-interest pleaders speak for an interest group and address issues that best meet that group's needs. Blockers are negative, resistant, and disagreeable without apparent reason and bring issues back to the floor after the group has rejected them. Self-confessors use the group to voice personal feelings, whereas help seekers express self-deprecation, insecurity, and personal confusion to elicit sympathetic responses. Playboys lack involvement in the group process and appear nonchalant. A high incidence of dysfunctional role playing in a group requires self-diagnosis to suggest what group training efforts are needed. Having a trained observer record who is acting out what roles during a meeting can be revealing. An observer records each time a participant plays a certain role. Use of a form with a list of roles down the left side and columns with the names of participants across the top can be helpful (Marquis & Huston, 2006; Roussel, Swansburg, & Swansburg, 2006; Sullivan & Decker, 2005).

"In our age, independence and the ability to get things done are often mutually exclusive." —John Dilenschneider

---

TEAM DEVELOPMENT

"An investment in knowledge pays the best interest." —Benjamin Franklin

---

Just as there are differences between individuals and groups, there are differences between groups and teams (Robbins, 2000) (Box 12-9). Teams are clusters of people that function at a higher level than a group. Groups go through stages of development but are not yet a team (Drinka & Clark, 2000) (Box 12-10). Groups typically form, organize, solve problems, implement solutions, and disband. During the formation stage, individuals are likely to feel anxious, fearful, doubtful, and self-protective. The leader concentrates on putting the members at ease, explaining the purpose, developing a workable climate, and exerting leadership. During the organizing or storming stage, tension tends to be high; suspiciousness, hostility, and resistance are common; and disagreement emerges with the power struggles that occur. The leader needs to clarify goals, policies and procedures, code of conduct, and communication patterns to help the members' progress. Loyalty, trust, confidence, dignity, pride, and group cohesiveness develop during problem solving stage. The leader seeks to approve recommendations by consensus through a systematic and logical approach.

BOX 12-9 Differences between Groups and Teams

GROUP
Information sharing
Possible absence of common objectives shared by all members
Tendency to have majority and minority opinions
Destructive criticism
Concealment of personal feelings
Little discussion about how the group is functioning
Actions by individuals to protect their roles and niches
Individual accountability
Members with varied and random skills
Neutral and sometimes negative energy
Leadership that is appointed or elected

TEAM
Collective performance goals
Objectives that are understood and accepted by members
Decision making by consensus with members heard and valued
Dialogue with resolution
Free expression accompanied by listening
Self-examination about team functioning
Understood roles
Individual and mutual accountability
Members with complementary skills
Synergy
Shared leadership

Modified from Robbins SP: *Organization behavior: Concepts, controversies, applications*, ed 9, Upper Saddle River, NJ, 2000, Prentice Hall.

A group in which individualism prevails is like a group of sprinters who are uncoordinated, all working toward a goal individualistically. A group working at the coordination level is like a relay team in which there is coordinated but independent effort. A group operating at the group dynamics level resembles a rowing crew that puts a concerted effort toward a goal (Robbins, 2000).

The team has structure and purpose, roles are clarified, and interpersonal relationships are stabilized during the performing stage. The

---

BOX 12-10 Stages of Group Development

Form
Storm
Norm
Perform
Adjourn

Data from Drinka TJK, Clark PG: *Health care teamwork: Interdisciplinary practice and teaching*, Westport, CT, 2000, Auburn House.

BOX 12-11 Key Components of Effective Teams

Clear sense of direction
Talented members
Clear and enticing responsibilities
Efficient operating procedures
Constructive interpersonal relationships
Active reinforcement system
Constructive external relationships

Data from Huszczo GE: *Tools for team excellence: Getting your team into high gear and keeping it there*, Mumbai, 2005, Jaico Publishing House.

---

leader should help the team focus on issues, behaviors, or problems, not on a person. The leader should encourage team members to help build self-confidence and self-esteem of others, maintain constructive relationships, and take the initiative to make things better. The leader should lead by example. Members may have positive or negative feelings about disbanding. The leader should express appreciation and give positive reinforcement (Drinka & Clark, 2000; Marquis & Huston, 2006; Roussel, Swansburg, & Swansburg, 2006; Sullivan & Decker, 2005).

The team is empowered to do what is required. The team members need to know the purpose of the team, the goals, and the targets for accomplishment. Setting goals and planning strategies to meet the goals are important. There should be plans to measure accomplishments (Box 12-11).

The leader should recruit and hire talented people. The inventory of talent on the team should be known. Team members should know each other's strengths and weaknesses. Team members need to continually develop their knowledge and skills. Although the organizations should use selection procedures and provide training and educational opportunities, individual team members have responsibility for updating their own knowledge and skills as well. Team members should know their roles and develop themselves to fulfill those roles. Active listening, problem solving, conflict management, communication skills, assertiveness, and basic teamwork are important skills to learn.

Teams need policies and procedures defining a disciplined but not overly rigid way to get things done. Ground rules help facilitate group process and may include rules such as the following: One person speaks at a time by waiting for a person to finish speaking and not interrupting others. Keep comments to the point by staying on the topic. Avoid lengthy stories and examples. Express views openly and honestly. Speak for yourself and use "I" statements. Maintain confidentiality of opinions expressed in the meeting. Focus on issues, not on individuals. Encourage everyone to participate. Respect differences of opinion (Brounstein, 2003; Payne, 2001).

It is also helpful for team members to be familiar with their own and each other's personalities. This helps people understand better how to work with each other. Self-assessment is a first step in career development because it is important for individuals to know who they are before they figure out what they want to do. Use of the *Myers-Briggs Type Indicator* can help individuals understand themselves better and can help team members plan strategies for resolving conflicts among themselves. The four dichotomous Myers-Briggs indicators are based on Carl Jung's work. They are extroversion and introversion, sensing and intuiting, thinking and feeling, and judging and perceiving (Table 12-4). Extroverts prefer to focus on other people and things and the energy flow is outward, whereas introverts prefer to focus on their own thoughts and ideas and the energy flow is inward. The sensing individual prefers to receive data primarily from the five senses, whereas the intuiting person prefers to receive data from the subconscious and

TABLE 12-4 Myers-Briggs Type Dichotomous
Indicators

Extroversion	Introversion
Sensing	Intuiting
Thinking	Feeling
Judging	Perceiving

sees relationships through insights. The thinking judgment function uses logical true-false or if-then connections, whereas the feeling judgment function uses "more or less" and "better or worse" evaluations. Thinkers use their heads, whereas feelers use their hearts. *Judging* does not mean *judgmental*, and *perceiving* does not mean *perceptive*. Rather, people who engage in judging are extroverted and tend to use the left brain to work step by step, usually following external rules and procedures, and want quick closure. People who engage in perceiving are introverted, tend to use the right brain, and may desire subjective judgments and want to leave options open (Barr & Barr, 1989)

The extrovert deals with the outside world, people, and things, and prefers active interaction. The extrovert is usually talkative and outgoing, refers to others as friends, and is sociable with many other people. Extroverts like meeting new people and having new experiences. They are energized by activity and react to stress primarily by increasing their activity. They make quick decisions, like brainstorming, gathering information quickly, and stimulate communications. They are able to switch gears easily, don't mind interruptions, and give good spontaneous responses. They are good at interacting socially in groups, stimulating ideas, and instigating action.

Introverts deal with the inner world of ideas, thoughts, and meanings, and prefer to be reflective. They are usually quiet and reserved. They are introspective, have a few friends, and refer to others as acquaintances. They are likely to avoid meeting new people and undergoing new experiences. They react to stress primarily by decreasing activity and are energized by depth and intimacy. Introverts gather information thoroughly, engage in deep concentration, and

make decisions that are well thought out. They have responsible, in-depth opinions, use discretion in talking, focus on subject matter, and bring talk back to the topic. They are tenacious, serious, and focused with long attention spans. They are good at one-on-one interaction and persuasive with sound logic. They have a calm, quiet manner in developing ideas and keeping confidences.

Extroverts can improve their communications with introverts by respecting privacy, giving introverts time to think about ideas and decisions, and not putting them in the spotlight. Introverts should be asked questions because they are not likely to volunteer information. Their confidences should be kept. Extroverts should think before they speak, give more substantive information and engage in less small talk, let introverts know when they are considering ideas or making decisions, and identify what they intend to do. They should pay attention to what the introverts are doing and saying, because introverts give subtle signals that are easy for an extrovert to overlook.

Introverts can improve communication with extroverts by showing interest, emotion, and involvement, and by giving feedback. They can respond more both verbally and nonverbally, control their annoyance with nonpurposeful talk, and add value from the process of interacting rather than the quality of the ideas. Introverts need to be more spontaneous, respond more quickly, not talk too long, and invite an extrovert to an active event.

Sensers are practical, concrete, realistic, and focused on the present; prefer factual interpretations; and tend to be physically competitive. Sensers are results-oriented, produce steadily, and do not like change, long-range planning, or ambiguity. They are sensible, prefer specific step-by-step routines, and prefer concrete examples and facts. Sensers take notes, make a list, write, organize and outline, analyze facts, and set priorities, goals, and objectives. They observe body language, compare, and judge. They separate the parts of a problem and put them back in order, look for details, and focus on the facts of the situation. They use machines, look at clocks, and shake hands. They are idea driven, factual, and idea testers. They prefer to make improvements incrementally, have strong expectations, have preprogrammed viewpoints based on norms and experiences, and see details in a linear fashion.

Sensers' strengths are that they like observable facts; like information explained step by step; prefer the practical, the realistic, and the present; prefer the tried and tested; demand proof; like to get things done; command others; and like competition. Sensers' weaknesses are they may overlook implications and meanings, may not see the guiding principle behind the information, may reject new or innovative ideas, may not see future demands in time, may use obsolete methods or techniques, may miss opportunities while waiting for proof, many cut too many corners, may push too hard, may do things too quickly, may not discuss or ask enough questions or take the time to build group support, and may compete over unimportant issues, become driven, and translate noncompetitive activities into a win-lose situation.

Intuitors are abstract, conceptual, idealistic, focused on the future, prefer interpretating things in terms of possibilities, and tend to be intellectually competitive. Intuitors see patterns, picture the meaning, and integrate the big picture. They respond to body language, feel the subtle relationships, discover convergent and divergent points of view, and find innovative approaches. They draw, use symbols to picture ideas, and arrange ideas, things, or spaces. They see the relationships between people and the parts of the whole problem and relate to their presence. They tend to unfocus and get an intuitive feel for the situation and check the meanings, the flavor, and the general feel of the situation. Intuitors are improvement driven, instinctual, idea generators. They make conceptual leaps. They prefer to make improvements by changing systems, structure, and procedures. They scan for general impressions, reject preprogrammed viewpoints, look for new views, and act simultaneously.

The intuitors' strengths are thinking quickly, reading between the lines, using "big picture"

thinking while synthesizing random data, conceptualizing easily, seeing possibilities, recognizing patterns, and developing systems for achieving work. Intuitors are visionary and individualistic, and works in burst of energy with good productivity. Intuitors' weaknesses are that they may skim information and therefore miss essential variables and omit facts, may leave things dangling, may include too many topics, and may be scattered and unfocused. They may overrate possibilities and see secondary instead of primary patterns, and may be impractical, too independent, and ego centered. They may be unrealistic about the time required to do the work and may find routine tasks tedious and get bored easily.

Thinkers have not developed feeling awareness in their judgment process and are critical, skeptical, cold, insensitive, and judgmental. Thinkers' strengths are that they prefer the analytical, logical, and expressive; value logic; handle emergencies logically; explain thoroughly and probe deeply into an issue; and prefer to keep remarks objective and impersonal. Their weaknesses are that thinkers may analyze instead of internalizing while trying to avoid emotional expression; may undervalue the role of feelings in motivating people; may appear cold and insensitive; may overexplain and ask too many questions; may try to force feelings to be what they should be or suppress them so they do not interfere with objective, rational expression; may appear insincere and unaffectionate; and may be overly formal.

Feelers have not developed thinkers' awareness and are confused, gullible, moody, overly sensitive, and unpredictable. Feelers' strengths are that they like to support and give to others, share emotional sensitivity, behave demonstratively and expressively, see the people perspective, interpret events as they affect people, charm and persuade, can identify people's initial interest, give descriptive accounts of a situation or event, willingly overextend to help, identify with people's feelings, and like to communicate. Feelers' weaknesses are that they may give and support indiscriminately; may collect too much emotional data and become overloaded with feelings that distort perceptions; may give away too much information, time, and energy; may oversimplify and overpersonalize; may rely too much on charm and not enough on preparation; may take too long getting to the main point; may be too imprecise to get the message across; may be too disorderly in presenting information; may tell too many anecdotes and stories; may burn out and drop into self-pity; may overreact and hold grudges; and may spend too much time in conversations.

Judgers want closure, want to finish, prefer advance notice, like to do things ahead of time, like scheduling and working according to the plan, control time, prefer decisiveness, are goal directed, and want only essential information for the plan.

Perceivers want to "hang loose," want to stay open for something new, enjoy spontaneous challenges, control their own participation, like to start the process and adjust it as needed, like to do things at the last minute, prefer to postpone decisions to see if they really need to be made, want ample information to explore options, adapt and change, and are process oriented (Barr & Barr, 1989).

The *Keirsey Temperament Sorter* can also help in understanding people. The Myers-Briggs Type Indicator focuses on how people think and feel, whereas the Keirsey Temperament Sorter focuses on how people behave. Keirsey identified four temperaments: (1) Artisans are observant and pragmatic. Their greatest strength is their skill in tactical variation. They are good at expediting and improvising. (2) Guardians are observant and cooperative. Their greatest strength is logistical intelligence good for organizing, checking, facilitating, and supporting. (3) Idealists are introspective and cooperative. Their strengths are clarifying, individualizing, inspiring, and unifying. They make good healers, counselors, and teachers. (4) Rationals are introspective and pragmatic. Their greatest strength is strategic intelligence. They make good masterminds and inventors. One can find Jungian, Myers-Briggs Type Indicator, and Keirsey Temperament Sorter assessment forms on the Internet.

Validating different values and motives, building respect for diverse points of view, and integrating a range of perspectives into decision making by ensuring that all team members participate are important. Symbols such as shirts, jackets, or hats can be used to emphasize team identity.

Team members should respect and appreciate each other. It is also important for the organization to have an evaluation and reward system for reinforcing desirable behaviors. Team members need to understand that they should not badmouth each other. They also need to develop diplomatic ties with key players outside their own team (Huszczo, 2005).

Organizational cultures that are people oriented, goal directed, and quality driven are conducive to team development (Box 12-12). The role of the manager in the development of self-managing teams is as follows:

- Show a willingness to help establish teams.
- Set goals and expectations.
- Monitor performance.
- Give the team feedback to help it self-correct as it proceeds.
- Build relationships.
- Train and educate team members.
- Acquire needed resources, such as education, consultation, supplies, and equipment.
- Allow processing time.
- Protect the team from the political obstacles and roadblocks that may occur when people in the hierarchy feel threatened because they believe they are losing decision-making power (Box 12-13).

BOX 12-12 Characteristics of Cultures That Support Teams

Value employees' interpersonal requirements
Promote cooperative rather than competitive relationships
Encourage individual accountability and responsibility
Recognize individual contributions
Have positive visions of the future
Have short- and long-term goals
Have quality standards
Believe in their products and services
Are people oriented
Support the community

BOX 12-13 Benefits of Self-Managed Teams

Increased productivity
Commitment to the organization
Commitment to the job
Common commitment to goals and values
Increased effort toward stated goals
Shared ownership and responsibility for tasks
Proactive approach to problems
Faster response to change
Increased employee development
Flexible work practices
Motivation through peer pressure rather than management mandates
Less need for management interventions
Increased employee satisfaction
Better work climate
Synergy

The manager can help ensure the team's success during its infancy by selecting members who work well together, are mature problem solvers, have positive attitudes, are future oriented, are willing to take risks, and are interested in working on a self-managing team. The leader should meet privately with an ineffective team player and confront the person about the undesirable behavior. The leader should listen to understand the other person's point of view, reestablish team norms, and negotiate an agreement on a new behavior. Positive reinforcement should be given for desirable changes. If the person's behavior remains ineffective, reassignment for a better fit and dismissal are options.

Building a successful experience is also important. Documenting and communicating success make it easier to take the next steps. Verbal feedback to the organization about the successes of the team is very powerful. The manager should make sure that the commitment, time, and resources are available for success. The manager should encourage the team to go slowly enough to do things right so that it can move faster in the long run. Employees should then start feeling autonomy, responsibility, accomplishment, and belongingness, which contribute to job satisfaction and synergy. The leader can educate team members so they know what to do, enable them so they know how to do it, and empower them by authorizing them to do it.

It is appropriate to do a needs assessment to plan for staff development. First, the desired knowledge and skills are identified. Then the present level of knowledge and skill is defined and the discrepancy is determined. Next, the resources available to meet the needs are identified, appropriate learning strategies are planned and implemented, and the results are evaluated. How did the learners react to the learning process? Was there behavior change indicating learning occurred? Was there an impact on the organization? Was the staff development cost-effective? Possible benefits of staff development are improved job performance, less cost for repeating work and fixing errors, lowered supervision costs, enhanced service reputation, increased job security, increased job enrichment, enhanced cross-training, higher morale, lower attrition, less expense for recruitment, more use of technology, faster implementation of strategic directions, and a more competitive strategic advantage (Marquis & Huston, 2006).

Diversity should be considered when planning learning activities. Learners have diverse learning styles, so it is advisable to use a variety of teaching methods. Cultural variables should also be considered. People raised in a traditional hierarchical system may regard the teacher as an unquestionable authority and may be reluctant to speak in class. Nonnative speakers of English may feel insecure about speaking in group discussions or activities. Requesting their views may help them speak out. Leaders and managers should not underestimate the power of talk. A story is a good way to convey meaningful knowledge. Organizations should probably shift their focus from documents to discussions. People structure their reality with language. Consequently, Hammond (1998) recommends appreciative inquiry, which recognizes and values the best of what is, envisions what might be, dialogues about what should be, and then innovatively introduces what will be. What people focus on becomes their reality. The use of successful history, tradition, and facts distinguishes appreciative inquiry from other visions based on dreams and wishes. People feel more comfortable taking what they know into the future. Dialogue is a powerful tool. It differs from debate, which uses power and knowledge of answers to prove and win a point. Dialogue uses questions to find out through respectful sharing and listening. Dialoging with others can help build bonds and personal relationships (Marquis & Huston, 2006).

Knowles (1984) differentiates pedagogy (Greek for "child leading") from andragogy (Greek for "adult leading"). In teaching children, it is appropriate to create an authoritative climate in which the teacher makes the decisions, sets the goals, lectures, evaluates, and encourages competition. A more relaxed and informal climate is used with adults, in which the teacher and the students make decisions, set goals, process activities, evaluate together, and encourage collaboration (DeYoung, 2007).

There are several principles of learning and transfer of knowledge. People need to be able to attach what they are learning to what they already know. They need underlying knowledge and skills. They also need confidence to believe they can learn and must be willing to try new skills. They are more motivated to learn if they believe the learning will lead to desirable outcomes. Immediate and specific feedback improves performance. Self-monitoring and feedback become important as people increase their competency. Content can be taught in a concentrated or distributed way. Complex material that is learned over time is usually retained longer than material taught in a concentrated way. Storage of knowledge and skills in long-term memory is necessary for transfer of training to practice. Presenting identical elements or training in a context similar to the real-work environment facilitates application in practice, as does stimulus variability, which incorporates into the training a variety of situations one would encounter on the job. Delineation of general principles also enhances transfer of knowledge by helping learners apply principles to a variety of situations they might encounter in the workplace. Relapse prevention then facilitates long-term maintenance of learned behaviors. People can identify high-risk situations and plan coping strategies to deal with them and can use "what if" scenarios to practice new knowledge and skills.

Numerous teaching methods and tools are available. These include, but are not limited to, lecture, discussion, role playing, case studies, simulations, games, small group activities, movies, audiotapes, videotapes, overhead projections, models, graphic materials, still pictures, drawings, graphs, posters, cartoons, and handouts. Technology has made possible the Internet, Web pages, e-mail, listservs, chat rooms, telephone calls, telephone bridges, conference calls, voice mail, faxing, audio conferencing, videoconferencing, virtual instrumentation, interactive video, and multimedia. The use of videoconferencing, videotelephone (a form of videoconferencing or desktop conferencing), video/image mailboxes, image/fax transmission, and desk-to-desk conferencing or integrated voice/data communications is increasing (Bastable, 2007; Billings & Halstead, 2004; DeYoung, 2007; Wilson, 2005).

CHAPTER SUMMARY

Good leadership and management in the recruitment and development of personnel are important so that the right people, who share the institution's values and meet the requirements of the job description, will be hired. Nurse leaders and managers need to be familiar with the laws. Legislation governing equal employment opportunity, affirmative action, and treatment of Americans with disabilities is among the most important related to recruitment. Once people are hired, they must be continuously helped to develop their skills and abilities. Career mapping, succession planning, and staff development, including preceptorships and mentorships for both beginning and experienced nurses, are important processes. Individual dynamics influence groups. A group is a collection of individuals with a common interest. Groups go through phases of development and become teams when they are highly functioning.

CASE STUDY

You are responsible for hiring staff for your unit. You have one staff nurse position available. You have four applicants. They have all graduated from the same school of nursing, have the same level of education, and have had similar clinical experiences. Three are whites and one is an African-American. What criteria will you use to make your decision? What is the affirmative action policy at your institution? What is the diversity mix on your unit? What is the cultural background of the clients you serve? What will your decision be, and why?

CRITICAL THINKING ACTIVITY

Reflective Journal: Make observations in a clinical setting or reflect on past experiences. Discuss the hiring or staffing process in an organization. What criteria are used in making hiring decisions? Who makes the decisions? Identify strengths and weaknesses of the process. Describe the continuing education and certification requirements for nurses working in the organization. What is the manager doing to ensure that these objectives are met? Reflect on your career stage and developmental activities. Compare your stage with the usual career stages.

ONLINE RESOURCES

evolve Additional critical thinking activities, worksheets, and case studies are available online at http://evolve.elsevier.com/Marriner/guide8e.

REFERENCES

Americans with Disabilities Act (ADA). 1990 (website): www.dol.gov/esa/regs/statutes/ofccp/ada.htm. Accessed February 14, 2007.

Anderson N, Smit-Voskuijl O, Voskuijl O, et al: *Personnel selection*, Washington, DC, 2006, Blackwell Publishing.

Armstrong v Flowers Hospital, Inc., 33 F 3d 1308 A-1, 1994.

Baggot D, Hensinger B, Parry J, et al: The new hire/preceptor experience: Cost-benefit analysis of one retention strategy, *J Nurs Adm* 35(3):138-145, 2005.

Baggot DM, Dawson C, Valdes MS, et al: Rethinking nurse recruitment: A return-on-investment approach, *J Nurs Adm* 35(10):424-427, 2005.

Barr L, Barr N: *The leadership equation: Leadership, management and the Myers-Briggs*, Austin, TX, 1989, Eakin Press.

Bastable SB: *Nurse as educator,* ed 3, Boston, 2007, Jones & Bartlett.

Benner P: *From novice to expert,* Reading, MA, 1984, Addison-Wesley.

Bennis W, Spreitzer GM, Cummings TG, editors: *The future of leadership: Today's top leadership thinkers speak to tomorrow's leaders*, San Francisco, 2001, Jossey-Bass.

Bennis WG: Leading for the long run, *Harv Bus Rev* 84(5):23-24, 2006.

Bennis WG, Thomas RJ: *Geeks and geezers: How era, values, and defining moments shape leaders*, Boston, 2002, Harvard Business School Press.

Beyers M: Nurse executives' perspectives on succession planning, *J Nurs Adm* 36(6):304-312, 2006.

Billings DM, Halstead JA: *Teaching in nursing: A guide for faculty*, ed 3, Philadelphia, 2004, Saunders.

Blouin AS, McDonagh KJ, Neistadt AM, et al: Leading tomorrow's healthcare organizations: Strategies and tactics for effective succession planning, *J Nurs Adm* 36(6):325-330, 2006.

Bonczek ME, Woodard EK: Who'll replace you when you're gone?, *Nurs Manage* 37(8):30-34, 2006.

Brounstein M: *Managing teams for dummies*, Hoboken, NJ, 2003, Wiley.

Cadmus E: Succession planning: Multilevel organizational strategies for the new workforce, *J Nurs Adm* 36(6):298-303, 2006.

Cahn SM: *Affirmative action debate*, ed 2, New York, 2002, Routledge.

Casey K, Fink R, Krugman M, et al: The graduate nurse experience, *J Nurs Adm* 36(6):303-331, 2004.

Cheung R, Aiken L: Hospital initiatives to support a better-educated workforce, *J Nurs Adm* 36(7–8):357-362, 2006.

Cody v Cigna Healthcare of St. Louis, Inc., 139 F 3d 595 (8th Cir), 1998.

Cox T: *Creating the multicultural organization: A strategy for capturing the power of diversity*, San Francisco, 2001, Jossey-Bass.

DeYoung S: *Teaching strategies for nurse educators*, ed 2, Upper Saddle River, NJ, 2007, Prentice Hall.

Doverspike D, Taylor MA, Arthur W: *Affirmative action: A psychological perspective*, Huntington, NY, 2000, Nova Science Publishers.

Drenkard K, Swartwout E: Effectiveness of a clinical ladder program, *J Nurs Adm* 35(11):502-506, 2005.

Drinka TJK, Clark PG: *Health care teamwork: Interdisciplinary practice and teaching*, Westport, Conn, 2000, Auburn House.

Goldberg B: *Age works: What corporate America must do to survive the graying of the workforce*, New York, 2000, Free Press.

Goodhouse v. Magnolia Hospital, 92F, 3d 248, 1996.

Goudreau K, Hardy J: Succession planning and individual development, *J Nurs Adm* 36(6):313-318, 2006.

Grohar-Murray ME, DiCroce HR: *Leadership and management in nursing*, Stamford, CT, 2003, Appleton & Lange.

Guido GW: Legal and ethical issues. In Yoder-Wise PS, editor: *Leading and managing in nursing*, ed 3, St Louis, 2007, Mosby.

Guion M, Highhouse S: *Essentials of personnel assessment and selection*, Hillsdale, NJ, 2006, Lawrence Erlbaum Associates.

Hammond SA: *The thin book of appreciative inquiry,* ed 2, Plano, Tex, 1998, Thin Book Publishing.

Hargrove R: *Masterful coaching fieldbook: Grow your business, multiply your profits, win the talent war!,* San Francisco, 2000, Jossey-Bass/Pfeiffer.

Harris K, Huber D, Jones R, et al: Future nursing administration graduate curricula. Part I: Call to action, *J Nurs Adm* 36(6):435, 2006.

Hart S: Generational diversity: Impact on recruitment and retention of registered nurses, *J Nurs Adm* 36(1): 10-12, 2006.

Howard v North Mississippi Medical Center, 939 F. Suppl 505, 1996.

Huber DL, editor: *Leadership and nursing care management,* ed 3, St Louis, 2006, Saunders/Elsevier.

Huszczo GE: *Tools for team excellence: Getting your team into high gear and keeping it there*, Fort Mumbai, 2005, Jaico Publishing House.

Jacobs RL, Osman-Gani AM: *Workplace training and learning: Cases from cross-cultural perspectives*, Upper Saddle River, NJ, 2006, Prentice Hall.

Jessie v Carter Health Care Center, Inc., 926 F Supp 613 (ED Ky), 1996.

Jones v Kerrville State Hospital, 142, F 3d 263 (5th Cir), 1998.

Karp H, Fuller C, Sirias D: *Bridging the boomer Xer gap: Creating authentic teams for high performance at work*, Palo Alto, CA, 2002, Davies-Black Publishing.

Kasoff J: How do hospitals represent the image of nursing on their web sites?, *J Nurs Adm* 36(2):73-78, 2006.

Kelly K: Recruiting the next generation into nursing: No negativity allowed! *J Nurs Adm* 36(2):55-57, 2006.

Kinderman KT: Retention strategies for newly hired Filipino nurses, *J Nurs Adm* 36(4):160-172, 2006.

Knowles M: *Andragogy in action*, San Francisco, 1984, Jossey-Bass.

Krugman M, Smith K: Goode CJ: A clinical advancement program: Evaluating 10 years of progressive change, *J Nurs Adm* 30(5):215-225, 2000.

Laborde SA, Lee JA: Skills needed for promotion in the nursing profession, *J Nurs Adm* 30(90):432-439, 2000.

Lancaster LC, Stillman D: *When generations collide: Who they are, why they clash, how to solve the generational puzzle at work*, New York, 2002, HarperCollins.

Laurin v Providence Hospital and Massachusetts Nurses Association, 150 F 3d 52 (1st Cir), 1998.

Lee R, Mills ME: International nursing recruitment experience, *J Nurs Adm* 35(11):478-481, 2005.

Little Forest Medical Center of Akron v Ohio Civil Rights Commission, 631 NE 2d 1068, 1993.

Luthy M, Feathers A: *Recommendation letter tips, tricks, and advice,* 2007 (website): www.writeexpress.com/recommendation-letters.html. Accessed August 12, 2007.

Lynn M: Mentoring the next generation of systems researchers, *J Nurs Adm* 36(6):288-291, 2006.

Madel v PCI Marketing, Inc., 116 F 3d 1247 (8th Cir), 1997.

Marquis BL, Huston CJ: *Leadership roles and management functions in nursing: Theory and application*, Philadelphia, 2006, Lippincott Williams & Wilkins.

Mauro v Borgess Medical Center, 4:94 CV 05 (Michigan), 1995.

McConnell CR: *Umiker's management skills for the new health care supervisor,* ed 4, Boston, 2006, Jones & Bartlett.

McNally D, Lukens R: Leadership development: An external-internal coaching partnership, *J Nurs Adm* 36(6):1555-1561, 2006.

Nelson D, Godfrey L, Purdy J: Using a mentorship program to recruit and retain student nurses, *J Nurs Adm* 34(12):551-553, 2004.

NetDoctor: *Work and ADHD*, 2007 (website): http://premium.netdoktor.com/uk/adhd/adult/living/article.jsp?articleIdent = uk.adhd.adult.living.uk_adhd_xmlarticle_004630. Accessed August 27, 2007.

O'Keefe ME: *Nursing practice and the law: Avoiding malpractice and other risks*, Philadelphia, 2001, FA Davis.

Payne V: *The team-building workshop: A trainer's guide*, New York, 2001, American Management Association.

Raines C: *Connecting generations*, Menlo Park, CA, 2003, Crisp Learning.

Raines C, Hunt J: *The Xers & the boomers: From adversaries to allies—A diplomat's guide*, Menlo Park, Calif, 2000, Crisp Publications.

Redman RW: Leadership succession planning: An evidence-based approach for managing the future, *J Nurs Adm* 36(6):292-297, 2006.

Robbins SP: *Organization behavior: Concepts, controversies, applications,* ed 9, Upper Saddle River, NJ, 2000, Prentice Hall.

Roussel L, Swansburg RC, Swansburg RJ: *Management and leadership for nurse administrators,* ed 4, Boston, 2006, Jones & Bartlett.

Silvestri LA: *Saunders comprehensive review for the NCLEX-RN examination*, Philadelphia, 2005, Saunders/Elsevier.

Sullivan EJ, Decker PJ: *Effective leadership and management in nursing,* ed 5, Upper Saddle River, NJ, 2005, Prentice Hall.

Thompson v Holy Family Hospital, 122 F 3d 537 (9th Cir), 1997.

Thorgrimson D, Robinson NC: Building and sustaining an adequate RN workforce, *J Nurs Adm* 35(11):474-477, 2005.

Tulgan B: *Managing generation X: How to bring out the best in young talent*, New York, 2000, WW Norton.

Tulgan B, Martin CA: *Managing generation Y: Global citizens born in the late seventies and early eighties*, Amherst, MA, 2001, HRD Press. p 63.

UAW v Johnson Controls, Inc., 55 Sup Ct 356, 1991.

U.S. Equal Employment Opportunity Commission. 2002 (website): www.ada.gov/q&aeng02.htm. Accessed February 14, 2007.

Walrath J, Theodoropoulos MS: Take the workforce development challenge, *Nurs Manage* 35(11):14, 2004.

Webb v Mercy Hospital, 102 E 3d (8th Cir), 1996.

Weiss L, Drake A: Nursing leadership succession planning in Veterans Health Administration: Creating a useful database, *Nurs Adm Q* 31(1):33, 2007.

Wilking v County of Ramsey, 983 F Supp 848 (D Kan), 1997.

Wilson JP: *Human resource development: Learning and training for individuals and organizations*, London, 2005, Kogan Page.

Winfeld L, Spielman S: *Straight talk about gays in the workplace*, ed 2, New York, 2001, Harrington Press.

Wolf G, Bradle J, Nelson G: Bridging the strategic leadership gap: A model program for transformational change, *J Nurs Adm* 35(2):54-60, 2005.

Workman LL: Staff recruitment and retention. In Huber DL, editor: *Leadership and nursing care management,* ed 3, Philadelphia, 2006, Elsevier, pp 625-648.

Zamudio v Patia, 956 F Supp 803 (ND Ill), 1997.

Zemke R, Raines C, Filipczak B: *Generations at work: Managing the clash of veterans, boomers, Xers, and nexters in your workplace*, New York, 2000, American Management Association.

Zimmer M: Rationale for a ladder for clinical advancement in nursing practice, *J Nurs Adm* 2(6):18-24, 1972.

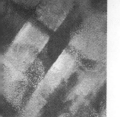

Staffing and Scheduling

13

"No person was ever honored for what he received. Honor has been the reward for what he gave." —Calvin Coolidge

Chapter Overview

Chapter 13 discusses the nursing shortage, assignment systems for staffing, staffing schedules, and magnet organizations.

Chapter Objectives

- Identify at least three causes of the nursing shortage.
- Recommend at least three strategies to decrease the nursing shortage.
- List at least five patient care delivery modes or assignment systems.
- Compare and contrast at least three patient care delivery modes or assignment systems.
- Discuss the relationship between case management and managed care if any.
- Identify at least six policy issues related to staffing schedules.
- Discuss at least three pros and cons of each centralized and decentralized scheduling.
- Discuss the pros and cons of at least three different staffing patterns.
- Explain how to calculate the number of full-time staff needed for vacation, holiday, and absentee coverage per year.
- Describe at least three ways the characteristics of magnet organizations affect recruitment and retention of nurses.

Online Resources

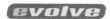

Critical thinking activities, worksheets, and case studies are available online at http://evolve.elsevier.com/Marriner/guide8e.

Major Concepts and Definitions

Case method *assignment of each patient to a nurse for total patient care*

Functional nursing *hierarchical division of labor*

Team nursing *system in which registered nurses (RNs) supervise auxiliary nursing staff*

Modular nursing *district nursing, specific to a geographic area*

Primary nursing *system in which RNs provide total patient care to a few patients*

Managed care *delivery of comprehensive health care services through established networks of hospitals, physicians, and other health care providers to give population-wide access to economical, high-quality care*

Case management *management and coordination of the care a patient receives in all settings during an episode of illness*

Collaborative practice *cooperative interdisciplinary practice*

Differentiated practice *nursing practice that distinguishes between professional and technical personnel*

Partners in practice *interdisciplinary team*

Staffing schedules *work schedules for personnel*

Centralized scheduling *scheduling done in one location*

Decentralized scheduling *scheduling done in local areas*

Self-scheduling *staff coordination of their own work schedules*

Rotating work shifts *alternation of work hours among days, evenings, and nights*

Permanent shifts *shift system in which personnel work the same hours repeatedly*

Block scheduling *use of the same schedule repeatedly*

Variable staffing *determination of the number and mix of staff based on patient needs*

Patient classification systems *systems for categorizing the acuteness of patients' conditions to determine staffing needs*

Staffing formulas *calculations used to determine staffing needs*

Magnet status *a gold standard for nursing that is correlated with high recruitment and retention of nurses and excellent quality of care through good leadership, decentralized structures, participative management, and professional delivery models*

DEALING WITH THE NURSING SHORTAGE TO PROVIDE STAFFING

Nurses are the main source of care for patients during the most vulnerable times in their lives, so the shortage of nurses is a serious problem. Facility restructuring for economic reasons, budget and staffing cuts, heavy workloads, mandatory overtime, nurse-to-nurse hostility, poor doctor and nurse relations, poorly prepared managers, changing legislation, and negative media stereotyping are some of the factors contributing to the shortage. Improved scheduling, safer staffing, a larger voice for nurses in their work, collaborative teaching of doctors and nurses, diversity training, use of best practice methods for preventing nurse-to-nurse hostility, management development, and involvement of nurses in public communications to tell what they know may be helpful strategies (Bartholomew, 2006; Buresh & Gordon, 2006; Nelson & Gordon, 2006; Porter-O'Grady & Malloch, 2006; Wilson, 2005).

Hospitals are the delivery system's most complicated setting for care and greatest consumer of resources. However, the shortage of nurses is also a grave concern for long-term care organizations, home health agencies, other delivery systems, and educational institutions. An aging baby boomer population with increasing numbers of chronic conditions, greater acuteness of care, greater complexity of care, and demands for care that exceed capacity are issues. The nursing workforce is also aging at a rate of more than twice that of other workforces in the United States. The nursing shortage impacts patient safety, diminishes hospitals' capacity to treat patients, and contributes to emergency department overcrowding, diversion of emergency department patients to other facilities, reduced numbers of staffed beds, cancellation of elective surgeries, and discontinuation of services. Complications such as urinary tract infection, pneumonia, and metabolic derangement are common in hospitalized patients. Failure to rescue is a concern and is defined as death due to one of five conditions: deep venous thrombosis, pneumonia, shock or cardiac arrest, sepsis, or upper gastrointestinal bleeding (Cho, Ketefian, Barkauskas, et al, 2003; Kovner, Jones, Zhan, et al, 2002).

Conversely, when nursing levels are optimized, there is a positive effect on quality, outcomes, and costs, with fewer adverse events; fewer complications such as catheter-related infections, nosocomial infections, and decubitus ulcers; fewer complaints in general; shorter length of stay; lower mortality; higher levels of patient, physician, and staff satisfaction; and less turnover of staff (Aiken, Clark, & Sloane, 2002; Aiken, Clark, Sloane, et al, 2002; Seago, Williamson, & Atwood, 2006).

Aiken, Clarke, Sloane, and others (2001) found that nurses in five countries (United States, Canada, England, Scotland, and Germany) expressed similar concerns about work environments. Nurses were performing nonnursing tasks such as delivering and retrieving food trays, carrying out housekeeping chores, ordering ancillary services, and transporting patients, while nursing activities such as comforting patients, developing and updating care plans, providing oral hygiene and skin care, and teaching patients and their families had been left undone in the last shift the nurses worked. The nurses indicated that manifestations of lower quality of care such as medication errors, nosocomial infections, patient falls with injuries, complaints from

patients and families, and verbal abuse directed at nurses do not occur infrequently. A shortage of nurses, high levels of job dissatisfaction among hospital nurses, and uneven quality of hospital health care are not unique to the United States. Low morale and dissatisfaction with jobs was common except in Germany.

Turnover of staff is expensive. It is costly to recruit, orient, and train new nurses. Financial losses are incurred above the routine costs of hiring temporary nurses or paying overtime. Revenue is lost when beds are closed or elective procedures are deferred. When it is difficult to acquire sufficient staff, the patient-nurse ratios may increase. That can lead to less safe care and nurse burn-out. It may be more economical to invest money in improving working conditions to retain nurses. Nurse managers can build a case for nurse retention (Atencio, Cohen, & Gorenberg, 2003; Jones, 2004, 2005). A nursing turnover calculator can help identify costs such as outlays for marketing, job fairs, application screening, interviews, testing, reference checks, recruitment firm fees, relocation, sign-on bonuses, salary and benefit differences, formal orientation, special nursing orientation, on-the-job-training, contract nurses, agency nurses, per diem nurses, and overtime per new hire as well as lost revenue due to closed beds and educational offerings for departing employees (QHR, 2007).

The Joint Commission on Accreditation of Healthcare Organizations (JCAHO; now known as The Joint Commission [TJC]), in its publication *Health Care at the Crossroads: Strategies for Addressing the Evolving Nursing Crisis* (JCAHO, 2002), advocates (1) creating cultures of retention in organizations, (2) bolstering the nursing educational infrastructure, and (3) establishing financial incentives for investing in nursing.

To develop a culture of retention the commission recommends providing management training; delegating authority to nurse executives and managers and to staff nurses to make decisions regarding patient care resource deployment; recognizing and rewarding hospitals that adopt the basic characteristics of "magnet" hospitals, including: high nurse/patient ratios, nurse autonomy, control over the practice setting, nurse participation in organizational policy decisions, good nurse-physician relationships, and strong nursing leadership; setting staffing levels based on competency and skill mix appropriate to the patient mix and acuteness; measuring, analyzing, and improving staffing effectiveness; adopting zero tolerance policies for abusive behaviors; minimizing paperwork; limiting the use of mandatory overtime to emergency situations; diversifying the workforce to improve patient care for patients of all backgrounds; adopting information, ergonomic, and other technologies to improve work flow; and adopting fair and competitive compensation and benefit packages. Nursing managers play a pivotal role in the retention of nurses (Anthony, Standing, & Glick, 2005).

Nurses have left hospital nursing to work for managed care organizations, insurance companies, pharmaceutical firms, health care technology vendors, medical device vendors, consulting firms, and so on. Many seek regular hours, no night work, no weekend work, and no mandatory overtime. However, some nurses like to get overtime work with advance notice. Some states and the federal government have started limiting mandatory overtime. The health care product giant Johnson and Johnson launched a campaign to use advertising to raise the image of nursing and to provide scholarships for students and faculty.

Nurses are also exiting nursing positions for work outside of health care. Nursing can be a stepping stone to other careers. Many of the nurses surveyed pursued additional studies after leaving nursing and moved into management positions. Few reported having difficulty adapting to nonnursing positions. Most agreed that their nursing skills had assisted them in locating new positions (Duffield, Aitken, O'Brien-Pallas, et al, 2004). Non–health care employers have found that nurses can work effectively both independently and in teams, even under immense pressure. They are able to make quick and effective assessments while adapting to change. Their training is likely to be less costly than that for other new employees (Duffield, Pallas, Aitken,

et al, 2006). Bowles and Candels (2005) found that 30% of registered nurses (RNs) having their first job experience left the position in 1 year and 57% left by 2 years. At the same time, the U.S. Bureau of Labor Statistics has predicted that registered nursing is the occupation that will experience the largest growth from 2002 to 2012. Nursing care issues, especially unsafe nurse/patient ratios, were the most frequent reasons nurses gave for leaving. The highest turnover is among nurses employed for 3 years or fewer. Consequently, maintaining a stable workforce will require finding ways to retain new employees (Lacey, 2003).

Some hospitals use sign-on bonuses to lure nurses away from other hospitals. However, sign-on bonuses do not create employee loyalty. They encourage job hopping to get higher levels of income. There has also been recruitment of foreign nurses, which leads to a brain drain and nursing shortage in the countries from which nurses are recruited. This practice is also complicated by federal and state certification requirements (Dikaya & Appelt, 2004). Temporary staffing agencies and traveling nurse services allow people to earn more money and choose their own hours. This can cause dissatisfaction among the regular staff who are making less and have little control over their work schedules. Although temporary nurses may be well-educated and experienced, they may not be familiar with the hospital's policies and practices. Nursing managers are responsible for screening and orienting temporary nurses. The Healthcare Integrity and Protection Data Bank and the National Practitioner Data Bank are two databases available for researching adverse actions taken against nurses (Sloan, 2004).

Attracting people into nursing seems to be the best option. Some hospitals are targeting high school students for recruitment, using student volunteers, providing shadow-a-nurse opportunities, partnering with schools of nursing, creating on-site programs, and developing mentoring programs for new graduates (West, Hallick, Schaal, et al, 2006). Others are considering how to recruit retired nurses and retain nurses who would otherwise retire. Although remarkably few differences were noted between older and younger RNs, the percentage of RNs working in acute care declines as the nurses' age increases. Older new nursing graduates may choose to be employed in hospitals, but older practicing RNs tend to choose other health care delivery settings in which the demands are not so intense. Changes in the work environment seem necessary to retain aging nurses in hospitals, and some of these changes are different from those that need to be made to retain younger nurses (Andrews, Manthorpe, & Watson, 2005; Institute of Medicine, 2006; Norman, Donelan, Buerhaus, et al, 2005; O'Brien-Pallas, Duffield, & Alksnis, 2004).

The average age of RNs working in hospitals increased by 5.3 years between 1983 and 1998, whereas the average age of the general workforce increased by fewer than 2 years. It is anticipated that the average age of the RN workforce will rise by about 4 years between 2000 and 2010, reaching 45 years of age and remaining there through 2020. Between 2010 and 2020 over 40% of the RN workforce will be over 50 years of age and is expected to retire or otherwise withdraw from the workforce. Nurses tend to leave hospital nursing around age 55 to 58 instead of waiting until retirement age of 65 or 66. This makes retention of the older nurse very important for dealing with the nursing shortage. The average age of new RN graduates was 31 years in 2006. It remains important to recruit older people who may be entering the workforce or starting a second career into nursing, even though they will have a shorter work life in nursing than new high school graduates. Then they need to be mentored through those first years of practice to advance from novice to expert nurse. It has become critically important to meet the needs of RNs over 50 years of age to diminish the nursing shortage.

Older nurses indicate that they leave the workforce because of challenging work schedules such as shift work, 12-hour shifts, and rotation shifts; high patient census; and physical demands of the work environment, such as long hallways, centralized workstations, and inconsistent use or lack of lifting devices and other

technologies. They are also concerned about the lack of advancement over the course of their careers, lack of recognition for their contributions, lack of valuing of the older RN, and absence of fair compensation.

Some of the corrective measures identified in the Institute of Medicine's *Wisdom at Work* report (2006) include implementing flexible work schedules, using shorter shifts, decreasing patient/nurse ratio, fostering a professional nurse practice environment, promoting respect for people in general and older nurses specifically, developing career paths, modifying the work environment, implementing ergonomics in health care facility designs, structuring decentralization, decentralizing workstations and storage of supplies and equipment, improving lighting at the bedside, providing adequate training in the use of technology, exploiting technology, using larger type and more readable fonts in printed materials, installing raised toilets, purchasing adaptive beds, using mechanical patient lifts, installing softer floors, providing waist-high electrical outlets, changing the organizational culture to appreciate the differences in younger and older nurses, allowing more autonomy and participation in decision making, assessing training, providing continuing education, increasing benefits, developing human resource policies on the retention of senior nurses as well as the recruitment of younger nurses, and developing new professional roles such as mentor, research assistant, and safety officer. Older nurses could also do telephone triage or work at the help desk, staff the holding or waiting areas for patients, conduct audits, do patient education, serve as staff educator for newly employed nurses, act as ombudsman for the unit or service, work for the employee assistance program, provide relief staffing for peak times, or serve as the medicine nurse (Barclay, 2006; Mion, Hazel, Cap, et al, 2006). It is also important to make changes to retain other nurses to improve quality of care while reducing recruitment costs (Jones, 2005).

Letvak (2003, 2005) found that higher levels of job satisfaction, greater control over practice, and lower job demands increased the physical health of nurses over the age of 50, and that they reported higher levels of physical and mental health than the national norm. However, nurses with higher job demands and those employed in hospital settings were more likely to experience an injury. Despite facing the stressors of intergenerational conflict with younger nurses, less respect from patients and families, and inequity in pay, older nurses continued to work because they care, are confident in their abilities, and are able to meet the demands of hospital nursing. Consequently, the nurse's ability to provide safe and competent care and the nurse's personal preferences should be considered in making assignments.

To bolster the nursing education infrastructure, the commission recommends funding nurse faculty positions and student scholarships at all levels of nursing education; increasing federal funding for nursing education; providing fast-track and low-cost opportunities for nurses to get higher levels of education; establishing standardized postgraduate nurse residency programs and providing funding to support the programs; emphasizing team training in undergraduate and postgraduate nursing education programs; enhancing hospital budgets for nursing orientation, inservice, and continuing education; and creating nursing career ladders that reflect educational levels.

To establish financial incentives for investing in nursing, the commission recommended making new federal monies available to invest in nursing services; requiring demonstrated achievement of criteria and goals for continued federal funding; basing new reimbursement incentives on evidence-based, nursing-sensitive indicators; and aligning private payer and federal reimbursement incentives to reward effective nurse staffing. If quality of nursing service, patient safety, and clinical outcomes are linked to funding, nursing should move from the cost side to the asset side of the balance sheet. This would recognize and reward good nursing care (JCAHO, 2002).

During the 2000s, research indicated that mortality and failure to rescue patients who had complications from common surgical procedures declined when the number of baccalaureate-prepared nurses providing care increased. There was a renewed effort to recruit people into nursing and to promote lifelong learning. Still, there were a disproportionate number of hospitals employing a workforce of nurses with less than a baccalaureate degree. The highest percentage of baccalaureate-prepared nurses was found in teaching hospitals and somewhat fewer in community hospitals (Aiken, Clarke, & Cheung, 2003; Aiken, Clarke, & Sloane, 2002).

ASSIGNMENT SYSTEMS FOR STAFFING

Changes in assignment systems are a response to changing needs. In the 1920s, the case method and private duty nursing were popular. By 1950, functional nursing was predominant in response to the shortage of nurses. During that decade team nursing was introduced to maximize use of the knowledge and skills of professional nurses and to provide supervision to auxiliary workers. The late 1960s and 1970s witnessed a shift back to care of the patient by a professional nurse through primary nursing. Case management became popular during the 1980s, and managed competition emerged as an economic strategy guiding health care reform during the 1990s. It stimulated the use of partners in practice, which is an interdisciplinary team. Each system involves leaders and managers (Table 13-1) and has advantages and disadvantages (Table 13-2) (Grohar-Murray & DiCroce, 2003).

STAFFING LEADERSHIP AND MANAGEMENT

The leader should be knowledgeable about staffing and scheduling, is accountable for safe staffing, communicates the need for a staff mix, and considers the impact of extraneous factors on staffing. The leader examines the unit standard of productivity periodically, encourages discussions of workload issues, encourages a team approach to staffing, and enables self-scheduling. The manager develops and disseminates fair

TABLE 13-1 Staffing Leadership and Management

Leader	Manager
Is knowledgeable about staffing and scheduling	Develops and disseminates fair scheduling policies
Is accountable for safe staffing	Assumes accountability for fiscal control and quality of staffing
Communicates the need for a staff mix	Negotiates staff mix coverage
Considers the impact of extraneous factors on staffing	Provides staffing to meet patient needs
Examines the unit standard of productivity periodically to determine if changes are needed	Schedules staff in a fiscally responsible way
Encourages discussion of workload issues	Facilitates discussions of workload issues
Encourages a team approach to staffing	Keeps policies in compliance with laws
Enables self-scheduling	Matches staff to patient needs

Modified from Huber DL, editor: *Leadership and nursing care management*, ed 3, Philadelphia, 2006, Elsevier; Marquis BL, Huston CJ: *Leadership roles and management functions in nursing: Theory and application*, ed 5, Philadelphia, 2006, Lippincott Williams & Wilkins.

scheduling policies, assumes accountability for fiscal control and quality of staffing, negotiates staffing and staff mix coverage, provides staffing to meet patient needs, schedules staff in a fiscally responsible way, and determines if changes are needed. The manager facilitates discussion of workload issues, keeps policies in compliance with the law, and matches staff to client needs (Finkelman, 2001; Huber, 2006; Kongstvedt, 2003; Marquis & Huston, 2006) (Table 13-3).

Case Method

The total patient care or case method was the primary care delivery model before the 1930s and had a resurgence during the 1980s. In the case method, each patient is assigned to a nurse for total patient care while that nurse is on duty. Continuity of care is guaranteed only for one shift. The patient has a different nurse each shift and no guarantee of having the same nurses the next day. The quality of care is considered higher than with functional or team nursing but not as high as with primary nursing. The patient care coordinator, who has no obligation to assign nurses to the same patient, supervises and evaluates all care given on the unit. Popular during the 1920s along with private duty nursing, the case method emphasized following physicians' orders. Now case management uses a multidisciplinary approach to provide and document care

to better coordinate care in complex health care systems. It may no longer be as cost effective as it once was because of the use of a higher percentage of RNs in managed care environments. The case manager is a client advocate who coaches, coordinates care, and negotiates with other professionals, clients, and families to improve the efficiency of care and use of resources, and to improve the quality of care. Patient satisfaction has been high with continuity of care and good communications among nurses. Some nurses complain that their time and skills are not well utilized because they perform patient care tasks that people with less education and skill could do (Grohar-Murray & DiCroce, 2003; Tiedeman & Lookinland, 2004).

Functional Nursing

In the 1950s, when few registered nurses and only some practical nurses were available, nurses' aides gave much of the physical patient care. In functional nursing, a hierarchical structure predominates, and personnel of different skill levels are used according to the complexity of the patients' care needs. Team members provide care to a specific group of patients under the supervision of an RN. The team leader may depend on the charge nurse for some clinical decision making and influences whether the care will be task or patient centered. The medication

TABLE 13-2 Pros and Cons of Various Assignment Systems

Assignment System	Pros	Cons
Case method	Total patient care is provided by one nurse on each shift.	Different nurses provide care on different shifts and different days.
Functional nursing	Efficiency is increased.	Nurses do managerial work. Nurses' aides perform patient care.
Team nursing	Care is provided through team effort. Patient care coordinator is freed to manage the unit. Nursing care conferences help problem solve and develop staff. Nursing care plan is developed.	Time is needed to coordinate delegated work.
Modular nursing	System is useful when there are few registered nurses (RNs). RNs plan care.	Paraprofessionals perform technical aspects of care.
Primary nursing	RNs give total patient care. Primary nurse has 24-hour responsibility. Associate nurse works with patient while the primary nurse is off duty. Accountability is in place. Continuity of care is facilitated. Number of errors from relay of orders is reduced. There are fewer patient complaints. Hospital stays are shorter.	Nurse's talents are confined to a limited number of patients. Associate nurse may change care plan without discussing with primary nurse.
Managed care	Case management is incorporated. Method can be used with any nursing care delivery system. Standard critical paths are used. Efficiency is increased. Cost is reduced.	Continuity of care is questionable.
Case management	Entire episode of illness is the focus. Achievement of outcomes is emphasized. Care is coordinated by a case manager. Care is provided by second-generation primary nursing. Critical paths are used. Variation analysis is conducted. Intershift reports are created. Health care team meetings are held. Interdisciplinary approach is used.	Coordination requires effort.

nurse, treatment nurse, and bedside nurse are all products of this system. The functional method implements classic scientific management principles, which emphasize efficiency, division of labor, and rigid controls. It is an efficient system that is the least costly because it requires few RNs. Procedural descriptions are used to define the standard of care, and psychological needs typically are slighted. Care tends to be fragmented and depersonalized. RNs may keep busy with managerial and nonnursing duties, and nurses' aides deliver the majority of patient care.

Although superficially cost efficient because it uses the smallest number of staff, the functional assignment method does not encourage patient and staff satisfaction. Research indicates that

TABLE 13-3 Leaders for Managed Care and Managers for Case Management

Leaders for Managed Care	Managers for Case Management
Facilitate the development of a managed care strategic vision and mission	Give and/or coordinate care
Facilitate the development of a managed care strategic plan	Emphasize outcomes in time frames
Communicate with and educate stake holders in the integrated network	Serve as impartial patient advocates
Develop a continuum of care	Educate patients and families
Develop contracts with providers of care and develop financial risk-sharing contracts	Work across agencies
Facilitate continuous quality improvement	Maintain relationships with referral sources
Facilitate use of critical paths and care maps with management development of staff	Serve as liaison for insurance claims
Support case management and use of alternative care delivery as a way to control costs	Perform variance analysis and evaluate outcomes
Facilitate development of integrated information management capabilities	Use case consultation as necessary
Lead a flexible organization that can make changes rapidly to meet quickly changing needs	Conduct team meetings as necessary.

Modified from Cesta TG: *Survival strategies for nurses in managed care,* St Louis, 2002, Mosby; Finkelman AW: *Managed care: A nursing perspective,* Upper Saddle River, NJ, 2006, Prentice Hall; Kongstvedt PR: *Essentials of managed health care,* ed 4, Gaithersburg, MD, 2003, Aspen Publishers.

outcomes are better with more educated staff. Regimentation of tasks may bore nurses because they do not have the satisfaction of seeing the effects of their total patient care. On the other hand, the functional system may work satisfactorily during critical staffing shortages. Routinized patient care for patients with similar needs may meet those needs more consistently than do other systems, and some staff members may be satisfied by doing repetitive jobs well (Bonczek, 2007; Marquis & Huston, 2006; Roussel, Swansburg, & Swansburg, 2006; Tiedeman & Lookinland, 2004).

Team Nursing

After World War II, RNs were still scarce, although the number of auxiliary personnel had increased. Team nursing was introduced during the 1950s to improve nursing services in hospitals and nursing homes by using professional nurses, with their greater knowledge and skills, to supervise the increasing numbers of auxiliary nursing staff. By 2000, interdisciplinary teams had become more popular. The result was an improvement in patient and staff satisfaction. Team nursing is based on a philosophy that supports the achievement of goals through group action. Each team member is encouraged to make suggestions and share ideas. When team members see their suggestions implemented, their job satisfaction increases, and they are motivated to give even better care.

The nursing team is led by a professional or technical nurse who plans, interprets, coordinates, supervises, and evaluates the nursing care. Team leaders assign team members to patients by matching patient needs with staff's knowledge and skills. They also do the work other members of the team, including the RNs, licensed practical or vocational nurses, and unlicensed personnel, are not qualified to perform, such as giving some medications, doing complicated treatments, making assessments, and teaching. They set goals and priorities for patient care; centralize information through the use of a Kardex; direct the planning of care through care conferences and development of care plans; assign responsibility for the work; provide for coverage during absences, such as breaks, meals, and conferences; and coordinate and evaluate team activities. Team members report to the team leader, who reports to the charge nurse or patient care coordinator. This is a form of decentralization that frees the charge nurse or patient care coordinator to manage the unit.

One of the main features of team nursing is the nursing care conference. Team conferences are now used in a variety of staffing systems. The primary purpose is the development and revision of nursing care plans or the multidisciplinary team's plans by providing an opportunity to identify and solve problems. Precision in the identification of problems is increased through information sharing. The belief that the total group has more information about a topic than does any one person enhances the staff's appreciation of group work. A resulting consensus increases the commitment to the decisions made. Identification of the problem and determination of goals early in the conference necessarily precede planning of interventions. During the conference, one care plan can be developed or the care plans for a caseload can be updated. Team conferences can be used in a variety of staffing systems, and more recently have become implemented in the form of multidisciplinary team conferences.

Team conferences also provide the opportunity to identify and work through staff educational needs. Nurses can review standards of care by comparing the condition of an actual patient with a textbook example. They can review procedures and learn specialized nursing care and the operation of infrequently used equipment. By studying critical incidents, they may prevent problems from recurring and identify the components contributing to excellent care. Team conferences also provide an opportunity to discuss and resolve interpersonal problems and may prevent future ones. Consequently, team spirit is fostered.

The team leader is responsible for planning and conducting the team conference, which should be limited in time and scope. Meeting for 15 to 30 minutes at the same time each day helps the conference become a part of the daily routine. A time that least interferes with other activities and a place away from the hub of activity are preferable. The team leader must arrange for coverage of the unit during the conference because relief from patient care responsibilities is essential to prevent interruptions. Staff should be informed of the time, place, and purpose of the conference, so that they can plan their other work around the conference and be well prepared on arrival. Interest can be stimulated by allowing the staff to decide which patient they wish to discuss at the next conference and by having one of the team members record patient problems and solutions during the conference.

Preparation of the meeting area is also a responsibility of the team leader. Temperature, ventilation, lighting, and chair arrangements should be controlled. Serving refreshments may be appropriate. The team leader introduces the topic and starts the meeting on time to motivate late comers to be more prompt. A brief review of the patient's condition is appropriate. The team leader monitors the group process, records problems and solutions on the nursing care plan or delegates that task, does appropriate teaching, and summarizes the major points. The nursing care plan is then available to the staff. The team leader serves as a role model by referring to the care plan while receiving and giving reports, giving out assignments, and administering nursing care.

The nursing care plan is another main feature of team nursing. A care plan identifying present and potential problems and long- and short-term objectives should be developed for each patient. The care plan should be realistic to prevent morale problems that result from setting unattainable objectives. Care plans should be individualized, reflecting the interrelatedness of psychosocial and physiologic needs, as well as input from patients and families. Problems, mutually acceptable goals, objectives, actions, and responses are identified. The care is evaluated in terms of how well the objectives are met. Staff can identify their contributions and the correlation between their work and patient outcomes. The closer interaction of staff contributes to esprit de corps.

Quality tends to be high because the nurse has responsibility and accountability for fewer patients, knows the patients better, and can better match the staff's skills to the patient's needs. Unfortunately, the most educated staff is responsible for supervising the less skilled personnel rather than giving care themselves. The experts are limited to a defined group of patients. The time it takes to communicate among the team members can decrease the direct care time. The team nursing model becomes ineffective when there is short staffing.

Changing team membership makes it difficult for the team leader to know team members well enough to match their talents with patient needs. Team nursing is similar to functional nursing when the team leader administers medications and treatments other team members are not qualified to give. Team conferences are often omitted because they are difficult to fit into busy days, and care plans (if created) usually note functional duties related to the physician's orders. Care plans rarely depict the patient as a total person and consequently are not comprehensive. Medication precautions, fluid intake requirements, dietary and environmental adaptations, protective measures, psychological support, teaching, rehabilitation, and referrals are seldom mentioned. In reality the key features of team nursing—nursing care conferences and nursing care plans—often receive inadequate attention, which results in routinized care. Team nursing is considered expensive because more personnel are needed, but research has yielded conflicting results. Findings related to the quality of team nursing care and patient and staff satisfaction have also been inconsistent. No differences were found in absenteeism, tardiness, or turnover between team and primary nursing (Dadich, 2007; Grohar-Murray & DiCroce, 2003; Marquis & Huston, 2006; Tiedeman & Lookinland, 2004).

Modular, or District, Nursing

Modular, or district, nursing is a modification of team nursing and primary nursing in which the nurse gives total patient care. In this method, smaller teams care for patients who are grouped geographically. Modular nursing is sometimes used when there are not enough RNs to practice primary nursing. Each RN, assisted by paraprofessionals, delivers as much care as possible to a group of patients. The RN assesses needs, plans the care, delivers as much of it as possible, and directs the paraprofessionals in performing the more technical aspects of care. The RN's role is that of a coordinator and information processor.

Modular nursing decreases the sense of isolation and unrealistic expectations often associated with primary nursing. When nurses are consistently assigned to the same module, continuity and quality of care can increase. More time may be spent in direct care. Closer monitoring is possible. Morale can improve when staff knows they are making a difference. Modular nursing is less costly than primary nursing but more costly and less efficient than team nursing.

Some physical changes may be necessary to implement modular, or district, nursing. For example, a medication cart may be placed in the hall instead of a medication room being used. Kardexes may be kept on the medication cart. Charts may be moved to the patient's room. Patient Kardexes and staff identification badges may be color coded (Marquis & Huston, 2006).

Primary Nursing

Before the advent of intensive care units, private duty nursing was common. It was a precursor of primary nursing. During the late 1960s and early 1970s, primary nursing as conceptualized by Marie Manthey was instituted in some hospitals by professional nurses who were unhappy with fragmented care and lack of direct patient contact. Based on the philosophy that patients, instead of tasks, should be the focus of professional nurses, primary nursing features an RN who provides total patient care to four to six patients. The RN remains responsible for the care of those patients 24 hours per day throughout the patients' hospitalization. An associate nurse cares for the patient by using the care plan developed by the primary nurse while the primary nurse is off duty. The associate nurse is expected to contact the primary nurse regarding changes in the care plan. The aim was to provide the patient and the family with continuous, coordinated, and comprehensive care. The number of patients assigned to one nurse varies depending on the length of hospitalization, complexity of care, number of medical and paramedical personnel involved in the patient's care, availability of support systems, and shift worked. Day-shift nurses are assigned the highest number of patients; evening nurses have some patients; and night nurses are primarily auxiliary nurses because of their reduced contact with patients and families.

Although primary nursing was designed for hospitals, it lends itself to home nursing, hospice nursing, and other health care delivery models. The primary nurse does the admission interview and develops the nursing care plan, including teaching and discharge planning, which is shared with the associate nurse. Primary nurses have autonomy and authority for the care of their patients. Consequently, accountability is placed with the primary nurse, and continuity of care is facilitated. Primary nursing decreases the number of people in the chain of command and reduces the number of errors that can result from a relay of orders. Other advantages include mobile use of auxiliary workers and increased satisfaction of both nurse and patient. Nurses can identify patient outcomes as a result of their work. Patients have the security of knowing that the nurse is available and has to cope with fewer people than in other assignment systems. Research suggests that patients have fewer complications and a shorter hospital stay when cared for by a primary nurse. Consequently, there tends to be improved continuity and coordination of care and increased patient, nurse, and physician satisfaction.

Unfortunately, primary nursing confines a nurse's talents to a limited number of patients. Other patients cannot benefit, and if a patient has a nurse who is not capable, the patient may be worse off than if cared for by numerous people, some of whom might meet the patient's needs. Another problem occurs when the associate nurse changes the care plan without discussing the reasons with the primary nurse. Thus it is critical that the primary nurse communicate verbal and written plans to the associate nurse. Primary nursing is further complicated by the use of 12-hour shifts, because the primary nurse only works 3 days a week, which interferes with continuity of care. Studies of the cost, time spent with patients, and patient satisfaction are inconclusive. The success of primary nursing seems to depend on the quality of the nursing staff and administrative support (Dadich, 2007; Grohar-Murray & DiCroce, 2003; Marquis & Huston, 2006; Sullivan & Decker, 2005; Tiedeman & Lookinland, 2004).

Case Management

The case management method has its roots in psychiatry and social work, which focused on long-term outpatient care in the 1920s. It was used by community health nursing in the 1930s and was adapted to acute care settings and outpatient services during the mid-1980s in response to the prospective payment system. It focuses on an entire episode of illness, including all settings in which the client receives care. A case manager identifies, coordinates, and monitors services for the patient and family. Options for alternative health care, living arrangements, and community and social services are considered. Arrangements with nonpreferred providers may be negotiated to reduce claim costs. Case management can cross departmental and disciplinary boundaries.

There are a variety of models for case management. The nurse may give care and coordinate it or just coordinate the care. The nurse may work across agencies, such as in ambulatory clinics, acute care facilities, and long-term care facilities, or may make site visits to the home or health care agencies. Case management emphasizes achievement of outcomes in designated time frames with limited resources. It is sometimes called *second-generation primary nursing.*

Case management may involve critical paths, variation analysis, intershift reports, case consultation, health care team meetings, a multidisciplinary action plan, and quality assurance.

Critical paths visualize outcomes within a time frame and have been developed for various diagnoses. Variation analysis notes positive or negative changes from the critical path, the cause, and the corrective action taken. This information is reported in intershift reports. Case consultation may be indicated when the client's condition differs from the critical path as noted in the intershift report. Case consultation is conducted about once each week for a few minutes immediately after the intershift report is submitted to deal with variations in acute care and, less frequently, in long-term care. It can also be conducted informally whenever a staff member identifies a variation and consults others. The problem solvers focus on the variation and the desired outcomes, brainstorm ideas for achieving desired outcomes, and use open communication to evaluate a plan. A summary can be used to close the session.

Health care team meetings provide an interdisciplinary approach to problem solving. The case manager needs to identify no more than three priority goals and decide what team members should be present after considering the patient, family, physician, social services, various therapists, and others involved. The case manager should set the time and place for the meeting, make the arrangements, and post the date, time, place, and people to attend in the Kardex. The case manager calls the meeting to order, states the goals, initiates discussion, documents the plans, and sets time limits for follow-through. The variance between what is expected and what happens is assessed for quality assurance. Collaboration is important.

Case management may also be called *outcomes management* or *clinical resource management.* The nursing care manager is typically assigned patients on admission based on the nurse's specialization. The case manager's responsibilities are assessment, planning, facilitation, and advocacy. Assessment batteries, questionnaires, and telephone or electronic communication assessment methods may be used. Health behaviors, beliefs, values, and cultural influences are considered to negotiate goals, identify potential barriers, and

consider alternatives. The nurse then works with an interdisciplinary team including the patient/client, family, physician, and other health care providers to develop a multidisciplinary action plan or critical path based on the diagnosis-related group, implements the plan or path by coordinating parts of the service delivery system, and monitors the progress until discharge. The nurse case manager advocates for the client by educating the client and family about the plan, using referrals to get appropriate and timely treatment, and locating funding (Case Management Society of America, 2002; Cesta, 2002; Cesta & Tahan, 2003; Cohen & Cesta, 2005; Dadich, 2007; Grohar-Murray & DiCroce, 2003; Huber, 2006; Marquis & Huston, 2006; Roussel, Swansburg, & Swansburg, 2006; Sullivan & Decker, 2005).

Collaborative Practice

Collaborative practice can include interdisciplinary teams, nurse-physician interaction in joint practice, or nurse-physician collaboration in caregiving. Collaboration is cooperative and synergistic. The interaction between nurses and physicians or other health care team members in collaborative practice should enable the knowledge and skills of the professions to influence the quality of patient care.

The American Nurses Association (ANA) and the American Medical Association established the National Joint Practice Committee in 1972 with funding from the W. K. Kellogg Foundation. The committee's report supported collaborative practice and suggested that increased collaboration results in improved quality of care, increased patient and nurse satisfaction, and a decreased need for physician supervision of nurses. Primary nursing, nurse decision making, integrated patient records, a joint practice committee, and a joint record review were found to enhance nurse-physician collaboration.

During the 1990s there was a rapid movement of health care from the hospital to the community. With the rapidly aging population and accompanying increase in chronic diseases, use of interdisciplinary teams, and advancing technology, creation of a computer-based and network-based community infrastructure became increasingly important. A prototype of an information system in community nursing was developed in a Delphi programming environment. Then an international classification of nursing practice was published and was copyrighted by the International Council of Nurses.

A common diagnostic classification system became increasingly important for communication. The first nurse-developed classification system was initiated in 1973 and is known as the North American Nursing Diagnosis Association (NANDA) system. Nurses have worked at refining it over the decades. The Nursing Diagnosis and Extension Classification research team at the University of Iowa was formed to refine, extend, validate, and classify nursing diagnoses in collaboration with NANDA to produce a comprehensive and validated taxonomy of nursing. Researchers have been leading the classification work through the Center for Nursing Classification at the University of Iowa College of Nursing. Treatments listed in the Nursing Interventions Classification have been linked with NANDA nursing diagnoses and Omaha System problems and are being linked with outcomes in the Nursing Outcomes Classification (NOC). The NOC has been recognized by the ANA Congress of Nursing Practice Steering Committee on Databases to Support Clinical Nursing Practice as useful for clinical nursing practice and has been included in the Unified Medical Language System of the National Library of Medicine (Johnson, Bulechek, Dochterman, et al, 2001; Johnson, Maas, & Moorhead, 2004; McCloskey & Bulechek, 2003).

Staff and supervisors of the Visiting Nurse Association of Omaha developed the Omaha classification system. The three components—problem classification, intervention scheme, and problem rating scale for outcomes—were developed for community health nursing. The 1999 ANA House of Delegates passed a recommendation calling for the timely implementation of ANA-recognized standardized nursing languages, including the Nursing Management Minimum Data Set, to establish comparability of nursing data across clinical settings, populations, geography, and time (ANA, 1999a).

During the 1990s primary care became a focus of health care. Nurse practitioner programs showed a marked increase in enrollment, and advanced practice nurses played a key role in primary care. Medical education made some shift from specialties to general medicine. The number of health maintenance organizations, preferred provider organizations, and integrated health care systems increased.

Differentiated Practice

Differentiated nursing practice takes into account the competency, education, and skill level of nurses. The aim is to match patient needs with nursing competencies to facilitate the effective and efficient use of nursing resources. It can be used in a variety of settings to improve patient care, increase patient safety, make effective and efficient use of scarce resources, increase patient and nurse satisfaction, and compensate nurses fairly based on their education, experience, and productivity (American Association of Colleges of Nursing, 2002; Blais, Hayes, & Kozier, 2005).

The competency model of differentiated practice can use the levels of practice defined by Benner (1984)—(1) novice, (2) advanced, (3) competent, (4) proficient, and (5) expert—and the ANA's eight standards of practice: (1) quality of care, (2) performance appraisal, (3) education, (4) collegiality, (5) ethics, (6) collaboration, (7) research, and (8) resource utilization. The 21 competencies for the twenty-first century set forth by the Pew Health Professions Commission (1998) can also be a useful tool.

The education differentiated practice model is based on the difference between professional nurses (who hold master of science in nursing and bachelor of science in nursing degrees) and technical nurses (who hold associate degrees). Complexity of decision making, timeline of care, and structure of the setting are the main distinctive features. Professional nurses give direct care to patients with complex interactions based on nursing diagnoses and relate to their families from preadmission to postdischarge in a variety of settings. Until the 1990s the technical nurse received a diploma or an associate degree and gave nursing care to patients with common conditions and to their families in structured settings. With the movement of health care into the community and an attempt to lower health care costs, technical nurses, licensed practical nurses (LPNs), and unlicensed personnel are used in the community and in less structured situations as well.

The original Integrated Competencies of Nurses (ICON) model addressed entry into practice roles by developing a differentiated practice model. Baccalaureate-prepared nurses assess, plan, and evaluate care. Nurses with an associate degree implement the care plan. One professional and two or three associate nurses care for 10 to 15 patients during the day. ICON II responded to the shortage of nurses by grandfathering all RNs into the professional role. LPNs then fill the technical role, which involves giving the physical nursing care (American Association of Colleges of Nursing, 1995).

Manthey's Primary Practice Partners model responded to the nursing shortage by recommending that former military corpsmen, emergency medical technicians, and registered certified technicians with special technical training become nurse extenders. These and other job categories may expand differentiated practice models (Manthey, 1988).

Under the partners in practice models of the 1990s, cleaning personnel, who had less down time than previous nurses' aides, were cross-trained to be nursing assistants. Use of unlicensed personnel increased during the 1990s, but many have not found that very satisfactory (Dadich, 2007; Grohar-Murray & DiCroce, 2003; Huber, 2006; Marquis & Huston, 2006; Roussel, Swansburg, & Swansburg, 2006; Sullivan & Decker, 2005).

LEVEL OF STAFF

The educational level of the staff available greatly influences the assignment system used. When there are a few RNs and a few practical nurses, many aides are quickly oriented and used. This is an expensive and relatively dangerous mix because aides do not have the educational background to do most of what is required or to recognize what should be reported. After the aides have done all they can, there is still much work to be done. Consequently, there is considerable downtime. This staffing mix lends itself best to functional nursing.

Team nursing is appropriate when there are some RNs, even more practical nurses, and fewer aides. The RNs plan and direct the care, pass medications, and perform the more complicated treatments. Although this provides better physical care, the staff is still not adequately educated to understand the pathophysiologic basis of symptoms, to plan nursing interventions, and to detect changes in the status of the patient at an early stage so that staff members may promptly call a rapid response team, implement a critical pathway, or report pertinent information to the physician. There may be a dearth of patient education and lack of response to psychosocial needs because technical nursing focuses more on physical care.

Modular nursing is appropriate when more RNs are available, and primary nursing works best with a staff of only RNs. Research examining care by staffs that are exclusively RNs indicates higher levels of staff, patient, and physician satisfaction. There is an increase in professional orientation, greater personal liking of colleagues, and increase in cooperation with others. Collegial relationships are more common, and there is more mobility on units because nurses can cover for each other. There may be greater skills competence, more creative interventions, more personalized care, and better continuity of care.

All-RN staffing is economical. It has been found to save money through a decrease in turnover, sick leave, unpaid absences, float hours, and overtime. RNs can give better care in fewer hours. Patients have fewer complications such as postoperative infections, pneumonia, urinary track infections, and pressure ulcers; shorter hospitalizations; and lower readmission rates. Hospitals also generate more revenue when patients have shorter stays with a concentration of treatments. Unfortunately, frequent shortages of nurses make all-RN staffing unlikely (ANA, 2000; Clark, 2005).

Pure applications of the case method, functional method, team nursing, modular nursing, and primary nursing are possible, but they seldom exist in pristine form. Rather, it is common to find elements from more than one assignment system combined and used at the same time. Case management is used across settings. During the 1980s, managed care was considered unit based. During the 1990s, disease management and case management became a part of managed care through community-focused, collaborative arrangements and structures such as health maintenance organizations. During the 2000s, health care became more globalized.

STAFFING SCHEDULES

Staffing policies have a large influence on staffing schedules. To determine staffing policies, one must consider the following questions (Marquis & Huston, 2006; Roussel, Swansburg, & Swansburg, 2006):

- What is the best organization for staffing—centralized or decentralized to clinical areas or nursing units?
- Who is responsible for the original scheduling or daily adjustments?
- Where are nursing hours posted and an accurate copy kept?
- For what period will schedules be prepared—1, 2, 4, or 6 weeks?
- How far in advance will personnel know their work schedules?
- Will there be an adjustment in staffing based on the identification of patient needs?
- Will there be shift rotation?
- If there is shift rotation, how often will it shift—daily, weekly, monthly?
- How much time should elapse between rotated shifts?
- What day starts a calendar week—Sunday or Monday?
- Will there be 2 days (for 8-hour shifts) or 4 days (for 12-hour shifts) off each week or an average of 2 or 4 days each week?

- How often are weekends off guaranteed?
- What days does a weekend include—Friday, Saturday, Sunday?
- Will days off be split or consecutive?
- What are the maximum and minimum work spans?
- How many holidays and vacation days are allowed?
- How far in advance of scheduling should employees request time off?
- How will holiday time off be determined?
- Will part-time help be used?
- If so, what is the most economical ratio between full- and part-time personnel?
- Will part-time help be allowed to specify when they can and cannot work?
- Will part-time help be required to work weekends? If so, how often?
- Will float personnel be used?
- What are the low-census procedures?
- Is there a policy for trading days off?
- What is the emergency request policy?

Centralized Scheduling

Two major advantages of centralized scheduling are fairness to employees through consistent, objective, and impartial application of policies, and opportunities for cost containment through better use of resources (Table 13-4). Centralized scheduling also relieves nurse managers from time-consuming duties, freeing them for other activities. Centralized scheduling is not without its critics, however. Lack of individualized treatment of employees is a chief complaint, and centralized scheduling has brought to the surface previously unrecognized organizational and managerial problems.

Organizational and managerial problems may be reduced when (1) the philosophy and goals of the agency are identified; (2) the goals, objectives, and organizational structure are defined; (3) scheduling policies are stated; (4) standards of nursing care practice are set; (5) acuteness of care as it relates to staffing needs is determined; (6) patient needs, personnel policies such as vacation and personal leave, and staff development are taken into account in

TABLE 13-4 Pros and Cons of Centralized and Decentralized Scheduling

Scheduling Method	Pros	Cons
Centralized	Fairness is promoted. Cost containment is facilitated. Frees some managerial time	There is no individualized treatment.
Decentralized	Managers have authority. Staff get personalized attention. Staffing is easier. Staffing is less complicated.	Schedule can be used to punish and reward. Staffing is time consuming for managers. Resources are used less efficiently. Cost containment is more difficult.

setting personnel schedules; and (7) quality of care is measured.

Resistance to centralized scheduling may be reduced when nurse managers prepare and control their own budgets, understand and approve the scheduling policies, and have open communication with the scheduler. Line and staff accountability should be carefully defined to prevent confusion over responsibility and authority when staff personnel make decisions for which line managers are accountable. Line authority is accountable for decisions, whereas staff provides support to help line managers make decisions.

The staff functions of the scheduler include scheduling employees according to staffing policies, implementing procedures for position control and reallocation of staff, maintaining records for line managers, gathering information and preparing reports to help line authority prepare personnel budgets, and maintaining communications with other appropriate departments, such as personnel and payroll.

Line responsibilities of managers include developing a master staffing pattern; establishing procedures for adjustment of staff; clarifying requirements for each job description and staff position; hiring, developing, promoting, disciplining, and firing employees when appropriate; and defining and controlling the personnel budget.

Computers can be used for centralized or decentralized scheduling, can increase effectiveness, and can help match competencies to patient needs (Donovan, 2004; Fabre, 2004). Before a computerized scheduling system is implemented,

policies and procedures are analyzed and baseline data are collected. Agency policies regarding the nature of the schedule—straight, alternating, or rotating shifts; frequency of alternating or rotating shifts; work stretch; weekends-off sequence; and use of part-time help—are constants in the information-processing system. Variables such as census, acuteness of patient conditions, special requests, special assignments, vacations, and holidays can be fed into the computer.

Advantages of centralized computer scheduling include cost-effectiveness through the reduction of clerical staff and better use of professional nurses by decreasing the time they spend in non–patient care activities; unbiased, consistent scheduling; equitable application of agency policies; production of an easy-to-read work schedule developed in advance so employees know what their schedules are and can plan their personal lives accordingly; and availability of data for monitoring the effect of staff size and composition, quality of care, and cost. However, staff may not trust the automated system. Nurse managers may feel a loss of control and may resist the use of technology (Bonczek, 2007; Englebardt & Nelson, 2002; Saba & McCormick, 2000).

Decentralized Scheduling

When nurse managers are given authority and assume responsibility, they can staff their own units through decentralized scheduling. Personnel feel that they get more personalized attention with decentralized scheduling. Staffing is easier and less complicated when done for a small area instead of for the whole agency. Each manager learns the responsibility and challenges of scheduling staff. With a philosophy of sharing and mutual trust, managers can work together to solve persistent staffing problems. Because of their knowledge and experience, managers can form a support system and offer each other informed advice. Computerization of scheduling can be helpful. When computers are used for staff scheduling, nurse managers and charge nurses have a lightened load from staffing responsibilities and have more time for other tasks.

Unfortunately, some staff members may receive individualized treatment at the expense of others, and work schedules can be used as a punishment-reward system. Scheduling staff, which is very time consuming, takes managers away from other duties or forces them to do the scheduling while off duty. Individual nurse managers will not have the "big picture" of staffing across units and may inadvertently create a staffing shortage. Decentralized scheduling may use resources less efficiently and consequently make cost containment more difficult (Bonczek, 2007).

Self-Scheduling

Self-scheduling is a scheduling system that is coordinated by staff nurses. It is a process by which nurses and other staff collectively develop and implement work schedules, taking into consideration policies and variables affecting staffing. The number of nurses needed per shift must be determined. Then typically a grid is developed so nurses can sign up for the shifts they want to work in conformity with the policies. The process might allow about 2 weeks for staff to indicate the days, shifts, weekends, holidays, and vacation days that they want. An additional 2 weeks are needed for negotiations to finalize a schedule that accommodates both the staff's and the unit's needs. Staff may negotiate before and after work and during break and lunchtime. They may also write notes to each other and wait for responses. The nurse manager needs to examine the work sheet and approve it or have the staff negotiate changes to ensure adequate staffing coverage.

Self-scheduling can help create a climate in which professional nursing can be practiced.

It saves the manager considerable scheduling time and changes the role of the manager from supervisor to coach. It increases the amount of time the staff spends on scheduling but helps develop a more accountable and professional staff. It also increases staff members' ability to negotiate with each other. Self-scheduling has been associated with increased perception of autonomy, improved professionalism, increased job satisfaction, more cooperative atmosphere, improved team spirit, improved morale, decreased absenteeism, reduced turnover, and shortened scheduling time. It has also been effective in recruitment and retention. Self-scheduling requires worker participation in the decision making and management flexibility. Staff do need negotiation and conflict resolution skills (Bard & Purnomo, 2004; Bonczek, 2007; Huber, 2006; Hung, 2002; Marquis & Huston, 2006; Roussel, Swansburg, & Swansburg, 2002; Shullanberger, 2000; Sullivan & Decker, 2005) (Table 13-5).

Alternating or Rotating Work Shifts

Although straight shifts are used by some institutions or for some personnel within institutions, rotating work shifts are common for staff nurses. The frequency of alternating between days and evenings or days and nights, or rotating through all three shifts varies among institutions. Some nurses may work all three shifts within 7 days.

Alternating and rotating work shifts create stress for staff nurses. Environmental cues, such as sunrise and sunset, fluctuate in a predictable cycle. Instruments that designate hours, minutes, and seconds correspond to the natural daily cycle and allow knowledge of one's location in that cycle. Social and work routines synchronize with the internal circadian rhythms as the body rhythms are timed to coincide with the usual activities. Thus, when environmental conditions are changed by altering work hours, sleep time, hour for arising, mealtimes, and social and recreational activities, the body must make accommodations for the environmental changes. Body rhythms need time to adjust to the discrepancy between the person's activity cycle and the new demands of the environment. The ability of body

TABLE 13-5 Advantages and Disadvantages of Various Scheduling/Staffing Methods

Method	Pros	Cons
Self-scheduling	Coordinated by staff nurses Saves manager scheduling time Helps develop accountability Increases perception of autonomy Increases job satisfaction Improves team spirit Improves morale Decreases absenteeism Reduces turnover Effective for recruitment and retention	Increases amount of time staff spends on scheduling
Rotating work shifts	Allows rotation of teams	Rotates personnel among shifts Increases stress Affects health Affects quality of work Disrupts development of work groups Leads to high turnover

Permanent shifts	Allows personnel to participate in social
	  activities
	Promotes job satisfaction
	Promotes commitment to the organization
	Leads to few health problems
	Reduces tardiness
	Decreases absenteeism
	Reduces turnover
		Most people want day shift
		New graduates predominantly staff
		  evening and night shifts
		Difficult to evaluate evening and
		  night staff
		Makes it harder for nurses to
		  appreciate the workload or
		  problems of other shifts

Block, or cyclical,
  scheduling
	Sets same schedule repeatedly
	Leads to less exhaustion
	Reduces sick time
	Allows personnel to know schedule in
	  advance
	Permits personnel to schedule social
	  events
	Decreases time spent on scheduling
	Treats staff fairly
	Decreases floating
	Promotes team spirit
		Rigid

Variable staffing	Uses census to determine number and
	  mix of staff
	Results in little need to call in
	  unscheduled staff	

functions to adjust varies considerably among individuals. It may take from 2 to 3 days to 2 weeks for a person to adjust to a different sleep-wake cycle.

Alternating and rotating work shifts affect the health of nurses and the quality of their work. The rapid shift of work schedules causes stress. The effect is further complicated by long shifts, short staffing, overtime, and multiple caregiving roles. Nurses complain of restlessness and nervousness while trying to sleep, wakefulness or sleepiness at inappropriate times, anorexia, digestive disturbance, disruption in bowel habits, fatigue, slower reaction time, lower job performance, and error proneness. Changes occur in the patterning of temperature, blood pressure, and urine excretory cycles, and resistance to disease is possibly lowered. Resultant increases in medication errors, equipment failures, and errors in problem solving are probable (Dean, Scott, & Rogers, 2006; Grosch, Caruso, Rosa, et al, 2006; Rogers, Hwang, & Scott, 2004; Rogers, Hwang, Scott, et al, 2004; Scott, Hwang, & Rogers, 2006; Seago, Spetz, & Mitchell, 2004; Sveinsdóttir, 2006; Trinkoff, Geiger-Brown, Brady, et al, 2006).

To guarantee that nurses work their share of weekends, holidays, and unpopular evening and night hours, alternating and rotating assignments currently focus on the time patterns of an individual nurse rather than on those of well-integrated work groups. The rotation of personnel on an individual basis is disruptive to the development of work groups.

The Federal Aviation Agency's (FAA's) rotation of teams of airport personnel might be used as a model by nursing services. The FAA rotates entire teams consisting of four or five controllers plus trainees and a leader, chosen because of their qualifications, amount of experience, and anticipated compatibility. Their schedules are planned 1 year in advance so that team members can plan their personal lives with confidence. Coverage for emergencies and vacations is handled within the team. Absenteeism affects the workload of the peers with whom one must continue to work; therefore team identification reduces absenteeism because of team pressure. Controllers have a low turnover rate.

In hospitals, rotation of teams instead of individuals could contribute to team development. If a group of personnel work together consistently, they can help each other through the dependence of the orientation phase of group development and the conflict experienced during the organizational phase, when the role negotiations determining who will be responsible for what occurs. The staff has a chance to become an interdependent, cohesive group with good communication and effective problem-solving abilities. Unfortunately, there is often a high turnover among nursing personnel, which complicates team development. Perhaps more attention to team development would reduce turnover.

Permanent Shifts

Permanent shifts relieve nurses of the stress and health-related problems associated with alternating and rotating shifts. They also provide social, educational, and psychological advantages. When nurses are able to choose the shift that best suits their personal life, they can participate in social activities (such as hobbies, sports, and community, professional, or church organizations) even when these require regular attendance. They may be able to continue their education by planning courses around their work schedule. Child care arrangements can be more stable. Nurses may develop a sense of belonging to a shift and feel and work better because the shift suits them. In studies of nurses in Montreal, those working permanent shifts had higher average scores on psychological scales such as those assessing mental health, job satisfaction, social involvement, and commitment to the organization. They had fewer health problems and lower rates of tardiness, absenteeism, and turnover (Sveinsdóttir, 2006).

Although the day shift is not always the preferred shift, it is likely to be. Consequently, assignment to a preferred shift may have to be done on a seniority-priority basis. This usually results in a predominance of new graduates staffing the evening and night shifts. Managers may have difficulty evaluating the evening and night shift personnel unless they make some observations during those shifts; therefore it may be easier for evening and night supervisors to evaluate permanent staff on those shifts. One disadvantage of permanent shifts is that nurses may not develop an appreciation for the workload or problems of those working other shifts.

Block, or Cyclical, Scheduling

In block, or cyclical, scheduling the same schedule is used repeatedly. One type is a 6-day forward rotation, in which personnel are scheduled to work 6 successive days followed by at least 2 days off. The schedule repeats itself every 6 weeks. It is also possible to schedule personnel with every other weekend off and 1 day off during the week so that there are no more than

4 consecutive days of work. Several types of blocks are possible. Because nurses are not exhausted by working too many consecutive days, sick leave can be reduced. By having one team member at a time on vacation and by rotating holidays among workers, vacations and holidays can be scheduled to avoid changes in the block. However, some nurses fear that 1 day off at a time is not adequate to feel rested. Nevertheless, nurses who do not work more than 4 consecutive days report that 1 day is adequate to refresh themselves.

There are several advantages to established rotations. Personnel know their schedules in advance and consequently can plan their personal lives. Absences because of social events decrease because staff can plan their social activities around their work schedules. There is a decrease in preoccupation with staffing, time spent in scheduling, time spent in maintenance of the schedule, and conflict over preferred days off. Staff are treated more fairly by equitable distribution of popular and unpopular days on duty. The scheduling of an appropriate number and category mix of personnel is simplified. Once the appropriate mix is determined, it is repeated. This helps establish stable work groups and decreases floating, which promotes team spirit and continuity of care. The initial schedule development is time consuming, and a decrease in flexibility of staffing may be perceived as a disadvantage, especially by people who need flexibility.

Eight-Hour Shift, Five-Day Work Week

The 5-day, 40-hour work week became popular during the late 1940s. It was a radical change from the 10-hour day and 5-day work week that contained split shifts and few holidays. The shifts are usually 7 AM to 3:30 PM, 3 PM to 11:30 PM, and 11 PM to 7:30 AM, which allows for a half-hour lunch break and a half-hour overlap time between shifts to provide continuity of care (Grohar-Murray & DiCroce, 2003).

Ten-Hour Shift, Four-Day Work Week or 7/70

A 10-hour-day, 4-day work week staffing pattern has been used. The main problem is fatigue, but it was not found to be as serious a problem as

anticipated. The long weekends and extra days off are attractions. In addition, there is time to finish work, peak workloads can be covered, and there is decreased overtime and related costs. The use of ten-hour shifts has been associated with reduced sick time, less turnover, and more requests to work nights. Ten-hour days are considered long workdays to some, however, and there is overlap of workers during the 24 hours. Consequently 10-hour shifts can increase salary expenditures and are not cost-efficient for many specialty units such as emergency departments, operating departments, and postanesthesia recovery rooms. There is also a 10-hour-day, 7-day work week known as 7/70. One works for 7 days and then has 7 days off (Grohar-Murray & DiCroce, 2003; Roussel, Swansburg, & Swansburg, 2006).

Twelve-Hour Shifts

The 12-hour shift, starting at 7 or 7:30 AM and ending at 7 or 7:30 PM, has been adopted by many institutions. Some work 3 days or 36 hours a week. Others work 7 days or 84 hours in 2 weeks and are paid 4 hours of overtime. Another pattern is six 12-hour days and one 8-hour day or 80 hours in 2 weeks. The better use of nursing personnel lowers staffing requirements, which consequently lowers the cost per patient-day. Nurses find they get to know their patients better because they have more time to review documentation and can visit patients more frequently. They have more time to get new admissions settled before the change of shift and feel that they can give better patient care because they are not so rushed. They find that there are fewer communication gaps. Consequently, nurse-patient relations, job satisfaction, and morale are improved.

Working relations are improved when personnel work with the same group of people, so team development is possible. There is less friction and no 3 to 11 PM shift to blame for problems. Less daily reporting results in less confusion about physicians' orders and changes in procedures and routines. Less time is required for staffing, which frees supervisors and head nurses for other duties.

Total time off is increased, with an increased usefulness of time. Total travel time is reduced.

There is less personal expense for babysitting, gas, and meals. Nurses find they have more time to relax and enjoy their days off and are able to return to work refreshed. Flexibility for personal schedules improves staff morale.

Overtime pay has been of some concern. The 1966 amendments to the Fair Labor Standards Act permit agencies to calculate overtime pay on a work period of 14 consecutive days. Consequently, overtime pay is required only for more than 80 hours of work in a 2-week period.

Some nurses complain that the extra time they have that could be used for learning and research becomes boring. Nurses also complain that their home and social lives suffer on the days they work. It can be more difficult for older nurses to manage longer shifts, and a day of absence results in greater complications. Nurses typically work longer than their scheduled 12-hour shift, and the risks of making an error are significantly increased when nurses work more than 12 hours, work overtime, or work more than 40 hours a week (Rogers, Hwang, Scott, et al, 2004). The wide variety of staffing practices suggests that there is no right or wrong staffing schedule for a given situation (Grohar-Murray & DiCroce, 2003; Roussel, Swansburg, & Swansburg, 2006).

"I have not failed. I've just found 10,000 ways that won't work." —Thomas Edison

---

Weekend Alternative

Baylor University Medical Center in Dallas, Texas, started a 2-day alternative plan. Nurses had the option of working two 12-hour days on the weekends and being paid for 36 hours for day shifts or 40 hours for night shifts. Nurses could also choose to work five 8-hour shifts Monday through Friday. This plan required a larger nursing staff and a larger budget, but filled weekend positions and reduced turnover. Some hospitals have implemented the Baylor plan, considering that the extra pay on weekends compensates for vacations, holidays, and sick time. It is more difficult to implement with budgetary restraints, so

variations have been developed. Some hospitals have nurses work 12-hour shifts just when they work weekends. This way fewer people have to work weekends, and consequently staff can have weekends off more frequently. Although illness and absences were found to increase with this system, recruitment and staffing improved. Some institutions have established a premium day weekend that gives a nurse an extra day off for working one additional weekend within a 4-week schedule. A premium vacation night has also been used. In addition, extra working days of vacation have been used to reward nurses who work only nights for a specified period (Roussel, Swansburg, & Swansburg, 2006).

Flexible Options

Flexible options are important for recruiting and retaining nurses and for reducing absenteeism. It is particularly important for the younger generation of nurses to accommodate their lifestyles.

Cross-training can prepare nurses to work in more than one area to facilitate flexible scheduling. Nurses in these float pools do need a thorough orientation, staff development, job descriptions, clear policies, and performance evaluations. Some facilities also have their own staffing pool of temporary workers to use as needed.

Temporary strategic staffing can be used for seasonal work and short-term projects. Using temporary staff can be economical when these staff do not receive benefits. Their talents need to be matched to the job, and they need to be oriented. To get good temporary workers, it may be necessary to work with specialized temporary employment agencies. It is the responsibility of the employing agency to ensure the competency of temporary staff.

Some nurses have joined temporary staffing agencies to get more control over their schedules. Downsizing has led to more use of temporary workers. Use of temporary workers gives agency personnel time to evaluate the worker before deciding whom to hire to staff and thus reduces hiring mistakes. It also gives the worker time to evaluate what it would be like to work more permanently for that agency. Some temporary staffing agencies have no hire clauses. It is becoming more important for nurses to develop good reputations for their competence in more than one clinical area and in more than one functional area, such as clinical practice, teaching, research, and/or management.

Travel nursing has grown in response to the nursing shortage and involves more than just working for local staffing agencies. It can offer opportunities for personal growth and professional development. The nurse can choose location, assignments, and type of work from per diem to long-term assignments. Pay rates can be competitive, and benefits can be good. There may be a relocation reimbursement, housing subsidy, and licensing assistance and reimbursement. Travel nursing can be appealing to young nurses who do not yet have family responsibilities as well as to empty nesters who want a new experience. The travel nurse can give an agency the benefit of a new view, and the nurse can gain a variety of experiences (Roussel, Swansburg, & Swansburg, 2006).

Variable Staffing

Variable staffing is a method in which the number and mix of staff are determined by patient needs. The number and skill mix of staff should be adjusted up or down as the numbers of patients and the acuteness of their conditions change. A fixed staffing pattern may use one RN, two LPNs, and four unlicensed personnel. With variable staffing, that ratio could be changed to one RN, four LPNs, and only one or no unlicensed personnel when patients' conditions are very acute. When there are larger numbers of patients with less acute illnesses, more unlicensed personnel and fewer LPNs might be assigned. Time measures are used for direct and indirect patient care. A patient classification system is developed, and tables are designed to determine the number of nursing hours required based on the number of patients in each category. This provides the information to determine staff needs by skill levels. Nursing pools, floats, part-time help, temporary workers, and cross-trained staff can be used to supplement the regular staff to accomplish the variable staffing. With analysis of previous staffing needs, redistribution of peak routine work, and slight overstaffing in some areas to create float personnel to meet last-moment requirements, there may be little need to call in unscheduled staff (Table 13-6). During the 2000s most staffing patterns were variations of those used earlier (Roussel, Swansburg, & Swansburg, 2006; Sullivan & Decker, 2005).

Full-Time Staff

Full-time staff may be hired to meet the average staffing needs of an institution. The most common adjustment for an increased workload is to transfer staff from a less busy area to the overloaded area. This is economical for the agency but disrupts the unity of work groups, causes the transferred nurse to feel insecure, and contributes to job dissatisfaction and turnover. Some units require specialized knowledge and skill that not every nurse has. Cross-training is helpful.

In the companion floor system, personnel from two units relieve each other. Staff nurses are oriented to the second unit and know that if they are transferred, it will be to the companion unit. Thus staff aggravation is minimized, flexibility is possible, and quality of care is maintained.

At best, a complementary, or float, staff is composed of full-time staff nurses who are oriented to many areas and like the challenge of different types of patients and settings. Unfortunately, most nurses prefer stability. Consequently, the float staff is likely to be part-time staff or new personnel waiting for a permanent assignment.

Letting full-time staff work double shifts, extra shifts, and overtime is another option. The nurse is already oriented to the area, and continuity of care is facilitated. There are also disadvantages, however. Institutional costs increase. The nurses may become fatigued, errors are likely to increase with fatigue, and overtime may interfere with the nurses' personal lives (Roussel, Swansburg, & Swansburg, 2006; Sullivan & Decker, 2005).

Mandatory overtime is requiring staff to stay on duty after their scheduled shift ends. Some managers may believe that a fatigued nurse is better than no nurse at all. The ANA and other professional organizations oppose mandatory

TABLE 13-6 Pros and Cons of Variable Staffing

	Pros	Cons
8-Hour shifts	Traditional	Longer workweek
10-Hour shifts	Time to complete work	Fatigue
	Long weekends	Overlap
	Extra days off	Difficulty finding substitute
	Decreased overtime	
	Cover peak workloads	
	Decreases costs	
12-Hour shifts	Lower staffing requirements	Greater exhaustion at end of work week
	Lower cost per patient-day	Increase in tension at end of work week
	Increased knowledge of patients	Increase in minor accidents
	Ability to get new admissions settled	Increase in medication errors
	Less feeling of being rushed	Home and social life suffer the week
	Better continuity of care	worked
	Possibility for team development	
	Less daily reporting	
	Less time spent in staffing	
	Reduced travel time	
	Lower personal expenses for gas, meals, babysitting	
Baylor plan/ weekend option	Decrease in number of people who need to work weekends	Increased illness
	More frequent weekends off	Higher absenteeism
	Fewer hours of work for higher pay	
	Improvement in staffing	
	Higher morale	

overtime. There is fear that tired, overworked nurses may have compromised decision-making abilities and be more prone to making mistakes. Nurses fear litigation and risk of losing their nursing license. Mandatory overtime is a political issue and is often a negotiating point for unionized nurses. Some states have adopted legislation prohibiting mandatory overtime. Organizations often have policies about their right to mandate overtime. Some specify that refusing to work required overtime constitutes patient abandonment and is punishable. Some states have clarified that refusing mandatory overtime is not patient abandonment (ANA, 1999a; Bonczek, 2007).

Part-Time Staff

Flexible working hours can be an incentive for inactive nurses to start part-time employment and can thus help to reduce staffing shortages. Most nurses are women who have to combine their nursing role with many other roles, such as wife, mother, and homemaker. A part-time job can broaden the woman's horizons beyond her home, increase her income, give her ego satisfaction, and help her maintain her nursing skills. It is not uncommon for nurses to want to work part time while continuing their education. Part-time nurses tend to work more than their share of unpopular hours, and some prefer evening and night duty exclusively. When part-time nurses' other responsibilities decrease, they are likely candidates for full-time work. It is sometimes possible for two people to share a job.

There are, of course, disadvantages to the use of part-time nurses. Educational and administrative expenses are proportionately higher for part-time than for full-time help. For example, it is likely to cost as much to orient a part-time nurse as a full-time nurse, so that the cost per hour worked is higher. Maintaining continuity of care is complicated, because two or more part-time people may fill budgeted full-time positions.

There are also disadvantages for the employee. The part-time nurse may not receive benefits, such as paid sick or vacation days, and is not likely to be considered for promotion. Sometimes benefits are prorated for part-time workers.

Temporary help is another option. Some institutions hire temporary help for the summer to provide coverage for staff vacations. Temporary bed and bath teams or premium days have been used to reduce weekend staffing shortages. Staff nurses get an extra day off (a premium day) if they work one additional weekend in a 4-week schedule. Some nurses may be willing to work on an on-call basis year-round.

External agencies providing temporary help are available in some areas. The use of such agencies can greatly reduce the amount of time middle management must spend on staffing. The manager merely calls the external agency and requests a certain number of nurses, and the agency makes the necessary contacts. The agency has a registry of available nurses, who are allowed to have highly flexible, self-determined schedules. This allows some nurses to work who could not do so otherwise and consequently helps those nurses maintain their skills. It is then more likely that those nurses will return to nursing practice on a full-time basis than if they had remained inactive. Their availability may boost morale, and they may introduce new ideas and stimulate creativity among the regular staff.

Unfortunately, there are also disadvantages to temporary help agencies. The matching of the nurses' credentials and qualifications with assignments and orientation to assignments are severe problems. Although some temporary help agencies do keep on file orientation information and procedures manuals for their client institutions, their use may still be optional. It is likely to take considerable time for the regular staff to orient the temporary help, errors are likely to increase, and continuity of care is jeopardized. The temporary nurses might get preferred schedules, which leaves the regular staff with more of the less-attractive hours if the staffing was not managed well. Consequently, morale could be lowered for the regular staff. A central placement service run by the state board of nursing or the state nurses association could be useful for matching nurses' qualifications and interests with actual or anticipated vacancies throughout the state.

There are many variables to consider when planning staffing schedules. The more accurately those variables are assessed, the better one is able to contain costs while providing high-quality care (Grohar-Murray & DiCroce, 2003).

Managers have several relatively undesirable options for handling a called-in absence or otherwise uncovered shift. They can consider the following:

- Using a float, per diem, or agency nurse
- Asking a nurse to work for the sick nurse and canceling a shift for that person later in the week
- Asking a part-time person to work an extra shift
- Substituting a person of one classification for another, such as an LPN for an RN
- Asking one staff member to work a few hours of overtime and another to come in a few hours early
- Doing without a substitute
- Covering the shift themselves

VARIABLES AFFECTING STAFFING

Although institutional and nursing service philosophy and objectives guide staffing, various patient, staff, and environmental factors also affect staffing patterns. The types of patients, their expectations, fluctuations in admissions, length of stay, and complexity of care complicate staffing (Finkler & Kovner, 2000) (Box 13-1). Personnel policies, educational and experience levels of staff, job descriptions, the mix of work titles or career ladder leveling, hour and rotation policies, absenteeism, and the competitive market also affect staffing. Environmental factors, such as the floor plan of the unit and hospital, number of patient beds, availability of supplies and equipment, organizational structure, and availability of support services from other departments and agencies are also considered when planning staffing patterns.

BOX 13-1 Variables That Affect Staffing

Workload budgets indicate the amount of work produced by a unit in terms of units of service, which are used to calculate expense budgets.

Activity reports provide statistics about current activity centering on the number of units of service given compared with the capacity.

Average daily census is the average number of patients cared for per day for a period of time.

Average length of stay is the average number of days that patients receive care in the institution.

Adjusted units of service allow budgeting based on expected workload units of service adjusted for the expected mix of patients.

Care hours calculation determines the average required care hours per patient per 24 hours for each classification level and the sum or total hours of care needed for all patients.

Personnel expense budget is the budget for all personnel assigned to a unit.

Fixed staff are employees whose work hours do not vary with the patient volume.

Variable staff are employees whose work hours change in response to the projected number of care hours needed.

Positions should be established based on the manager's judgment regarding the use of full-time and part-time personnel to achieve the number of full-time equivalents required to meet patient care needs.

Labor costs are determined by calculating the dollar outlays for straight-time salary, differentials, overtime, raises, and fringe benefits for each person employed by the unit.

Expense budget (not including personnel) is a combination of the direct unit expenses plus the indirect overhead expenses.

Revenue budget is the unit's income.

Modified from Finkler SA, Kovner CT: *Financial management for nurse managers and executives,* Philadelphia, 2000, Saunders.

Budget submission is done periodically by providing a summary of the revenue and expense sections of the budget for review. A narrative justification is used to negotiate changes in the budget. Managers are responsible for implementation of the budget to meet the staffing needs of the unit, including weekend, holiday, vacation, and sick leave coverage through busy and slow periods (Bonczek, 2007).

Staffing Studies

Three major types of staffing studies are used to predict the number, level, and mix of personnel required for staffing. Nursing care needed may be predicted from patient classification systems by assigning patients to categories according to diagnosis, acuteness of care, or amount of self-sufficiency. Number, level, and mix of staff needed can be determined by noting the number of patients in each category. Then a cost-effective nursing personnel budget based on the needs of patients and the qualifications of nursing personnel can be determined. Patient classification systems can be combined with nursing care plans, and costs for individual patients can be determined. Systems that charge patients for the care they receive can be designed.

Time standards can be determined for nursing procedures by listing and analyzing the procedures required by each patient. The time required for each patient and the sum for all patients on a unit can then be calculated. Formulas deduced from statistical analysis of work sampling data can be used to predict the number of nursing care hours needed and to negotiate for increases in staffing despite financial pressures. However, staffing is a function of fiscal factors, market availability, creativity, and innovation (Beglinger, 2006).

"It is better to light a candle than to curse the darkness." —Eleanor Roosevelt

Principles of Nurse Staffing

The ANA (1999b) identified the following principles for nurse staffing related to unit patient care: Staffing levels should reflect individual and aggregate patient needs. The concept of nursing hours per patient-day should be questioned. Functions to support quality patient care should be considered when determining staffing levels.

Principles related to staff include the following: Patient needs should determine the required

RESEARCH Perspective 13-1

Data from Seago JA: A comparison of two patient classification instruments in an acute care hospital, *J Nurs Adm* 32(5):243-249, 2002.

Purpose: The purpose of this study was to compare the time spent in caring for patients predictive validity of two types of patient classification instruments commonly used in acute care hospitals in California.

Methods: Two general types of patient classification systems commonly used are the summative task type of classification system and the critical incident or criterion type of classification system. One study shift was used, the first day after the patient had been hospitalized a full 24 hours. The predictor score was determined before each shift that day, and the actual score was determined at the end of each shift that day. Data were collected using medical record review only.

Both types of data collection instruments, criterion and summative, were completed for all 349 patients at both collection points. A before and after shift core was determined for each patient using each instrument. Three hundred forty-nine medical records for inpatients meeting the inclusion criteria were examined.

Results/conclusions: The most significant finding of this study was that there were virtually no differences in the predictive ability of the summative and criterion patient classification instruments. For the same set of patients, there was agreement between the predictor and the actual scores more than 78% of the time.

clinical competencies. Nurses need nursing management support as well as representation at both the operational and executive levels. Clinical support for less proficient RNs should be readily available from experienced RNs.

Principles related to the organization include the following: Organizational policy should reflect the valuing of employees. All organizations should have documented competencies for staff. Organizational policies should recognize the needs of both patients and staff.

Time Standards

When figuring time standards for nursing care, one should consider both direct and indirect care. Direct care involves the patient and includes feeding, bathing, treating, and giving medications. Indirect care includes all activities that are not direct care, such as preparation for and cleaning up after medication administration and treatments, coordination of clinical care, reporting, communications, documentation of care, and coffee and lunch breaks.

Once the number and kind of care activities required by each patient are identified and the length of time required to carry out the activities

is calculated, one can add up the time required by all patients on a unit and divide by the number of productive work hours on a shift to determine the number of personnel needed. The mix of nursing personnel can be predicted by categorizing the care according to the qualifications required to deliver it, adding the time in each category, and dividing by productive hours on a shift to obtain the number of specific types of personnel required to meet patient needs. Once this is accomplished, patients can be charged by the level of care required.

Public health nurses deal with health needs of aggregate groups and individuals in the community, whereas visiting nurses provide care to clients in their own homes. There are also health care clinics and nurse practitioner clinics in the community. For visiting nurse services and home health agencies, staffing is determined by the number of clients who need to be seen in a day. A standard amount of time is often allocated per visit. A standard of 45 minutes per visit for four to six clients depending on the amount of driving has been used, but the acuteness level of clients treated at home has increased. Thus a system based on acuteness is merited.

Patient Classification Systems

Patient classification systems were introduced when managers realized that nurse staffing needs were related more to the patient's dependency on care than to the medical diagnosis. The three basic types of patient classification systems are (1) narrative description, (2) checklist, and (3) time standard or relative value unit. In the descriptive type, the nurse classifies the patient into the category that most closely describes the care received. The tool used is a narrative on a concise acuteness table. Category 1 may be self-care and category 4 complete care, including feeding, frequent skin care, complete bathing, complete bed rest, and frequent positioning. The patient does not have to receive all the care in a category to be classified in that category. The nurse chooses the category that best describes the patient. The major problem with this type of system is low interrater reliability, caused by subjectivity in the nurse's interpretation of degree of care required by the patient. The descriptive type is a quick-check guide, but poor interrater reliability leads to a wide range of requested nurse/patient ratios. Many administrators have moved away from this subjective type of patient classification.

The checklist-type acuteness table divides elements of care routines into activity categories, such as eating and bathing. Activity levels are described in each category. Levels in the eating category might be self-care, help setting up, feeding, and frequent feeding. Each activity is assigned an activity level point score, such as 1 for routine care or self-care and 4 for comprehensive care. The nurse checks the activity level for each patient in each category and totals the points for each patient to determine the level of care. This is usually done at each shift or daily. It, too, is a subjective system.

A time standard, or relative value unit, system assigns a value unit (usually a measure of time) to various activities of patient care. These activities are usually clustered according to categories, such as diet, bathing, and mobility. There is considerable variation in the complexity of these systems.

Medicus was one of the first patient classification systems developed and was introduced in the late 1960s. It is still being used. It clusters patients into five categories, with 5 indicating the greatest intensity of care. Indicators and the average hours of nursing care required determine the level. It reflects both direct and indirect care.

GRASP (Grace Reynolds Application and Study of PETO) was introduced in 1970 and has been commonly used for decades. It identifies about 50 direct and indirect patient care activities. Time studies are performed to validate that the time estimates are accurate for the given organization. Interrater reliability is checked. Calculations are to be made every 12 hours and may be done using a computerized form or manually with paper and pencil. Although GRASP is time consuming, it is commonly used today. It is a multidimensional nursing management information system that includes staffing/scheduling, cost identification, budgeting, and quality evaluations. It determines total hours of care and required staff.

The Therapeutic Intervention Scoring System (TISS) determines illness severity by assessing the time and intensity of the required interventions for patient care. This is done by classifying numerous conditions and treatments into categories assigned 1, 2, 3, or 4 points. The points are then summed to yield one of four classifications: class I—fewer than 10 points; class II—10 to 19 points; class III—20 to 39 points; and class IV—more than 40 points. The system works well for acute medical-surgical areas. Other classification systems have been developed for specialty areas such as hospice care and long-term care.

The Expert Nurse Estimation Patient Classification System (ENEPCS) is a contemporary model that is customized by the caregivers in the agency. It identifies unique patient characteristics in eight categories: (1) cognitive status, (2) self-care status, (3) emotional and psychosocial support needs, (4) comfort/pain management needs, (5) family information and support needs, (6) treatment needs, (7) interdisciplinary coordination and patient teaching, and (8) transition needs. It can be used in multiple clinical settings to calculate the skill mix and cost of labor for each patient (Malloch & Krueger, 2006).

The matrix system had become increasingly popular by the early 2000s. Census may be recorded as the number of patients down the left-hand column. Then there may be columns for the number of licensed staff (RNs, LPNs) and unlicensed staff (aides, technical personnel) needed, including the unit secretary, for days and nights for 12-hour shifts. With increasingly sophisticated technology, computers can incorporate time-and-motion data plus expert nurse judgment to use in predicting the cost of achieving certain patient outcomes, matching patient needs with caregiver profiles, and tracking and monitoring patient-caregiver interactions.

There are advantages to patient classification systems. They can be used to help nurse managers establish the amount of care required, determine the unit staff and skill mix needed, prepare the unit budget based on need, determine the cost of patient care, and refine the daily staffing requirements. There are also disadvantages. The reliability and validity of self-reported data can be questioned. There can be observer-induced biases as well as self-reporting biases. However, computerized real-time systems that record direct and indirect nursing care activities are available. Leaders and managers may worry about being able to meet the staffing levels indicated by the patient classification system and the related liability. Consequently, some agencies have stopped using patient classification systems.

Clinical outcomes can be used to assess the adequacy of staffing. The following indicate a need for better staffing: adverse drug reactions, family complaints, injuries to patients, long length of stay, patient complaints, patient falls, postoperative infections, shock/cardiac arrest, skin breakdown, upper gastrointestinal bleeding, and urinary tract infections. Nurse-sensitive indicators include nursing hours per patient-day, use of on-call or per diem personnel, overtime, sick time, staff satisfaction, staff turnover rate, staff vacancy rate, and failure to achieve the levels in the institution's staffing plan (Bonczek, 2007).

Staffing Formulas

When determining the number of staff to hire, one must consider the hours for which coverage is required, vacations, holidays, absenteeism, and staff development time. If nurses work 5 days per week and coverage is needed for 7 days, it takes 1.4 nurses to have one nurse on duty for 7 days and 2.8 nurses to have two nurses on duty for 7 days. This can be calculated by multiplying the number needed on duty by the number of days per week for which coverage is required and dividing by the number of days each employee works per week to determine the number of personnel needed for coverage (Table 13-7). This figure does not allow for vacations, holidays, absenteeism, or staff development time.

To calculate vacation coverage, multiply the number of vacation days per year by the number of people at the given skill level. Then divide the total number of vacation days per skill level by the total days worked per year per person to determine the number of people needed for vacation coverage. For example:

$$\begin{matrix} \text{Number of} \\ \text{vacation days} \\ \text{per year} \end{matrix} \times \begin{matrix} \text{Number of} \\ \text{full-time people} \\ \text{at given skill level} \end{matrix} = \begin{matrix} \text{Total vacation} \\ \text{days by} \\ \text{skill level} \end{matrix}$$

$$\begin{matrix} \text{Total vacation} \\ \text{days by} \\ \text{skill level} \end{matrix} \div \begin{matrix} \text{Total days} \\ \text{worked per} \\ \text{person per year} \end{matrix} = \begin{matrix} \text{Number of} \\ \text{full-time people} \\ \text{needed for} \\ \text{vacation} \\ \text{relief coverage} \end{matrix}$$

To determine holiday coverage, multiply the total number of personnel required (7-day coverage per skill level) by the number of holidays to determine the number of holiday days to be staffed. Then divide the total holiday relief days by the total days worked per year per person to obtain the number of personnel required per skill level for holiday coverage per year.

$$\begin{matrix} \text{Number of} \\ \text{personnel} \end{matrix} \times \begin{matrix} \text{Number of} \\ \text{holidays} \end{matrix} = \begin{matrix} \text{Number of} \\ \text{holiday relief days} \\ \text{needing coverage} \end{matrix}$$

$$\begin{matrix} \text{Number of} \\ \text{holiday} \\ \text{relief days} \end{matrix} \div \begin{matrix} \text{Number of} \\ \text{days worked} \\ \text{per year} \\ \text{per person} \end{matrix} = \begin{matrix} \text{Number of} \\ \text{personnel} \\ \text{required for} \\ \text{holiday} \\ \text{coverage per year} \end{matrix}$$

The percentage of absentees is used to calculate absentee relief coverage:

$$\frac{\text{Weeks}}{\text{per year}} \times \frac{\text{Days worked}}{\text{per week}} \times \text{Percent absent} = \frac{\text{Absentee days per person per year}}{}$$

$$\frac{\text{Number of personnel}}{(7 \text{ days per week})} \times \frac{\text{Absentee days per person per year}}{} = \frac{\text{Number of absentee days requiring coverage}}{}$$

$$\frac{\text{Number of absentee days}}{} \div \frac{\text{Total days worked per person per year}}{} = \frac{\text{Full-time personnel required for absentee coverage per year}}{}$$

Personnel required for staff development relief per year can also be calculated:

$$\frac{\text{Number of hours required or recommended for staff development}}{} \times \text{Number of staff} = \frac{\text{Number of hours per year for staff development needing relief coverage}}{}$$

$$\frac{\text{Number of staff development hours needing coverage}}{} \div \frac{\text{Hours worked per day}}{} \div \frac{\text{Total days worked per person}}{}$$

$$= \frac{\text{Full-time personnel required for staff development coverage}}{}$$

A staffing slide rule can be developed to save time when computing the number of budgeted positions needed to meet staffing standards by preparing a table that identifies the number of persons needed on duty, number of persons needed to cover days off, and number of persons needed to cover additional days off for vacation, holiday, sick, and personal leaves. Table 13-8 provides examples.

One full-time equivalent (FTE) position is equal to 40 hours per week for 52 weeks. That equals 2080 hours per year. One person or a combination of personnel can fill an FTE. For example, two people could share a job by together working for 80 hours every 2 weeks. Fixed FTEs are for employees scheduled to work no matter what the volume of work is. Variable FTEs are for

TABLE 13-7 Staffing Formulas

Number Needed	Days of Week	Number of Days Each Work Week	Number of People Required
1 ×	7 ÷	5 =	1.4
2 ×	7 ÷	5 =	2.8
3 ×	7 ÷	5 =	4.2
4 ×	7 ÷	5 =	5.6
5 ×	7 ÷	5 =	7.0

employees such as temporary part-time workers who are scheduled according to workload needs (Bonczek, 2007; Huber, 2006; Marquis & Huber, 2006; Roussel, Swansburg & Swansburg, 2006; Sullivan & Decker, 2005). Computers are being used with increasing frequency to determine nurse staffing depending on factors such as system availability, reliability, capital resources, revenue resources available, resource consumption, system benefits, training, and implementation of a computer program (Fralic, 2000).

Reductions in Force

Budget cuts, declining inpatient activity, and changing patient care patterns have caused some institutions to "rightsize" or downsize. Proactive rightsizing measures may eliminate or minimize the need for downsizing. Rightsizing is a comprehensive and systematic process that studies ineffective, costly programs and generates ideas for replacing them with revenue-generating programs. Units that should be investigated include those where the occupancy rate is below 60%, where caregiver hours worked per patient have increased by several percentage points in a year, where fixed staffing levels have increased by a small percentage of the FTEs, where productivity goals are not met, and where costs exceed revenues, as well as units that have been out of service.

Finding new work for present employees can delay the need for downsizing. Examples are contracting out continuing education and laundry services and attracting work by expanding services or initiating new services, such as geriatrics services. Slow times can be used for providing inservice education for personnel to increase competence, for cross-training personnel to work

TABLE 13-8 Staffing Formulas*

Number Needed on Duty	Number Needed to Cover Usual Days Off	15.6 Extra Days + 6%	18.2 Extra Days + 7%	20.8 Extra days + 8%	23.4 Extra Days + 9%
1	1.4	1.46	1.47	1.48	1.49
2	2.8	2.92	2.94	2.96	2.98
3	4.2	4.38	4.41	4.44	4.47
4	5.6	5.84	5.88	5.92	5.96
5	7.0	7.30	7.35	7.40	7.45

*For 5-day work week and variable numbers of days off for vacation, holidays, and sick and personal leave.

in more than one area, for carrying out special projects, and for updating policies and procedures. Reducing overtime; encouraging use of holidays, vacation time, and leaves of absence without pay; reducing temporary help; and deferring hiring can decrease the budgetary deficit.

Use of attrition, temporary offers of early retirement, and conversion of full-time to part-time positions may be considered before job terminations. When it becomes necessary to implement layoffs, many issues must be considered: Will layoffs be based on seniority, job skills, job classification, or a combination of these factors? It is beneficial to involve managers from the patient care coordinator position on up in deciding the criteria for layoffs. If seniority is used, is there a bumping policy? Bumping through transfers, demotions, and layoffs makes layoffs much more complicated and time consuming and involves about five times more people than originally targeted. People who know their positions are in jeopardy may experience more stress than those who have actually been bumped. Nurses may be angry and frustrated that they are transferred outside their specialty area. They may not be suited to their new positions and may file grievances that are time consuming and costly to both staff and management. Many nurses would rather be laid off and be eligible for unemployment compensation than work in areas in which they do not feel qualified. Orientation and training for the new positions also cost time and money. Nurses may be too angry to orient the people who will replace them. Those who are staying may worry about being responsible

for inexperienced nurses placed on their units. Those who retrain may leave the institution as soon as they find another position in their area of interest. Many qualified people may leave voluntarily but will discuss their unhappy experiences in the community.

There are also communication issues. Many people prefer to be informed about a layoff by personal communication rather than in writing. It is common to have a public meeting with immediate written follow-up. Many want information about why cuts are needed, the extent of the cuts, and the potential effects. They may want to be informed as soon as possible so they can make necessary arrangements.

Attention must be given to morale building through increased communication and input into decision making. Designating a central communication office may be helpful by providing a place for personnel to call or where they can stop in for clarification or information. A meeting may be scheduled to explain rules, present facts, and answer questions in an attempt to reduce anxiety. Discussion of the organization's bumping policy and procedures is particularly appropriate. Recall policy should also be discussed so that retained and laid-off personnel know their rights and responsibilities concerning future vacancies. Support groups can be formed to allow for venting anger and sharing feelings. Stress management workshops are appropriate.

A placement committee may be formed to match affected personnel to openings, or a review process may be implemented to respond to objections. Job skill evaluation and job counseling may be offered to affected personnel.

Clear-cut procedures for matching personnel skills and openings are essential. Training opportunities to prepare people for new jobs should be provided, and prospective employees should be informed of the organization's layoff policies before they are hired. Public relations efforts to address community image will require attention.

Productivity

Productivity is the amount of product or work produced by a specific amount of resources, measured as outputs divided by inputs. For example, productivity can be measured as required staff hours divided by provided staff hours multiplied by 100. Improvements in productivity involve obtaining more work or product for less overall cost. Productivity can be increased by decreasing the staff hours provided while holding the required staff hours constant or increasing them. Many actions can be taken to increase outputs while maintaining or reducing inputs. Outputs are often measured through the patient classification system: average daily census, number of patient-days per month, number of patients treated, and number of procedures performed are productivity measures.

Hours per patient-day is an indicator often used by hospitals to measure productivity. It is a direct method of patient classification–related staffing in which the number of staff hours is divided by the number of patient-days. It assumes a direct relationship between hours per patient-day and salary expenses per patient-day to measure costs. However, many factors affect time requirements, so that averages do not account well for outlier situations.

Such things as recognizing the need to do better, involving the staff, seeking staff ideas and recommendations, creating challenges, demonstrating management interest in staff achievements and concerns, and providing praise and rewards for good performance can help increase productivity. Evaluating the problems, resources, and realities in the organization; using work flow analysis and work simplification procedures; and improving the use of time by helping personnel keep and analyze time diaries and decreasing waiting time can make a difference. There are many ways to improve productivity: set a climate for productivity by asking personnel what would help them be more productive and implementing their ideas; set targets for increasing outputs; have personnel set personal objectives and measure performance against them; seek new approaches to old problems and improve products and services. Staff development and attention to process, ethics, and aesthetics enhance productivity through emphasis on doing the right things the right way (Roussel, Swansburg, & Swansburg, 2006).

Magnetism

During the early 1980s, the American Academy of Nursing appointed a task force to study the shortage of nurses. Many problems had been recognized, but factors that correlated with successful settings had not been identified (McClure, 2005). In 1982 to 1983, the ANA sponsored a study to identify variables related to recruitment, retention, and job satisfaction of nurses. Forty-one of 165 institutions nominated by Fellows of the American Academy of Nursing based on their reputations for attracting and retaining nurses were sampled. Most of them were private, nonprofit institutions affiliated with an educational program in nursing. Predominately professional nursing staff provided the care, and at least 85% of the budgeted registered positions were filled on an annual basis (McClure, Poulin, Sovie, et al, 1983). The original study stimulated a series of further studies that added variables, developed and refined instruments, and expanded the scope to include facilities besides hospitals, such as nursing homes, and facilities in other countries. In particular, Marlene Kramer and Claudia Schmalenberg researched characteristics essential for magnetism starting in the mid-1980s; Linda Aiken studied the impact of magnetism on patient outcomes, including morbidity and mortality; and Margaret McClure and Ada Sue Hinshaw synthesized research findings (Kramer, 2005; Kramer & Schmalenberg, 2005; McClure & Hinshaw, 2002).

RESEARCH Perspective 13-2

Data from Williams KA, Stotts RC, Jacob SR, et al: Inactive nurses: A source for alleviating the nursing shortage? *J Nurs Adm* 36(4):205-210, 2006.

Purpose: The United States experienced a shortage of 110,000 registered nurses (6% of the number needed) in 2000. It is projected that the shortage of registered nurses will reach 29% of the required number by 2020. The purpose of this study was to learn why inactive registered nurses chose to become inactive and to examine what they would want to return to nursing.

Methods: A quantitative cross-sectional survey was used to collect data from 428 inactive nurses younger than age 60 in one southern state. Descriptive and inferential statistics were used to analyze the data.

Results/conclusions: Many (27.6%) left nursing because of conflicts between parenting responsibilities and work, and 13.5% left because of scheduling requirements at work. Respondents indicated that they would return to active nursing if given an opportunity to work part-time, with flexible and shorter shifts. The pool of inactive registered nurses younger than age 60 is one source for potentially alleviating some of the nursing shortage. Employers may encourage many of them to return to active duty by providing more flexible schedules, including part-time work and shorter shifts, and by decreasing workloads.

The American Nurses Credentialing Center (ANCC) launched a program to promote and recognize hospitals based on standards of nursing service administration and nursing care in 1990. Urden and Monarch (2002) defined the 14 characteristics of magnetism as follows:

1. Quality of leadership: knowledgeable risk takers with articulated philosophy for advocacy and support
2. Organizational structure: flat, decentralized structure in which unit-based decisions prevail and the nursing leader serves at the executive level in the organization and reports to the chief executive officer
3. Management style: participative management at all levels of the organization with visible and accessible leaders who value and encourage communications
4. Personnel policies and programs: competitive salaries and benefits, promotional opportunities, flexible staffing with minimal rotation of shifts, and staff involvement in policy development
5. Professional models of care: RNs who are responsible and accountable for their patient care and the coordination of care
6. Quality of care: a priority for the organization; nursing leaders develop the environment for

providing a high quality of care, and nurses believe they are giving it
7. Quality improvement: participation of staff nurses in this educational activity to improve quality of care
8. Consultation and resources: availability of knowledgeable experts and supportive peers
9. Autonomy: expectation that nurses will exercise independent judgment consistent with professional standards in the context of a multidisciplinary approach to patient care
10. Community and the hospital: ongoing long-term outreach programs that result in the perception of the hospital as a positive, strong, productive community corporate citizen
11. Nurse as teacher: incorporation of teaching into nursing care
12. Image of nursing: view of nursing services as integral and essential to the quality of care
13. Interdisciplinary relationships: mutual respect among all disciplines
14. Professional development: value for personal and professional growth and development and emphasis on orientation, inservice education, continuing education, formal education, and career development.

In 2005, the 14 forces of magnetism became the conceptual framework for the magnet program (Brady-Schwartz, 2005).

Goode, Krugman, Smith, and others (2005) described how University of Colorado Hospital personnel achieved and are striving to maintain magnet status. They indicated that magnet recognition starts long before the actual preparation of the application to the ANCC for magnet status. The executive team affirmed that magnet status was a strategic hospital goal. A multidisciplinary team was formed. Each committee member received a notebook of published articles and background materials. Standards were assigned to teams of one nurse leader and one staff nurse. The committee members were responsible for educating other staff. After the written documentation was submitted, two nurse appraisers representing the ANCC verified the written documentation through a site visit. Efforts were made to sustain the magnet culture by structuring shared governance, orienting new personnel to the culture, writing magnet-level standards into performance appraisals, setting research standards, and developing and integrating a system of evidence-based practice to improve the clinical and management outcomes. Ellis and Gates (2005) also described committee selection, education, team building, and planning and development of a process inspired by a mission to provide excellent, safe patient care to achieve magnet status. Drenkard (2005) described how one health system achieved redesignation of magnet status for its flagship hospital through a culture of shared governance with participation in decisions about clinical practice. Jasovsky, Dornan, Geisler, and others (2005) recommended a cost-effective on-line system for demographic data collection to generate the ANCC report. Shirey (2005) described a professional certification drive to provide evidence of magnetism.

There have been a vast number of publications about magnet hospitals during the 2000s. The paradigm shift in the Magnet Recognition Program has been identified as involving a shift in the appraisal process from tradition to best practice and evidence based practice; from colleague review to peer review; from passive learning to learning community; from low technologic level to high technologic level; from a small business model to a professional business model; from a competency-based model to a performance management model; from a static compensation model to pay for performance; and from blind to transparent activities (Triolo, Scherer, & Floyd, 2006). Results of a study of 470 staff nurses at both magnet and nonmagnet hospitals supported other evidence that nurses at the magnet hospitals demonstrate significantly more job satisfaction, and this is linked to retention (Brady-Schwartz, 2005).

Baldrige National Quality Award

In 1987, Congress established the Baldrige National Quality Award (BNQA) program to recognize organizations in the United States for achievement in quality and performance. The award was named after Malcom Baldrige who was the Secretary of Commerce from 1981 to 1987. He saw quality management as a key to the country's success. Many government and industry leaders noted that quality was needed for businesses to compete in a demanding and expanding market. Manufacturing, small businesses, and service were the first award categories. Education and health care were added in 1999 and some health care providers have been recognized. The organizations have to meet seven areas of excellence: (1) leadership, (2) strategic planning, (3) customer and market focus, (4) information and analysis, (5) human resources focus, (6) process management and (7) business or organizational performance results. Some states have started developing awards based on the BNQA criteria (Huber, 2006).

CHAPTER SUMMARY

The nursing shortage has a deleterious effect on staffing and the quality of care. Nurses need to be active in recruiting people into nursing and encouraging the retention of nurses. There are many strategies available to recruit and retain nurses. Several assignment systems for staffing have evolved over time, but institutions mainly employ variations on the basic types. There are a number of possible staffing schedules. Flexibility has become increasingly important.

Magnet status is a gold standard for nursing that is correlated with high recruitment and retention of nurses and excellent quality of care through good leadership, decentralized structures, participative management, and professional delivery models. Competitive salaries and benefits help attract nurses. Availability of consultation and resources, and quality improvement through evidence-based practice that leads to autonomous decision making can help retain nurses. Nurses incorporate teaching into their practice. In magnet organizations there is professional development and interdisciplinary relationships with nurses, who are viewed as essential to patient care. Some health care providers have also been acknowledged for excellence with the Malcolm Baldrige National Qualtiy Award.

CRITICAL THINKING ACTIVITY

Reflective Journal: Make observations in a clinical setting or reflect on past experiences. Identify the nursing model and staffing schedules used in the facility. What factors determine the assignment of personnel? How is the work of the unit or department organized? Identify the responsibilities of key persons in the unit. Describe the patient classification system used, if any. How does the patient classification system relate to staffing, budgeting, and quality assurance?

CASE STUDY

You are responsible for the budget on your unit. You have a registered nurse vacancy that you may fill with one registered nurse or two unlicensed personnel. What will you do, and why?

ONLINE RESOURCES

evolve Additional critical thinking activities, worksheets, and case studies are available online at http://evolve.elsevier.com/Marriner/guide8e.

REFERENCES

Aiken LH, Clarke SP, Cheung RB, et al: Educational levels of hospital nurses and patient mortality, *JAMA* 290(12):1617-1623, 2003.

Aiken LH, Clarke SP, Sloane DM: Hospital staffing, organization, and quality of care: Cross-national findings, *Int J Qual Health Care* 14(1):5-13, 2002.

Aiken LH, Clarke SP, Sloane DM, et al: Nurses' reports on hospital care in five countries, *Health Aff* 20(3):43-53, 2001.

Aiken LH, Clarke SP, Sloane DM, et al: Hospital nurse staffing and patient mortality, nurse burnout, and job dissatisfaction, *JAMA* 288(16):1987-1993, 2002.

American Association of Colleges of Nursing: Hallmarks of the professional nursing practice environment, *J Prof Nurs* 18(5):295-304, 2002.

American Association of Colleges of Nursing: *A model for differentiated nursing practice,* Washington, DC, 1995, Author.

American Nurses Association: House of Delegates materials, Washington, DC, 1999a, The Association.

American Nurses Association: *Principles for nurse staffing with annotated bibliography*, Washington, DC, 1999b, American Nurses Publishing.

American Nurses Association: New ANA study provides more proof of link between RN staffing and quality patient care, Washington, DC, 2000, The Association (press release).

Andrews J, Manthorpe MA, Watson R: Employment transitions for older nurses: A qualitative study, *J Adv Nurs* 51(3):298-306, 2005.

Anthony MK, Standing TS, Glick J, et al: Leadership and nurse retention: The pivotal role of nurse managers, *J Nurs Adm* 35(3):146-155, 2005.

Atencio BL, Cohen J, Gorenberg B: Nurse retention: Is it worth it?, *Nurs Econ* 21(6):262-268, 2003.

Barclay L: *Retaining older nurses in hospital practice: A newsmaker interview with Barbara J. Hatcher*, 2006 (article online): http://medscape.com/viewarticle/537115. Accessed February 15, 2007.

Bard JF, Purnomo HW: Preference scheduling for nurses using column generation, *Eur J Oper Res* 164:510-534, 2004.

Bartholomew K: *Ending nurse-to-nurse hostility: Why nurses eat their young and each other*, Marblehead, MA, 2006, Opus Communications.

Beglinger JE: Quantifying patient care intensity: An evidence-based approach to determining staffing requirements, *Nurs Adm Q* 30(3):193-202, 2006.

Benner P: *From novice to expert: Excellence and power in clinical nursing practice*, Menlo Park, CA, 1984, Addison-Wesley.

Blais KK, Hayes JS, Kozier B: *Professional nursing practice: Concepts and perspectives*, Upper Saddle River, NJ, 2005, Prentice Hall.

Bonczek ME: Staffing and scheduling. In Yoder-Wise PS, editor: *Leading and managing in nursing*, ed 4, St Louis, 2007, Mosby.

Bowles C, Candels L: First job experience of recent RN graduates: Improving the work environment, *J Nurs Adm* 35(3):130-137, 2005.

Brady-Schwartz D: Further evidence on the Magnet Recognition Program: Implications for nursing leaders, *J Nurs Adm* 35(9):397-403, 2005.

Buresh B, Gordon S: *From silence to voice: What nurses know and must communicate to the public*, ed 2, Oxford, England, 2006, ILR Press.

Case Management Society of America: *Standards of practice for case management*, Little Rock, AR, 2002, The Society.

Cesta TG: *Survival strategies for nurses in managed care*, St Louis, 2002, Mosby.

Cesta TG, Tahan HA: *The case manager's survival guide: Winning strategies for clinical practice*, ed 2, St Louis, 2003, Mosby.

Cho S, Ketefian S, Barkauskas V, et al: Multilevel models in health outcomes research. Part II: Statistical and analytic issues, *Applied Nursing Research* 19(2):113-115, 2003.

Clark SP: The policy implication of staffing-outcomes research, *J Nurs Adm* 35(1):17-19, 2005.

Cohen EL, Cesta TG: *Nursing case management: From essentials to advanced practice applications*, ed 4, St Louis, 2005, Mosby/Elsevier.

Dadich KA: Care delivery strategies. In Yoder-Wise PS, editor: *Leading and managing in nursing*, ed 4, St Louis, 2007, Mosby.

Dean GE, Scott LD, Rogers AE: Infants at risk: When nurse fatigue jeopardizes quality care, *Adv Neonatal Care* 6(3):120-126, 2006.

Dikaya Z, Appelt H: Foreign registered nurses: Successful landing in turbulent waters, *J Nurs Adm* 34(7–8):379-383, 2004.

Donovan L: Matching a blueprint to match competency, *JONA* 34, (IT solutions supplement): 14, 2004.

Drenkard K: Sustaining magnet: Keeping the forces alive, *Nurs Adm Q* 29(3):214-222, 2005.

Duffield C, Aitken L, O'Brien-Pallas L, et al: Nursing: A stepping stone to future careers, *J Nurs Adm* 34(5):238-245, 2004.

Duffield C, Pallas LO, Aitken LM, et al: Recruitment of nurses working outside nursing, *J Nurs Adm* 36(2):58-62, 2006.

Ellis B, Gates J: Achieving magnet status, *Nurs Adm Q* 29(3):241-244, 2005.

Englebardt SP, Nelson R: *Health care informatics: An interdisciplinary approach*, St Louis, 2002, Mosby.

Fabre J: IT solutions: Advancing healthcare through information technology, *JONA* 34, (IT solutions supplement): 12-14, 2004.

Finkelman AW: *Managed care: A nursing perspective*, Upper Saddle River, NJ, 2001, Prentice Hall.

Finkler SA, Kovner CT: *Financial management for nurse managers and executives*, Philadelphia, 2000, Saunders.

Fralic M, editor: *Staffing management and methods: Tools and techniques for nursing leaders*, San Francisco, 2000, Jossey-Bass.

Goode CJ, Krugman ME, Smith K, et al: The pull of magnetism: A look at the standards and the experience of a western academic medical center hospital in achieving and sustaining magnet status, *Nurs Adm Q* 29(3):202-213, 2005.

Grohar-Murray ME, DiCroce HR: *Leadership and management in nursing*, Stamford, CN, 2003, Appleton & Lange.

Grosch JW, Caruso CC, Rosa RR, et al: Long hours of work in the US: Associations with demographic and organizational characteristics, psychosocial working conditions, and health, *Am J Ind Med* 49(11):943-952, 2006.

Huber DL: Staffing and scheduling. In Huber DL, editor: *Leadership and nursing care management*, ed 3, Philadelphia, 2006, Elsevier, pp 713-754.

Hung R: A note on nurse scheduling, *Nurs Econ* 20(1):37-38, 2002.

Institute of Medicine: *Wisdom at work: The importance of the older and experienced nurse in the workplace*, Princeton, NJ, 2006, Robert Wood Johnson Foundation.

Jasovsky DA, Dornan L, Geisler L, et al: Magnet demographic data: Creating a system to streamline the process, *J Nurs Adm* 35(11):490-496, 2005.

Johnson M, Bulechek G, Dochterman, et al: *Nursing diagnoses, outcomes, and interventions: NANDA, NOC and NIC linkages*, St Louis, 2001, Mosby.

Johnson M, Maas M, Moorhead S: *Nursing outcomes classification (NOC)*, St Louis, 2004, Mosby.

Joint Commission on Accreditation of Healthcare Organizations (JCAHO): *Health care at the crossroads: Strategies for addressing the evolving nursing crisis*, Oakbrook Terrace, IL, 2002, Joint Commission.

Jones CB: The costs of nurse turnover. Part 2: Application of the nursing turnover cost calculator methodology, *J Nurs Adm* 35(1):41-49, 2005.

Jones CB: The costs of nurse turnover. Part 1: An economic perspective, *J Nurs Adm* 34(12):562-570, 2004.

Kongstvedt PR: *Essentials of managed health care*, ed 4, Gaithersburg, MD, 2003, Aspen Publishers.

Kovner C, Jones C, Zhan C, et al: Nurse staffing and postsurgical adverse outcomes: Analysis of administrative data from a sample of US hospitals, 1990-1996, *Health Serv Res* 37(3):611-629, 2002.

Kramer M: Revising the essentials of magnetism tool: There is more to adequate staffing than numbers, *J Nurs Adm* 35(4):188-198, 2005.

Kramer M, Schmalenberg CE: Best quality patient care: A historical perspective on magnet hospitals, *Nurs Adm Q* 29(3):275-287, 2005.

Lacey LM: Called into question: What nurses want, *Nurs Manage* 34(2):25-26, 2003.

Letvak S: Health and safety of the older registered nurse, *Nurs Outlook* 53(2):66-73, 2005.

Letvak S: The experience of being an older nurse, *West J Nurs Res* 25(1):45-56, 2003.

Malloch K, Krueger J: Expert Nurse Estimation Patient Classification System, 2006 (website):, www.enepcs. com. Accessed November 28, 2006.

Manthey M: Primary practice partners (a nurse extender system, *Nurs Manage* 19(3):58-59, 1988.

Marquis BL, Huston CJ: *Leadership roles and management functions in nursing: Theory and application*, ed 5, Philadelphia, 2006, Lippincott Williams & Wilkins.

McCloskey JC, Bulechek GM, editors: *Nursing interventions classification (NIC)*, St Louis, 2003, Mosby.

McClure M: Magnet hospitals: Insights and issues, *Nurs Adm Q* 29(3):198-201, 2005.

McClure ML, Hinshaw AS: *Magnet hospitals revisited: Attraction and retention of professional nurses*, Washington, DC, 2002, American Nurses Publishing.

McClure M, Poulin MS, Sovie MD, et al: *Magnet hospitals: Attraction and retention of professional nurses*, Kansas City, MO, 1983, American Nurses' Association.

Mion L, Hazel C, Cap M, et al: Retaining and recruiting mature experienced nurses: A multicomponent organizational strategy, *J Nurs Adm* 36(3):148-154, 2006.

Nelson S, Gordon S: *Nursing against the odds: How health care cost cutting, medical stereotypes, and medical hubris undermine nurses and patient care*, Oxford, England, 2006, ILR Press.

Norman LD, Donelan K, Buerhaus PI, et al: The older nurse in the workplace: Does age matter?, *Nurs Econ* 23(6):282-289, 2005.

O'Brien-Pallas, Duffield C, Alksnis C: Who will be there to nurse? Retention of nurses nearing retirement, *J Nurs Adm* 34(6):298-302, 2004.

Pew Health Professions Commission: *Twenty-one competencies for the 21st century*, 1998 (website): www.futurehealth.ucsf.edu/pewcomm/competen. html. Accessed November 28, 2006.

Porter-O'Grady, Malloch K: *Managing for success in health care*, St Louis, 2006, Mosby.

QHR: Nursing turnover calculator smart tools, 2007 (website): www.qhr.com. Accessed March 3, 2007.

Rogers AE, Hwang WT, Scott LD: The effects of work breaks on staff nurse performance, *J Nurs Adm* 34(11):512-519, 2004.

Rogers AE, Hwang WT, Scott LD, et al: The working hours of hospital staff nurses and patient safety, *Health Aff* 23(4):202-212, 2004.

Roussel L, Swansburg RD, Swansburg RJ: *Management and leadership for nurse administrators*, ed 4, Boston, 2006, Jones & Bartlett.

Saba VK, McCormick KA: *Essentials of computers for nurses*, ed 3, New York, 2000, McGraw-Hill/Appleton & Lange.

Scott LD, Hwang WT, Rogers AE: The impact of multiple care giving roles on fatigue, stress, and work performance among hospital staff nurses, *J Nurs Adm* 36(2):86-95, 2006.

Seago JA: A comparison of two patient classification instruments in an acute care hospital, *J Nurs Adm* 32(5):243-249, 2002.

Seago JA, Spetz J, Mitchell S: Nurse staffing and hospital ownership in California, *J Nurs Adm* 34(5):228-237, 2004.

Seago JA, Williamson A, Atwood C: Longitudinal analysis of nurse staffing and patient outcomes: More about failure to rescue, *J Nurs Adm* 36(1):12-21, 2006.

Shirey M: Celebrating certification in nursing: Forces of magnetism in action, *Nurs Adm Q* 29(3):363-395, 2005.

Shullanberger G: Nurse staffing decisions: An integrative review of the literature, *Nurs Econ* 18(3):124-136, 2000.

Sloan A: How's your travel nurse quality control?, *J Nurs Adm* 34(suppl):10-11, 2004.

Sullivan EJ, Decker PJ: *Effective leadership and management in nursing*, Upper Saddle River, NJ, 2005, Prentice Hall.

Sveinsdóttir H: Self-assessed quality of sleep, occupational health, working environment, illness experience and job satisfaction of female nurses working different combinations of shifts, *Scand J Caring Sci* 20(2):229-237, 2006.

Tiedeman M, Lookinland S: Traditional models of care delivery: What have we learned? *J Nurs Adm* 34(6):291-297, 2004.

Trinkoff A, Geiger-Brown, Brady B, et al: How long and how much are nurses now working? *Am J Nurs* 106(4):60-71, 2006.

Triolo PK, Scherer E, Floyd J: Evaluation of the Magnet Recognition Program, *J Nurs Adm* 36(1):42-48, 2006.

Urden LD, Monarch K: The ANCC Magnet Recognition Program: Converting research findings into action. In McClure ML, Hinshaw AS: *Magnet hospitals revisited: Attraction and retention of professional nurses*, Washington, DC, 2002, American Nurses Publishing.

West MM, Hallick SM, Schaal MG, et al: A rural academic-service partnership, *J Nurs Adm* 36(2):63-66, 2006.

Williams KA, Stotts RC, Jacob SR, et al: Inactive nurses: A source for alleviating the nursing shortage? *J Nurs Adm* 36(4):205-210, 2006.

Wilson A: Impact of management development on nurse retention, *Nurs Adm Q* 29(2):137-145, 2005.

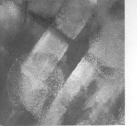

Evaluation and Discipline of Personnel

14

"Love truth, and pardon error" —Anonymous

Chapter Overview

Chapter 14 explains methods of performance management, appraisal interviews and reports, legal implications, principles of disciplinary action, penalties, components of a disciplinary action program, modification of employee behavior, problem employees, employee counseling, and outplacement counseling.

Chapter Objectives

- Recall at least five purposes of personnel evaluation.
- Explain at least four common effects in performance evaluation.
- Describe five methods of personnel evaluation.
- Define 360-degree evaluation.
- Describe at least two kinds of appraisal interviews.
- Explain at least two ways to arrange a room for performance evaluations.
- Defend at least five principles of disciplinary action.
- Relate at least three components of a disciplinary action program.
- Compare discipline without punishment with progressive discipline.
- Explain behavior modification.
- Describe at least three types of problem employees.
- Identify at least three types of employee counseling.
- Explain outplacement counseling.

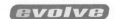

Major Concepts and Definitions

Evaluation *valuation, appraisal, determination of worth*
Anecdotal note *recording of objective description of behavior*
Criterion *a standard on which a judgment can be based*
Forced distribution *evaluator rates the individual according to all individuals that manager evaluates*
Peer review *group evaluation of a group member*
Appraisal interview *verbal evaluation*
Appraisal report *written evaluation*
Discipline *to train, control, punish*
Penalties *punishment; negative consequences*
Behavior modification *changes in behavior*
Reinforcement *actions that strengthen a behavior or increase its probability*
Shaping *reinforcing successive attempts at achieving the desired behavior*
Extinction *annihilation, destruction*
Substance abuse *misuse of drugs*
Angry *furious, raging, tumultuous*
Withdrawn *retreated, isolated*
Productivity *results*
Absenteeism *absence from work*
Due process *procedural requirements to ensure fairness*
Termination *end of something*
Directive counseling counselor *telling one what to do*
Nondirective counseling *client deciding what to do*
Outplacement counseling *helping dismissed personnel find another job*

LEADERSHIP AND MANAGEMENT FOR EVALUATION AND DISCIPLINE OF PERSONNEL

Leaders inspire high performance, encourage peer review, promote motivation and growth through performance appraisal, reduce the anxiety related to it, and develop trust by being honest and fair. Leaders facilitate two-way communication, facilitate growth through coaching, and support employees attempting to correct performance deficiencies. Managers evaluate performance, use a formalized system, document standards, gather fair and objective data, determine educational and training needs, follow up on performance deficiencies, maintain documentation of the appraisal process, and give frequent informal feedback

(Marquis & Huston, 2006; Nemeth, Harris-Eaton, & Weaver, 2006) (Table 14-1).

PURPOSES

Performance appraisal is a periodic formal evaluation of how well personnel have performed their duties during a specific time period. Purposes of the evaluation are as follows: (1) determine job competence; (2) provide feedback to enhance staff development and motivate personnel toward higher achievement; (3) discover the employee's aspirations and encourage and recognize accomplishments; (4) improve communications between managers and staff associates and to reach an understanding about the objectives of the job and agency; (5) improve performance by examining and encouraging better

TABLE 14-1 Leadership and Management for
Evaluation and Discipline of Personnel

Leader	Manager
Encourages peer review process	Uses a formalized system for performance appraisal
Promotes motivation and growth through the appraisal process	Uses documented standards as bases for performance appraisal
Reduces anxiety inherent in the appraisal process	Gathers fair and objective data for performance appraisals
Develops trust by being honest and fair	Determines education and training needs from appraisal process
Facilitates two-way communications through appraisal interviews	Follows up on performance deficiencies
Encourages growth through coaching	Maintains documentation of the appraisal process
Supports employees attempting to correct performance	Provides frequent informal feedback
Inspires high performance deficiencies	Evaluates performance

Modified from Nemeth LS, Harris-Eaton KY, Weaver K: Performance appraisal. In Huber DL, editor: *Leadership and nursing care management,* ed 3, Philadelphia, 2006, Elsevier; Marquis BL, Huston CJ: *Leadership roles and management functions in nursing: Theory and application,* ed 3, Philadelphia, 2006, Lippincott.

relationships among nurses; (6) aid the manager's coaching and counseling; (7) determine training and developmental needs of personnel; (8) inventory talent within the organization and reassess assignments; (9) select qualified staff members for advancement and salary increases; and (10) identify unsatisfactory employees (Finkelman, 2006; McConnell, 2006; Nemeth, Harris-Eaton, & Weaver, 2006).

COMMON ERRORS/EFFECTS IN EVALUATION

Criteria leading to judgments are used for performance evaluation. Because human judgment is flawed by the potential for prejudice, bias, and other subjective and extraneous factors, the attempt to arrive at objective, accurate evaluations is extremely difficult. A number of errors/effects may affect performance ratings. The manager should be aware of the most common ones and try to minimize them.

The *halo effect* is the result of allowing one trait to influence the evaluation of other traits or of rating all traits on the basis of a general impression. A logical error occurs when a rating for a person is high on one characteristic because the person possesses another characteristic that is understandably related. Sometimes employees are given a good rating because they did good work in the distant past, or outstanding performance on a recent job may offset a mediocre performance during the rest of the evaluation period. A manager is likely to rate personnel who are compatible with the manager higher than they deserve and may not see certain types of weaknesses that are like the manager's. The person who does not complain is likely to have higher ratings than the person who does.

The *horns effect* is the opposite of the halo effect. The evaluator is hypercritical. Managers who are perfectionists may rate personnel lower than they should and may compare how a person previously performed with how that person presently performs. Evaluators are more likely to rate people doing jobs with which the evaluator is familiar lower than those with jobs with which one is not familiar. Good workers on weak teams are more likely to get lower ratings than if they were working on a better team. Persons who are not well known may be judged by the company they keep. A recent mistake may offset a year's good work. If the worker is contrary, managers may vent their irritation by lowering the rating. The nonconformist or person with a personality trait that is not appreciated is likely to be rated lower than that person's work merits.

The *contrast effect* is produced by the tendency of the evaluator to rate the employee opposite from the way the evaluator perceives oneself. A small range of scores may be a result of the *central tendency effect.* When the rating on a preceding characteristic influences the rating on the following trait, a *proximity effect* exists. Because raters tend to have their own built-in set of standards or frame of reference on which to make evaluations, it becomes a major problem comparing different raters' scores. Some evaluators may be lenient, whereas others may be restrictive and severe in their judgments.

The manager can take precautions to minimize judgment errors. For instance, a forced-distribution technique may be used to overcome leniency and central tendency errors. A critical incident checklist can reduce the halo effect and logical rating errors. Ranking systems, paired comparisons, and forced-choice techniques may be used, but all of them also have disadvantages. They could be used privately by the evaluator to do a self-evaluation of potential common errors in evaluation, thereby minimizing judgment errors (Sullivan & Decker, 2005).

METHODS OF PERFORMANCE MANAGEMENT

Anecdotal Notes

Anecdotal records are objective descriptions of behavior recorded on plain paper or a form. The notations should include who was observed, by whom, when, where, and doing what. The notation comprises a description of the setting or background and the incident. Interpretation and recommendations may be included. Value-laden words such as *good* and *bad* should be avoided. Accurate coverage of facts is essential.

Characteristic behavior cannot be determined without several incidents depicting similar behavior. The director or patient care coordinator may use time sampling to accumulate observations. The time that is set aside specifically for observations may be divided by the number of staff members to be observed. The manager then concentrates on the scheduled staff member for a short time. It is advisable to make several brief observations over a period of time to allow for temporary variables and to identify patterns of behavior.

An advantage of anecdotal recordings is that the description is not coerced into a rigid structure. However, this latitude becomes a problem when the interpreter tries to develop relationships between notations that may have little or no relationship to each other. Although anecdotal records provide a systematic means for recording observations, they do not guarantee that observations will be made systematically or that specific, relevant behaviors will be observed. It also takes considerable time to record the observations.

Checklists

With a checklist, the manager can categorically assess the presence or absence of desired characteristics or behaviors. Checklists are most useful for tangible variables, such as inventory of supplies, but they can be used for evaluation of skills as well. It is advisable to list only the behaviors essential to successful performance, and it is advantageous to determine the behavior to be observed in advance. The same criteria can then be used in each situation. A *simple checklist* uses words or phrases to describe behaviors. They may be categorized by concepts such as assertiveness skills. A *forced checklist* requires the evaluator to select a desirable and an undesirable behavior for each person. The behaviors are given a quantitative value that results in a score that may be used for employment decisions. The *weighted checklist* gives weighted scores for each behavior. The overall performance appraisal score is determined by the behaviors chosen. Unfortunately, checklist use neither guarantees that the observed behavior is a persistent one in a representative situation nor facilitates evaluation of interpersonal relations (Marquis & Huston, 2006; Sullivan & Decker, 2005).

Rating Scales

The *rating scale* does more than just note the absence or presence of desirable behavior. It locates the behavior at a point on a continuum and notes quantitative and qualitative abilities. The *numerical rating scale* usually includes numbers against which a list of behaviors are evaluated:

Observation of working hours	1 2 3 4 5
Ability to get along with others	1 2 3 4 5

A numerical rating scale is not a very reliable tool because of the inconsistent value attributed to the number. That fault can be partially overcome by adding a few quantitative terms (Box 14-1).

The numerical rating scale can be made even more reliable by developing a standard scale using comparative examples to promote a common understanding of the values. The difficulty for the manager is finding appropriate comparative standards. A nurse-to-nurse comparison scale might be developed where the personnel are rated in highest, above average, average, below average, and lowest categories (Figure 14-1).

As long as the managers can agree on the qualifications of a few nurses known to all of them, a comparison scale that gives a common reference for rating the rest of the staff nurses can be developed.

The *graphic rating scale* differs from the numerical rating scale in that words rather than numbers are used (Figure 14-2). Graphic rating scales usually list extremely broad and general personal

characteristics that are to be rated from poor to excellent or from low to high. Raters are given little if any guidance about what work behavior qualifies a person for a particular rating. Consequently, raters must use their own judgments about how to classify the behaviors. The *descriptive graphic rating* scale is similar to the graphic rating scale except that it presents a more elaborate description of the behavior being rated (Figure 14-3).

BARS is an acronym for *behaviorally anchored rating scales,* sometimes known as *BES,* or *behavioral expectation scales.* They are similar to graphic rating scales in that a person is rated on a series of dimensions or qualities. However, BARS differ from graphic rating scales in the ways that the criteria are identified and the alternative responses along the rating scale are anchored or described. BARS evaluate behavior relevant to the specific demands of the job and provide examples of specific job behaviors corresponding to good, average, and poor performances. These descriptions reduce the amount of personal judgment needed by the rater.

The major disadvantage of BARS is the time and expense required to involve large numbers of employees in determining the dimensions of effective performance and behavioral examples of various levels of performance for each variable. Separate BARS are needed for each job. They are primarily applicable to physically observable behaviors rather than to conceptual skills. However, they should reduce rating errors and provide more reliable, valid, meaningful, and complete data. Employees give more acceptance and commitment to this appraisal

---

BOX 14-1 Rating Scale

Rate the staff member on the items below.
Responses have the following values:
1 = Never
2 = Sometimes
3 = About half the time
4 = Usually
5 = Always

A. Observation of working hours   1 2 3 4 5
B. Ability to get along with others   1 2 3 4 5

| Nurse | Observation of working hours | | | | |
	Lowest (1)	Below average (2)	Average (3)	Above average (4)	Highest (5)
Betty Green	X				
Sara Smith		X			
Pam Peterson			X		
Sue Jones				X	
Anita Anderson					X

Figure 14-1 • Nurse-to-nurse comparison scale.

system because of their involvement in designing it. They have full knowledge of the requirements of the job, and they evidence less defensiveness and conflict because people are evaluated on the basis of specific behaviors rather than personalities. This system thereby identifies performance deficiencies and needs for development.

BOS is an acronym for *behavioral observation scales* (Box 14-2). This system capitalizes on some of the strengths of BARS while avoiding some of the disadvantages. BOS also use critical incidents of worker behavior. The evaluator lists a number of critical incidents for each performance dimension and rates the extent to which the behavior has been observed on a five-point scale ranging from almost never to almost always. BOS too are relatively reliable, well accepted and understood, and provide useful data. The drawback of BOS is that they are relatively time consuming and expensive to develop.

Instead of a descriptive choice, a *percentage rating scale* provides a quantitative choice. The manager may rank the employee's behavior on any given criterion as among the bottom 10% of a specific category of personnel, next 20%, middle 40%, next 20%, or top 10% of that category of personnel (Figure 14-4).

To maintain perspective, the manager may list staff member names down the side of a paper and the behavior to be rated across the top. Rating one behavior at a time, the manager checks for variation in evaluations because one expects variation in performance. Forced distribution should be used cautiously. It is based on a normal bell-shaped curve with a few people ranked high, a few ranked low, and the majority ranked in the middle. However, forced distribution assumes that a group is representative of the total population, which is not true for a group of nurses that are well educated.

Ranking

> *"He who spares the guilty threatens the innocent."*   —Legal maxim

Ranking forces managers to position staff members in descending order from highest to lowest even if the evaluators do not think there is a difference. Ranking implicitly requires the manager to compare each staff member with others, but that comparison is not systematically built into the method. *Paired comparison* forces the manager to compare each nurse with another nurse (Table 14-2). If managers are ranking four nurses, they must deal with six possible pairs; this number can be calculated as follows:

$$N(N-1)/2 = 4(3)/2 = 12/2 = 6$$

Each pair is then presented to the manager, who must determine which of the two is better

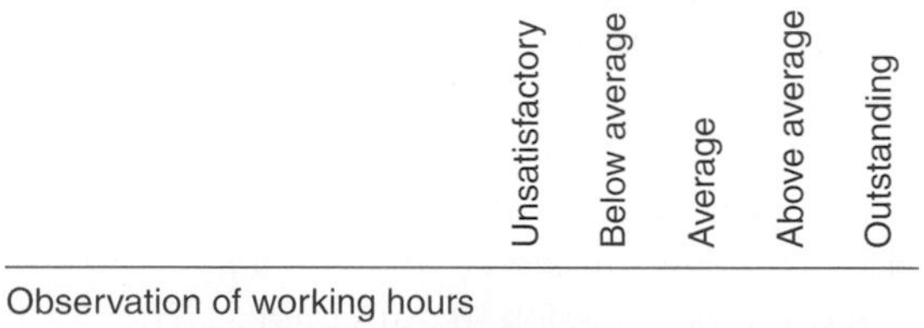

Observation of working hours

Figure 14-2 • Graphic rating scale.

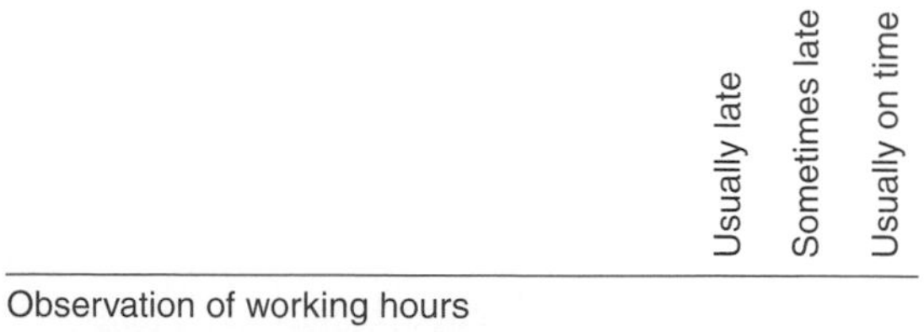

Observation of working hours

Figure 14-3 • Descriptive graphic rating scale.

BOX 14-2 Behavioral Observation Scale

Circle the number that most closely approximates your assessment of the staff member on the following qualities:

| Punctual | Almost never | 1 2 3 4 5 | Almost always |
| Gets along well with co-workers | Almost never | 1 2 3 4 5 | Almost always |

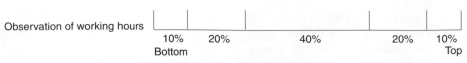

Figure 14-4 • Percentage rating scale.

TABLE 14-2 Example of Ranking Using Paired Comparison

Nurses	Possible Pairs	
Anita Anderson	AA with SJ	SJ with PP
Sue Jones	AA with PP	SJ with SS
Pam Peterson	AA with SS	PP with SS
Sara Smith		

Figure 14-5 • Paired comparisons.

based upon some characteristic or criterion. Choices should be marked (Figure 14-5). Tally marks can be placed in a matrix to help visualize the ranking (Figure 14-6). The major disadvantages of paired comparisons are that they do not lend themselves to large numbers of staff members and that they demand a considerable amount of the manager's time (Shepard, 2006).

Forced Distribution Scale

With the forced distribution scale, the evaluator is to rate all individuals reporting to that person in order from the best performer to the weakest performer. This is not a bell curve because it just rates the individuals reporting to a manager. This gives a visual of how each person ranks with all others reporting to that manager. This method fosters competitiveness versus cooperation, undermines morale and group cohesiveness, may stifle creativity, and does not take into account the uniqueness of the individuals and their special gifts (Twedell, 2007).

Management by Objectives or Outcomes

"Success comes in cans; failure in can'ts."
—*Anonymous*

Management by objectives (MBO) or outcomes is a tool for effective planning and appraisal. It emphasizes the achievement of objectives or outcomes instead of demonstration of personality characteristics. It focuses attention on individual achievement, motivates individuals to accomplishments, and measures performance in terms of results. MBO is a managerial method whereby the manager and staff person identify major areas in which the staff person will work, set standards for performance, and measure results against the mutually agreed upon standards. It determines the outcomes that the staff member is to achieve within a given time frame (Box 14-3).

To develop MBO, personnel should first review the mission of the agency or unit and group objectives or outcomes. The mission and objectives or outcomes can be determined by analyzing what staff does or what staff members think they should do. People describe their jobs and clarify its purposes. This process helps identify major job responsibilities. Next, personnel list their major job responsibilities. Expected outcomes, rather than activities, should be listed. While many agencies are not using MBO, many performance systems are built on an organization's missions, annual goals, and job descriptions plus job requirements. The Joint Commission (TJC) and other important accreditation bodies require job performance appraisals consistent with the job descriptions be in place and specifically outline human resources personnel and mandatory education related to patient safety, quality programs, etc.

Major job responsibilities of a nurse manager are related to productivity, quality of care, morale, turnover, staff development, self-development,

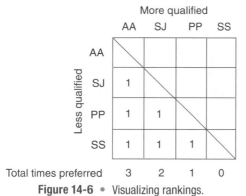

More qualified

Figure 14-6 • Visualizing rankings.

BOX 14-3 Management by Objectives or Outcomes Process

Review the agency mission.
Review the group objectives or outcomes.
Determine the major job responsibilities.
Determine the expected levels of accomplishment.
Meet with the manager to establish priorities.
Develop plans for the accomplishment of the outcomes.
Manager determines if the outcomes are compatible with the organization's goals.
Manager and staff member meet periodically to check progress and make adjustments.
Annual review should compare actual results with expected levels of accomplishment and plan the outcomes for the next period.

and affirmative action. Once the major job responsibilities are identified, expected levels of accomplishment are determined. Criteria for expected levels of accomplishment should be outcomes oriented, established before the fact, time bound, realistic and attainable, measurable and verifiable, written, and agreed on by both the manager and the staff member. Common errors to avoid when developing outcomes are writing too many outcomes or too complex outcomes; having too high or too low standards; using too long or too short a time period; and identifying outcomes that are not measurable, or outcomes for which the cost of measurement is too high.

After staff members have reviewed the mission and group objectives or outcomes and determined their major job responsibilities and the expected levels of accomplishment, they should meet with the manager to establish priorities and to develop plans for the accomplishment of the outcomes. The manager will determine whether the outcomes are compatible with the overall goals of the organization. The manager and staff member should hold periodic reviews to check the progress and make adjustments. An annual review should be held to compare the actual results with the expected levels of accomplishment and to set the outcomes for the next period.

The underlying philosophy of management by objectives or outcomes is a belief that people perform best and develop most in an environment of participative management, high performance standards that build on individual strengths, prompt feedback that accentuates the positive, and appropriate rewards. Staff members are encouraged to "do their thing" while maintaining a team orientation and individual accountability. The manager is a listener and clarifier who readjusts staff members' responsibilities on the basis of individual differences.

Higher frequencies of appraisal are associated with a more favorable attitude toward MBO, higher goal success, improvement of manager–staff member relationships, clarity of goals, an opinion that the manager was helpful and supportive, the attitude that staff associates had influence in matters affecting them, and esteem for and satisfaction with the manager. More praise and less criticism of the outcomes by the manager are associated with higher goal success. It is advisable to use an incentive system that rewards effective planning, as well as goal achievement, when using MBO.

Advantages of MBO for nurses are that the standard of evaluation is based on the characteristics of a specific person and job; nurses have input and some control over their future; nurses know the standard by which they will be judged; nurses have knowledge of the manager's goals, priorities, and deadlines; nurses have a greater understanding of where they stand with the manager in relation to relative progress; there is a better basis for evaluation than personality traits; MBO emphasizes the future, which can be changed, instead of the past; and it stimulates higher individual performance and morale.

Advantages for the manager include a reservoir of personnel data and performance information for updating personnel files; an indication of personnel development needs within the agency; a basis for promotion and compensation; a relationship with the staff that makes the manager a coach rather than a judge; and better managerial planning and use of the employee. MBO directs work activities toward organizational goals, facilitates planning, provides standards for control, provides objective appraisal criteria, reduces role conflict and ambiguity, and uses and motivates human resources.

MBO is limited because it is not an easy system to implement and requires hard work for maintenance; the process must be taught and reinforced for managers to become and remain proficient in applying the principles of the system; the MBO system assumes that staff members and managers will define suitable standards that will serve the agency; it presumes that managers understand their limitations; managers are responsible for assessing actual results rather than activities that seem to indicate results; some managers are unable to manage by objectives; some staff nurses may not want to be involved in setting goals; managers and staff may give lip service to MBO,

although managers really set the goals; staff nurses may set their goals according to what they know their managers expect; MBO stresses results but does not supply the methods for achieving them; nurses can become frustrated if they believe that increasingly higher goals will be expected of them; overlapping objectives are difficult to evaluate; MBO lends itself to quantitative assessment but may neglect qualitative factors; and MBO does not provide comparative data for promotions and salary increases (Marquis & Huston, 2006; Odiorne, 1978, 1982; Twedell, 2007).

Self-Appraisal

Self-appraisal promotes dignity and self-respect. It is a less structured approach used in participative organizations that promote employee acceptance of plans for improvement and uses the manager as a coach instead of a judge. Personnel are the best source of information about their work. Self-appraisal ensures that the person is prepared for the discussion, and it increases the perception of fairness. Personnel may be fearful of punishment; rate themselves low to avoid disagreement with the boss; or evaluate themselves high to influence the supervisor. Sometimes employees undervalue their achievements or feel uncomfortable giving themselves high ratings. If used alone, self-appraisal could provide an inaccurate picture. If the self-appraisal is not consistent with other available data, the manager should confront the

---

 RESEARCH Perspective 14-1

Data from Meretoja R, Leino-Kilpi H: Instruments for evaluating nurse competence, *JONA* 31(7/8):346-352, 2001.

Purpose: The purpose of this study was to review the literature to help nurse administrators locate and evaluate existing instruments to ensure safe and qualified nursing care.

Methods: Data collection procedures included literature searches from MEDLINE and CINHAL.

Results/conclusions: Of the studies reviewed, seven were conducted to develop or to test a new instrument; six were conducted to differentiate job performance by education, experience,

and career commitment; four reported development of new instruments; and two dealt with item identification for performance standards and assessment models, and were regarded as early stages of instrument development. All the instruments were designed to assess practicing nurses. The method of nurse competence assessment was nurses' self-evaluation in 11 studies; supervisor, preceptor, or manager evaluation in 7 studies; and the single method in 2 studies. Patient evaluation was used in 1 study.

differences (Grote, 2006; Marquis & Huston, 2006; Roussel, Swansburg, & Swansburg, 2006).

Peer Review

Peer review is a process whereby a group of practicing registered nurses (RNs) evaluates the quality of another RN's professional performance. It provides a feedback mechanism for sharing ideas, comparing the consistency of the staff member's performance with standards, recognizing outstanding performance, and identifying areas in which further development is required. This process can increase personal and professional growth and job satisfaction because of the recognition from peers.

Once it has been decided that an institution will use peer review, appraisal tools must be developed. A review of the evaluation tools currently used and the literature on evaluation tools is necessary. Various standards may also be reviewed. The tool developed may address technical competence, human relationships, communications, organizational leadership, and other skills. The process must also be determined, and then staff members must be oriented to the system. Self-governance is often a part of a peer review process. Clinical ladders are used to set standards especially in magnet organizations.

The staff members should be oriented to the components of the peer review before it is implemented and thereafter during orientation. It is appropriate to give them copies of the peer review process and forms used for peer review. Opportunities to learn how to complete the forms, how the peer review committee uses the materials, and what questions are to be expected during the peer review interview should be provided.

The peer evaluation process typically includes a review of an employee's self-evaluation form (including short- and long-term goals or outcomes), reference letters, committee work, special projects, additional education, and contributions to nursing; a performance evaluation by the nurse's immediate manager; a review of past performance; care plans and charting done by the nurse; assessment; observation of the nurse; interviews with clients; a summary of the findings; a presentation of the findings; and recommendations to the nurse. It is appropriate to allow the candidate some compensation or agency time to prepare a review folder. A leader is assigned to the nurse to help clarify policy and procedures and to check the documents for completeness.

Who will evaluate whom must be determined. A committee may be appointed, elected, or randomly selected, but it should represent a number of job titles and a wide variety of specialty areas. The members should become familiar with committee responsibilities. The committee's recommendations should be made by consensus, with dissenting opinions recorded.

Once the candidate has been evaluated, there should be a peer review interview for feedback. All feedback must be well documented in the review materials. Hearsay reports are not permitted. The review committee chairperson or designee is responsible for arranging the interview and helping the candidate feel welcome and comfortable. The interview may provide recognition of outstanding performance, identification of areas in which further development is required, recommendations regarding learning needs, and possibly a recommendation for classification.

Peer review can be threatening and time consuming. There is a risk of rating candidates too high or too low. Friends may inflate evaluations. Peers may omit suggestions for improvement for people with whom they work. Managers may feel threatened. However, staff members will be held accountable and responsible for their performance when they are measured against realistic and attainable standards (Marquis, Huston, 2006; Roussel, Swansburg, & Swansburg, 2006).

Customer or Subordinate Evaluation

Student evaluation of teachers is common in education, and customer feedback in the workplace has become common. Managers need to use staff's performance evaluations to impact the customer feedback. Staff performance evaluations should increase excellence in patient care and satisfaction that leads to better patient evaluation of care. Managers are often evaluated on the results of patient evaluation of care. Staff members can evaluate their managers and leaders.

360-Degree Feedback

The 360-degree feedback is a multisource system of assessment including self-appraisal and subordinate, peer, and administrative feedback. It creates credible information, reduces supervisor bias, supports a team environment, supports career development, moves from a seniority to a performance system, and substantiates rewards for high performers. Unfortunately, recipients may resist feedback; friendships or competition may bias the process; some people may conspire for or against an employee; some respondents are more critical than others; some teams are harder than others; some evaluators may not be completely honest to avoid hurting feelings; and it is time consuming. Computers with safeguards for confidentiality can be used for online assessment (Grote, 1996; McConnell, 2006) (Table 14-3).

Appraisal Interview

There are several kinds of appraisal interviews. They include *tell and sell, tell and listen, problem solving,* and *goal setting* (Maier, 1976). When using the tell-and-sell technique, the manager does most of the talking while the staff member listens. The manager reports the results of the evaluation to the employee and tries to persuade the staff member to improve. This approach assumes that managers are qualified to evaluate staff members and that staff members will want to correct their weaknesses. In this role of judge, the interviewer risks losing the loyalty of the employee and inhibiting independent judgment. Face-saving problems are created as the interviewer has to justify the negative ratings. Employees usually suppress defensive behavior and attempt to cover their hostility to protect themselves (Table 14-4).

The tell-and-sell method uses positive and negative extrinsic motivation and is most likely to be successful when the employee respects the interviewer. It tends to perpetuate existing values and practices. The tell-and-sell method works best with young or new employees or individuals who are new to an assignment. These employees may want advice and assurance from an authority figure. Under these conditions, managers are most likely to be respected because of their position, knowledge, and experience. Unfortunately, the tell-and-sell method fosters dependent, passive-aggressive, docile, or rebellious behavior. After a tell-and-sell style evaluation, the employee often feels like looking for another job.

When using the tell-and-listen method, the manager speaks for about half the time and lets the staff member speak for the remainder. The interviewer outlines the strong and weak points of the staff member's job performance and then listens to the interviewee's response. Although still in the role of judge, the interviewer listens to disagreement and allows defensive behavior without attempting to refute any responses. This method tends to remove defensive behavior. The employee expresses concerns or frustrations and feels accepted while the interviewer listens, reflects, and summarizes. Thus resistance to change is reduced, and the staff member develops a more favorable attitude toward the manager. Although this method fosters upward communication and allows the interviewer to learn and change views, the need for change may not be developed in the employee. Tell and listen works best when there is a good relationship between the interviewer and interviewee. Interviewers can learn about staff members' needs and aspirations, but the latter may not know where they stand. There are no plans for personnel development.

With the problem-solving method, the interviewer assumes the role of helper to stimulate growth and development in the interviewee. It assumes that change can occur without correcting faults and that discussing problems can lead to improvements because the discussion develops new ideas and mutual interests. The staff member does most of the talking while the interviewer listens, reflects ideas and feelings, asks exploratory questions, and summarizes. Intrinsic motivation is stimulated through increased freedom, increased responsibility, and problem-solving behavior; thus change is facilitated. Both the manager and staff member learn from each other. Staff members may view their

TABLE 14-3 Pros and Cons of Various Methods of Performance Appraisal

Appraisal Method	Pros	Cons
Anecdotal notes	Objective description of behavior No rigid structure Systematic means for recording observations	Latitude becomes a problem regarding relationships of observations Doesn't guarantee relevant observations Is time consuming
Checklists	Can categorically assess the presence or absence of behaviors Determine behavior to be observed in advance Consistent use of criteria	Behavior observed may not be representative
Rating scales	Locates behavior on a continuum Notes qualitative and quantitative abilities	Not very reliable Use own judgment Little understanding of what behavior qualifies for what rating
BARS (behaviorally anchored rating scale) or BES (behavioral expectations scales)	Evaluates behavior related to specific demands of the job Gives examples of specific job behaviors Reduces the amount of personal judgment needed Reduces rating errors Is more accepted by staff Identifies performance deficiencies and needs for development	Takes time Is expensive to use Separate BARS is needed for each job Is applicable to physically observable behaviors rather than conceptual skills
BOS (behavioral observation scales)	Uses critical incidents Is relatively reliable Is well accepted and understood	Is time consuming Expensive to develop
Ranking	Compares workers with each other	Doesn't lend itself to large numbers Can lead to competition vs. cooperation
MBO (management by objectives)	Tool for effective planning and appraisal Focuses attention on individual achievement Motivates individuals to accomplish Measures performance in terms of outcomes Staff have input and some control over their future Staff know the standard by which they will be evaluated Staff have knowledge of the manager's goals, priorities, and deadlines Emphasizes the future that can be changed Indicates personnel development needs Is a basis for promotion and compensation Manager is coach vs. judge Better managerial planning Better use of employees	Not easy to implement Is hard to maintain Process must be taught and reinforced Assumes staff will define suitable standards Too many outcomes identified Too complex outcomes identified Too high or too low standards Too long or too short time periods Imbalanced emphasis Nonmeasurable outcomes or outcomes that are too costly to measure

Continued

TABLE 14-3 Pros and Cons of Various Methods of Performance Appraisal—cont'd

Appraisal Method	Pros	Cons
Self-appraisal	Promotes dignity and self respect Promotes acceptance of plans for improvement Staff are the best source of information Ensures preparation for discussion Increases perception of fairness	Staff may be fearful of punishment May rate self low to prevent disagreement with the boss May evaluate self high to influence the manager May undervalue own achievements May feel uncomfortable giving self high ratings Could provide inaccurate picture if used alone
Peer review	Provides feedback for sharing ideas Compares consistency of performance with standards Recognizes outstanding performance Identifies areas needing development Increases professional growth Increases job satisfaction from receiving recognition	Staff need to be oriented to the process Committee needs to be formed It takes time to prepare the folder for review Recommendation should be made by consensus It can be threatening It can be time consuming
360-Degree feedback	Is a multisource system Creates credible feedback Reduces manager bias Supports team environment Supports career development Focuses on performance Substantiates reward for high performance	Friendships or competition may bias the process Some raters or teams are more critical than others Friends may inflate evaluations Peers may omit suggestions Managers may feel threatened People may conspire for or against someone Recipients may resist feedback

job in relation to others more accurately, and managers gain insights into staff members' working conditions. Unfortunately, the employee may lack ideas, and change may be other than what the interviewer had planned. Although this method is excellent for problem solving and personnel development, it does not warn staff members or let them know where they stand, evaluate them for lateral transfers or promotional purposes, provide a rating or furnish an evaluation record, or supply top administration with an inventory of talent.

Goal setting is future oriented. It focuses attention on the employee's achievement and consequently stimulates accomplishment. The philosophy behind MBO or by outcomes is teamwork. Top administration sets the organization's objectives, and employees set individual objectives. This method integrates institutional and personal achievement goals. It clarifies objectives or outcomes and, because it focuses on results and not methods, encourages the person closest to a job to decide how to do it. MBO or by outcomes involves participative management. An autocratic leader is likely to dictate goals to a staff member. Although that is not consistent with a participative management philosophy, it is better for staff members to know what is expected of them than not to know.

Which appraisal interview style is used largely depends on the purpose of the evaluation, the manager's philosophy of management, and the institutional guidelines. The manager can create an atmosphere during the interview that is consistent with the appraisal interview style, often by the way the room in which the evaluation is done is arranged. To create an authoritative

TABLE 14-4 Appraisal Interview Methods

	Tell and Sell	Tell and Listen	Problem-Solving Method	Goal/Outcome Setting
Objective	To communicate evaluation To persuade employee to improve	To communicate evaluation To release defensive feelings	To stimulate growth and development in employees	To plan future objectives/outcomes
Psychological assumptions	Employee desires to correct weaknesses if the person knows them To persuade employee to improve	People change if defensive feelings are removed	Growth can occur without correcting faults Discussing job problems leads to improvement of performance	People tend to do what they plan to do
Role of interviewer	Judge	Judge	Helper	Facilitator
Attitude of the interviewer	People profit from criticism and appreciate help	One can respect the feelings of others if one understands them	Discussion develops new ideas and mutual interests	People can control their own behaviors
Skills of the interviewer	Salesmanship Patience	Listening Reflecting feelings Summarizing	Listening Reflecting feelings Using exploratory questions Summarizing	Listening Reflecting feelings Using exploratory questions Summarizing
Reaction of the employee and motivation to change	Suppresses defensive behavior Attempts to cover hostility Some positive and some negative incentives Extrinsic motivation	Expresses defensive behavior Feels accepted Positive incentive Extrinsic and some intrinsic motivation Resistance to change reduced	Problem solving behavior Increased freedom Increased responsibility Intrinsic motivation Increased chance of changing	Sets goals/outcomes Stimulates accomplishments Intrinsic motivation Increased chance of change
Possible gains	Success most probable when the employee respects the interviewer	Employee develops favorable attitude toward the manager, with increased probability of success with change	Almost guaranteed of some improvement	Almost guaranteed of some accomplishment
Risk of interviewer	Loss of loyalty Inhibition of independent judgment Face-saving problems Loss of personnel	Need for change may not be developed	Employee may lack ideas Change may be other than what the manager wanted	Employee may lack drive or interests in accomplishments Employee may not want to accomplish according to the agency goals/outcomes
Probable results	Perpetuates existing practices	Allows the interviewer to change views because of employee's responses Some upward communication	Both learn Change is facilitated Employee feels like an important part of the process	Both learn Change is facilitated Employee feels empowered

Adapted from Maier RF: *Appraising performance: An interview skills course*, La Jolla, CA, 1976, University Associates.

image for the tell-and-sell method, managers should have the interview in their office and sit behind a desk, preferably looking down on the staff members (Figure 14-7).

To create an atmosphere of equality for the tell-and-listen, problem-solving, or goal-setting style, the interviewer and employee may sit at a corner table looking at each other (Figure 14-8). Sitting at a table helps create a working situation for problem solving and goal setting, and sitting either side by side or at the corner of the table helps create a sense of equality and a working relationship (Figure 14-9).

Nonverbal communication is important and should be consistent with verbal communication. Active listening can be expressed through eye contact, a responsive posture, and facial expressions and lets the interviewee know that the interviewer is trying to understand the employee's attitudes and feelings. Pauses give the employee time to think and respond. The interviewer may restate what the employee said. Although this helps the interviewee know the interviewer is listening, it does not guarantee that the meaning of the message was understood. Paraphrasing states the message in fewer and simpler words. If the interviewee says, "I don't understand! One minute she tells me to do it this way, and the next minute she tells me to do it that way," the interviewer may paraphrase, "She confuses you." One should ask for clarification if the intent is not clear or say, for example, "Do you mean…?" Reflection of feelings, such as "You sound proud of that," helps show understanding. Summarizing what has been said at the end of the interview is particularly important.

The manager's assessment of the staff member's performance should be continuous rather than annual. Ongoing assessment maximizes feedback for learning. The manager and staff member should set an appointment to do the appraisal interview when both are unhurried and where privacy is ensured. They should allow adequate time and minimize interruptions. The purpose of the interview should be clear; both should enter it ready to compare notes, knowing that the counseling notes will not become part of

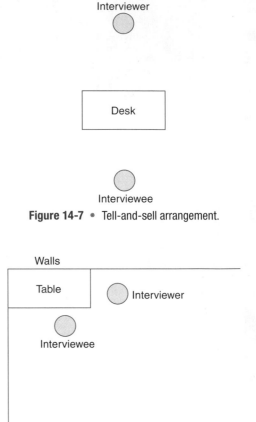

Figure 14-7 • Tell-and-sell arrangement.

Figure 14-8 • Problem-solving arrangement.

the personnel file. Emphasis should be on the growth of the staff member and on accomplishments related to specific outcomes. Actual, observed behavior rather than broad personality traits should be discussed during the exchange of ideas between the manager and the staff member. The staff member should be encouraged to take the initiative in setting goals for improving performance, with the manager supporting, guiding, and validating the staff member's plans.

If managers find it necessary to make unfavorable comments, they should insert them between favorable comments. It is important that managers not create an atmosphere in which they appear to be sitting in judgment. When a manager enumerates needed improvements, this threatens the staff nurse's self-esteem, and the

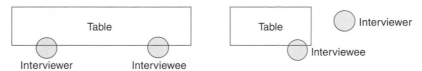

Figure 14-9 • Goal-setting arrangement.

nurse may become defensive. The greater the threat to the self-image, the poorer the attitude toward evaluations will be, thus resulting in less improvement in job performance. If the staff nurse becomes defensive or aggressive, the manager should accept comments and defuse the situation. Keeping quiet and not exposing issues at that time can help the staff member save face.

Before the interview is terminated, ways in which the manager can help the staff nurse accomplish goals should be explored. Staff members will probably approach their work with more enthusiasm and confidence if they believe they have the respect and support of the manager (Green, 2006; Maier, 1976; Max & Bacal, 2003).

Appraisal Reports

The appraisal report is to be written jointly by the manager and staff nurse. It should be reliable, valid, and accurate, showing progress made by the nurse and giving illustrations to substantiate value judgments. If both have kept notes that they have periodically assessed, and if the staff member believes the manager's intent is to help rather than to blame, the staff member will feel freer to be honest in an evaluation of strengths and weaknesses. If staff members have not been functioning satisfactorily, they will most likely already be aware of it. If their performance has not improved adequately since previous interviews, they should be informed that the weakness will be included in the report. Any improvements are to be noted, and staff members should know exactly where they stand. It may be necessary to tell them they have to make certain improvements within a definite time period or they will be terminated.

Permanent, cumulative evaluation records can be used to assess how the nurse can best be matched to agency needs. They can be used as a basis for pay increases and promotions or terminations.

Legal Implications for Performance Appraisals

The Equal Pay Act of 1963, which prohibits paying personnel of one gender at a different rate from personnel of the other gender for the same work; the Civil Rights Act of 1964, which prohibits discrimination on the basis of race, color, religion, gender, or national origin; and the Age Discrimination in Employment Act of 1967, which prohibits discrimination against persons 40 to 70 years of age, all require that employers document the quality of employee performance before making decisions about selection, training, transfer, retention, and promotion.

The most legally defensible content of performance appraisals should be based on job analysis; and should be objective, verifiable, specific, and job related rather than global. Individual traits such as attitudes should not be evaluated. Performance standards, performance results, the appeal process, and antidiscrimination laws should all be communicated to personnel. Raters should have written instructions for how to do an unbiased appraisal. Using more than one rater is desirable, and raters should observe the worker firsthand. Documentation requirements should be consistent for all personnel within a job category, documentation of critical incidents for extreme ratings should be required, and a thorough written record of evidence should be collected including evaluations, counseling about performance deficits, and methods employed as corrective actions before termination decisions are made (Margrave, 2001; Sullivan, Decker, 2005).

DISCIPLINE OF PERSONNEL

Need for Discipline

*"Don't be afraid of opposition. Remember,
a kite rises against, not with, the wind."*
—Anonymous

Lack of knowledge about policies and procedures is a major cause of the need for disciplinary action. Management should provide orientation from the first day of employment. Nurses cannot be expected to follow rules that are unknown to them, vague, or loosely enforced. Consequently, each new employee should be given an employee handbook. The handbook itemizes the rules and procedures of the agency and specifies the type of discipline that will be imposed for infractions. New employees should be encouraged to read the handbook and ask questions about it.

During orientation the manager should explain in detail the most frequently violated rules and discuss their significance and rationale. It is recommended that the manager conduct regularly scheduled meetings with staff to discuss changes or to review policies. Rules and regulations also may be posted in a consistent and conspicuous manner.

Most employees are not disciplinary problems, but some individuals require more than positive stimuli. These few cases are potentially explosive. About one half of the grievance cases appealed to an arbitrator by labor unions involve disciplinary action. In about one half of those cases, management either reversed or modified its decision when the individual's appeal was upheld. Consequently, it is of utmost importance that disciplinary action be undertaken in a judicious manner. The disciplinary action program and grievance procedure must be uniform for all personnel of a specific grade or classification. A standard disciplinary action program with procedures outlined and forms provided should be available to managers (McConnell, 2006).

Principles of Disciplinary Action
Have a Positive Attitude

The manager's attitude is very important in preventing or correcting undesirable behavior. If personnel are treated as suspect, they are more likely to provide the trouble that the manager anticipates. People tend to do what is expected of them; therefore it is the manager's duty to maintain a positive attitude by expecting the best from the staff.

Investigate Carefully

The ramifications of disciplinary action are so serious that managers must proceed with caution. They should collect the facts, check allegations, talk to witnesses, and ask accused employees for

---

 RESEARCH Perspective 14-2

Data from Potylycki MJ, Kimmel SR, Ritter M, et al: Nonpunitive medication error reporting: 3-Year findings from one hospital's primum non nocere initiative, *JONA* 36(7-8):370-376, 2006.

Purpose: The purpose was to identify practices and attitudes in medication error occurrences and reporting practices.

Methods: A pre- and post-initiative questionnaire to measure staff practices and attitudes on medication error reporting was developed and administered to staff in one hospital. Pre- and post–comparative analysis was used following a baseline post-implementation design.

Results/conclusions: Medication errors with more serious outcomes are more likely to be reported than those with less serious outcomes. Staff reporting carries the risks of disciplinary action, and this was identified as a primary barrier to the likelihood of reporting. Evaluation of the initiative indicated that a multicomponent approach facilitates positive movement in the direction of a nonpunitive culture toward reporting medication errors.

their side of the story. Managers should accept the employee's account until and unless the allegations are proven. The manager may wish to consult other managers or the director. If the situation is serious enough to require action before a full investigation can be conducted, it is better to suspend the employee subject to reinstatement after investigation than to take more drastic action.

Be Prompt

Managers should not be so expeditious that they neglect to be thorough in ascertaining the facts. If staff members are disciplined unfairly or unnecessarily, the effects on the entire staff may be severe. However, if the discipline is delayed, the relationship between the punishment and the offense may become less clear. Because of the distastefulness of disciplinary action, the manager may tend to postpone the disciplinary action as long as possible. The longer the delay, the more the staff members forget their actions, and the more likely they are to feel that the discipline is not deserved. Positive educational effects for the future are optimized when disciplinary action takes place in a timely fashion.

Protect Privacy

Disciplinary action affects the ego of the staff nurse. Thus it is better to discuss the situation in private. By helping the nurse save face, there is less possibility of future resentment and a greater chance for future cooperation.

Focus on the Act

When disciplining a staff nurse, the manager should emphasize that it was the act that was unacceptable, not the employee. If the employee is not acceptable (e.g., dishonest, abusive, addicted with no plans for recovery), the person should be terminated.

Enforce Rules Consistently

Offending employees should be treated equally and consistently for similar transgressions. Equal treatment is based on rules with specific penalties for various acts and the number of offenses. Consistency reduces the possibility of favoritism, promotes predictability, fosters acceptance of penalties, and defeats allegations of discrimination.

Be Flexible

Consistent implementation is complicated by the fact that individuals and circumstances are never the same. A penalty should be determined only after the entire record of the employee is reviewed. The manager should consider length of service, past accomplishments or problems, level of skill, and expendability to the organization. The intent of the staff nurse, the extenuating circumstances, and whether this situation constitutes a test case and will set precedent for the future should also be taken into consideration. If managers enforce identical penalties for seemingly similar offenses, they may be excessively severe with one person and lenient with the other if they have not considered the varying circumstances.

Advise the Employee

The employees must be informed that their conduct is not acceptable. Personnel files containing anecdotal notes can be a useful management tool, but they are of little value in upholding disciplinary action if the staff member is not informed of the contents promptly.

Take Corrective, Constructive Action

The manager should be sure that the staff nurse understands that the behavior was contrary to the organization's requirements and should explain why such regulations are necessary. The staff nurse should be counseled as to what behavior is required and how to prevent future disciplinary action.

Follow up

The manager should quietly investigate to determine whether the staff nurse's behavior has changed. If the staff nurse continues to invite disciplinary action, the manager should reevaluate the situation to try to determine the reason for the staff member's attitude. The manager must try to come to terms with the offender and the reasons for the transgression. The staff member could be referred to the agency's employee assistance personnel to help support attitudinal adjustments.

Penalties
Verbal Reprimand

For minor violations that have occurred for the first time, managers may opt to give a verbal warning in private. They might tactfully correct the deviation by telling the staff member the proper way to deal with the situation or by reprimanding the staff person. A verbal reprimand is of limited value beyond alerting the nurse in a relatively friendly way to a need for correction. Because nothing is in writing and the reprimand is given in private, it is difficult to prove that a warning was given. Over time the manager may become unsure and inexact about what was said to whom and under what conditions. When a verbal warning is given, the manager is advised to make an anecdotal note of the time, place, occasion, facts, and the gist of the reprimand. Spoken comments may be easily forgotten, but too formal handling of initial minor offenses can be counterproductive.

Written Reprimand

If the offense is more serious or repeated, the reprimand may be written. It is suggested that the manager and staff member develop a written plan for improvement that defines what the staff member will do to make the performance acceptable and what the manager will do to change the environmental situation if appropriate. A time limit should be set for implementation. Additional penalties or consequences may be defined to address a situation in which the employee's behavior does not adequately improve during the allowed time period. The written notice should include the name of the worker, the name of the manager, the facts and behaviors describing the problem, the plan for correction, and the consequences of future repetition. It is recommended that the worker sign the report to indicate that the person read it, received a copy of it, or both. A copy should be given to the employee and one retained for the personnel file. If the employee believes that signing such a document would be considered an admission of guilt and hence refuses to sign, the manager may ask another managerial person to sign as witness to the fact that the document was discussed with the worker and that a copy was given to the worker. It is appropriate for higher management and the personnel department to review this report. At the end of the designated time, the manager and worker should have another conference to determine if the terms of the agreement have been met. It is hoped that the nurse can be complimented for having made progress and that no further action is deemed necessary. However, if no change or inadequate change has occurred, the continuing nature of the problem should be identified and documented. Additional penalties will probably be necessary. The manager needs to keep the director informed, and continuing consultation with the agency's human resources department is essential for any disciplinary and especially termination process from the beginning to ensure legal aspects are in order. It is also helpful to have a representative from the human resources department present during the final phases of a disciplinary situation leading up to termination.

Other Penalties

Layoff, demotion, and discharge are the most serious penalties and require approval beyond the manager. Layoff may be appropriate in situations where it is best to remove the staff member while an investigation is conducted. The staff member may be reinstated with no loss of pay if cleared through the investigation or may be suspended if found guilty of a serious offense. Demotion is a questionable solution. It creates hard feelings, which may be contagious, and more than likely places offenders in a position for which they are overqualified. Termination becomes necessary as a last resort (Marquis & Huston, 2006).

Components of a Disciplinary Action Program
Codes of Conduct

Employees must be informed of the nature and meaning of codes of conduct. Agency handbooks, policy manuals, and orientation programs may be used. The staff member must understand that the rules are reasonable and directly related to efficient, effective operation of the agency.

Authorized Penalties

During disciplinary action the personnel record should indicate that a fair investigation was made of charges before the assessment of guilt and determination of penalties. The agency's disciplinary action program should indicate that the current action is being administered without bias and is directly related to the offense.

Records of Offenses and Corrective Measures

Records are of utmost importance when disciplinary action is appealed. The personnel record should clearly indicate the facts surrounding the offense, management's efforts to correct the problem of the employee's noncompliance with corrective measures, and resulting penalties.

Right of Appeal

Formal provision for the right of employee appeal is a part of each disciplinary action program. Appeal beyond the manager ensures equitable treatment and encourages more employee acceptance of the disciplinary process. At the same time, managers who have been fair need not fear a review of their actions by others. Grievance procedures should be readily available to all staff members so they can use them if they feel they have been mistreated. If others have not followed policies and procedures, a grievance may be in order.

Discipline without Punishment

"Justice is better when it prevents rather than punishes with severity." —Legal maxim

Progressive discipline starts with a verbal reprimand, followed by a written reprimand, and then suspension without pay. If no corrective action is taken, the last step is termination. Discipline without punishment gives disciplinary suspension with pay to demonstrate that management is sincere in the desire to see the worker change and stay. It starts with complete documentation to recognize and reinforce desirable performance, to confront the few who do not meet the standards, and to support workers to correct problems while maintaining self-esteem. The system is designed to influence the worker to accept responsibility, to change behavior, and to return to an acceptable standard of performance. Without punishment, there is a verbal reminder, a written reminder, and a leave during which the employee makes a decision about taking responsibility for one's behavior, but no punishment. This allows for solving problems and enhancing relationships. It focuses on personal responsibility and decision making. The manager initially lets the employee know what is expected and the employee's responsibility to do what is expected. A memo is used to document the interaction. By making the correction, the employee can "wipe the slate clean" and have information about the incident removed from the record. Otherwise, the employee gets one day with pay to take responsibility for his or her behavior and do what is best for him or her and the organization or face termination. That helps reduce the anger associated with the final step. If necessary, the employee is discharged from the organization fairly, humanely, and permanently. The decision to perform well or poorly and to follow the rules or not are the employee's. Requiring employees to take responsibility for their own behavior is more effective than punishing. Punishment can produce compliance but not commitment. Seeking agreement about why a problem must be solved and the logical consequences to the employee if it is not helps get commitment (Grote, 2006).

MODIFICATION OF EMPLOYEE BEHAVIOR

Can an employee's behavior be changed by changing the manager's behavior? Is behavior that recurs in the presence of the manager being reinforced by the manager? Is it possible that doing nothing is doing something? In all three instances the answer is yes. Behavior leads to consequences, and the consequences that follow the behavior affect the probability of recurrence of that behavior. Because behavior is a function of the consequence, it is important for nurse managers to identify the contingency relationship.

Consequences may be favorable, punitive, absent, or insufficient. Positive consequences increase the probability of recurrence of the behavior that preceded them. Absence of consequences decreases the probability, and insufficient consequences have little effect. Punishing consequences have varied and unpredictable effects. Punishment is not the opposite of a favorable consequence. Having no consequence is the opposite of a favorable one.

Reinforcement

Positive reinforcement increases the probability of a recurrence of desired behavior. It is more effective the sooner it follows the desired behavior, and it should be clearly connected to the behavior that the manager wishes to increase. Positive reinforcement may be as subtle as a smile or a nod of the head when someone speaks. Whatever is being said when the manager smiles or nods is reinforced and will recur with increasing frequency. Recognition is a powerful reinforcer. "Mr. Jones must feel so much better now since you have completed his morning care" and "You collected a lot of valuable information during your interview with Mrs. Smith" are examples. "I'm glad to see you here today" reinforces attendance, whereas "I see you were absent again yesterday" gives attention to the absence.

The nurse manager can even stimulate new behavior by verbal acknowledgment of the desired response. Words are used to describe the behavior the nurse manager wants to encourage. A comment such as "I really appreciate nurses attending in-services" is likely to increase attendance at in-services. A number of stimuli—such as feedback, attention, praise, avoidance of punishment, merit pay increases, special assignments, assistance with tuition, or tickets to a ball game or play—can be used to reinforce behavior. However, nurse managers must consider that any stimulus can be reinforcing or aversive depending on the person and the situation, so they should carefully select stimuli that are reinforcers for the individual in a given situation. For example, tickets to a ball game may be reinforcing to some and aversive to others. Recognition is one of the easiest, cheapest, and most universally effective reinforcers.

Shaping

Shaping is a behavior-modification technique used when the response does not meet the criteria. By systematically reinforcing successive approximations, the nurse manager can shape the responses into the desired behavior and get the staff member to do something new. The manager provides favorable consequences after any attempt at the desired behavior and then withholds consequences until improvement is made. When working with the staff member who is chronically absent or late, the manager may acknowledge that the person is at work: "I see you were only 30 minutes late today." Later, "I see you were only 15 minutes late today." Still later, "I noticed you were only 5 minutes late today." The manager may initially praise a new employee for attempting a new task and then note improvements in skill as they occur. Once the level of desired performance has been reached, it can be maintained by providing favorable consequences intermittently. Too many positive consequences cause satiation, and they lose their effect on the behavior. Performance that has been intermittently reinforced is most resistant to extinction.

Extinction

Withholding reinforcers will decrease the probability of the occurrence of the behavior and contribute to its extinction. Therefore, if the manager does not mention or otherwise reward undesirable behavior, the lack of action should contribute to extinction. Conversely, any reinforcer that is presented frequently but not paired with another reinforcer will lose its effectiveness. Promises of "raises" or "hiring more help and getting some relief" become meaningless if not paired with a pay increase or recruitment and selection of personnel. Managers who praise everyone for everything all the time will find that their words lose their effectiveness as reinforcers. When the consequences are not worth the effort, the desirable behavior will decrease also.

Punishment

The manager can decrease the probability of a response by pairing the behavior with an aversive stimulus, but that must be consistent across pay grades and with agency policy. Employees who do not meet work standards will be terminated. Termination of a few workers who were not meeting standards can have an immediate impact on the remaining personnel, who initially work harder to avoid losing their jobs. However, if management does nothing to reinforce the more productive work behavior, avoidance behavior is likely to occur. Employees may cover up for each other, steal from the agency what they rationalize is theirs, or resign. By using aversive stimuli to control behavior, management pairs itself with those stimuli and becomes viewed as aversive.

Once managers have started an aversive stimulus, they should not stop it until the behavior has been corrected or the cessation may act as a positive reinforcer. Absences, tardiness, excuse making, rationalizing, placing blame elsewhere, and other avoidance behaviors will increase if they successfully reduce the aversive stimuli. If the manager gruffly asks a nurse why some work has not been done (aversive stimulus), and the manager backs off when the staff member replies that she thought someone else was doing it, blaming others is reinforced. Although punishment causes behavior to occur less frequently, it does not teach new behaviors and is likely to increase avoidance behaviors. Most motivation problems are caused by punishment, absence of consequences, or insufficient consequences (Sullivan & Decker, 2005).

Behavior Modification for the Employee with a Performance Problem

Besides being aware of the subtle ways that one's behavior may reinforce, shape, or reduce behavior of others, the nurse manager may apply behavior modification to personnel with performance problems. First, one must identify the performance problem and analyze the antecedent behavior, and consequence. What happened before the behavior occurred? Each time person A was late to work, person A had worked the prior evening shift. Each time person B yelled at staff, an emergency treatment was being performed. Nurse manager C was condescending to a staff member after a physician had scolded nurse C. What happened after the behavior occurred? Someone had already done part of person A's work by the time he or she got to the unit. Staff members responded quickly when person B yelled at them during an emergency procedure. Nurse C was avoided by staff members.

Once the performance problem has been identified, the baseline frequency is determined. The baseline measure is the frequency before any attempts to change it have been taken. If people are interested in modifying their own behavior, they may collect the baseline data themselves. The behavior must be precisely defined, observable, and consequently countable. Written records should be kept, preferably on a portable recording system that is present when the behavior occurs, so the person can record it immediately. A tailor-made tally sheet is useful because one can see data in relation to time. If the behavior occurs daily, it should be recorded for one week. If there are large variations in the behavior from one day to the next, observations should be recorded for two weeks. A time-sampling technique can be used by busy managers by randomly selecting short periods to observe and tally behaviors. This technique is effective only for high-frequency behavior. The manager must consider if the period of data collection was representative of the typical situation and use a stable baseline rate as a cue to start the intervention (Figure 14-10).

If one transfers the information from the tally sheet to a graph that depicts frequency over time, it is easy to visualize the effect of the intervention. One can put a wavy vertical line on the graph to depict the point where intervention was started (Figure 14-11).

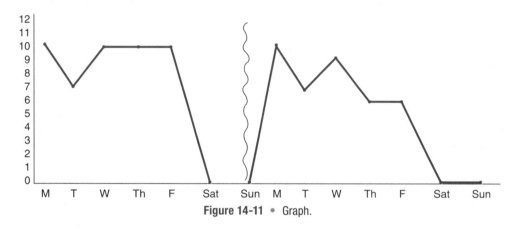

	7:00	I I I	I I	I I	I I I	I I		
	8:00			I				
	9:00	I I			I	I		
	10:00		I		I			
	11:00			I		I		
	12:00				I	I		
	1:00		I	I		I		
	2:00	I I	I	I I	I I	I		
	3:00	I I I	I I	I I I	I I	I I I		

Figure 14-10 • Tally sheet.

Figure 14-11 • Graph.

After identifying the relevant variables, the manager and staff member select appropriate reinforcement, extinction, punishment, or any combination of intervention strategies to decrease the frequency of the undesirable behavior. If the desired performance is punished, the punishment should be removed because the desired performance should not be punished . Instead of making fast workers finish everyone else's work, they can be allowed time to do what they choose, such as read in the library, meditate in the chapel, receive a bonus day at a specified frequency, or be given a merit pay increase specifically for doing more than their share of the work. If undesirable behavior is rewarded, the reward should be removed because undesirable behavior should not be rewarded. Instead of having slow employees' work completed by others, the manager should inform the workers that they are

responsible for their assignments. Further they must have that work completed before leaving, and will receive no overtime pay for completion of the normal workload (if that is legal).

If desired behavior has not been rewarded, the manager should arrange a consequence. This effect may be as simple as verbally acknowledging a nurse's accomplishment occasionally. Nurses' accomplishments could be acknowledged in the agency's newsletter. Awards can be created to recognize desirable behavior.

If obstacles are identified, they should be removed. Nurses can be referred to professional counseling to help them work through situational crises that are interfering with their work performance. The manager can try to get the resources nurses need to do their jobs. Nurses should also have the necessary education to do what is expected of them. They may need formal education, on-the-job training, practice sessions, or simply feedback. The staff member is the best source of information for what can serve as a positive reinforcer because what may be desirable for the manager may be aversive to the staff member.

Once the intervention strategy has been planned, it should be implemented and the response frequency recorded. The strategy should be evaluated for effectiveness. If it is not working, it should be analyzed and revised. Once the desired behavior is obtained, it should be maintained through intermittent reinforcement (Marquis & Huston, 2006; Sullivan & Decker, 2005).

PROBLEM EMPLOYEES

Substance abusers, angry or withdrawn workers, personnel with excessive absenteeism, and employees who are being terminated provide challenges to nurse managers. In each case the manager must be alert to symptoms of problems, help the employee solve the problem, and evaluate the results.

Substance Abusers

Substance abuse is not uncommon among health professionals. It affects all socioeconomic classes, cultures, and races. Among alcoholic nurses studied, most had been in the top one third of their class, held advanced degrees, held responsible and demanding jobs, and had an excellent work history.

Nurses with alcohol or other drug addictions often exhibit psychosocial problems (Box 14-4). Personality changes may be noted as the nurse becomes more irritable, withdrawn, and moody. Because of a decreased interest in outside activities, isolation increases. Related social changes include eating alone and avoiding social gatherings. Changes in personal appearance become apparent. Changes in dress, an unkempt appearance, flushed complexion, red eyes, swollen face, and hand tremors are common. Mental status changes include forgetfulness, confusion, and decreased alertness.

General behavior changes too. Inappropriate responses and irritability occur more frequently. Excuses for behavior become more elaborate. Intolerance and suspicion of others and nervousness increase. Avoidance of others is noted. Work efficiency drops, there is a decline in the quality and quantity of work, and the work pace becomes uneven. Some assigned tasks are forgotten. Arriving late, leaving early, and extended lunch hours and break times become patterns of behavior. Practice errors increase. The alcoholic staff member is more likely to miss work because of hangovers, whereas the drug-addicted health professionals are likely to work overtime to have additional access to drugs and to earn money to cover the costs to maintain the habit. It is important for staff members to know the importance of their reporting chemical abuse, because it is often not the manager who identifies the problem, especially if the manager supervises more than one unit.

When a staff member reports to work in a state of acute intoxication, the manager notes the signs objectively and asks a second person to validate the observations. The odor of alcohol, slurred speech, unsteady gait, and errors in judgment are symptoms of intoxication. The intoxicated staff person is removed from the situation, confronted briefly and firmly about the behavior, and sent home to rest and recuperate. Typically agencies have specific policies and specific follow through procedures. Some agency policies require that a blood sample be evaluated for alcohol concentration to validate or refute the suspicion. Then the incident is recorded. The manager describes the observation, states the action taken, indicates future plans, and has the employee sign and date the memo after returning to work. Refusal to sign and date the memo should be noted by the manager and a witness.

Chronic performance problems are more common than acute intoxication. Each time performance problems are observed, they should be documented, including date, time, who was observed by whom, and a description of the incident and circumstances. At a prearranged

---

BOX 14-4 Signs and Symptoms of Possible Substance Abuse

SIGNS

Psychosocial problems:
  Irritability
  Moodiness
  Tendency to isolate self
Social changes:
  Eating alone
  Avoiding social gatherings
Changes in personal appearance:
  Changes in dress
  Unkempt appearance
  Flushed complexion
  Red eyes
  Swollen face
  Hand tremors

Mental status changes:
  Forgetfulnes
  Confusion
  Decreased alertness
General behavior changes:
  Inappropriate responses
  Elaborate excuses for behavior
  Intolerance of others
  Suspiciousness
  Nervousness

SYMPTOMS
Odor of alcohol
Slurred speech
Unsteady gait
Errors in judgment

---

conference, the staff member is confronted with the observations and how they affect job performance and patient care. The staff member is allowed to respond. Alternatives are explored, and a course of action is planned. When substance abuse is identified as the problem, the offender is encouraged to take voluntary action. The manager refers the staff member to a local treatment facility and meets with the person periodically to monitor progress. The manager is not to serve the role of therapist.

Instead of disciplining and firing personnel whose job performance is impaired, more and more health care organizations are trying to help them regain their health and productivity through employee assistance programs (EAPs). At first EAPs focused on alcohol and drug abuse, but the services have broadened to include financial, legal, and marital problems; gambling; work addiction; and eating disorders. EAPs have increased productivity, reduced absenteeism, and lowered insurance costs. Assessment, diagnosis, and early intervention benefit the employee and the organization.

Many state nurses associations have started peer assistance programs. Ideally the association intervenes early in the addiction process before legal action is necessary. Reports of impairment are often made through a confidential telephone call or as a referral to the chairperson of the peer assistance program. The chairperson verifies that an impairment exists and may coach the nurse manager about documentation, verification, and intervention. A regional representative or local intervener contacts the person in question and makes an appointment.

The local intervener typically outlines the purpose of the visit with the impaired person, presents information about chemical abuse, and identifies behavior and circumstances in which the impairment has been evident. The fact that the disease is progressive is stressed. Various treatment options are presented. Issues such as hospitalization, insurance coverage, use of sick time and accrued vacation time, and family responsibilities are discussed. If the person denies impairment or refuses treatment, the impaired nurse may be reported to the state board of nursing by the employer. The majority of RN license suspensions are related to practicing nursing while impaired.

When an impaired nurse participates in a peer assistance program, an advocate is assigned. The advocate maintains contact with the impaired nurse during treatment and until a solid recovery is established. A contract made by the peer review program advocate and the impaired nurse typically identifies employment restrictions, random urine screens, attendance at Alcoholics Anonymous or Narcotics Anonymous meetings, attendance at nurses' support groups, and contacts with the advocate.

When alcoholic or drug-abusing staff members refuse counseling or fail to follow the plan of care, they are told treatment is mandatory for continued employment. If they still refuse mandatory participation in the treatment, they are terminated in accordance with the agency's policies (Marquis & Huston, 2006).

Angry or Withdrawn Employees

Nurse managers often deal with angry or withdrawn employees. Anger and withdrawal are the fight and flight responses to anxiety. The angry nurse is more likely to be considered a troublemaker. The withdrawn person may be viewed as nice. However, both need help.

Anxiety occurs from the frustration of unmet expectations or loss of self-respect. The anxiety is transformed into feelings or actions, and relief is felt. Angry, hostile, and destructive behavior is a primary response to frustration. It is intended to gain mastery over the situation. The angry employee may become hostile and use critical, sarcastic, and obscene language with others. Consequently, interpersonal relationships suffer, and productive work may be impaired. Anger can also be displaced to patients and others.

Withdrawn persons do not invest emotional energy in others. Fear of self-disclosure or having others become attached to them is frightening. Withdrawal is a protective mechanism to avoid hurt. Withdrawn persons sit through meetings without becoming involved. They are not assertive and do not protect their rights. They may be delegated more than their fair share of the work because they are so cooperative and polite. This cycle leads to more feelings of use, abuse, and helplessness.

Nurse managers need to recognize aggressive and passive behaviors among employees, teach and display assertive behavior, and encourage problem solving. They should help personnel understand themselves and their job responsibilities, develop trust, and promote group harmony. Employees should be encouraged to express themselves without fear of reprisals. Managers should be sincere, firm, and fair. Job expectations should be clear and personnel rewarded liberally and disciplined justly.

Decreased Productivity

Decreased productivity is a side effect of personnel problems. Managers should make sure that desired performance is not being punished or undesirable behavior rewarded. Expectations are clarified. Employees are taught how to do what they are expected to do. If boredom is a problem, job rotation and special projects are considered.

Absenteeism

Absenteeism is also a side effect of personnel problems. Ineffective management, poor working relationships, boredom, lack of control over decisions affecting one's life, and overwork are contributing factors. Some workers are immature and lack the self-discipline to get themselves to work. Others stay away to avoid an unpleasant or boring job. Some are poorly motivated, do as little as necessary to prevent being terminated, and do not see their jobs as means toward ends. The hypochondriacal employee uses absenteeism to get attention and sympathy from others. Abusive absenteeism may be used to get even with a manager. Some personnel are exhausted from overwork, have lost their enthusiasm for the job, or are burned out.

Managers should make sure that there are attendance policies, that the policies do not reward nonattendance, and that they are enforced consistently. Attendance records should be maintained, and grievance procedures should be established.

Documented attendance policies greatly influence absence rates. Traditional sick leave policies have rewarded employees for absenteeism and have encouraged them to be dishonest to collect sick pay or be punished by losing it. Employees who receive sick pay are absent considerably more than those who do not. They use the sick pay benefits while those that do not have the benefits may come to work ill. Some agencies have required a physician's excuse before an employee can receive sick pay to decrease the dishonest use of sick time. Because most people are sick only one or two days at a time, some hospitals do not compensate for the first two days of any sickness. The third and successive days are compensated. Other agencies have gone to paid time off (PTO). Each employee receives a certain amount of paid time off inclusive of holiday, vacation, and sick leave with few restrictions as to its use. It is typically collected at a rate calculated by length of continuous service. It simplifies record keeping but provides incentive to use the days whether sick or not.

Absenteeism data should be collected and analyzed to determine trends and patterns of individuals and personnel in general. Recording the date of absence, the reason and whether excused or unexcused, day of the week, preceding or following a day off, the employee's job classification, shift, tenure, age, gender, marital status, or any other information thought to be useful provides information to detect trends and pinpoint problems. Absenteeism often occurs more frequently in certain job classifications or departments, on specific days or shifts, or among a group working under a specific manager. Problems need to be identified so managers can develop control measures. Baseline data are also useful to determine the success of the control program.

A progressive discipline policy that imposes increasingly severe penalties is appropriate. Such a policy allows employees to know in advance the consequences of their behavior. Progressive discipline often starts with a verbal reprimand that is documented and progresses through a written warning, suspension with or without pay, and dismissal. The manager needs to investigate circumstances, objectively formulate a judgment based on fact, adhere to standards, policies, and behaviors of professional performance (Hader, 2006).

Terminating Employees

Although not many RNs are terminated, during economic recessions the incidence of reduced workforces increases. Outplacement counseling can be used to minimize the emotional and professional scarring that results from being dismissed from one's position.

Poor job performance, tardiness, absenteeism, substance abuse, inappropriate behavior, and staff reduction are the most common reasons for discharging nurses. A termination of this nature is usually a progressive process. However, for some offenses nurses can be terminated immediately. These are likely to include abuse of patients and visitors, insubordination, intoxication,

possession of drugs, theft, gambling, disorderly conduct, willful destruction of property, sleeping on duty, or falsification of records.

A termination checklist can help the manager through the termination process (Box 14-5). Typically the terminated employee is not allowed on the work site after all institutional property has been collected, or the employee is allowed to collect personal effects in the company of the manager at a prearranged time. Confidentiality must be maintained in a disciplinary or termination situation even though rumors may be rampant. Outplacement and career counseling are best conducted by the human resources department.

It is not uncommon for employees who are being terminated to detach themselves from the job and do little for some time before the termination. The manager can assign tasks that are considered important that can either be finished or transferred to someone else at the time of the employee's termination. Rituals such as best wishes cards and going away parties serve to acknowledge the termination and provide a rite of separation that facilitates the termination process (Roussel, Swansburg, & Swansburg, 2006).

Support services are needed by people who are terminated. The agency should have termination policies regarding severance pay, terminal vacation, accrued holidays and sick time, and insurance. The person may need information about unemployment. This is an opportune time for a counselor in personnel to help terminating employees reassess their location and vocation. Where do they want to live? What type of climate do they like? What type of work interests them and provides the most satisfaction? What do their educational background and skills prepare them to do? What can they do to prepare themselves better to reach their goals? How important are salary, fringe benefits, retirement plans, work hours, and opportunities for advancement?

Once employees who are being terminated decide what they want to do and where, they may need assistance to locate job openings. Professional journals, employment agencies, and college placement services are sources of information.

BOX 14-5 Termination Checklist

DATE COMPLETED	ACTION TAKEN
_____	Review termination plan for consistency with laws, policies, and procedures with Human Resources.
_____	Get supervisor's approval for termination.
_____	Have witness present for termination conference.
_____	Terminate access to information technology.
_____	Notify security.
_____	Collect department's property, such as keys, disks, manuals, and so on.
_____	Collect agency's property, such as employee badge, handbooks, parking pass, and so on.
_____	Complete necessary forms.
_____	Arrange for employee to remove personal property from the premises.
_____	Advise employee he or she will not be permitted back on the premises.
_____	Advise employee of employee assistance program.
_____	Advise employee that the final paycheck will be mailed. Confirm mailing address.
_____	Forward employee file to Human Resources.

---

focus on the knowledge and skills they have learned on the last job that they can transfer to the new one. They should not be critical of the last employer.

The sooner one accepts the fact that one has been terminated, the sooner one can put the pieces back together and move on. The boss should be very clear about the reason. The termination should not come as a surprise. With the progressive process the employee should know the consequences of not meeting the performance standards. Any reduction in workforce should be done with fair warning and target dates. Employees should be informed of the grievance policy and procedure when reflecting if they have been fairly treated. The outplacement counseling can help the person know what questions to ask about pay and benefits, how to tell the family, how to solicit help from friends and acquaintances, and how to budget to protect securities until another job can be obtained. Career counseling and job placement counseling are useful. Being terminated initiates stress and can be quite devastating. Outplacement counseling can help reduce the related personal and professional scarring that inevitably results from being dismissed.

"Keep away from people who try to belittle your ambitions. Small people always do that, but the really great make you feel that you, too, can become great." —Mark Twain

---

EMPLOYEE COUNSELING

Counseling helps improve employees' mental health, thus enhancing understanding, self-control, self-confidence, and consequently their ability to work effectively. Counseling accomplishes several activities on a directive to nondirective scale. It provides an opportunity to give advice, offer reassurance, improve communication, release emotional tension, clarify thinking, and reorient to appropriate behavior.

When giving advice, a counselor tells the employee what the counselor thinks the employee should do. Unfortunately, it is almost impossible

Recruiters are often present at professional meetings. Friends, relatives, and acquaintances may help locate positions, and employers can be contacted directly.

Employees who are being terminated are likely to need help preparing resumes, writing marketing letters, and interviewing. They do not need to state the reason that they left the last job on this marketing letter, resume, or job application. However, they should be prepared to address the issue during an interview. They should be honest about the reason for termination, speak about the treatment they have had, if any, and

to understand another person's complicated problems, and consequently the advice may not be sound. Advice may foster feelings of inferiority and dependence on the counselor.

Reassurance provides courage to face a problem and confidence that one is handling the situation appropriately. False reassurance, however, is dangerous. It may prevent the employee from getting the professional help needed. It offers little comfort when the counselee knows that the counselor cannot predict the outcome. Even if there is some comfort obtained, it tends to dissipate when the person faces the problem again.

Counseling improves both upward and downward communication. It allows employees to express their feelings to management. Although individual names must be kept confidential, feelings can be grouped into categories and interpreted to higher management. The counseling session allows the counselor to explain company policies and activities to the employee, thus achieving downward communication.

Catharsis, or the release of emotional tension, often occurs when people have the opportunity to talk about their frustrations. They become more relaxed, and their speech becomes more coherent and rational as they explain their problems to a sympathetic listener. Then, as emotional blocks to clear thinking are eliminated, thinking becomes more rational. People may realize that their emotions are not appropriate for the situation. This may help people recognize and accept their limitations and bring about a reorientation or change in values and goals.

Directive counseling occurs when the counselor listens to the employee's problems, decides how to solve the problems, and tells the employee what to do. The counselor predominantly gives advice. This type of counseling does give some emotional release, can be reassuring, and fosters communication. Thinking may be clarified in a limited way. Reorientation seldom occurs.

Nondirective counseling is client centered. The counselor listens and encourages employees to explain their problems, identify alternatives, explore the ramifications of each option, and determine the most appropriate solution. Emotional release occurs more frequently in nondirective than in directive counseling. Clear thinking and reorientation are fostered. Reassurance may be used, but advice should be limited. This approach can be very beneficial, but managers must be cautious not to neglect their normal directive leadership responsibilities.

Nondirective counseling is more time consuming and costly than directive counseling. To be effective, the employee must have the intelligence to identify problems and assess solutions, and the emotional stability to deal with them. The nondirective counselor must be cautious not to allow emotionally dependent employees to avoid their work responsibilities.

Cooperative counseling is a compromise between directive and nondirective counseling. It is the cooperative effort by the counselor and employee through an exchange of ideas to help solve the problem. The cooperative counselor starts by listening, as would a nondirective counselor. As the interview progresses, however, the cooperative counselor offers information and insight and is likely to discuss the problems with a broad knowledge of the organization's point of view. This may help change the employee's perspective. Cooperative counseling combines the advantages of both directive and nondirective counseling and avoids most of the disadvantages.

Because of employees' rights to privacy, it is appropriate for the manager to refer an employee to the human resources department or to professional help when personal problems are interfering with job performance, or when a person needs reorientation (Roussel, Swansburg, & Swansburg, 2006).

CHAPTER SUMMARY

Managers are responsible for performance appraisals. Therefore it is important for managers to know the legal implications of doing appraisal interviews and reports. It is helpful for managers to know how to modify problem employee's behavior, the principles and components of disciplinary action, and employee and outplacement counseling. It is important to include the human resources department in any disciplinary and especially the termination process to ensure legal aspects are in order.

CRITICAL THINKING ACTIVITY

Reflective Journal: Make observations in a clinical setting, or reflect on past experiences. Answer the following questions: When and how are personnel evaluated? Is there a process for disciplinary action in place? If so, what is it? Discuss how the agency handles chemically impaired employees. What are the policies and procedures regarding chemically impaired employees in the agency? What is the manager's role? What are the criteria for notification to the nursing administration and board of nursing? Who is responsible for notifying them?

CASE STUDY

You do appraisal interviews with appraisal report follow-ups once per year with the personnel who work with you. You want to create an atmosphere of equality for planning and problem solving. What will you do to create that atmosphere?

ONLINE RESOURCES

evolve Additional critical thinking activities, worksheets, and case studies are available online at http://evolve.elsevier.com/Marriner/guide8e.

REFERENCES

Finkleman AW: *Leadership and management in nursing*, Upper Saddle River, NJ, 2006, Pearson/Prentice Hall.

Green ME: *Painless performance evaluations*, Upper Saddle River, NJ, 2006, Prentice Hall.

Grote D: *The complete guide to performance appraisal*, New York, 1996, American Management Association.

Grote D: *Discipline without punishment*, New York, 2006, American Management Association.

Hader R: Put employee termination etiquette to practice, *Nursing Management* 37(12):6, 2006.

Maier RF: *Appraising performance: An interview skills course*, La Jolla, CA, 1976, University Associates.

Margrave A: *The complete idiot's guide to performance appraisals*, Royersford, PA, 2001, Alpha.

Marquis BL, Huston CJ: *Leadership roles and management functions in nursing: Theory and application*, ed 3, Philadelphia, 2006, Lippincott.

Max D, Bacal R: *Perfect phrases for performance reviews: Hundreds of ready-to-use phrases that describe your employees' performance*, New York, 2003, McGraw-Hill.

McConnell CR: *Umiker's management skills for the new health care supervisor*, ed 4, Boston, 2006, Jones and Bartlett Publishers.

Meretoja R, Leino-Kilpi H: Instruments for evaluating nurse competence, *JONA* 31(7/8):346-352, 2001.

Nemeth LS, Harris-Eaton KY, Weaver K: Chapter 30: Performance appraisal. In Huber DL, editor: *Leadership and nursing care management*, ed 3, Philadelphia, 2006, Saunders/Elsevier.

Odiorne GS: *Management decisions by objectives*, Englewood Cliffs, NJ, 1978, Prentice Hall.

Odiorne GS: *Management by objectives: A system of managerial leadership*, Belmont, CA, 1982, Pitman Publishing.

Potylycki MJ, Kimmel SR, Ritter M, et al: Nonpunitive medication error reporting: 3-Year findings from one hospital's primum non nocereinitiative, *JONA* 36 (7-8):370-376, 2006.

Roussel L, Swansburg RC, Swansburg RJ: *Management and leadership for administrators*, Boston, 2006, Jones and Bartlett Publishers.

Shepard G: *How to make performance evaluations really work: A step-by-step guide complete with sample words, phrases, forms, and pitfalls to avoid*, New York, 2006, Wiley.

Sullivan EJ, Decker PJ: *Effective leadership and management in nursing*, Upper Saddle River, NJ, 2005, Prentice Hall.

Twedell D: Chapter 17: Selecting, developing and evaluating staff. In Yoder-Wise PS: *Leading and managing in nursing*, ed 4, St. Louis, 2007, Mosby/Elsevier, pp. 289-302.

Continuous Quality Improvement, Risk Management, and Program Evaluation

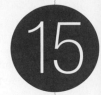

"The greater the difficulty the more glory in surmounting it. Skillful pilots gain their reputation from storms and tempests." —Epicurus

Chapter Overview

Chapter 15 discusses the history of regulatory influences and continuous quality improvement including the Institute of Medicine reports, program evaluation, magnetism, risk management, and liability issues.

Chapter Objectives

- Compare and contrast the roles of leaders and managers regarding quality improvement.
- Indicate trends in the history of continuous quality improvement.
- Identify three quality management heroes and their contributions to the field.
- Select at least three recommendations from the Institute of Medicine reports.
- Outline a process for continuous quality improvement.
- Describe at least five tools that can be used to facilitate continuous quality improvement.
- Define evidence-based practice.
- Itemize activities that could be on a calendar of events for program evaluation.
- Explain at least six internal and six external sources of invalidity.
- Identify at least six research designs and identify which sources of invalidity the design controls and which could still be a problem.
- List the five steps in the risk management process.
- Identify at least three sources for identifying potential risks.
- Discuss the importance of customer satisfaction in relation to risk management.
- Describe the research process as applied to quality improvement.
- Determine the relationship among torts, negligence, and malpractice.
- Evaluate at least one liability issue.
- Identify at least five characteristics of a magnet hospital.

Online Resources

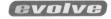

Critical thinking activities, worksheets, and case studies are available online at http://evolve.elsevier.com/Marriner/guide8e.

Major Concepts and Definitions

Evidence-based practice *problem solving approach to the delivery of care that integrates the best evidence from well-designed studies, a clinician's expertise, and patient preferences and values*

Continuous quality improvement *preventive problem solving that results in exemplary service*

Risk management *development and implementation of strategies to prevent patient injury, minimize financial loss, and preserve agency assets*

Customer satisfaction *risk management of public relations that strives for customer satisfaction*

Evaluation *valuation*

Validity *measurement of what is to be measured*

Internal invalidity *extraneous variables that confound the effects of the experimental variable*

External invalidity *factors that reduce the findings' generalizability*

Statistics *facts or data of a numerical kind that are assembled, classified, and tabulated so as to present significant information about a given subject*

Sentinal event *an unexpected outcome involving a death or serious injury*

Root cause *the underlying problem*

Torts *legal wrongs*

Negligence *unintentional tort where harm results by not behaving in a reasonable and prudent manner*

Malpractice *negligent acts of people with professional education*

Legally liable *legally responsible*

Plaintiff *complaining party*

Defendant *answering party*

Magnet hospitals *facilities that usually have improved patient outcomes, better nurse recruitment and retention, enhanced nurse work environments, and use of evidence-based practice and research*

LEADERSHIP AND MANAGEMENT FOR QUALITY IMPROVEMENT

Leaders envision high-quality care, model quality care management, encourage others to be involved in quality improvement, encourage setting high standards, are proactive, facilitate interdisciplinary quality, consequently build a culture of quality, and enable interdisciplinary quality improvement. They also foster development of infrastructure and processes for quality improvement, encourage the use of electronic systems, communicate the quality findings to others, and act as a role model. Managers organize quality-driven services; monitor quality of care; select standards and tools to measure them with others; facilitate collecting and analyzing data; determine discrepancies between care provided and standards; facilitate ongoing quality improvement, and evaluate quality of care. They also use the infrastructure and processes with their staff for quality improvement, use electronic systems for quality control, assess the sources of information, and keep informed about government, accrediting bodies, and licensing regulations regarding quality improvement (Pelletier & Albright, 2006; Marquis & Huston, 2006) (Table 15-1).

TABLE 15-1 Quality Improvement Leadership and Management

Leader	Manager
Envisions high-quality care	Organizes quality-driven service
Models quality care management	Monitors quality of care
Encourages others to be involved in quality standards improvement	Selects standards and measures of those with others
Encourages setting high standards	Selects tools with others
Is proactive versus reactive	Facilitates collecting and analyzing data
Facilitates interdisciplinary quality improvement	Determines discrepancies between care provided and standards
Builds a culture of quality	Facilitates ongoing quality improvement
Enables interdisciplinary quality improvement	Evaluates quality of care
Fosters development of infrastructure and processes for quality improvement	Uses the infrastructure and processes with employees for quality improvement
Encourages use of electronic systems	Uses electronic systems for quality control
Communicates the quality findings to others	Assesses the sources of information
Acts as a role model	Keeps informed about the government, accrediting bodies, and licensing regulations regarding quality improvements

Modified from Huber DL: *Leadership and nursing care management*, ed 3, Philadelphia, 2006, Elsevier; Marquis BL, Huston CJ: *Leadership roles and management functions in nursing: Theory and application*, ed 3, Philadelphia, 2006, Lippincott.

HISTORY OF REGULATORY INFLUENCES

Health insurance can be traced to the seventeenth century in London where workers could pay to ensure that their family members would receive health care if needed. That worked well until the cholera epidemic in 1831, when there were insufficient funds to meet the needs of so many sick people.

Health care in the United States was simple before the depression of the 1930s. Most of the medical practices were simple remedies, because there were few medicines and no advanced technologies. The fee for service was typically paid at the end of the visit and may have been a trade, such as a chicken, for the health care. Most people before the depression could afford medical care. Hospitals were supported by charitable donations, but people who received charitable care often got less quality of care than those who paid. However, during the Depression most people in the United States could not afford medical care, and many hospitals closed because of the drop in charitable donations. There was no insurance or local, state, or federal funding to defray costs.

There was some disability insurance where the employer continued to pay a portion of a sick employee's salary, but there was no assistance for medical costs.

Technological advances and the development of antibiotics during the 1940s advanced the ability to improve health, but unfortunately the cost was prohibitive for most people in the United States. A prepaid payment system that would relieve the burden on the sick person during an illness and ensure that the physician and hospital expenses were paid was envisioned. The first known insurance in the United States was in Oklahoma in 1927 when a physician had people in the community buy shares from the physician to build the hospital in order to qualify to receive any needed medical care at that hospital. A prepaid program for teachers was started at Baylor University Hospital in Dallas in 1929. A prepaid program for municipal employees under written by a Kaiser insurance company was also started that year in Los Angeles. Although physicians, hospitals, and legislators resisted prepaid health care programs, the American Hospital Association (AHA) developed national standards to govern those programs in 1933. Physicians, legislators, and hospitals collaborated to introduce the Blue Cross Plan in 1939.

A period of health care expansion from the 1940s through the 1960s was supported by the federal government. The Hill-Burton Act (The Hospital Survey and Construction Act of 1946) was the beginning of extensive federal subsidization for health care resources. These acts facilitated medical education, research, and technological progress. Policies developed at this time focused on an increase in access to quality health care. The Hill-Burton Act also resulted in more hospitals being built. The Social Security survey of 1963 found that about one half of the retirees had no private health insurance, and it was common for a worker to lose employer-sponsored health insurance upon retiring. Thus Medicare and Medicaid were introduced in 1965 to support the right to quality health care for individuals who were elderly, poor, or 65 years or older and entitled to Social Security or a railroad retirement.

Legislation was passed to extend Medicare coverage to permanently and totally disabled people in 1973. Part A is totally funded by federal funds and covers inpatient care. Part B is voluntary, is partially funded, and covers outpatient services. Large enrollment, inflation, and increasing technology increased the costs to the federal government. Medicaid, which aids states in providing health care to the poor, is a companion to Medicare. Although it provides federal funding to states, states are responsible for the administrative operation.

By the early 1970s the federal government understood that it could not afford unlimited coverage for unlimited numbers of enrollees in Medicare. Cost containment policies such as utilization review, rate control, and control of capital expenditures were addressed. In 1972 the Social Security Act was amended to create the professional standards review organization (PSRO). Physicians reviewed Medicare patient's charts to control health care utilization and costs. The Economic Stabilization Program, which was a federal program to control rates with individual states responsible for rate control, was in effect

from 1971 to 1974. The National Health Planning and Resources Development Act of 1974 authorized and established a national certificate-of-need (CON) program to control capital expansion in health care.

The federal government could not meet the health care costs by regulations alone, so it started combining market and regulatory strategies in the early 1980s through the Omnibus Budget Act of 1981 and the Tax Equity and Fiscal Responsibility Act (TEFRA) of 1982. These laws permitted health maintenance organizations (HMOs) to offer competitive medical plans and encouraged competition. The TEFRA Act of 1982 set operating cost per case and required development of a prospective pricing system. The Peer Review Improvement Act of 1982 repealed the PSRO program and started the peer review organization (PRO). The Social Security Amendment of 1983 encouraged prospective pricing based on diagnostic-related groups (DRGs) to control utilization and costs. The National Health Planning and Resource Development Act was repealed in 1986, consequently repealing the CON requirement. Civilian Health and Medical Programs of the Uniformed Services (CHAMPUS) was given authority to reimburse institutional providers based on DRGs in 1984. The Consolidated Omnibus Budget Reconciliation Act of 1985 required all Medicare-participating hospitals to accept patients from CHAMPUS starting in January 1987. Legislation was facilitating competition among health care services.

For nearly a century various groups have recommended proposals for health care reform. In 1915 one group recommended a focus on prevention and sharing of health care costs by employers, employees, and the government. In 1932, a commission encouraged doctors to form group practices to share responsibility for cost-effective, high-quality health care. In 1933, President Franklin Roosevelt initiated the Social Security Act, in which he intended to include national health insurance, but that was left out of the bill. In 1946, President Harry Truman introduced a plan for national health reform, declaring that health is a right, not just a privilege. His plan met with public and special interest group opposition; the "Red Scare" and the "Cold War" took the priority. In 1971, President Nixon submitted a comprehensive National Health Strategy to congress and in 1972 he advocated that employers take responsibility and contribute to their workers' health care. Congress only implemented parts of the plan.

In 1993, President Bill Clinton advocated more health care reform. He outlined six principles basic to the Health Security Act: (1) security—guaranteeing comprehensive benefits to everyone in the United States; (2) simplicity—cutting red tape and consequently simplifying the system; (3) savings—controlling the costs of health care; (4) quality—making health care better; (5) choice—preserving and increasing the options available; and (6) responsibility—making everyone responsible for health care. Security would be accomplished by providing every person in the United States with a comprehensive health benefits package that could not be taken away. Simplicity would be achieved by reducing paperwork, which wastes time and costs billions of dollars. Savings would be achieved through group purchasing. Quality would involve emphasizing health and giving consumers information to judge the quality of health care themselves. Choice means the right to choose one's health care provider to protect the doctor-patient relationship. Responsibility means that every employee and every employer contribute to the cost of health care (White House Domestic Policy Council, 1993). In 1994, Hillary Clinton gave testimony about the complex proposal to several congressional committees on health care. The proposal was criticized for being too bureaucratic and received extensive criticism. Other democrats offered competing plans instead of supporting the President's proposal. None of the proposals were passed.

Quality standards are often set by professional bodies and promulgated through codes of ethics, standards of care, standards of performance, and practice guidelines, which can be monitored through accreditation, peer review, and certification processes. State boards of nursing help enforce standards under each state's nurse practice act. However, multiple associations in nursing have developed standards using different criteria and formats that have lead to confusion. The American Organization of Nurse Executives (AONE), American Association of Colleges of Nursing (AACN), National League for Nursing (NLN), and the American Nurses Association (ANA) have joined efforts to coordinate and standardize formats and criteria for certification and practice standards. The ANA has a set of nursing standards, including *Standards of Clinical Nursing Practice* and standards for areas of nursing such as addictions, nurse administrators, advanced practice, cardiac rehabilitation, college health, community health, continuing education and staff development, correctional facilities, developmental disabilities or mental retardation, diabetes, forensics, genetics, gerontological nursing practice, home health, nursing informatics, oncology, otorhinolaryngology, parish nursing, pediatric clinical nursing, psychiatric-mental health, and respiratory nursing. The ANA outlines standards of care including the following: (1) assessment, (2) diagnosis, (3) identification of outcomes, (4) planning, (5) implementation, and (6) evaluations. The ANA standards of professional performance include the following: (1) quality of care, (2) performance appraisal, (3) education, (4) collegiality, (5) ethics, (6) collaboration, (7) research, and (8) resource utilization. The ANA (1995, 1996a, 1996b, 1998) has also published *Nursing Quality Indicators: Definitions and implications; Nursing Quality Indicators: Guide for implications; Nursing Care Report Care for Acute Care;* and *Standards of Clinical Nursing Practice* to help assess risk and improve quality of care.

The three voluntary accrediting agencies for community health nursing are the Community Health Accreditation Program (CHAP) of the National League for Nursing, the National Home Caring Council, and Joint Commission on Accreditation of Healthcare Organizations (now The Joint Commission [TJC]). CHAP is one of two organizations nationwide authorized to provide home care accreditation, and in 1998 it became the first accrediting organization in the nation to be deemed an authority for Medicare hospices (National League for Nursing, 1998). TJC accreditation is also voluntary for long-term care. Nursing homes are required to meet state and federal licensing standards. Federal and state surveys and regulatory activities have increased since the Omnibus Budget Recognition Act (OBRA) was passed in 1987 and implemented in 1990.

HISTORY OF CONTINUOUS QUALITY IMPROVEMENT

In the late 1950s, planning, organizing, and evaluating health care services became a public concern. In 1951 the Joint Commission on Accreditation of Hospitals (JCAH) was formed. The American Nurses Association (ANA) and the National League for Nursing (NLN) both published manuals in 1959 to establish standards for health care.

During the 1960s the ANA started a division of nursing practice to develop standards for nursing practice, which became the basis for quality assurance programs. The ANA also developed a process to evaluate the quality of patient care.

In October 1972, Congress passed Public Health Law 92-603, an amendment to the Social Security Act that mandated the establishment of PSROs to review the quality and cost of care received by clients of Medicare, Medicaid, and Maternal Child Health programs. Health care facilities were to develop quality control programs by 1976, or the government would do it for them. Consequently, quality assurance received considerable attention. The ANA developed guidelines for standards of nursing practice under the PSRO system; the American Hospital Association (AHA) and JCAH developed a retrospective review of care. Individuals and agencies developed criteria and processes for the measurement of quality of care.

The JCAH required audits of care, delivered in its initial quality assurance standards, and increased the number of multidisciplinary audits required in 1975. Nursing then became a major contributor for evaluation of documentation. During the 1990s, the Joint Commission on Accreditation of Healthcare Organizations (JCAHO; later TJC) examined a nursing care problem each quarter, documented an assessment of the problem, developed and implemented the plan for correction, and evaluated the effectiveness of the implemented actions.

Instruments for measuring nursing care were developed during the 1970s, but limited data were generated or published in quality assurance studies. The quality assurance (QA) program recommended by JCAH was a retrospective review of patient care through a closed-chart audit that focused on patient-care outcomes.

Cost containment became a major issue in the 1980s. The federal prospective payment system (PPS), which used a series of DRGs to determine a hospital's reimbursement for care provided to Medicare patients, was introduced. Outpatient services that were often not covered in the 1970s became the preferred alternatives to health care in the 1980s. Outpatient services, long-term care, and home care were less expensive ways to deliver some treatments. The power in health care shifted from the provider to the consumer, primarily third-party payers and insurers (Koch, Fairly, 1993).

Total quality management (TQM), the philosophy of which was "the right thing to do the first time, on time, all the time" was introduced in industry in the 1940s in Japan. Japan called upon quality experts from the United States to train Japanese personnel as they had started to focus on quality through total workforce training and participation in quality improvement efforts. Deming and Drucker led the charge to change industrial standards and quality control; Juran also worked with the Japanese in quality management. In the 1980s the United States also began to adopt these standards of quality. Later, the respective work of Deming, Drucker, Juran, Crosby, Donabedian, and Berwick became instrumental in the adoption of quality control standards in health care.

Deming (1982) was primarily responsible for training engineers in the United States to improve the production and quality of military goods during World War II. After World War II, Deming, with his 14-point management philosophy, revitalized Japanese industry with his focus on total quality management (TQM) and Continuous Quality Improvement (CQI). The Deming chain reaction is as follows: (1) improve quality, (2) decrease costs with fewer mistakes, less rework, fewer delays, and better use of time and materials, (3) improve productivity, (4) capture the market with better quality at lower prices, (5) stay in business, and (6) provide jobs (Walton, 1990) (Box 15-1).

BOX 15-1 Fourteen Points of the Deming Management Method

1. Create constancy of purpose for improvement of products and services. Deming suggests that the purpose is to stay in business and provide jobs through maintenance, research, innovation, and constant improvement.
2. Adopt the new philosophy. Mistakes and negativism should be unacceptable.
3. Cease dependence on mass inspection. Deming maintains that quality arises from improvement in the process rather than from inspection and that workers should participate in improvement in the process. When quality is addressed at the inspection phase, workers are paid to make the mistake and then paid to correct it, which is very expensive.
4. End the practice of awarding business on the price tag alone. Buyers should get the best quality in a long-term relationship with a single supplier for any specific item, rather than purchasing the lowest-priced and often poor-quality items from the cheapest vendor.
5. Constantly improve the system of production and service. Management must always look for ways to reduce waste and improve quality.
6. Institute training. Workers cannot be expected to do their jobs well if no one tells them how to do so.
7. Institute leadership. Deming believes that people who do not do well are just misplaced. It is the leader's responsibility to identify workers who need individual attention, find an appropriate place for them in the organization, and help them do a better job.
8. Drive out fear. Many workers are afraid to ask questions or point out problems for fear of being blamed for the problem. They may continue to do something wrong or not at all. For the best quality and productivity, people need to feel secure.
9. Break down barriers between staff areas. Often departments compete with each other or have goals that conflict. It is better to have teamwork to solve problems.
10. Eliminate slogans, exhortations, and targets for the workforce. It is better for workers to develop their own slogans.
11. Eliminate numerical quotas because they deal with numbers, not quality. They often contribute to inefficiency and high cost because workers meet quotas at any cost to keep their jobs.
12. Remove barriers to pride of workmanship. People are eager to do a good job. Barriers such as faulty equipment, defective materials, and misguided managers should be removed.
13. Institute a vigorous program of education and retraining. Both managers and staff need to be educated about new methods and teamwork.
14. Take action to accomplish the transformation. Managers and staff need a plan of action to carry out the quality mission. A critical mass of people must understand the 14 points about continuous quality improvement.

Modified from Walton M: *Deming management at work*, New York, 1990, Putnam's Sons.

Deming introduced the plan-do-check-act cycle (PDCA), which is frequently used in health care settings yet today. The planning phase involves identifying customers, their needs, areas not meeting those needs, and improvement proposals. Deming identified the following seven helpful charts: cause-and-effect chart, flow chart, Pareto chart, histogram, run (trend) chart, scatter diagram, and control chart. Other tools that can be used to display information graphically include checklists, pie charts, time charts, decision matrices, affinity charts, tree diagrams, relationship diagrams, force-field analysis, and bar graphs. Processes that can be used to envision and make decisions include benchmarking, observations, interviews, questionnaires, record audits, nominal group technique, brainstorming, quality circles, focus groups, action planning, and voting.

PDCA cycle methods include the following (Cofer & Greeley, 1998):

Plan

Plan the change.

Identify opportunities.

Develop vision statement.

Collect data to define problems and opportunities.

Use CQI tools to organize data and thinking.

Decide on improvement initiatives.

Do

Implement the planned change.

Implement initiatives.

Test with a trial run.

Identify costs, people, and materials.

Educate staff and management about changes in the process.

Check

Observe the effect of the change.

Monitor progress of initiatives.

Meet with staff to discuss changes.

Delegate staff to monitor results.

Compare new data with original data, using CQI tools.

Use CQI tools to monitor results.

Act

Adjust as necessary.

Incorporate changes into department policies.

Inform and educate all involved.

Distribute new policies to key individuals.

Look for new opportunities.

Juran and his trilogy of interrelated processes of quality planning, quality control, and quality improvement were also used to train the Japanese. By the end of World War II, Juran was a highly regarded teacher and industrial engineering theorist. The Union of Japanese Scientists and Engineers asked him to teach them and help them rebuild their economy (Juran, 1981, 1988, 1989, 1992; Juran, Goyna, & Bingham, 1988) (Box 15-2).

Crosby, known for his zero defects concept, has 14 steps that emphasize training all employees,

---

> **BOX 15-2** Juran's Quality Trilogy
>
> **QUALITY PLANNING**
> 1. Determine who the customers are.
> 2. Determine the needs of the customers.
> 3. Develop product features that respond to the customers' needs.
> 4. Develop the processes that produce those product features.
> 5. Transfer the resulting plans to the operating forces.
>
> **QUALITY CONTROL**
> 1. Evaluate actual quality performance.
> 2. Compare actual performance with quality goals.
> 3. Act on the difference.
>
> **QUALITY IMPROVEMENT**
> 1. Establish the infrastructure needed to secure annual quality improvement.
> 2. Identify the specific needs for improvement, which become the improvement projects.
> 3. Establish a project team with responsibilities for bringing the project to successful closure.
> 4. Provide the resources and training needed by teams to diagnose the problems, develop a remedy, and establish controls to maintain the gains.

Modified from Juran JM: *Juran on leadership for quality: An executive handbook*, New York, 1989, Free Press.

---

using teams, setting goals, and recognizing employees for their involvement. Crosby defines quality as conformance to requirements. He believes that the system for creating quality is prevention of errors instead of appraisal (Crosby, 1989, 1992a, 1992b, 1995) (Box 15-3).

Donabedian and Berwick applied quality management principles to health care. Donabedian (1986) is known for his structure, process, and outcome criteria for quality assessment while Berwick (1989) stressed the importance of improving process toward quality improvement.

Quality became the issue in the 1990s. The objective became to provide quality health care in the most appropriate health care setting at the most economical cost. Customers started wanting involvement in decision making and wanted information about quality and costs. Safe care became a predominate issue during the 2000s as a result of the Institute of

---

BOX 15-3 Crosby's 14 Steps to Quality Improvement

1. Commitment from management
2. Use of quality improvement teams composed of people with process knowledge and commitment to actions
3. Quality measurement to identify areas that need improvement and change
4. Measuring the cost of quality and nonquality
5. Quality awareness by all personnel
6. Corrective actions through opportunities for improvement
7. Zero defects planning—do it right the first time
8. Employee education for quality improvement
9. Zero defect day as demonstration of commitment to quality
10. Goal setting toward zero defects
11. Error-causal removal by removing barriers
12. Recognition for meeting goals
13. Quality councils to assist people in quality improvement
14. Do it all over again

Modified from Crosby PB: *Let's talk quality*, New York, 1989, McGraw-Hill; Crosby PB: *Quality is free: The art of making quality certain*, New York, 1992, McGraw-Hill; Crosby PB: *Quality without tears: The art of hassle-free management*, New York, 1995, McGraw-Hill.

Medicine reports. This brought intense competition among health care providers, and quality improvement became the key to survival and success.

Institute of Medicine Reports

The Clinton Administration instituted the Institute of Medicine Reports with the President's Advisory Commission on Consumer Protection and Quality in the Health Care Industry in the late 1990s. The quality problems identified included wide variation in health care services, underuse and overuse of services, and an unacceptable level of avoidable errors. For example, the study found that only 21% of eligible patients received beta blockers while the mortality rate among recipients was 43% less than for the nonrecipients. There was also an estimate that one in six hysterectomies was inappropriate, and some services were provided when the potential for harm outweighed possible benefits. It was clear that the practice of health care was not current with the science of health care. A national commitment to quality improvement from the President and Congress through every level of the health care industry was needed.

The report *To Error Is Human: Building a Safer Health System* was released in November 1999. It reported that, according to a couple of research studies, as many as 44,000 to 98,000 people may die in hospitals each year as a result of medical errors that could have been prevented. Medical errors have been defined as implementation of the wrong plan or failure of a planned action to be completed as intended. Medical errors can include such events as adverse drug events, burns, death, falls, improper transfusions, mistaken patient identity, pressure sores, suicides, surgical injuries, restraint-related injuries, and wrong-site surgery. The report concluded that errors are more likely caused by system processes and conditions that lead people to make mistakes or that fail to prevent errors rather than by human carelessness. The focus was to prevent mistakes by designing health systems to make it harder for people to make mistakes, easier to do things correctly and consequently to be safer at all levels. The report recommended a four-tiered approach: (1) establish a national focus to create leadership, research, tools, and protocols to enhance the knowledge base about safety; (2) identify and learn from errors by developing a nationwide public mandatory reporting system and by encouraging health care organizations and practitioners to develop and participate in voluntary reporting systems; (3) raise performance standards and expectations for improvements in safety through the actions of oversight organizations, professional groups, and group purchasers of health care; and (4) implement safety systems in health care organizations to ensure safe practices at the delivery level. This report deals with accreditation, payment, policy, and regulation in a national agenda for patient safety.

Crossing the Quality Chasm: A New Health System for the 21st Century was released March 2001. It indicated that with the rapid changes in medical science, technology, and complexity of health care, the delivery system had not been able to translate knowledge into practice and to apply new technology appropriately and safely. The health care system still catered to acute, episodic care even though aging has caused an increased incidence in chronic diseases like asthma, diabetes, and heart disease, and more than 40% of people with chronic diseases have more than one chronic condition. There are cumbersome processes that waste resources, have voids in coverage and loss of information, and lack interdisciplinary and coordinated team efforts.

Consequently, members of the Committee on Quality of Healthcare in America suggested a comprehensive strategy and action plan for the next decade. The members believed that health care facilities that aim to meet the core needs for health care to be safe, timely, effective, efficient, equitable and patient centered care (known as the STEEEP Principles) would be better at meeting client needs through visits, telephone, and the Internet.

Ten rules of redesign were identified as: (1) care is based on continuous healing relationships; (2) care is customized according to client needs and values; (3) the client is the source of control; (4) knowledge is shared and information flows; (5) decision making is evidence based; (6) safety is a system issue; (7) transparency is necessary; (8) needs are anticipated; (9) waste is continuously decreased; and (10) cooperation among clinicians is a priority.

The six challenges of redesign imperatives identified were: (1) reengineered care processes, (2) effective use of information technologies, (3) knowledge and skills management, (4) development of effective teams, and (5) coordination of care across patient conditions, services, and sites of care over time. This report increased interest in applying evidence to practice, using information technology, aligning payment policies with quality improvement, and better preparing the workforce by emphasizing the six aims for improvement, stressing evidence-based practice, increasing interdisciplinary training, modifying professional regulation and accreditation, and increasing accountability among professionals and professional organizations.

Envisioning the National Health Care Quality Report was also published in 2001 and provided a framework for types of measures to use, criteria for selecting measures, and recommendations for how to reach intended audiences (for the annual reports on the national trends in quality of health care delivery in the United States that the Agency for Healthcare Research and Quality [IHRQ] started producing in 2003).

Leadership by Example: Coordinating Government Roles in Improving Health Care Quality was released on October 30, 2002. It described the federal programs and the populations they serve including Medicare for the elderly, Medicaid for low income people, SCHIP for children, VHA for veterans, TRICARE for military members, and HIS for Native Americans. It recommended focusing on performance measurement of clinical quality and patient perceptions of care, developing and pilot-testing measures, and creating an information infrastructure for comparing performance and disseminating results, and it proposed a research agenda to support quality improvement.

Who Will Keep the Public Healthy? Educating Public Health Professionals for the 21st Century was published in 2003. It recognized that the quality of health care is largely dependent upon the quality and preparedness of the public health workforce, which is dependent upon the quality and relevance of education. *Health Professions Education: A Bridge to Quality*, published in 2003, indicated that core competencies for health professionals are patient-centered care, interdisciplinary teams, evidence-based care, quality improvements, and informatics.

Priority Areas for National Action: Transforming Health Care Quality (2003) identified 20 priority areas for improvement that occur in small and large communities with about the same frequency in managed care and fee-for service systems. Impact (the extent of issues such as disability, mortality, and economic costs), improvability (the extent of the gap between current practice and evidence-based best practice, and the likelihood that the gap can be closed), and inclusiveness (the broad range of individuals regarding age, gender, socioeconomic status, race, and spectrum of health care and range of settings) were the criteria used. The priorities include: care coordination, self-management, asthma, cancer screening, children with special health care needs, diabetes, end-of-life care especially from congestive heart failure and chronic obstructive pulmonary disease, frailty associated with old age, hypertension, immunization of both children and adults, major depression, medication management, nosocomial infections, pain control in advanced cancer, pregnancy and childbirth, mental illness, stroke, tobacco dependence, and obesity.

Patient Safety: Achieving a New Standard for Care (2004) identified the need for a commitment by all stakeholders to a culture of safety and an improved information system to prevent errors and to learn from them.

Keeping Patients Safe: Transforming the Work Environment of Nurses (2004) revealed problems such as loss of trust in hospital administration, reduced clinical nursing leadership, unsafe workforce deployment with understaffing, long work hours, and unsafe work and workspace design. It recommended adopting evidence-based management and leadership practices, maximization of the capability of the workforce, design of work and workspace to reduce error, and create and sustain a culture of safety through governing boards that focus on safety, leadership and evidence-based management structures and processes, effective nursing transformational

leadership, adequate staffing, organizational support for ongoing learning and decision support, mechanisms that promote interdisciplinary collaboration, work design that promotes safety, and organizational culture that continuously strengthens patient safety. Major recommendations had numerous subrecommendations.

QUALITY ASSURANCE, TOTAL QUALITY MANAGEMENT, AND CONTINUOUS IMPROVEMENT

Continuous quality improvement differs from quality assurance but is used interchangeably with total quality management (Table 15-2). Continuous quality improvement is a process conducted by a team. Customer needs are identified and a needed change that will have the most impact is chosen for study. Then a multidisciplinary team representing a cross-section of people who are involved with the problem area is selected. The team establishes criteria, identifies relevant information, collects and analyzes data, judges quality, takes corrective action, reevaluates, and does public reporting (Box 15-4).

Establish Criteria

The team can establish criteria by developing standards and setting benchmarks. Standards are written value statements that define a predetermined level of expected performance. They are typically

TABLE 15-2 Comparison of Quality Assurance and Quality Improvement

Quality Assurance	Quality Improvement
Detection oriented	Prevention oriented
Reactive	Proactive
Narrow focus	Cross-functional
Getting by	Raising standards
Tradition and safety	Experimentation and risk
Busyness	Productivity
Leadership not vested	Leadership leading
Leader as director	Leader as empowerer
Employee as expendable	Employee as customer
Responsibility of few	Responsibility of all
Problem solving by authority	Problem solving by all
We-they thinking	Organizational perspective
Cynicism	New optimism

> **BOX 15-4** Continuous Quality Improvement Process
>
> - Identify the customers, their expectations, and the outputs using brainstorming, focus groups, and interviews.
> - Describe the current process using flow charts and focus groups.
> - Measure and analyze the discrepancy between desired expectations and reality using check sheets, logs, time charts, trend charts, histograms, and surveys.
> - Focus on an improvement opportunity using decision matrices, Pareto charts, and voting.
> - Identify root causes of inefficiencies through brainstorming, affinity charts, cause-and-effect diagrams, tree diagrams, relationship diagrams, force-field analysis, and focus groups.
> - Generate and select solutions to the problem by brainstorming and using decision matrices and tree diagrams.
> - Map out a trial run through brainstorming, force-field analysis, action planning, tree diagrams, and flow charting.
> - Implement the trial run using check sheets, logs, and histograms.
> - Evaluate the results using check sheets, logs, surveys, focus groups, histograms, and trend charts.
> - Draw conclusions using Pareto diagrams, focus groups, and force-field analysis.
> - Standardize the change using force-field analysis, brainstorming, action planning, tree diagrams, and flow charting.
> - Monitor holding the gains through check sheets, trend charts, surveys, histograms, and control charts.

about structure, process, or outcomes. Structure standards are typically about the physical environment, the structure, or the management. One structure standard could be "All nurse managers will have a master's degree in nursing." Process standards are related to the delivery of care. An example of a process standard could be "Every patient will have a discharge plan before being discharged." Outcome standards are the results of the care or administration and, as a result of the Institute of Medicine reports, are receiving considerable attention now. An outcome standard could be "No more than 20% of patients with a specific diagnosis will be readmitted for that diagnosis within 2 months of discharge."

Accreditating body standards, professional organization standards, and laws can be sources of standards. An indicator is the tool used to measure the standard. A chart audit could be done to check if a discharge plan was available before discharge or if patients were readmitted with the same diagnosis within 2 months. Benchmarking is measuring what exists against the best practice. The indicator allows for comparison of data. Best practice is a structure, process, or outcome that has produced superior results.

Identify Relevant Information

The team should identify relevant information from major regulatory and accrediting bodies that control health care organizations. The Joint Commission (TJC) is an accrediting body for hospitals, long-term care facilities, home health operations, ambulatory care programs, and psychiatric facilities. The Joint Commission on Accreditation (JCOA) was established in 1948 and became the Joint Commission on Accreditation of Hospitals (JCAH) in 1951. It was renamed the Joint Commission on Accreditation of Healthcare Organizations (JCAHO) in 1987. In 2007, it was renamed again and became The Joint Commission (TJC). This voluntary, independent accrediting organization published the first hospital accreditation standards in 1953. In 1965 the Health Care Financing Administration (HCFA) gave JCAH standards that benchmark quality for meeting most of Medicare standards. In 1970 the JCAH changed its standards from review of minimum requirements to optimum level of care, and in 1975 it required every hospital to have a plan for quality assurance using explicit, measurable criteria that could be used in retrospective audits of care documented in medical records. In 1979 the standards were written that stressed a coordinated, organization-wide program for medical and nursing quality assurance. The structure and process standards stressed quality assurance activities that focused on problems whose solutions would have a big effect on patient care outcomes. It established a quality assessment standard in 1980 that has since been revised. In 1982, JCAH started requiring quarterly evaluations of standards for nursing care measured against written standards. In 1985, standards replaced the broad, problem-based approach with narrower systematic monitoring and evaluation of important aspects of patient care. The standards focused on specific departments, with each conducting its own systematic monitoring and evaluations that were conducted by concurrent audits of both patient care processes and medical records so that problems could be resolved while the patient was still hospitalized. In 1988 the quality assurance standards for nursing were revised to be evaluated objectively against preestablished standards and criteria. The results needed to be analyzed to determine problem areas and a plan developed to correct practice deficiencies. Reevaluation of the effectiveness of the corrective action was expected. In 1991, JCAHO published a 10-step process for the assessment, measurement, and improvement of quality of care: (1) assign responsibility, (2) delineate scope of care, (3) identify important aspects of care, (4) identify indicators, (5) establish thresholds for evaluation, (6) collect and organize data, (7) evaluate care, (8) take action to improve care, (9) assess actions and document improvement, and (10) communicate information.

In the late 1990s, JCAHO shifted its focus from structure to outcomes that required the development of clinical indicators to measure the quality of care. In 1997, JCAHO approved ORYX technology performance measurement system to integrate outcomes and other performance measures into the accreditation process. Organizations could volunteer for ORYX Plus to create a national standardized database of several performance measures.

By 2000 there were enormous changes in response to a rapidly evolving environment and health care arena. There was a focus on continuous monitoring of performance; use of active, collaborative multidisciplinary teams; more randomized data selection for review; reporting of aggregate data; use of computers to manage and analyze data; linkages among patient, organization, and structure functions; sentinel events; root causes; performance improvement and sustained performance leading to continuous quality improvement; surveying physician practices that are part of a system; and random, unannounced surveys.

JCAHO responded to the IOM reports. The National Patient Safety goals and requirements and a new infection control standard that requires organizations to offer influenza vaccinations to staff and licensed independent practitioners became effective January 1, 2007. Online reporting of sentinal events and complaint reporting became mandatory for all health care organizations on January 1, 2007. TJC requires accredited hospitals to collect and submit performance data on three of the following four measures: (1) acute myocardial infarction, (2) health failure, (3) pregnancy and related conditions, and (4) community-acquired pneumonia.

The safety movement began in ancient times with the Egyptians, Greeks, and Romans; in the Middle Ages, guidelines were established regarding working conditions. The safety movement became a major force in industry during the industrial revolution. In 1913 the National Council for Industrial Safety (later renamed the National Safety Council, then the Health Care Financing Administration [HCFA], and still later renamed the Center for Medicare and Medicaid Services) was founded. It developed a forum for developing national standards. Other groups also formed and started keeping statistics on accident and injury rates in industry.

Occupational diseases and safety issues were identified, and methods to control hazardous and toxic materials and to protect the people who handle them were developed. On-the-job safety issues received serious attention. Since World War II, the safety movement not only has reduced injuries and deaths but also has shown administrators that money spent on safety measures returns a profit of up to several hundred percent. Changes in the workforce, new technologies and their hazards, environmental hazards, blood-borne diseases, and drug and alcohol abuse are safety challenges.

Home health agencies, nursing facilities, and skilled nursing facility units certified to participate in the Centers for Medicare and Medicaid Services (CMS) are required by federal regulations to collect, encode, and transmit the Minimum Data Set (MDS) Outcome Assessment Information Set (OASIS) to the State Repository at the Oklahoma State Department of Health (CMS, 2007). The Quality Improvement and Evaluation Services Division is responsible for coordinating activities and database functions that fall under the umbrella of the national QualityNet system. The CMS and its Conditions of Participation (CoP), introduced the Medicare Quality Initiative (MQI) in 2001 to conduct regulation and enforcement activities, to make information about the quality of care in target settings available to consumers through a variety of media, to maintain ongoing data for various quality initiatives, and to collaborate and partner with all stakeholders. This fostered making quality reports readily available to consumers (Harris, 2003).

The National Committee for Quality Assurance (NCQA) is a private, nonprofit organization that accredits managed care organizations. It has developed the Health Plan Employer Data and Information Set (HEDIS) to compare managed care organization access, quality of care, patient satisfaction, service utilization, and financial stability. It assigns a mean score for indicators and provides an analysis for each managed care organization's progress in meeting the goals of the U.S. Public Health Service's Healthy People health promotion initiative rather than to compare the managed care organizations. It contains much numerical and descriptive information. The measures are expected to increase, and the Medicaid and Medicare segments of the population enrolled in managed care have additional, more specific performance indicators. The accreditation is voluntary and only about half of managed care organizations have been participating, but since 1999, Medicare and Medicaid have contracted their managed care plans only with NCQA-accredited managed care organizations.

The Multistate Nursing Home Case Mix and Quality Demonstration has developed quality indicators for long-term care settings. It attempts to develop and implement a case mix classification system to be the basis for Medicare and Medicaid payment as well as to serve as a quality monitoring system.

In the early 1990s, California mandated the development of report cards, and other states such as Ohio and Pennsylvania passed similar laws. Most states have laws requiring some form of reporting. Not all report cards use the same measures, and the report cards may not be readily accessible to the public or easy for the public to understand.

Collect Information

Nursing audits are a basic form of data collection. They may be structure, process, or outcome audits and may be retrospective or concurrent audits. Structure audits may be done with a check list that can note the presence or absence of policies, procedures, medical records, physical facilities, equipment, organizational structure, caregivers' knowledge and experience, adequate staffing, and the patient's ability to reach call lights, food, and water.

Process audits are related to care such as implementing the physician's orders, observation of symptoms, implementation of nursing procedures, teaching, discharge planning, and appropriate charting. Critical pathways and standardized clinical guidelines are examples of standardization of the process of care. Procedure manuals, nursing protocol statements, and nursing care plans can be used for process standards. Observational studies and work flow analysis can be used with process audits.

Outcome audits observe the result of the care or how the patient's health status changed as a result of the interventions. Outcome standards may be related to physical health status, mental health status, physical function, social function, health knowledge, health behaviors, utilization of services, and satisfaction with the service received. Until the 2000s most audits were focused on structure and process. Outcomes are now considered to be the most valid indicator of the quality of care. Consequently, interdisciplinary teams of physicians, nurses, pharmacists, dietitians, social workers, and finance experts develop evidence-based practice models. Care is redesigned based on the analysis of the outcomes. Then new processes are designed, implemented, and reevaluated. Many standards and measures have already been tested for reliability and validity, pilot tested, and are available in the literature. Measures from the literature can be adopted or adapted for various services.

Retrospective audits are done after the patient is discharged. That is usually done by examining the medical records of many discharged patients. Comparisons are made across cases. Recommendations are made based on the experiences of many patients with similar care problems. Concurrent audits are conducted while the patient is receiving care. Consequently, care can be modified if the observations indicate the need to make changes.

Peer reviews are done when practicing nurses determine the standards and criteria they believe indicate quality of care and assess the performance of nurses against those standards. Utilization reviews have been mandated by The Joint Commission are not specific to nursing care but can provide information about nursing practices that need further investigation (Huber, 2006; Marquis & Huston, 2006; Roussel, Swansburg, & Swansburg, 2006; Sullivan & Decker, 2005).

Analyze Information

A *bar graph* is a series of bars representing successive changes in the value of a variable or different data sets. A simple bar graph can measure one set of data that does not need to be subcategorized (Figure 15-1). The cluster bar graph can divide simple bar graph totals into subtotals (Figure 15-2). The histogram and Pareto chart are bar graphs (Cofer & Greeley, 1998).

Benchmarking is a process of identifying best practices and comparing them with the agency's practices to improve performance. It is learning and borrowing from others. The process is as follows: (1) identify the benchmark team, (2) identify what to benchmark, (3) gather information through search of the literature, (4) survey benchmark partners through written or telephone surveys or site visits, (5) compare benchmark data with organization's current practices and outcomes, (6) borrow ideas from the best and adapt them to important processes within the organization, and (7) monitor the results (Roussel, Swansburg, & Swansburg, 2006).

Brainstorming is the process of creating a free flow of ideas without fear of criticism and then thinking about the good in the wild ideas that were generated (Cofer & Greeley, 1998) (see Chapter 3).

A *cause-and-effect diagram*, or *fishbone diagram*, is used to identify the root causes of a problem or outcome. One can first identify a problem and then use brainstorming to identify root causes. First, identify causal categories, such as facilities or equipment, materials or supplies, methods, and people, and items within those categories that cause the problem. One would then ask "why" four or five times. Identify first-, second-, and third-level causes until the causes become narrow enough to address. This can be outlined to look like a fish skeleton or can be done as hierarchical outlining on the computer (Folse, 2007; Pelletier & Albright, 2006; Roussel, Swansburg, & Swansburg, 2006) (Figure 15-3).

Check sheets are grids that can be used to collect and classify raw data. They are good tools for

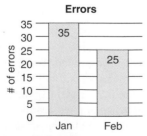

Figure 15-1 • Simple bar graph.

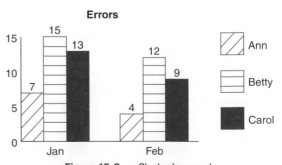

Figure 15-2 • Cluster bar graph.

monitoring key performance indicators. The raw data can be used to generate histograms, Pareto charts, run charts, and other tools that display information graphically (Roussel, Swansburg, & Swansburg, 2006) (Table 15-3).

A *decision matrix* is a grid that helps prioritize options. First, there is brainstorming to identify options. Those options are then evaluated, and unfeasible options are eliminated, leaving viable alternatives. The viable options are then listed down the left side of the grid. Criteria for evaluating each option are identified at the top of columns. How well the item meets the criterion can be rated as follows: 1=poorly, 2=adequately, and 3=well. The criterion can be weighted as follows: 1=unimportant, 2=important, and 3=very important. Then a weighted score can be calculated by multiplying the score by the criterion weight. The score can be recorded to the left of the diagonal dividing the score box, with the weighted score to the right of the diagonal (Cofer & Greely, 1998) (Table 15-4).

A *histogram* is a bar graph that can be used to compare patterns of occurrence over time. It displays the frequency with which comparable events occur and illustrates the variations in the occurrences. It can be used to identify trends and analyze variations. The measurement should occur at least 25 times during the period studied to get useful data. Raw data are gathered possibly using a checklist to plot the histogram. The range of the data is calculated by subtracting the smallest from the largest data point. The square root of the total number of data points collected will determine how many bars to use in the histogram. Divide the overall range by the number of bars to determine the interval for each bar. Use the check sheet to group the raw data by intervals. The number of data points per interval determines the height of the bar for that interval. A histogram that peaks in the middle with a narrow base indicates little performance variance. A histogram that peaks in the middle with a wide base indicates much performance variance. Histograms that peak to the right or left are skewed histograms and probably indicate that something unexpected happened during the process. Histograms with two peaks are bimodal and probably contain incompatible data sets that should be separated. Histograms visualize the data's distribution, symmetry, and any extreme data values. One should recalculate abnormal histograms before considering defective processes (Cofer & Greely, 1998; Folse, 2007; Pelletier & Albright,

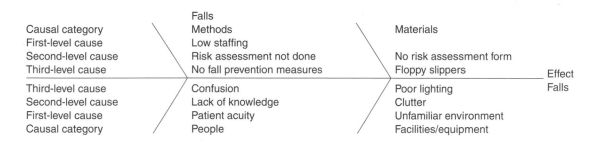

Figure 15-3 • Cause-and-effect diagram, or fishbone diagram.

TABLE 15-3 Check Sheet

Staff/Day	Sunday	Monday	Tuesday	Wednesday	Thursday	Friday	Saturday	Weekly Total/ Person
Ann		///	//	/	/		/	8
Betty	/	//	//	//	//			9
Carol		//	///	///	////	///		15
Daily total	1	7	7	6	7	3	1	32

2006; McLaughlin, Kaluzny, 2004; Roussel, Swansburg, & Swansburg, 2006) (Figure 15-4).

A *process flow chart* helps analyze how a task is being performed (Figure 15-5). Process flow chart symbols include ○ for operation, → for transportation, □ for inspection, D for delay, and △ for storage. An operation is the actual performance of the work, such as giving an injection. Transportation represents physical movement—the relocation of a person or thing from one place to another, such as movement of the syringe from the medication room to the patient's bedside. Inspection is to determine whether the necessary work has been properly performed. Nurses make sure that they are giving the right medication to the right patient and using the right mode at the right time. A delay is an unplanned interruption in the flow of the process. Storage is an anticipated interruption in the process or at the end of it. When making a flow process chart, one must decide whether to follow the flow of material or

the activities of the worker because they may not be the same. As a result of process improvement, one should eliminate activities or combine steps when possible and change the sequence of activities as necessary to improve the performance of various steps. The newly proposed method or process is then analyzed using a flow chart. The potential impact on people is considered. Trial runs are conducted, and debugging is done (Pelletier & Albright, 2006; Cofer & Greeley, 1998; Roussel, Swansburg, & Swansburg, 2006).

A *Gantt chart* is a grid with a timeframe across the top that could be in minutes, hours, days, weeks, months, years, or decades, depending on the time frame of the process. Tasks to be accomplished are listed down the left side of the grid. An X is put in the cell when a certain task is to be done. A line is drawn through cells when the task takes a period of time. This tool is used for managing production activities to complete a project (Roussel, Swansburg, & Swansburg, 2006) (see Chapter 3).

TABLE 15-4 Decision Matrix

	Criteria						
	Ease of Implementation 2	Cost 3	Timeliness 2	Value Added 3	Quality Impact 3	Weighted Score	Rank
Surveys	3/6	3/9	3/6	2/6	3/9	36	1
Interviews	1/2	1/3	1/2	3/9	1/6	22	2
Observations	1/2	1/3	1/2	2/6	2/6	19	3

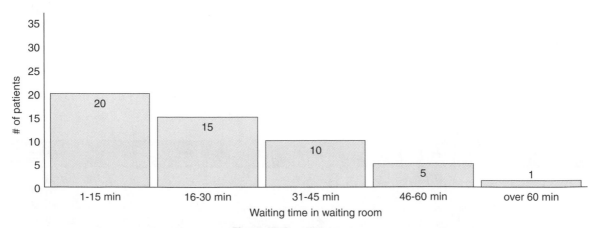

Figure 15-4 • Histogram.

Procedure: Injection		Distance traveled			Present ☐ Proposed ☐	

Person ☐

Material ☐

	Present		Proposed		Savings	
	No	Hr	No	Hr	No	Hr
Operation	8					
Transportation	2					
Inspection	2					
Delay	0					
Storage	1					

Steps in procedure	◯ → ▪ D ▲	Distance (ft)	Time (hr)	Remarks
Read medication order	◯ → ▪ D ▲			
Collect vial and syringe	◯ → ▪ D ▲			
Open vial	◯ → ▪ D ▲			
Open disposable syringe	◯ → ▪ D ▲			
Draw up solution	◯ → ▪ D ▲			
Recheck medication order	◯ → ▪ D ▲			
Put vial in medication drawer	◯ → ▪ D ▲			
Take shot to patient	◯ → ▪ D ▲			
Check patient identification	◯ → ▪ D ▲			
Administer shot	◯ → ▪ D ▲			
Return to medicine room	◯ → ▪ D ▲			
Dispose of syringe	◯ → ▪ D ▲			
Chart medication	◯ → ▪ D ▲			
Store chart	◯ → ▪ D ▲			

Key:
◯ Operation
→ Transportation
▪ Inspection
D Delay
▲ Storage

Figure 15-5 • Flow process chart.

Nominal group technique is a process for developing team goals and priorities. Individuals list ideas that are silently generated. Each participant may give one idea at a time during a round-robin session. The ideas are written onto a chalkboard or paper and are expressed around and around the circle until all ideas have been expressed. Then there is a discussion for clarification before the preliminary vote. Participants may rank the first five to seven items, with the highest number being the highest weighting. Then the votes are weighted by multiplying the number of votes with the priority for each item. If one item received 10 votes for a priority of five, the weighted score would be 50. If more than nine items surface as priorities, there can be further discussion and a second vote weighting the top items. Once items have been identified, brainstorming can be used to address the issues (Cofer & Greeley, 1998; Roussel, Swansburg, & Swansburg, 2006) (see Chapter 3).

A *Pareto chart* is a bar graph that displays categories of data in descending order of frequency or significance from the left to the right. It is named after Pareto, an economist who noticed that 80% of the wealth in Italy in the nineteenth century was controlled by 20% of the population. The Pareto principle states that most effects come from a few causes (Figure 15-6). Once the major cause of a problem is identified, it can be solved, leading to considerable impact (Folse, 2007; Pelletier & Albright, 2006; Cofer & Greeley, 1998; McLaughlin & Kaluzny, 2004; Roussel, Swansburg, & Swansburg, 2006).

Pie charts compare the relative size of different data sets in a circle instead of as bars on graphs. Data are collected and assigned percentages of the whole (Figure 15-7). A circle is drawn and divided into proportional pieces equal to the percentage of each indicator subtotal. Different segments can be shaded differently (Cofer & Greeley, 1998).

Program evaluation and review technique (PERT) is a system model for planning that identifies key activities in a project and sequences those activities in a flow diagram with the duration of each phase of the program assigned (Roussel, Swansburg, & Swansburg, 2006) (see Chapter 3).

Radar charts are circular displays of before-and-after data to demonstrate progress made or lost. Decide what indicators to measure. Draw a circle and divide it into equal segments numbering the number of indicators. Establish the rating scale. Rate each indicator using the rating scale, and post the finding on the segment line for that indicator. Draw a line connecting the posted ratings. Repeat the process later, use a different type line to connect the second posted ratings, and compare the old and new ratings (Cofer & Greeley, 1998) (Figure 15-8).

A *run chart* is a line graph that displays the variations in data over time. It allows a quick assessment of patterns and trends. It is good for monitoring time-related trends and shifts in processes (Cofer & Greeley, 1998; McLaughlin & Kaluzny, 2004) (Figure 15-9).

Scatter diagrams help determine relationships between two variables. They reflect correlations

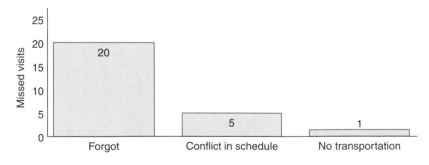

Figure 15-6 • Pareto chart.

but do not explain causation. Identify two variables to compare. Collect the data, and note the highest and lowest values for each variable. Draw axes for each variable ranging from the lowest to the highest value for each variable. Plot each data point where the two measurements intersect, and analyze the pattern. If the points are clustered together from the lower left to the upper right, there is a positive correlation. If the points are clustered together from the upper left to the lower right, there is a negative correlation. If the points are scattered randomly, there is no correlation between the variables (Cofer & Greeley, 1998; Pelletier & Albright, 2006) (Figure 15-10).

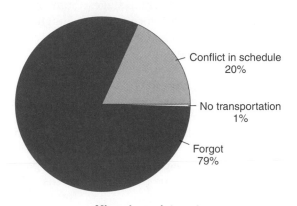

Missed appointments

Figure 15-7 • Pie chart.

Judge Quality, Take Corrective Action, and Monitor

The implemented plan needs to be evaluated to determine if the outcome standard was met. If not, revisions may be needed. Unanticipated problems could have been created. Solving one problem can create new problems. The interdisciplinary team may need to meet periodically to reassess the outcomes and make adjustments as necessary (Folse, 2007). Problems can be identified from the analysis and reporting of the evaluation data. Then problems can be prioritized according to the severity of the problem, its frequency, cost effectiveness, professional liability, and effect on accreditation. Corrective actions can be delegated to appropriate services. Then the process needs to continue to be monitored to continue to set standards of care, measure care according to the standards, evaluate care from many sources, recommend continuing improvement, and implement the improvements (Roussel, Swansburg, & Swansburg, 2006).

Public Reporting

Not only should the interdisciplinary team discuss the results, but stakeholders should be informed of the evaluation results. Results can be disseminated through mass media, computer announcements, department meetings, and discussion groups. Sharing information by such means as The Joint Commission's ORYX process

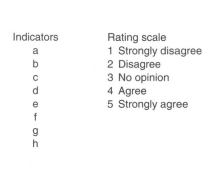

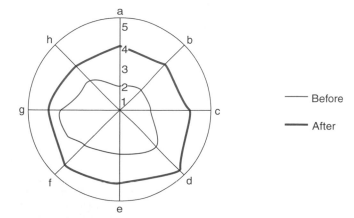

Figure 15-8 • Radar chart.

and the CMS system increases the power of findings. Multiinstitutional studies help make it possible to generalize findings.

Quality improvement is a management tool to improve systems and outcomes of a specific health care facility population rather than to generate generalizable knowledge, while research is intended to contribute to generalizable knowledge for populations and administrators beyond the setting of the research. Research requires more rigorous circumstances than quality improvement or some evidence-based practice. Research requires an Institutional Review Board (IRB) for the protection of human subjects. Development of a research program in a health care facility needs a strategic plan to put the infrastructure in place; a commitment from the facility administration; informed leaders; mentorship of staff; a nursing approval process as well as the protection of human subjects; statistical consultation for analysis of data; space to store research data in a confidential area; and time for staff to conduct studies (Newhouse, 2006). See Chapter 8 for a discussion of evidence-based practice.

PROGRAM EVALUATION

Program evaluation is an essential part of effective administration. It is the evaluation of a set of activities designed to determine the value of the program or of the program elements. Evaluative research is the use of scientific research methods to make an evaluation. Program evaluation may be formative or summative. Formative evaluations provide information about the program during the developmental stages. Summative evaluations provide information for judging a developed program. Evaluation may be descriptive or comparative.

Programs are evaluated for any number of reasons. Federal, state, or local agencies may require program evaluation. Program evaluation can be used to improve programs systematically or to determine the state of the programs. It can be used to evaluate the effect of new technologies on programs and help determine if parts responsible for success in one program can be used in other parts of the system.

Once the program to be evaluated and the purpose for its evaluation have been decided, someone should be made accountable for the evaluation. Credibility is the major argument in favor of an external evaluator. A person who is part of the program may have difficulty in being objective about the program's strengths and

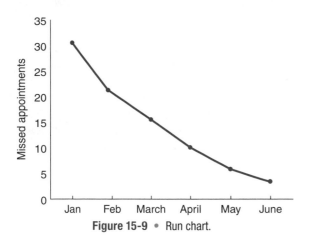

Figure 15-9 • Run chart.

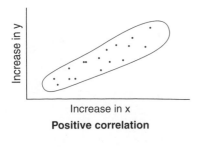

Positive correlation

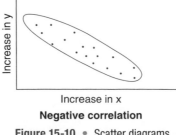

Negative correlation

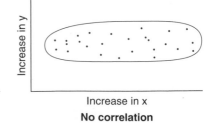

No correlation

Figure 15-10 • Scatter diagrams.

weaknesses because of pride, loyalty, or job security. On the other hand, an internal evaluator may be as objective as an external one and has knowledge about the program, its history, and circumstances; such knowledge facilitates the evaluation (McDavid & Hawthorn, 2006).

Calendar of Events

One of the first things the evaluator should do is develop a calendar of events that depicts the tasks to be done, the schedule, and organization of the project. A calendar of events for program evaluation itemizes activities to be done down the left margin and projected dates across the top. The projected date for each activity is estimated. This is a valuable tool for planning and judging the progress of the program evaluation (Table 15-5).

Committee Selection and Functions

Each agency needs multidisciplinary committees to establish criteria and a process for continuous quality improvement and to evaluate care, make recommendations, and do follow-up work. A chairperson with enthusiasm and attention to detail helps ensure a successful program. Members also need to be interested in quality assurance and knowledgeable about channels of communication, hospital resources, patient population, and nursing needs. Representation of nurses, physicians, pharmacists, therapists, nutritionists, and housekeepers from various units helps produce a wide variety of ideas. Preset meeting times allow for staffing to accommodate attendance, and large committee membership supplies personnel to do the work.

Conceptual Framework

Structure, process, and outcome, or any combination of these, is the common approach to evaluation. The structure approach focuses on the delivery system by which nursing care is implemented. Committee members evaluate policies, procedures, job descriptions, orientation schedules, in-service schedules, and charting. The process approach measures what the health professional does while delivering patient care. Both nurse and patient may be interviewed to collect evidence of professional judgment and functions. The outcome approach measures the results of the care administered to the patient and evaluates whether the goals were reached by considering clinical manifestations, patient knowledge, and the client's self-care. Outcomes became the focus of accreditation standards during the 1990s.

Audits may be concurrent or retrospective. Concurrent audits evaluate care as it is being administered and may include observation of staff; inspection of patient; open-chart auditing; staff and patient interviews; and group conferences including participation from the client, family, and staff. Retrospective audits judge care

TABLE 15-5 Calendar of Events

	Jan-Feb	March-April	May-June	July-Aug	Sept-Oct	Nov-Dec
Inform personnel of purpose of the evaluation and who is responsible	×					
Define goals	×					
Determine criteria	×					
Develop instrument		×				
Train data collectors		×				
Pilot test			×			
Collect data			×			
Analyze data				×		
Report findings				×		
Correct deficiencies					×	
Reassess (follow up)						×

after it has been delivered through the study of patient charts or care plans after the patient has been discharged, postcare questionnaires, patient interviews, or all of these.

Review of the Literature

A review of the literature locates instruments, criteria, and standards that have been developed and allows committee members to benefit from others' accomplishments and mistakes.

Program Evaluation Model

The formulation of program goals is essential for program evaluation. The goals should be clear, specific, and measurable. The evaluator will need to develop indicators to measure the extent to which the goals are achieved. These program-outcome indicators are the dependent variables of the study. The standards set by accrediting agencies such as the American Nurses Association (ANA), the National League for Nursing (NLN), and TJC can be used to determine goals and criteria (American Nurses Association, 1996a, 1996b).

Methods of data collection should be decided next. There are numerous sources for the collection of data, including questionnaires, interviews, observations, ratings, government statistics, instructional records, policy and procedure manuals, financial records, documents such as minutes of meetings or transcripts of trials, and tests.

Instrument Development

An operational definition of quality of care gives direction to instrument development. Instruments may be general and appropriate for all patients or structures, or applicable only to a specific process or to a homogeneous group in which differences in scores are due to variations in the concept being evaluated, rather than to other factors. Medical diagnosis, symptoms, acuity, age, and health care settings often are used to determine homogeneity. A taxonomy of nursing diagnoses is evolving. Identification of homogeneous patient groups for the development and application of instruments necessitates the development of numerous tools.

Once the patient group or specific process has been identified, selection of goals, criteria, and items is the priority. The goal is a statement of the end that one strives to attain. Criteria are the standards or scales against which judgments are made. Criteria describe what is implied in the goal in concise, measurable statements of desired structure, process, or outcome. They are written for a specific condition and are understandable, clinically sound, and achievable.

Brainstorming is a common approach for identifying items. Actual problems (those that patients generally experience) and potential problems (those with a high risk of occurring) are identified, and the structure, process, or outcome to resolve or prevent them is determined. The generation of as many ideas as possible without immediate evaluation is recommended initially. Later, items can be eliminated, checked for comprehensiveness, put into a uniform format, precisely defined, and quantified. A pilot study to collect data with the instrument can clarify which items should be retained, discarded, or rewritten.

Scales and measurements must be developed. A checklist to determine whether a characteristic is present; ratings to give each item a measure of worth such as good, average, or poor; and ranking by comparison, such as more or less than the standard, are common measurements. Scales are nominal, ordinal, interval, or ratio. The simplest type is the nominal. Its categories are collectively exhaustive, and each is mutually exclusive, meaning that there is a category for all the observations and that each observation can fit only one category. Gender, marital status, and the presence or absence of a condition are examples of nominal data. Ordinal scales classify observations into a specific order of more or less, such as good, average, or poor. Interval scales are ordered with equal measurement between each class, but the unit of measurement is determined arbitrarily. Examples of interval scales are the thermometer and sphygmomanometer. Ratio scales contain the properties of the other scales plus an absolute-zero point. Multiplication and division are possible because each number has a relationship to any other number. Currency systems are examples of ratio scales.

Sources of Internal and External Invalidity

Establishment of validity and reliability is important. Validity is the measurement of what is supposed to be measured and is difficult to establish. Face validity is an analysis of the instrument's appearance as valid. Someone simply looks at an instrument and decides if it has face validity. It is the easiest assessment of validity but is a questionable criterion because of its high degree of subjectivity. Content validity is a judgment that the content of the instrument is appropriate and closely related to what is to be measured. It is best determined by a jury of experts.

The construct is a hypothetical definition that clearly defines observable phenomena. Construct validity is particularly important when phenomena or concepts that are not directly observable, such as intellectual skills, human characteristics, and personal adjustment, are involved. Construct validity is theory oriented. An instrument contains predictive validity to the extent that it predicts future behavior. It can be determined by checking the prediction after a period of time. Concurrent validity reveals the behavior that is being demonstrated presently and is particularly important for concurrent audits.

When designing research, the evaluator gives careful consideration to sources of internal and external invalidity. Extraneous variables can confound the effects of the experimental variable and are therefore sources of *internal invalidity*. Factors that reduce the generalizability are sources of *external invalidity*.

There are several sources of *internal invalidity*. *History* is a problem when an event extraneous to the purpose of the study occurs between the pretest and posttest and confounds the effect of the experimental variable. It is a hidden treatment or a change-producing event that occurred in addition to the treatment. With a longer elapsed time between pretests and posttests, the explanation of the change being due to the problem of history becomes more plausible as there is more time for hidden treatments to occur. The internal invalidity caused by history can be controlled with experimental isolation, which can almost never be used when human subjects are involved. For example, a group-training technique to reduce racial prejudice against African Americans has been developed. A group of prejudiced individuals is convened, pretested, trained, and posttested. If an African American political leader is assassinated during that time, one would suspect that history confounded the experimental effect. The reduced prejudice could be attributed to sympathy for the assassinated African American politician rather than to the therapy.

Maturation is another internal invalidity problem. It is a systematic change over time in a person's biological or psychological condition, including growing older or becoming tired or hungry. Prescribed planned activities to promote walking for 12- to 15-month-olds or bladder control for 2- to 3-year-olds would be questionable because children normally learn those skills during those times.

Testing is a practice effect or the effect on the scores of taking a pretest. The practice effect is larger for the same test than for an alternative form of the test. The practice effect is a form of test-wiseness that lasts about 3 months. People taking an achievement, intelligence, or personality test for a second time within a 3-month period will usually do better than people taking it for the first time, although it is unlikely that they have become brighter or better adjusted.

Instrumentation becomes a problem when there are changes in the measuring instrument over time. Changes in tests, judges, measuring devices, or calibrations cause instrumentation problems. Results from one test cannot usually be compared with results of a different test. Instrument decay or the fatiguing of spring scales causes invalidity problems. Observations produce instrumentation problems. There are intrahuman differences of the observer through fatiguing, the process of learning, the process of increased skill with practice, and learning to establish rapport. There are differences in observations by the same person at different times. One may be more lenient at one time than at another. One becomes more skillful with experience. There are also interhuman differences, such as knowledge and skill. Researchers observing disruptive behavior in psychiatric patients before and after a treatment may become more aware of disruptive behavior by the second observation and record more behaviors, or they may record fewer minor disruptions the second time because of the high level of disruptive behavior they had observed. In either case, the treatment effect is difficult to determine.

Statistical regression becomes a problem when groups have been selected because of their extreme scores. The phenomenon of regression toward the mean is the inevitable tendency of persons whose scores are extreme (far above or below the norm) on the first test to be less extreme on the second test. Patients chosen for a therapy group because of their high anxiety would usually show less anxiety on a second test regardless of the treatment.

Selection is a problem when the experimental group differs from the control group. For example, a selection problem may exist when one is trying to compare a control unit with an experimental unit because patients were assigned as a function of systematic characteristics, such as presenting symptoms or histories. Randomization is a control for selection. This problem often occurs when the subjects are already formed into groups for reasons other than the study.

Experimental mortality is a differential loss of subjects from comparison groups. It includes lost cases, cases for which only partial data are available, and cases who refuse to participate. For example, people who smoke or drink heavily are more likely to be the first to drop out of therapy groups to reduce smoking and drinking, leaving the remaining clients to appear successful with the therapy.

Researchers must also be aware of *external invalidity* problems that complicate the generalizability of the findings. Subjects who are available to the experimenter may not represent the population, and consequently the results of the research are not generalizable. Random *sampling*

solves this problem. The independent variable needs to be operationally defined so that replication of the research is possible. Multiple-treatment interference, Hawthorne effect, novelty effect, and experimenter effect are considered. When two or more treatments are given consecutively to the same subjects, it is difficult, if not impossible, to know the cause of the results, and *multiple-treatment interference* occurs.

The person who knows he or she is a subject may change behavior, not because of the treatment, but because the person knows he or she is being observed. This is the *Hawthorne effect*. The subject may react either positively or negatively because of the newness of the treatment, thus producing the *novelty effect*. The *experimenter effect* occurs when the subject is influenced by the experimenter. Such subtle behavior as smiling and nodding one's head during an interview may unintentionally influence the subject.

Pretest sensitization is the same as an internal validity problem. However, an external validity problem may exist. It relates to generalizability of the results. Identification of the dependent variables and selection of instruments to measure those variables are necessary for external validity. One must also consider if the effect will last, or if one is likely to get different results at different times. For example, in the situation where an African American political leader is assassinated, thereby reducing prejudice against African Americans among those in group therapy, we may have a history internal validity problem. Now we have an *interaction-of-treatment-with-time* external validity problem. The racial prejudice may have been temporarily reduced as a result of the assassination but will probably not be maintained for long. Treatments to reduce smoking may appear most successful right after a cancer scare but not as successful later. One must have internal validity to obtain external validity, which is the ability to generalize the research results. With program evaluation there may be little intent to generalize the results.

Reliability is repeatability and is easier to determine than validity. Scores obtained by different raters' observations of the same event at the same time or by the same rater at different times can be compared. The *test-retest method* involves administration of the same test again after a period of time with the hope that the results will be consistent. The fact that people may remember items from the first administration or that people change over time is a problem. This method is appropriate for stable characteristics but is problematic for unstable traits. The *split-half method* compares halves of the test to determine internal consistency. Reliability is suggested when the results of both halves are similar. To use the split-half method, both halves need to contain enough items to be reliable. *Statistical methods* to check reliability include the Kuder-Richardson test for internal consistency and the Spearman-Brown formula for a coefficient for the total test (Campbell & Stanley, 2005).

Research Designs

Next, the evaluator should design the evaluation. Will the evaluation be one shot only or a continuous process? Will a program be assessed, or will programs be compared? Will an experimental or a quasiexperimental design be used? The pretest-posttest control group, posttest-only control group, Solomon four group design, and factorial design are experimental designs.

Experimental Designs

In the *pretest-posttest control group*, experimental subjects are randomly divided into two comparison groups as follows:

    R O X O
    R O   O

where:

> R = Randomly assigned individuals
> O = Observation
> X = Experimental treatment

The control and experimental groups are randomly assigned. The two groups are considered equivalent during initial observation. During final observation, the difference between groups should be the result of a variable being applied to one group but not to the other. The pretest-posttest control group true experimental design controls for history, maturation, testing, instrumentation, regression, selection, and mortality. One should consider the Hawthorne and novelty effects because the interaction of the testing and the experiment is not controlled.

In the *posttest-only control group*, experimental subjects are randomly divided into two groups to be compared as follows:

    R X O
    R   O

RESEARCH Perspective 15-1

Data from Burke TA, McKee JR, Wilson HC, et al: A comparison of time-and-motion and self-reporting methods of work measurement, *JONA* 30(3):118-125, 2000.

Purpose: The purpose of this study was to compare the results from a time-and-motion study with those using self-reporting.

Methods: A single observer observed eight nurses during five shifts or 40 hours per nurse. After completion of the time-and-motion study, participants were to self-report their work activities during their ensuing five shifts.

Results/conclusions: For analysis, 290 hours of time-and-motion study observations and 338 hours of self-reporting data were available. Comparable amounts of total time were reported within the various activity categories using time-and-motion and self-reporting methods. A significantly higher number of activities were reported using time-and-motion. Mean activity times were significantly longer using the self-reporting method compared with time-and-motion. The researchers concluded that nurse executives should consider continuous self-reporting as a low-cost means of quantifying allocation of time among nursing personnel. Self-reporting is not recommended for estimating the total number of activities or the mean time per activity because of perceptual differences between participants of what constitutes an activity.

The control and experimental groups are randomly assigned. A pretest is not administered. A treatment is applied to one group only. Because of the random selection, it is assumed that the groups are equivalent before the treatment is administered to one group and that the difference noted on the posttest is due to the treatment. This design controls for history, maturation, testing, instrumentation, regression, selection, mortality, and the interaction of the testing and the experiment. It is superior to the pretest-posttest control design unless there is a question about the randomness. This design is appropriate when a pretest is awkward and is convenient for maintaining anonymity.

The *Solomon four group design* is a better design but may not be worth more than double the effort. The Solomon four group design uses four randomly selected groups. It combines the pretest-posttest control group and the posttest-only control group designs as follows:

```
R O X O
R O   O
R   X O
R     O
```

It is considered the most desirable of the experimental designs because it allows the investigator to examine the effects of the treatment in four independent comparisons. The Solomon four group design controls for history, maturation, testing, instrumentation, regression, selection, mortality, and the interaction of testing and the experiment. However, it may not be worth the effort.

Factoral design allows for observation of some subjects at all levels of all experimental variables and can be used when the situation is under the complete control of the experimenter, which is rarely the situation.

Quasiexperimental Designs

The evaluator usually cannot control the time and subjects to whom experimental variables are applied. However, the evaluator may be able to select the time and persons on whom observations will be made and can consequently gain some control through the use of quasiexperimental designs.

A *time series* involves a series of measurements over a period of time with an experimental variable introduced at some point in the sequence as follows:

```
O O O O X O O O O
```

Maturation is controlled because it is not likely to cause the difference among each of the observations. Testing, regression, and selection are controlled. History is the most probable problem, and the longer the time over which the observations are made, the more probable the problem. Instrumentation is also a potential problem. It is important not to change the instruments or their calibration. It is best if this design is repeated by several researchers in separate situations.

When the *equivalent-time-samples design* is used, the time available for making the observations is divided into equal time periods as follows:

```
XO XO XO XO XO
```

The times to make observations are randomly selected. This design controls for history, maturation, testing, instrumentation, regression, selection, and mortality. The multiple-treatment effect is a problem, and generalization of the findings is limited to similar populations.

In the *nonequivalent control group*, the broken line (- - - -) means the groups are not equivalent samples:

```
O X O
- - - - -
O   O
```

For this design a control and an experimental group are both given a pretest and posttest. However, the groups are not randomly selected and do not have sampling equivalence. It is better than a one-group pretest-posttest design because it controls for history, maturation, testing, and instrumentation. Regression, mortality, and interaction between selection and maturation need to be considered as potential problems.

The *counterbalanced designs* are sometimes called Latin squares, switchover designs, crossover designs, and rotation experiments. The following is an example:

$X_1O\ X_2O\ X_3O\ X_4O$
$X_2O\ X_4O\ X_1O\ X_3O$
$X_3O\ X_1O\ X_4O\ X_2O$
$X_4O\ X_3O\ X_2O\ X_1O$

Four experimental treatments are applied in a random manner in turn to four individuals or groups. Counterbalanced designs control for history, maturation, testing, instrumentation, regression, selection, and mortality. Multiple-treatment interference is a problem. Strength can be obtained through replication.

For *separate-sample pretest-posttest design*, a pretest is given on one group and a posttest on another as follows:

R O (X)
R   X O

This simulated before-and-after design is weak, but it is better than a single-group pretest-posttest design because it controls for testing, regression, and selection. History, maturation, and mortality are not controlled, and the instrumentation needs to be questioned.

For the *separate-sample pretest-posttest control group*, two groups are pretested, one receives the experiment, and the two are posttested. This excellent design controls for history, maturation, testing, instrumentation, regression, selection, and mortality. Because it is an expensive design, it has probably never been used.

R O (X)
R   X O
R O
R O

For the *multiple time-series design*, a series of measurements is taken over a period of time on two separate groups with an experimental variable introduced at some point in the sequence of one of the groups as follows:

O O O X O O O
- - - - - - - - - - - -
O O O   O O O

This excellent design can be used to compare one agency with a similar one. Controlling for history, maturation, testing, instrumentation, regression, selection, and mortality, it is the best of the more feasible designs. Power is increased through repeated measures.

The *recurrent institutional cycle design* is a patched-up design that starts with an inadequate design and adds features to control for sources of invalidity. It becomes an accumulation of precautionary checks that approaches experimentation.

X O
- - - - - - -
    O X O

(Campbell & Stanley, 2005).

Methods of Data Collection

Observation, interviews, questionnaires, and content analysis of charts and care plans are the most common methods for data collection. When *observation* is used, the quality assurance committee determines what to observe, develops observational procedures, and trains observers. Observations should be planned and recorded systematically and subjected to controls. Observation is suitable for concurrent audits. Behavior is observed and recorded as it occurs, and the process can be noted. Because observation does not demand participation of the observed, it is relatively independent of the subject's willingness to cooperate and therefore makes subjects readily available. Observation is a comparatively inexpensive method that lends itself to simple data-gathering instruments and recording equipment. Although it can be stopped at any time, it is limited to the length of the occurrence. The timing of an event may be difficult to predict, and consequently the observer may waste time waiting for something to happen. The presence of an observer also may influence the subject's behavior. Observations may be difficult to record, are subject to observer bias, and may vary among observers. Consequently, observers need training. Specifications of observer tasks; detailed instructions; sharp, measurable categories; immediate, detailed recording; observation averaging; and the use of recording equipment such as cameras and tape recorders help overcome observer bias and variability.

Interviews of both clients and staff may be used to evaluate care. Interviews may be (1) nondirective—subjects talk about whatever they desire; (2) focused—the subject speaks to a list of topics; (3) nonstandardized—the interviewer makes up the questions; (4) semistandardized—the interviewer asks a specific number of questions and probes; or (5) standardized—the interviewer conducts each interview in exactly the same manner using the same wording without probing. The interviewer can minimize misunderstanding by probing, clarifying, pursuing topics in depth, and observing nonverbal communication. Subjects do not need to be literate. Interviewing provides more flexibility and a greater response rate than questionnaires. However, it can be time consuming and consequently expensive. The subject may be nervous or may attempt to please the interviewer, and the recording of answers is problematic.

Questionnaires are less time consuming and consequently less expensive than interviews. They are particularly useful when subjects are dispersed over a large geographical area. Less skill is needed to administer a questionnaire than to conduct an interview. Questionnaires put less pressure on the subject for immediate response, standardize instructions and questions, and offer anonymity. The participants, however, must be literate. Unfortunately, often only a small percentage of questionnaires are returned, and the effect of nonrespondents is difficult to evaluate. Items may be omitted or misunderstood. A forced choice may not be an actual choice while probing is not possible.

When preparing a questionnaire, the subjects' frame of reference and information level and the social acceptability of the item should be considered. Language should be gauged to the level of the subjects. Lengthy or leading questions and double negatives are to be avoided, and each question should contain only a single idea. Questions are arranged from general to specific. A pretest is helpful for identifying problems with the instrument. A high proportion of omissions, "other," "don't know," or all-or-none responses suggests poor questions. Added qualifications and comments and variation in answers when questions are reordered also suggest problems.

The percentage of returns of the questionnaires is influenced by a personal cover letter requesting cooperation, sponsorship by the health care agency, attractive format, short length, ease of filling out and returning, and inducements for replying. The best response is from people interested in the topic.

Content analysis of charts and care plans is a common method of data collection. It is a method of observation and measurement that is systematic, objective, and quantitative. Frequency of occurrences usually is noted on a check-off list. Descriptive statements can then be given about frequency of occurrences and changes in conditions. Unfortunately, it can take a long time to review records; classification systems may be too ambiguous for a phenomenon to fit a category; the chart chosen may not represent the phenomenon; and prejudices in the scoring method can bias the results.

Sampling

Sampling is a technique of selecting a sample from the whole population being studied. Evaluators want to be able to generalize their conclusions concerning the quality of care given the total population. Adequacy of sample size is important, especially with small samples, if the quality assurance committee members are to have confidence in their inferences. The more homogeneous the population, the smaller the sample size necessary to be representative. Budgetary and time restrictions greatly influence sample size.

The best sampling technique is *random sampling*, which allows each patient an equal chance to be included in the sample. A table of random numbers that can be located at the back of most statistics books is frequently used. To use this method, patient records are numbered. Evaluators close their eyes and point to a number on the table to start the selection. They then systematically progress by row or column until the appropriate number of records is selected. A roulette wheel can be used. The wheel is spun, and the charts of the patients whose numbers are chosen by the pointer are selected for review. The wheel is repeatedly spun until the desired sample size has been reached. A third possibility is to put pieces of paper with a chart number or patient name on each into a large container. The evaluator draws a piece of paper, rotates the papers, and draws another until the desired sample size is reached.

Systematic sampling consists of selecting every -nth subject. Selection can be according to admission, discharge, or an alphabetical listing. The evaluator makes a random start and then selects systematically. The size of the interval is determined by the percentage of the population desired in the sample size. For example, if one wants the sample to be 10% of the population, the evaluator chooses every tenth subject.

Stratified sampling divides the population into sections and then takes a random sample from each section to ensure that important variables are represented. For instance, patients may be classified according to body systems by the major diagnosis. If 30% of hospital admissions are classified as cardiovascular cases, 30% of the sample would be drawn from those cases.

Cluster sampling uses small samples from various sections of the population. A certain number of audits may be selected from each hospital unit. Instead of randomly selecting 100 patient charts, 10 charts may be randomly selected from each of 10 hospital units.

Multistage sampling randomly selects some percentage of the population and then randomly samples smaller subunits. For instance, in a large hospital system, the evaluator would randomly select which hospitals are to be audited. Next, the specialty area to audit within the selected hospitals is randomly selected. Finally, the specific units within those specialty areas and the specific patients on those units are randomly chosen.

Incidental or convenience sampling uses readily available subjects. The families of patients who happen to be in the coffee shop at a particular time or patients who happen to be in their rooms at a particular time may be interviewed.

The sample mean is not truly representative of the total population average. It is an attempt to approximate it. The difference between the mean or average of the sample and the total population is the sampling error (Rossi, Lipsey, & Freeman, 2004).

Analysis of Data

Simple scoring is preferred and can be subjected to descriptive measures. Frequency distribution indicates how many times observations were assigned to specific categories. Measures of central tendency can be calculated from the frequencies. The *mean* is the average. It is calculated by adding all the scores and dividing that sum by the total number of scores. The *mode* is the most frequently occurring score, and the *median* is the score in the middle with one half the number values above it and one half below it (Burns & Grove, 2005; Campbell & Stanley, 2005; Polit, Beck & Hunger, 2005).

Utilization of Research

"None of us is as smart as all of us."
—*Japanese Proverb*

Karkos and Peters (2006) found that the setting domain was the greatest barrier to nurses using research. Nurses needed education and communication, access and availability, practical application, and a supportive environment. There was a significant difference based on the nurses' level of education. Nursing faculty and clinical nurse educators have a responsibility to incorporate evidence-based nursing into clinical through learning activities. The current nursing culture, nurses' research knowledge and skills, learning opportunities, access to information and resources, and time complicate using evidence-based practice (Kelly & Bassendowski, 2006). It is helpful to have nursing faculty collaborate with nursing staff to do research. One organization used a collaborative research day to encourage collaborative projects and provided an opportunity for sharing the research findings. A collaborative research award was also given (Engelke & Marshburn, 2006).

Nursing students tend to energize nursing units by bringing a level of curiosity that helps keep staff members intrigued with their practices. Students encourage staff members to reexamine their practices that may be based on tradition rather than on evidence (Zuzelo, McGoldrick, Seminara, & Karbach, 2006). It is also important that knowledge gained through practice is shared to sustain changes (Allen, Bockenhauer, Egan, et al, 2006). Nurses are key to identifying, measuring, and improving processes through evidence-based practice (Newhouse, 2006). It is desirable to not research, but to lead interdisciplinary research as well (Bauer-Wu, Epshtein, & Ponte, 2006).

RISK MANAGEMENT

Health care risk management is relatively new. Losses were low before 1965, when the case of *Darling v. Charleston Community Memorial Hospital* set a precedent for holding hospitals directly liable for failure of administrators or staff to properly monitor and supervise health care delivery in the hospital. States also began to liberalize their workers' compensation laws into no-fault programs that facilitated an increase in claim settlements. Hospitals then started creating alternatives to commercial malpractice insurance including self-insurance. Medicare required self-insured hospitals to have risk management programs. JCAHO started requiring risk management programs in 1989. Several states require reporting of any event that resulted in harm to the safety or life of a patient or employee.

Risk management involves the development and implementation of strategies to prevent patient injury, minimize financial loss, and preserve agency assets. Risk management focuses on liability control. It assesses areas in which claims can be prevented. By reducing the frequency and severity of injuries to patients, the likelihood of litigation can be decreased and litigation costs lessened. The risk management process includes risk identification, analysis, treatment, evaluation, and follow-up. Health care risk management is a process that is designed to reduce or prevent practices or situations that pose a threat to the safety and well being of a patient, visitor, or staff member. The risk management process includes risk identification, evaluation, and reduction strategies. An effective risk management program will help to minimize financial loss for the organization by reducing the frequency of lawsuits (general liability/medical malpractice).

The goals for risk management are:

To provide patient, staff, and visitor safety and to prevent injury or harm to all concerned.

To avoid liability exposure by evaluating new and existing services, practices, and procedures including consultation with a professional liability carrier

To maintain an incident reporting system to identify trends and patterns of practice and occurrences that have the potential of causing an adverse occurrence and to implement measures to prevent such events

To maintain a quality improvement program to identify areas of risk in specific clinical applications, and reduce their untoward impact on patient care

Both the Risk Management Department and the Quality/Performance Improvement Department are involved with patient quality, safety, and prevention activities, so it is important for those two departments to work closely to develop plans for reduction or improvement. The first step in risk management is identifying potential or actual risks for accidents, injury, and financial loss. An error is failure of a planned action to be completed as intended or use of a wrong plan. An adverse event is an injury caused by medical management that resulted in a measurable disability. An unpreventable adverse event is an adverse event that resulted from a complication that could not be prevented given the current state of knowledge. A near miss is an event that could have resulted in an accident, injury, or illness but did not by chance or timely intervention. Identification can occur in a variety of ways including incident reporting, evaluation of patient grievances, litigation, quality referrals, and concerns identified by state and federal agencies. If the organization is going to be successful in identifying risk it is imperative that all staff members understand the process and feel comfortable with reporting issues or concerns. Leadership should foster an environment that encourages staff to report and to be involved in the process to make improvements.

Patient falls, medication errors, infections, operative and postoperative complications, wrong-site surgery, patient suicide, equipment failures, improper maintenance of utilities and patient protective systems, patient grievances, and noncompliance with regulations/laws historically have all been known to cause injuries to patients and should be given priority when determining risk indicators. Energy should be put into preventive activities such as providing a safe physical environment, fostering customer satisfaction, and providing high-quality service. The present institution-wide monitoring system should be reviewed. The completeness of the monitoring system should be evaluated, including audits, committee minutes, incidence reports, patient questionnaires, and oral and any other complaints. Whether additional systems need to be implemented to provide data for risk management control should be determined.

After data have been collected, they should be analyzed to determine the frequency and severity of problems in general categories. One should consider the severity or consequence of a failure, the occurrence or frequency of the problem, and the detection or the probability of detecting the problem before the impact of the effect is realized to set priorities. Then a plan to reduce the risks as much as possible should be developed and implemented. Review of problem-prone systems, policy and procedures, equipment safety, consents, and laws and regulations will be necessary when implementing plans for reducing or preventing risk. Corrective actions may include education, new policies and procedures, changes in policies and procedures, changes to systems, new equipment, and counseling/disciplinary action. Safety procedures should be reviewed and laws and codes related to patient care, consent, and safety should be monitored. Needs for personnel, patient, and family education should be identified and education implemented. The results of the risk management program should be evaluated and reported to appropriate groups. Risk management programs should include customer satisfaction, safety and security, continuous quality improvement, and liability control (Folse, 2007; Grohar-Murray & DiCroce, 2003; Lorah, M, personal correspondence, February 2007; Sullivan & Decker, 2005; Roussel, Swansburg, & Swansburg, 2006).

Nurses should be able to recognize sentinel events. A sentinel event is an unexpected outcome involving a death, serious physical or psychological injury, or permanent loss of function not related to the natural course of the patient's illness that needs immediate investigation and response. Accredited organizations are expected to identify and respond to all sentinel events occurring in the organization by doing a thorough and credible root-cause analysis, implementing improvement to reduce risk, and monitoring the effectiveness of the improvements. A thorough analysis involves identifying what factors are directly related to the sentinel event; analysis of the underlying processes and systems; identification of areas of risk that could potentially contribute to the sentinel event; and assignment of responsibility for implementation of necessary improvements. Credibility is established by having organizational leadership involved in the process; consistent analysis; explanation of the findings; and consideration of related literature.

Asking "why" at least five times helps discover underlying problems that might otherwise be overlooked. Sentinel events could include but are not limited to death or major permanent loss associated with a medication error; inpatient suicide; elopement; restraints/seclusion; any procedure performed on the wrong patient, wrong side, or wrong body part; perinatal death; unanticipated death of a full-term infant; abduction of any patient; discharge of an infant to the wrong family; assault or homicide; rape; patient falls; delays in treatment; or hemolytic transfusion reaction involving blood group incompatibilities (Folse, 2007; Joint Commission on Accreditation of Healthcare Organizations, *BOJ's Guide to 1990 Standards and Scoring,* 1990, p. 13).

Medical errors are believed to result in thousands of preventable events annually. A medical error is "the failure of a planned action to be completed as intended or the use of a wrong plan to achieve an aim" (Institute of Medicine, 1999). To improve the situation we need to create a culture of safety in the health care system instead of the culture of secrecy and the name, blame, and shame game that exists (Milstead, 2006). When one is punished for reporting an error the probability of reporting the error is decreased. In fact, errors are often an accumulation of several systematic factors such that if one element in the chain had been changed, the harm to the patient might have been prevented. A system error is not the result of an individual's actions but is the predictable outcome of a series of actions that comprise a diagnostic and treatment process. A safety culture assumes that to err is human, and good people often make errors in a flawed system. It distinguishes between blameworthy errors (those errors made out of vindication, carelessness, or recklessness) and those that are unintentional. Reporting of errors is rewarded instead of punished. Accountability involves acknowledging the error, apologizing, repairing the harm, uncovering the causes of the error, and correcting the process or system. There may be an error of planning that is the failure to determine the appropriate course of action or an error of execution that is the failure to implement the appropriate course of action through to completion. Many reported medical errors are medication related.

Pape (2001) reports the results of several research studies of medication administration errors. A medication error has been defined as "any preventable medication-related event occurring as a result of actions by a health care professional that may cause or lead to patient harm while the patient is in the care of the health care provider" (Pape, 2001, p. 154). Prescribing, transcribing, dispensing, and administering errors are common. Medication errors include omitting a medication, giving medication at the wrong time, to the wrong patient, in the wrong dose, by the wrong route, to a patient with a known allergy, giving repeated medication without an order, or discontinuing medication without an order. Illegible handwriting, improper abbreviations, not putting a zero before a decimal point or putting one after an unnecessary decimal point following a whole number contribute to errors. "D/C" could mean discontinue or discharge; "HS" could mean hour of sleep or half strength; "cc" for cubic centimeter has been mistaken for "u" for units;

and "1.0" often looks like "10." One should avoid using similar abbreviations such as QD for daily, QID for four times daily, and QOD for every other day. There can be confusion among drugs with similar names such as Celebrex for arthritis, Cerebyx for convulsions, and Celexa for depression. Those drugs should not be stored near each other. Hazardous medications should be stored away from patient care areas. Bar coding can help prevent and track medication errors.

Lack of knowledge or application of knowledge, use of wrong drug name, incorrect calculations or unit expressions, distractions, interruptions, identifying patients by room numbers instead of identification bands, and fatigue can contribute to errors. System factors that can contribute to errors include but are not limited to the following: excessive workloads, inexperience, crowded spaces, noise, distractions, interruptions while preparing medications, and failure to follow policies, procedures, and protocols. Staff should be oriented to the policies, procedures, and protocols that should also be readily available to staff in policy books in units and online. Computerized systems for a physician order entry system and drug compatibility check and including pharmacists in planning and prescribing patient care can be helpful. Availability of patient information such as allergies, age, weight, current diagnosis, lab values, and current medications should be available to the pharmacist before dispensing medications. Clarification is important for any illegible, incomplete, or otherwise questionable order. Pharmacist should double-check all mathematical calculations for neonatal and pediatric dilutions, parenteral nutrition solutions, and other compounded pharmaceutical products. Computer-typed medication orders and labels reduce the difficulty in reading orders and labels. Workspaces where medications are prepared should be kept clean, orderly, well lit, and relatively free from noise and other distractions. Drug reference texts should be readily available. There should be standardized methods for labeling, packaging, and storing medications. Unit-doses versus multiple-dose vials and ready-to-administer medications can decrease medication errors. High alert drugs such as chemotherapy, anticoagulants, insulin, and narcotics should be identified.

Barriers to reporting errors include fear of punishment, reduced self-esteem, and perceived decrease in level of professionalism. Sometimes doctors are relaxed about medication errors and write orders to erase the error. Teaching staff policies, procedures, and guidelines; labeling "medication error" as "drug variance"; and rewarding instead of punishing reporting may increase accuracy of reporting medication errors. Asking nurses to identify all causes of medication errors, doing a root-cause analysis, and using an interdisciplinary team approach to identify problems from different perspectives and to recommend solutions may help reduce errors through continuous quality improvement (Pape, 2001).

Wrong-site surgery occurs more commonly in orthopedic procedures than in other surgical specialties. The American Academy of Orthopaedic Surgeons recommends that surgeons sign their initials at the correct site of surgery with an indelible pen. The surgeon should not make an incision unless the initials are visible. "No" can be written in large letters on the side not to be operated on. An intraoperative radiograph and radiopaque marker can be used to determine the exact level of spinal surgery (Ogle, 1998). Operating staff should not rely totally on the surgeon for verifying the surgical site. Patients should confirm the location of the surgery. All of the operating room personnel should monitor procedures.

The Joint Commission on Accreditation of Healthcare Organizations (JCAHO, 1998a) identified multiple surgeons, multiple procedures, pressure to operate quickly, and unusual body characteristics to be particularly high risk.

Miscommunication has been identified as the primary root cause of the most common operative and postoperative complications including interventional imaging; endoscopy; tube or catheter insertion; head and neck, thoracic, abdominal, and orthopedic surgery. Incomplete preoperative assessment, failure to question inappropriate orders, failure to follow established procedures, and inconsistent postoperative monitoring procedures are common root causes. Direct communications between health care providers is paramount to preventing operative and postoperative complications. Staff orientation and training, clarification of communication channels, and monitoring consistency of compliance with procedures are preventive measures (JCAHO, 2000a).

The elderly are at highest risk for patient falls, especially those with altered mental status and with a history of falls. Elderly patients may have poor vision because of cataracts or glaucoma. Cardiovascular problems can result in syncope or postural hypotension and consequently poor balance. Lower extremity dysfunctions like muscle weakness, arthritis, or peripheral neuropathy make it difficult to ambulate. Nocturia may cause ambulation at night. Obstetrical patients are at higher risk for falls because of decreased sensation and mobility from the administration of epidural anesthesia. They may also have excessive blood loss and consequently postural hypotension. JCAHO (2000b) reported that root causes included communications most frequently and failure to obtain adequate information related to fall history, failure to report important information during shift reports, and failure to document changes in conditions in the medical record. Other root causes included lack of protocols, incomplete plan of care, environmental issues like nursing stations and door designs, malfunction or misuse of equipment especially bed alarms, inadequate staffing, staffing shortage, and decreased use of restraints without alternatives. Preventive measures include staff orientation and training especially regarding fall risk assessment and fall prevention protocols.

Most inpatient suicides have occurred in psychiatric hospitals, followed by general hospitals' psychiatric units and medical/surgical floors, then in residential care facilities. Root causes that have been identified include inadequate patient assessment and inadequate suicide risk assessment, inadequate and infrequent patient observations, deficient orientation and training, inadequate staffing, inappropriate assignment of the patient, inaccurate communication among caregivers, and information not available when needed. Environmental factors include presence of nonbreakaway bars, rods or safety rails, lack of testing breakaway hardware, and inadequate security. Risk reduction measures include adequate staffing, monitoring consistency of the implementation of observation procedures, revising information transfer procedures, having family and friends participate in contraband detection, and education about suicide prevention. Careful screening through the admission process and removing harmful items such as belts can help prevent patient suicide (JCAHO, 1998b).

Most delays in treatment occur in emergency departments, but they can occur in any health care setting. The most common delay in treatment is misdiagnosis, but delayed test results, physician availability, delayed administration of ordered care, incomplete treatment, overcrowding, poor staffing, and inability to find the entrance to the emergency department are also causes. The main cause contributing to delays is poor communication between physicians. JCAHO (2002) recommends implementing processes and procedures that improve timelines, completeness, and accuracy in communications; implementing face-to-face interdisciplinary change-of-shift debriefings; and reducing reliance on verbal orders and requiring a "read back" or verification when verbal orders are necessary.

A preventable adverse event or sentinel event is an event that causes an injury that cannot be related to the patient's underlying medical condition, such as the development of pneumonia after surgery caused by medical intervention or inaction like not washing hands. A nonpreventable adverse event could be pneumonia caused by age and comorbidities.

Changes in facilities have been made to address disasters, terrorism, and mass casualties including but not limited to advanced security/ lockdown systems; additional generator capacity; expanded emergency communications systems; enhanced air pressure control and isolation capabilities; and extra space for decontamination/ mass casualties.

Changes for increased flexibility include wireless infrastructures; extra cabling and conduit; power plant expansion capacity, decentralized nurses' stations; and added air treatment/air movement capacity. Evidence-based design grew during 2006. Consumer demand for privacy and family-centered care contributed to building larger private rooms with amenities like wireless technologies, in-room sinks, and individual room temperature controls. Like-handed or nonmirrored rooms and bar codes have also reduced the chances of errors. Healing gardens and indoor water features have been shown to increase patient satisfaction.

Additional features have included flex-up rooms from semiprivate to private provisions; 200 square feet or more for larger room size for single room and in-room family area; standard room design with same hookups and equipment integration; universal acuity-adaptable room design, specialty lighting for added comfort and safety, and rooms with a view of nature (Carpenter & Hoppszallern, 2007).

CUSTOMER SATISFACTION

"One enemy can harm you more than a hundred friends can do you good." —German saying

The dissatisfied customer is the one most likely to pursue litigation. Therefore it is important to identify incidents that might lead to claims, educate patients and their families about the care, and handle patient complaints. To handle complaints, listen and let the patients express themselves before speaking. Do not become defensive. Avoid reacting emotionally. Negotiate. Ask for the patient's expectations, and explain what you can or cannot do. Agree on actions to be taken and a time frame. Follow through. A caring attitude can be very effective. It is also important to teach personnel about customer relations and how to prevent and handle complaints. Patient satisfaction has not been correlated with improved patient outcomes, but it can reduce litigation (Ervin, 2006).

SAFETY AND SECURITY

A culture of safety is desirable. Common safety issues include medication errors, adverse drug events, falls, safe transfers, surgical site infections, central line infections, ventilator-associated pneumonia, care for acute myocardial infarction, etc. Fear of retribution, punitive actions, and professional humiliation have been identified as reasons some medication errors are not reported. Ordering, dispensing, transcription, and administration are where medication errors can occur (Force, Deering, Hubble, et al, 2006).

Nurses have a key role in monitoring, preventing, and treating adverse drug events (ADE). Increased legibility of drug orders, provision of decision support, and increased access to medical records can be helpful. While technology has helped provider order entry, bar code administration, automated drug-to-drug interaction checking, and allergy tracking, it has a negative effect because of the decreased access to nursing narratives (Weir, Hoffman, Nebeker, & Hurdle, 2005). One study found that with decreased staffing there was a greater number of reported medication errors among nurses (Moody, 2006). Some have tried to use unlicensed personnel to remove nonnursing duties from nurses to reduce errors without documented success. Additional contributions to medication errors that have been identified are: inadequate continuity of care between hospital and the community; multiple health care providers where medications can be prescribed by several people unknown to each other; keeping unnecessary medications, and confusion about generic and trade names; and misunderstanding label instructions. Review and Safety Committees may help reduce medication errors by increasing awareness of medication error reporting and prevention (Joanna Briggs Institute, 2006).

A medication error implies that the health care provider did something wrong or neglected to do something. Medical errors are adverse events, but not all adverse events are medical errors, negligence, or unethical behavior. However, failure to disclose and document adverse events may be negligence or unethical. One should document as soon as possible after the event by noting the date, time, location, individuals present, and relationship to the patient. One should describe the situation factually including questions and answers and use quotes as appropriate. Identify the follow-up plan and document follow-up discussions that occur later. Do not speculate, give opinion, blame others, or reference any incident reports, peer review activities, or risk management investigations (Monson, 2006).

Shifting from a culture of blame to a culture of safety changes the responsibility from the individual worker to the system. To make that change, Heinen, Coyle, and Hamilton (2004) recommend: (1) demonstrating patient safety as a top priority, (2) actively promoting a nonpunitive environment for sharing information and lessons learned, (3) routinely evaluating patient outcomes and identifying risk factors, (4) searching for collaborative partners from whom one can learn and share information, (5) analyzing adverse events using root cause analysis to identify system failures and plan corrections, (6) recognizing and regarding safety-driven decisions and reports, (7) fostering teamwork through training and support, (8) implementing care delivery processes that do not rely on memory, (9) engaging patients and caregivers in the redesign of care delivery processes, and (10) constantly looking for ways to improve. They also encourage close call reporting.

Most falls have an anticipated physiological cause that puts the person at increased risk for a fall. Teaching staff about those risks and how to minimize them by minimizing environment factors can decrease accidents. A scholars program of guest speakers about safety issues can increase staff competence. WalkRounds format can be used to identify problems, prioritize them, and problem solve to increase safety (Kruger, Hurley, & Gustafson, 2006).

Tourangeau (2006) found that nursing staff mix, continuity of care provider, proportion of baccalaureate-prepared nurses, use of care maps, and adequacy of resources were determinants of mortality for acute medical patients but not for surgical patients. Wertenberger and Wilson (2005) reported using patient follow-up in the home and interventions via a hand-held camera phone to reduce injuries across the continuum of care. Rabert and Sebastian (2006) described the service of a board-certified intensivist and technological advances such as a computerized physician-order entry system and an electronic medication administration record to deliver high quality care to critically ill patients throughout a network.

A safety and security program should provide safety for patients, their families, other visitors, and personnel. Risks from custodial negligence should be controlled. Screening practices to reduce workplace violence can reduce negligent hiring lawsuits (Bradley & Moore, 2004). There should be plans for natural disasters, fire, electrical shock, power loss, and bioterrorism. Hospital Emergency Incident Command Systems provides a template for responding to a disaster. It requires an understanding of situation awareness and a highly reliable team that needs education, training, and good communication systems (Autrey & Moss, 2006). There should be an equipment maintenance program.

Regarding terrorism, clinicians need necessary information to make diagnoses, manage care, prevent further problems, and report actions. They need to maintain their personal safety, manage scarce resources, isolate as necessary, treat acutely ill, and decide who needs treatment and who can wait. Public health officials have to interpret surveillance data, investigate outbreaks, use epidemiologic measures, and issue surveillance alerts.

The American Nurses Association encourages the development of policies that release registered nurses as part of organized medical rescue teams during disasters. The agency should keep a listing of all nurses who have been educated in disaster and emergency preparedness and who are members of emergency preparedness teams. The registered nurse should keep the employer informed of competency in disaster and emergency preparedness and give the employer copies of disaster/emergency preparedness education competence. The nurse should inform emergency teams if the employer denies or withdraws consent for emergency deployment (ANA, 2002).

"Anger is only one letter short of danger." —Anonymous

Occupational Safety and Health Act

The purposes of the Occupational Safety and Health Act of 1970 and the Mine Safety and Health Act of 1977 are to ensure safe and healthful working conditions and to preserve the nation's human resources. They established nationwide safety guidelines and standards for health and mining for the first time. The Secretary of Labor and the Occupational Review Committee are responsible for administration and enforcement of the acts. Research and education activities are the responsibility of the Secretary of Health and Human Services and are implemented by the National Institute for Occupational Safety and Health (NIOSH). The Assistant Secretary of Labor for Occupational Safety and Health acts as the chief of the Occupational Safety and Health Administration (OSHA). OSHA monitors the following: (1) development of standards about occupational health and safety, (2) development of health and safety regulations, (3) inspections and investigations to check the status of compliance, and (4) citations and proposals for penalties for noncompliance with the standards.

OSHA's primary responsibilities are as follows: (1) to promulgate, modify, and revoke health and safety standards; (2) to approve or reject state plans for programs; (3) to require employers to keep records of safety and health data; (4) to conduct investigations and inspections and to issue citations and propose penalties; (5) to petition the courts to restrain imminent danger situations; and (6) to provide educational programs, consulting, funding for state plans, and statistical records of illnesses, injuries, and accidents.

The Occupational Safety and Health Review Commission (OSHRC) is a three-member quasijudicial board that hears cases when OSHA actions are contested by employees and employers. The committee decisions can be reviewed by state and federal courts.

NIOSH is the federal agency responsible for research, education, and training. The representatives can inspect agencies and ensure compliance but are not authorized to enforce OSHA regulations. The main functions of NIOSH are as follows: (1) to develop educational programs, (2) to develop occupational health and safety standards, and (3) to conduct research. The responsibility to establish research methods and conduct statistics surveys belongs to the Bureau of Labor Statistics.

With few exceptions, OSHA applies to every employer in all 50 states and all U.S. possessions who has one or more employees and who engages in business affecting commerce. Under OSHA the employer is responsible for providing a safe, healthful work environment and for complying with the applicable standards. The employees must comply with applicable standards. The employer is subject to state and federal sanctions for violating standards. Employees are subject to their employer's sanctions.

All standards promulgated by OSHA are published in the Federal Register. OSHA requires employers to keep records of all occupational illnesses and accidents and to report either to OSHA or to the state plan within 48 hours. OSHA can grant two types of variances from the standards: temporary and permanent. Employers must show just cause for either variance and inform the employees of the application.

Workplace inspections are usually conducted without prior notice. Investigations of imminent dangers are top priority, followed by catastrophic and fatal accidents, followed by employee complaints regarding hazards, and reinspections. General inspection procedures include an opening conference, a walk-through documenting alleged violations, interviews with workers, and a closing session. Citations and penalties vary according to the seriousness of the violation. Violation citations are to be posted near where the violation occurred. If an employer wants to contest a case, the area office that initiated the action should be contacted. OSHA encourages states to assume responsibility for administering and enforcing occupational safety and health laws. Areas needing regulations include but are not

limited to blood-borne pathogens, lifting guidelines, confined-space regulations, ergonomic guidelines, respiratory guidelines, and egress.

Administrators need to identify the tasks to be performed, identify the tools necessary, evaluate the environment in which the tasks will be performed, assess the organization in which this takes place, and make necessary changes to provide a safe work environment for the employee (Kavianian & Wentz, 1997).

SOURCES OF LAW

There are four sources of law and parallel systems at the state and federal levels. The four sources of law are constitutions, statutes, administrative agencies, and court decisions that contribute principles for common law.

The constitution is the highest law in the United States. It defines the structure, power, and limits of government, and it guarantees citizens certain fundamental rights. It is interpreted by the U.S. Supreme Court and gives authority to the other sources of law. It has little direct involvement in malpractice.

Statutory law or legislative law is law passed by local, state, or federal legislators, such as the U.S. Congress, state legislatures, and city councils, and must be signed by the mayor, governor, or president. Statutory law regulates employment issues like worker's compensation and health and retirement benefits, and can be expanded, amended, or repealed by action of the legislature. Nurse practice acts vary among states but must be consistent with provisions or statutes established at the federal level. Nurse practice acts define and limit the practice of nursing and determine what constitutes unauthorized practice. Before 1970, very few federal or state laws dealt with malpractice. Since then, many statutes affect malpractice.

Administrative agencies are given authority to act by legislative bodies. They create rules and regulations that enforce statutory laws. Administrative laws are valid only when they are within the scope of the authority granted to them by the legislative body. State boards of nursing are administrative

RESEARCH PERSPECTIVE 15-2

Data from Gates D, Fitzwater E, Succop P: Reducing assaults against nursing home caregivers, *Nursing Research* 54 (2):119-127, March/April 2005.

Purpose: The purpose of this research was to use Social Cognitive Theory to test the effectiveness of a violence-prevention intervention to increase knowledge, self-efficacy, and skills, and to decrease assaults among nursing assistants working in long-term care because they have the highest incidence of workplace assault among all workers in the United States.

Method: A baseline questionnaire regarding demographics, employment, and violence experience was administered to 138 nursing assistants in three intervention and three comparison nursing homes. For this quasiexperimental study, a pre-baseline, post-intervention, and 6 months follow-up administration of the State Trait Anger inventory, the Knowledge and Self-Efficacy Survey were done and an Assault log for 80 hours of work was completed. The subjects participated in a simulation exercise to assess violence-prevention skills. Tabulation, Poisson regression, and analysis of variance were done to analyze the data.

Results/conclusions: The intervention participants had significant increases in knowledge, self-efficacy, and violence-prevention skills. There was an interaction effect between the intervention and the number of preintervention assaults, without any significant main effect on the incidence of assaults. The intervention had a significant effect on the nursing assistants who had fewer than six assaults preintervention and no significant effect on those who had more than seven assaults preintervention. There were significant relationships between assaults and anger, state anger, and the number of residents assigned. The researchers state "Anger is a subjective emotional state and this emotional state may provoke aggression, which is a verbal or physical act of violence. Spielberger (1999) stated that whereas persons with high state anger are currently experiencing relatively intense angry feelings, persons with high trait anger frequently experience angry feelings and often feel that they are treated unfairly by others." It was the state anger rather than the trait anger that had a significant difference.

agencies created to implement and enforce the state nurse practice act. The state board members write rules and regulations and conduct investigations and hearings to ensure that law's enforcement. The National Labor Relations Board and health and safety boards can affect nursing practice.

Court decisions are called tort laws. Initial trial courts usually have a single judge or magistrate make the decision. Intermediary appeal courts have three justices, and the highest courts of appeal have nine justices. They interpret legal issues that are in dispute and set precedents. There are two levels of courts in the United States: trial court and appellate court. The Supreme Court is the highest appellate court and hears and determines appeals from the division courts and constitutional questions. The courts interpret most malpractice law (Marquis & Huston, 2006; Pozgar, 2004; Sullivan & Decker, 2005).

CATEGORIES OF LAW

Laws are categorized into two basic types: public law and private or civil law. Public law is composed of constitutional law, administrative law, and criminal law and deals with relationships between individuals and the government. Private or civic law deals with relationships between private persons and is classified into tort law, contract law, and protecting and reporting law (which is sometimes categorized as criminal law and involves theft, rape, and homicide and can result in imprisonment). The most common law affecting nursing practice is tort law.

Tort law is the branch of civil law that concerns legal wrongs committed by one person against the person or property of another. Tort law is categorized into two categories: unintentional and intentional. Negligence and malpractice, which is professional negligence, are considered *unintentional torts*.

Negligence is the failure of a person to perform an act (omission) or to perform an act (commission) that a reasonable person would or would not do in a similar situation. Negligence is an unintentional tort that involves harm resulting from the failure of people conducting themselves in reasonable and prudent ways. Carelessness is not thinking before one acts or not paying attention. One can be careful and still be negligent for not acting as prudently as others would in the same circumstances (Grohar-Murray & DiCroce, 2003; Guido, 2007; Marquis & Huston, 2006; O'Keefe, 2001; Pozgar, 2004).

Malpractice is negligent acts of people with specialized education. Malpractice reflects negligence, but not all negligence is malpractice. When people are held legally responsible for their negligent acts, they are legally liable and may be required to pay for damages. Medical malpractice refers to the negligent acts of any health care professional when conducting patient care responsibilities. Nursing malpractice refers specifically to nurses conducting their patient care responsibilities. Common causes of malpractice claims against nurses are medication errors from misreading the medication order, not clarifying an incomplete or ambiguous order, and technique in giving injections.

Negligent conduct depends on the act itself and the surrounding circumstances, including the following: (1) the nature of the nursing function, (2) the nurse's qualifications to perform the function, (3) the urgency of the situation, and (4) the foreseeable harm if the care is not implemented. The emergency room nurse is not held to the same standards of care expected under more normal circumstances. Being a minor does not exempt a nurse from liability for acts of malpractice, and the nurse's state of mind and physical condition are not considered relevant.

The rule of personal liability means that people are responsible for their own tortious conduct even when someone else may share that liability under some other law. Managers will not usually be held liable for the negligent acts of those they lead because all professional persons are held liable for their own negligent behavior. However, a manager may be found guilty of negligence for making an assignment beyond a worker's capabilities without giving adequate direction in carrying out the delegated functions. If a supervisor believes that certain staffing will jeopardize patient safety and potentially precipitate litigation, the position should be documented and the hospital administrator informed.

The doctrine of respondeat superior applies to the U.S. government because the government has agreed to be sued for negligent acts of its employees under the Federal Tort Claims Act (FTCA). By virtue of special statutory enactments, nurses employed by the Veterans Administration and the U.S. Public Health Service have complete immunity from personal liability for acts of negligence in the implementation of their government responsibilities. However, the aggrieved patients may sue the government for injuries they have sustained. Occupational health nurses are potentially exposed to a greater risk of being sued for negligent conduct than other nurses because of the joint effect of the doctrine of respondeat superior and workers' compensation laws. Workers' compensation laws usually prevent an employee from suing an employer, so the aggrieved employee can sue only the nurse.

A nurse is legally required to implement medical procedures ordered by a licensed physician or a physician assistant acting on behalf of the physician employer unless the nurse has reason to believe harm would result from doing so. Failure to carry out the physician's order will subject the nurse to liability for subsequent harm to the patient if there is no reason to question the order. Consequently, nurses must know how to implement the procedure and the effect of the procedure on the patient. When nurses question a physician's orders, they should tactfully question the physician. If the physician is insistent, the nurse should take the matter to the supervisor or responsible hospital official. Patient safety is of utmost concern. The nurse has a legal responsibility not to follow the order when there are reasonable grounds to believe that the action would harm the patient.

Malpractice is professional negligence that involves any misconduct or lack of skill in carrying out professional responsibilities. Duty, breach of duty, causation, and injury must be present for malpractice to exist. If one of these factors cannot be proved beyond a reasonable doubt, the malpractice claim maybe dismissed (Cooper, 2006; Grohar-Murray & DiCroce, 2003; Guido, 2007; O'Keefe, 2001; Roussel, Swansburg, & Swansburg, 2006).

Intentional torts have an intent to harm and include the following: assault, battery, false imprisonment, invasion of privacy, libel, slander, and defamation of character. *Assault* involves mental disturbance of personal integrity, including fright and humiliation and a threat to touch a person without justification such as "If you don't . . . I will force you." It does not include actual contact (O'Keefe, 2001; Pozgar, 2004; Roussel, Swansburg, & Swansburg, 2006).

Battery is an intentional tort involving unpermitted and intentional contacts with one's person or extension of the body such as clothing, object in the hand, car, and so forth. A hostile intent of the defendant is not necessary. It is the absence of the plaintiff's consent to the defendant's contact that is the issue. Battery may include touching in an embarrassing or wrongful way, causing injury, or without permission such as continuing a procedure after a person has asked that it be stopped. Direct contact with the plaintiff is not necessary, and the personal integrity exists even when the plaintiff is under anesthesia or asleep. The defendant is liable for all harm, including unforseeable consequences from the conduct (O'Keefe, 2001; Pozgar, 2004; Roussel, Swansburg, & Swansburg, 2006).

Grounds for civil actions regarding assault and battery include forcefully handling an unconscious patient, forcing a patient out of bed to walk, forcing a patient to submit to treatment even if a consent had been signed because resistance implies withdrawal of consent, lifting a protesting patient from bed to a stretcher or chair, threatening to strike or striking a child or adult unless in self-defense, and in some states performing alcohol, blood, urine, or other health tests for presumed drunken driving without consent. Some mental health patients and nursing home residents have brought suits

for assault and battery against their health care providers. Assault, battery, and false imprisonment are considered intentional torts. Intentional torts such as assault and battery often are not covered in malpractice insurance (O'Keefe, 2001; Pozgar, 2004; Roussel, Swansburg, & Swansburg, 2006).

False imprisonment is willful detention without consent or authority of law. It is an intentional infringement of the right of a person to move freely and without hindrance. Actual physical force is not necessary. All that is necessary is for a person who is physically confined to a given space to experience fear that force, which may be implied by words, threats, or gestures, will be used to detain the person or to intimidate him or her without legal justification. Most false-imprisonment cases in health care involve locking mentally ill patients in their rooms. An agency can be held liable for the conduct of a nurse-employee who unlawfully confines or detains a patient against the patient's will because of the doctrine of respondeat superior. A health care professional cannot detain a client who insists on leaving treatment against medical advice. The client has the right to leave even if that is harmful to that person unless the person is considered incompetent or committed through a legal process. That would be considered protecting the person from harm. Some mental health patients and nursing home residents have brought suits for false imprisonment against their health care providers (O'Keefe, 2001; Pozgar, 2004; Roussel, Swansburg, & Swansburg, 2006).

Privacy and confidentiality are very important. Invasion of privacy is a tort violation of a person's right to make personal choices without interference and to not be subjected to uninvited publicity. The information disclosed by patients is confidential and only to be available to authorized personnel. Nurses should be discreet about the release of information over the telephone because of the difficulty of identifying the caller and may not use photographs, videotapes, or research data without the explicit permission of the involved patient. The nurse must even obtain permission to release information to family members and close friends.

The patient can sue for invasion of privacy when confidential information is directly or indirectly communicated to unauthorized people.

The Health Insurance Portability and Accountability Act (HIPAA) was enacted by the federal government in 1996 to give people portability of their health care coverage and control over how their personal information is used and disclosed; it also made organizations that create or receive personal information accountable for protecting it. HIPAA is composed of three different sets of rules: (1) the Privacy Rule, effective April 14, 2003; (2) the Electronic Transactions/Code Sets Standards, effective October 21, 2005; and (3) the Security Rule, effective April 21, 2005. Some believe that you cannot keep information private if it is not secure.

Health care providers covered under HIPAA must follow strict guidelines to protect health information including the following:

1. Provide all patients with a written notice on how their information may be used or disclosed.
2. Restrict use and disclosure of health information except as permitted by law.
3. Establish safeguards to limit incidental disclosures of health information.
4. Establish policies and procedures to protect and safeguard protected health information.
5. Train all workforce members on safeguarding health information.

The privacy rule creates rights for individuals to do the following:

1. Request restriction on the use or disclosure of health information.
2. Inspect and obtain copies of protected health information.
3. Request changes in health information.
4. Request an accounting of disclosures of protected health information.

Telehealth raises challenges to privacy and confidentiality. It uses telecommunications and information technologies to provide care at a distance and to transmit health care information. Teleconferencing cameras can be used to diagnose, treat, monitor, and educate patients from a distance. X-ray films and electrocardiograms (ECGs) can be transmitted and viewed. Electronic dermoscopes and stethoscopes can allow health care providers to look at eyes, ears, skin, and wounds and to listen to heart, lung, and bowel sounds. This allows ready access to expert advice and patient information that is especially beneficial in rural areas. E-mail can be used to deliver health services, and the World Wide Web can be a valuable resource for health education (Saba & McCormick, 2005).

The Uniform Health Care Information Act of 1997 governs the flow of health care information. Under it, patients are to have access to health care information to make informed decisions, provide informed consent, and correct inaccurate or incomplete information in the record. The legal implications for telenursing, which uses communications technology to transmit health information from one location to another, includes the reasonableness standard for disclosure, nurses' potential for civil or criminal liability, and the elements necessary to obtain a valid disclosure authorization from the patient. The patient has a right to privacy via the telephone, cordless telephone, cellular telephone, and computer. Under the 1992 Amendment to the Federal Wiretap Statutes, cordless telephone communications are protected the same as land-based telephone communications. Unfortunately, unintended interceptions of cordless health care communication can happen through devices such as other cordless telephones, baby monitors, and FM radios. Cellular telephones are similar to cordless telephones in that they broadcast the communication to a receiving station that transmits the communication over a land-based telephone line. Unfortunately, cellular telephone communications are commonly intercepted inadvertently by other cellular telephones. Considering the ease with which cellular and cordless telephone communications can be intercepted, the provider must consider the risks of harm versus the benefits to the patient. When the risk of harm is greater than the benefit, the provider should inform the patient of the potential risks of disclosure of the health care information and get agreement in writing for the provider to use the telephone. The use of the Internet to communicate health care information also has an expectation of privacy.

A fax sent by computer or telephone between two providers is an electronic digital communication sent over a land-based telephone line and is subject to the right of privacy and confidentiality.

Confidentiality is the right to privacy of records. Patients have the right to believe that the information they disclose to health professionals will be used strictly for diagnosis and treatment and will not be shared with others without permission of the person.

There are a few exceptions to confidentiality. All 50 states require disclosure in cases of child abuse when certain professionals suspect abuse. The identified professionals vary from state to state but usually include nurses, physicians, child care providers, and school teachers. Elder abuse and abuse of the disabled may also require disclosure. Case law helps guide professional actions when clients are dangerous to themselves or others. In the case of *Tarasoff v. Regents of the University of California*, a 1976 decision created the Tarasoff duty, or the duty to warn. If a client revealed an intent to harm another person, the health care provider has a legal obligation to notify the intended victim. The *Gross v. Allen* (1994) decision informed mental health professionals that they must tell the patients' caregivers of any intent of suicide or intent to harm others. Although these cases involved psychologists, there is relevance to advanced practice nurses (American Bar Association, 2001; Grohar-Murray & DiCroce, 2003; Guido, 2007; Marquis & Huston, 2006; O'Keefe, 2001; Sullivan & Decker, 2005; Swansburg & Swansburg, 2002; Yount, 2001).

Defamation is verbal or written communication that injures someone's reputation. It usually involves hatred, contempt, or ridicule and may cause someone to be avoided or shunned. It often harms the reputation of another by lowering the estimation toward that person. Oral defamation is slander, and written defamation is libel. Defamation, slander, and libel as well as invasion of privacy are quasiintentional torts.

To be held accountable for the tort of libel, the plaintiff has to show that the defendant published a defamatory statement about him or her. However, the defendant may not have intended to communicate the defamatory statement to anyone or may not have intended the statement to be defamatory. The statement may not be defamatory until put together with facts unknown to the writer. The writer may have thought the information was factual or made a general statement that was taken personally by someone. In *Olson v. Molland* (1930) and *Weidman v. Ketcham* (1938), when the defendant did not intent to publish the statement, the law did not impose liability. However, when the truth of the statement is questioned, there are many rules that vary from state to state. Absolute privilege and qualified privilege may provide a defense to an action for defamation. The first, absolute privilege, attaches to statements made during judicial or legislative proceedings as well as confidential communications between spouses. The second, qualified privilege, attaches to statements that result from a legal or moral duty to speak in the interests of third parties when the statement is made in the absence of malice such as ill will, hatred, or monetary gain. The case *of Judge v. Rockford Memorial Hospital* (1958) demonstrates the defense of privilege. A director of nurses wrote a letter to a nurse's professional registry stating that the hospital did not want to have a specific nurse's services available to them because of losses of narcotics during times that nurse was on duty. The director of nurses' letter was considered a privileged communication because of the director of nurse's legal duty to write the communication in the interests of society.

There are fewer *slander* than libel lawsuits because slander is more difficult to prove, the awards are small, and the legal fees are high. A person bringing a slander suit usually must prove special damages. However, a professional does not need to prove that the words caused damage because it is presumed that slander toward one's professional capacity is damaging. However, if the person making an injurious comment cannot prove the statement is true, the person can be held liable. Consequently, health professionals should avoid making slanderous remarks about other health professionals. However, reporting alleged professional misconduct is not grounds for defamation because of qualified privilege to report complaints to the professional's supervisor (Killion & Dempski, 2000; O'Keefe, 2001; Pozgar, 2004).

While tort law duties and rights among individuals are not based on contracts, contract law enforces agreements.

LIABILITY CONTROL

"The palest ink is better than the best memory." —Anonymous

Policies and procedures for handling incidents and claims should be developed and implemented. Some incidents may relate to medication errors, falls, procedures (particularly invasive procedures), patient or family refusal of treatment, and patient or family dissatisfaction with care. Because of the negative connotation of the word *incident*, some agencies use *event*, *occurrence*, or *situation* instead. Filing an incident report is not admitting guilt. It is reporting something that is not a part of routine care.

It is preferable that incident report forms contain questions that can be answered yes or no or by multiple choice. Narrative should be limited. The observer should give a factual, nonjudgmental account of what was seen, heard, felt, or smelled. No impressions, interpretations, or opinions should be stated. All information needed should be in one place.

Documentation is critically important. When documenting, the nurse should use the appropriate form and black ink, putting the patient's name and identification number on each page. Each entry should be specific, record the date and time, and use only approved abbreviations. The nurse should document nursing actions taken in response to identified patient problems, patient's responses to medications and treatments, and safeguards to protect the patient. The nurse should write on every line without inserting notes between lines or leaving empty spaces. To correct an error, the nurse should draw a line through it and write "error" above it with the date, time, and nurse's initials. Never erase or obliterate an entry. The nurse should always follow the institution's policies and procedures and give care that is appropriate according to the standard of care as defined in the state nurse practice act. There should be no entry in the patient's record about the existence of an incident report, and the incident report should not be left in the chart. Incident reports that are inadvertently disclosed are no longer considered confidential and can consequently be subpoenaed in court (Marquis & Huston, 2006).

The quality of the documentation often determines the outcome of lawsuits. Medical records are legal documents that can be introduced in court. Nurses and other personnel must be well versed in accurate and comprehensive documentation. Nurses should also know how to testify in court and how to serve as expert witnesses (Holburn, Bond, Solon, & Burn, 2000).

LIABILITY ISSUES

Liability issues discussed here are related to three areas (Box 15-5).

Nurse Licensure

The usual organizational pattern for nurse licensing authority in each state is the establishment of a separate board that is organized and operated within the guidelines of specific legislation to license all professional and practical nurses; to determine eligibility through specific knowledge and skills to practice within a defined scope of practice for initial licensure and relicensure; to enforce licensing statutes, including suspension, revocation, and restoration of licenses; and to approve and supervise educational institutions (Pozgar, 2004). Members of the state board of nursing are typically appointed by the governor. Licensure is mandatory for employment. The employer and possibly the state board of nursing should be notified regarding issues of client safety, substance abuse, and health care fraud.

BOX 15-5 Liability Issues

Nurse licensure
Nurse practice acts
Nursing standards

Nurse Practice Acts

Nurse practice acts are the policing power of the state. These laws typically have rules and regulations that are implemented by state boards of nursing. The nurse practice acts define nursing, set standards for licensure, mandate licensure examinations, set standards for curricula of schools of nursing, regulate schools of nursing, regulate advanced practice nurses, and allow state boards of nursing to investigate reports of violations, and discipline violators. Discipline may include probation, revocation of license, and referral to criminal courts (Roussel, Swansburg, & Swansburg, 2006).

The nurse practice act typically defines nursing, delineates the scope of practice, and outlines the activities nurses licensed in that state can legally perform. Each state has a nurse practice act, and while they may differ one from another, all states require licensure in order to practice technical or professional nursing. The mutual recognition model allows jurisdictions to retain the rights to govern practice within the jurisdiction even with mutual recognition agreements with other compact states. The nurse practice acts outline requirements for initial licensure and renewal. Licenses are generally valid for 2 to 3 years. In 1976, California was the first state to institute mandatory continuing education for renewal of the nursing license. Several states now require continuing education, typically with a requirement of 20 to 40 hours of continuing education over 2 to 3 years. Some states require specific continuing education content such as specific health problems, and others allow the nurses wide latitude in meeting the requirements (Cherry & Jacob, 2002).

Nursing Standards

The standard of care is generally defined as the degree of care, expertise, and judgment used by a reasonable and prudent nurse under similar circumstances. It is established by expert testimony in nursing malpractice cases. Experts use a variety of sources. Not all the sources have the same information, and there is no single standard of care. Nurse practice acts, ANA standards, TJC standards, institutional policies and procedures, nursing literature, and physicians' orders may be used to establish standards for court cases. Common causes of nurse liability include failure to assess, failure to plan and implement a plan of care based on the patient's condition, and failure to follow the organization's policies and procedures (O'Keefe, 2001; Tucker, Canobbio, Paquette, et al, 2000).

The State Board of Nursing and often a private organization such as the National League for Nursing or the American Association of Colleges of Nursing evaluate and approve educational programs or services that meet predetermined standards. The State Board of Nursing must accredit all school of nursing programs in the United States. Accreditation of health care organizations and the managed care organizations is also important.

PATIENT CARE ISSUES

Patient's Bill of Rights

Patients retain their basic fundamental rights as identified in the Constitution and courts of law when they are admitted to a health care system. They are often given the Patient's Bill of Rights as they enter the health care system.

Informed Consent

Informed consent is given by patients who fully understand what is being consented to. It involves legal individual capacity to consent, voluntary freedom of choice, and access to understandable information. If the patient is not a competent adult, the following may give consent: a legal guardian; emancipated, married minor; mature minor; parent or legal guardian of a child; minor for diagnosis and treatment of specific disease states or conditions, and court order. Consent may be given orally or in writing. Both are legally effective, but it is advisable to get the consent in writing. The patient or legal consenter must be told the suspected diagnosis, nature of the proposed treatment, expected outcomes, benefits and risks, and alternative treatments possible. A statement that the patient can withdraw consent at any time should be provided, and the patient should be given an opportunity to ask questions (Guido, 2007; Marquis & Huston, 2006; O'Keefe, 2001; Pozgar, 2004; Sullivan & Decker, 2005).

Consent is not legally required when immediate care is necessary to save the life and consent cannot be obtained either from the patient or an authorized legal representative. Constructive consent or consent implied by law is effective. Minors are not legally capable of giving valid consent to medical treatment, but minors who live apart from their parents and are married are considered emancipated and are capable of giving consent. The law presumes every adult is mentally competent until adjudicated otherwise. After people have been declared mentally incompetent in a judicial proceeding, they cannot give valid consents. When patients have been deemed clinically incompetent but not legally incompetent, nurses should seek the participation of the patient's next of kin in making decisions. When family members cannot agree, treatment should be postponed until a legal guardian is appointed with the authority to make the necessary medical decisions.

Right to Refuse Treatment

Competent adults have the right to refuse treatment. That is guaranteed by the Constitution and has been tested in court cases. More recently, most states have passed statutory laws to protect the right to refuse treatment and to protect the health care provider who agrees to not treat even when treatment could be considered indicated. Those laws are related to advanced directives, living wills, and durable power of attorney (Sullivan & Decker, 2005).

Advance directives are documents that allow the competent person to make choices such as being put on life support, stopping treatment, or refusing treatment before the need for medical treatment arises. Advanced directives do not need to be signed by an attorney. However, they are to be signed by two witnesses preferably who are not heirs, relatives, or physicians. They are only effective when the patient is not able to make decisions and can be changed or cancelled at any time. A *living will* is a document signed by a competent adult indicating what health care the person wants in the future. Those decisions are to be upheld even if the adult's decision-making capacity is lost. The *durable power of attorney* permits a competent adult to appoint a proxy to make decisions for that person if that person becomes incompetent. It has broader applications than a living will because it can be applied to any injury or illness that leaves a person incapacitated. Health care providers are to follow the wishes stated in these documents. In the absence of these documents, family members are asked to make those decisions. However, the family members do not have the legal authority to make those decisions unless they are legally appointed as guardians or are the parents. The Patient Self Determination Act of 1990 is a federal law that requires all health care facilities that receive Medicare or Medicaid funds to provide written information to adult patients concerning their right to make health care decisions (Sullivan & Decker, 2005). The ANA supports the patient's right to self-determination and indicates the role of the nurse includes public education, education of the profession, in-service education of other health care providers, research, and patient care regarding advanced directives, living wills, durable power of attorney, health care proxy, and do-not-attempt-to-resuscitate orders. The ANA recommends that questions about advanced directives be part of the nursing admission assessment (see www.nursingworld.org).

Do-not-attempt-resuscitation (DNAR) orders state the patient will not receive cardiopulmonary resuscitation (CPR) or other aggressive treatments if the heart stops beating. The order should be given to family members, the physician, and designated proxy and taken to the health care facility during admission. In some states the physician can write DNAR orders in conjunction with the client's family or significant other even if the client does not have a living will. Nurses need to be familiar with the state and institutional requirements regarding DNAR orders because they can vary from place to place. The order should be placed where it can be easily found during an emergency. Families often call 911 during a medical emergency. However, emergency medical staff may not be required to follow the order in some states (American Bar Association, 2001).

Freedom from Chemical or Physical Restraints

The Omnibus Budget Reconciliation Act (OBRA) of 1987 also provides patients a right to be free from chemical or physical restraints for the purpose of convenience or discipline not required to treat medical symptoms. Restraining patients without consent and sufficient justification can be interpreted as false imprisonment. This law applies to health care organizations that receive Medicare or Medicaid funds. Health care providers are to consider alternatives to restraints. Physicians' orders are to specify duration and circumstances required when using restraints on a patient. No per rate needed (PRN) restraints are allowed. Patients are to be monitored and reassessed frequently to evaluate the continued need for the restraints. Physical restraints have been associated with injuries and deaths. Psychotropic drugs, often used as chemical restraints, are no longer legal for the purpose of controlling behavior. They may only be used for diagnosis-related conditions. Psychotropic drugs have caused patients to become deeply sedated, agitated, and combative (Sullivan & Decker, 2005).

Organ Donation

Congress enacted the National Organ Transplant Act (NOTA) in 1984. Consequently organ procurement organizations (OPOs) were created. They keep a list of possible recipients and train hospital staff about getting family consent. There are legal documents to consent to donate organs, and in many states, adults can

sign their desire to donate organs on the back of their driver's license. In some states, there is still a need for the client's family to give consent for organ donation after the person's death, and family can revoke the deceased person's consent to donate. Because of the shortage of organs for transplantation, a required request law was enacted. At the time of a person's death, a trained requestor must ask family members to consider organ or tissue donation. National Organ Transplant Act of 1984 prohibits the purchase or sale of organs and the Uniform Anatomical Gift Act deals with other issues involved in transplantation of organs. State laws determine if a nurse may serve as a witness to signing an organ donation consent document. Nurses need to be aware of the policies and procedures for organ donation in the institution and in the state. Hospitals usually act as donees of anatomical gifts, coordinate procurement of anatomical gifts, and have agreements with other hospitals and procurement organizations.

There are no costs to the organ donor for donating organs. However, the funeral and burial expenses are still the responsibilities of the donor's family. The United Network for Organ Sharing maintains a national computer list of patients waiting for transplants. Organs are offered to local patients first and then to the regional and national levels. Efforts are made to select patients regardless of their race, gender, religion, or other personal information.

Anatomical gift is the legal term for organ donations (kidneys, hearts, livers, lungs, pancreases) and tissues including corneas, eyes, bones, bone marrow, skin, and heart valves. Bone marrow and kidneys can be donated while the donor is still alive. If the person did not indicate whether organs were to be donated, the family makes the decision after the patient dies.

A child or incompetent person cannot consent to be an organ donor so that people needing organs will not be able to prey on vulnerable people. A person must be at least 18 years old and of sound mind to be an organ donor. Removal of anatomical parts involves a surgical procedure that rarely interferes with funeral or burial arrangements. Even if a person has signed an organ donor card or indicated organ donation in an advanced directive, the next of kin will probably be asked for permission to take parts. If the next of kin refuses, the authorities will probably not remove parts even if the patient has volunteered parts. A desire to donate organs should be discussed with the family and written into advanced directives, as well as put in a will. It is usually too late to donate organs by the time the will is located (American Bar Association, 2001).

Assisted Suicide

The ANA believes that nurses should not participate in assisted suicide or active euthanasia because such acts violate the Code for Nurses, ethical traditions, goals of the profession, and its covenant with society. Nurses have an obligation to provide compassionate and comprehensive end-of-life care that includes promotion of comfort, relief of pain, and sometimes forgoing life-sustaining treatments (see www.nursingworld. org). Hospice organizations do not endorse taking medications in doses that cause the patient's death. However, letting death come naturally does not mean the patient will not be given medication to ease the pain. Pain management is not the same as committing suicide by taking large doses of pain medications (American Bar Association, 2001). Euthanasia is classified as active or passive. Active euthanasia is intentional and thought of as suicide. If someone helps a person take his or her own life, the person assisting could be subject to criminal sanctions for aiding and abetting suicide. Passive euthanasia occurs when life-saving measures are withdrawn or withheld, allowing the person to die a natural death. Those acts are generally accepted pursuant to legislative acts and judicial decisions (Pozgar, 2004).

PERSONNEL ISSUES

"Hatred and anger are powerless when met with kindness."   —Anonymous

Employment-at-Will

Employment-at-will means that an employee is free to accept or not accept a job at will, and the employer is free to hire or discharge an employee at will for any reason. However, case law has provided exceptions to the employment-at-will doctrine for defamation, public policy issues, retaliatory discharge, contractual relationships, and fairness to the extreme that employment-at-will has little applicability today. Public policy exception is the first exception and involves cases in which an employer discharges an employee in direct conflict with public policy, such as for serving on a jury, whistle-blowing by reporting the employer's illegal actions, or filing a workers' compensation claim.

There have been several court cases related to retaliation for the employer for whistle-blowing, such as for speaking out against unsafe practices, reporting a violation of federal laws, or filing lawsuits against employers. In *Roulston v. Tendercare (Michigan) Inc.* (2000), a social services director was fired for confronting the director of nursing about patient abuse. The court supported the social services director's lawsuit against the nursing home for retaliation. In *UTMB v. Hohman* (1999), a nurse felt wrongfully discharged for reporting a physician's alleged abuses. In *Fleming v. Correctional Health-care Solutions, Inc.* (2000), a nurse was discharged for reporting financial mismanagement. Both courts upheld the right for the nurses to sue for retaliation.

In *Taylor v. Memorial Health Systems, Inc.* (2000), the conditions that must be present to file a valid employer retaliation lawsuit were enumerated as "(1) The whistleblower must disclose or threaten to disclose an allegation in writing and under oath to the state department of professional regulation. (2) The allegation must have been about the activity, policy, or practice of the employer that is or was a violation of a state or federal law, rule, or regulation. (3) The employee must have given the employer written notification and reasonable time to correct the problem. (4) The employee must have suffered retaliation in the form of some actual harm

(*Taylor v. Memorial Health Systems, Inc.*, 2000, p. 755)" (Guido, 2007, p.79). These may vary from state to state.

Courts may uphold implied contracts. In *Watkins v. Unemployment Compensation Board of Review* (1997) the court treated employee handbooks, company policies, and oral statements made at the time of employment as setting the employment relationship. In *Trombley v. Southwestern Vermont Medical Center* (1999) the court found the procedure for progressive discipline in the employee handbook must be followed before terminating a nurse for giving incompetent care.

Employee handbooks and departmental policy and procedure manuals are implied contracts if they are without disclaimers. Handbooks that do not contain disclaimers may alter an employer's or employee's at-will status. A disclaimer is the denial of a right that is alleged to belong to someone. In *Simonson v. Meader Distribution Co.* (1987) the court found the employer's disclaimers clear. The disclaimers included the following: Management can make any changes at any time by adding to, deleting, or changing any existing policy. The rules are as complete as we can reasonably make them, but they are not necessarily all-inclusive, because circumstances that we have not anticipated may arise. Some currently unanticipated circumstances may warrant the application of discipline, including discharge. Management may vary from the above policies if, in its opinion, the circumstances require (Pozgar, 2004).

The purpose of the good faith and fair dealing exception is to prevent unfair or malicious termination. In *Fortune v. National Cash Register Company* (1977) an employee was discharged just before a final contract was signed for which the employee was to receive a large commission. The court found that the discharge was in bad faith to prevent payment of the commission.

The nurse manager needs to know related state and federal laws. Managers should review employee handbooks, departmental policy and procedure manuals, and recruitment materials for unwanted statements and to consider adding disclaimer clauses. Managers should take corrective action to whistle-blowers' complaints and monitor the treatment of the employee after the complaint is filed, making sure that employee performance evaluations are performed according to the policies and that appropriate paperwork is in appropriate files (Guido, 2007; Pozgar, 2004).

COBRA

The Consolidated Omnibus Budget Reconciliation Act of 1985 (COBRA) is a federal law that amends the Employee Retirement Income Security Act of 1974 (ERISA), which is a federal law that controls how the employee benefit plan is administered. COBRA is a complex law that allows an employee and dependents to continue the group insurance coverage at about the same cost for a specific period of time after the employment status changed. The employer that employees 20 or more people on a typical business day and sponsors group health plans for the employees must inform the employee within 14 days of the qualifying event that the employee has the right to continue coverage under COBRA. COBRA must be elected for coverage within 60 days of the qualifying event and is retroactive to the qualifying event. Coverage by a spouse's health care plan does not disqualify a person if that person was covered before the qualifying event. If the new health care plan does not cover a preexisting condition, a person may still be able to continue on the former health plan under COBRA. Qualified beneficiaries qualify for COBRA when the employee dies, is fired except for gross misconduct, has hours reduced, becomes divorced or legally separated, becomes eligible for Medicare, or the child is no longer considered a dependent under the health plan. If the person lost a job or had hours reduced, continued coverage lasts for 18 months or until the person gets other insurance. In the event of death, the spouse and dependents may pay for coverage for another 36 months. In the cases of divorce or a child no longer being a dependent, continued coverage lasts for 36 months or until the spouse or child finds other insurance (American Bar Association, 2001).

Diverse Workforce

There are legal considerations to managing a diverse workforce. People are protected from overt and subtle discrimination by Title VII of the Civil Rights Act of 1964. People have a responsibility to be fair and just. Diversity in language, word meanings, accents, and dialects leads to misunderstanding. People from unassertive cultures may be reluctant to ask questions. Cultural differences can lead to conflict and unfulfilled expectations. Managers can learn about cultural diversity and increase their own sensitivity, role model cultural sensitivity, and develop a comprehensive cultural diversity program for staff (Marquis & Huston, 2006).

TESTIFYING

Testifying under oath can be a terrifying experience, but understanding procedures and a few rules can make the experience less stressful. Appearance is important. One should dress neatly and conventionally. A business suit is usually appropriate. If one is testifying just before, after, or during a shift, a uniform is appropriate.

A pleasant demeanor is also important. One should project a polite, sincere, and cooperative image. One should know the facts before testifying. It is appropriate to review the record, particularly the part one is responsible for. The health care agency record should never be falsified. It may be helpful to make a sketch or diagram if placement of persons and objects is important.

The court recorder records everything said, so one should enunciate clearly. Questions must be answered orally because nodding the head and other nonverbal responses are difficult to record and subject to interpretation. One is likely to be asked for personal and professional information, such as residence, age, marital status, educational background, grades received, and employment history. One should be sure the question is understood before answering it. Making an inaccurate response because the question was not understood can adversely affect the outcomes. Pausing before answering the question is appropriate to formulate an answer and to allow time for an attorney to raise objections. If the attorney objects to a question, one should refrain from re-

sponding until the issue is resolved. The lawyer will direct the witness if an answer is required. One should keep answers brief, tell the truth, and answer only the question asked. One should try to give favorable facts and avoid questionable words such as think, guess, and maybe. Sometimes matters of amount, distance, and time are crucial. One should not be forced into guessing. If unable to make a reliable judgment, "I don't know" is an appropriate response. When asked to identify an exhibit such as a medical record, one should scrutinize it carefully and indicate whether it is recognized or not. Whoever calls one as a witness has the first opportunity to ask questions. Afterward, the opposing party's attorney has the opportunity to ask questions (O'Keefe, 2001; Pozgar, 2004).

EXPERT WITNESSES

Because malpractice litigation has increased and physicians are serving as expert witnesses for nursing less than they did before the 1970s, nurses are increasingly acting as expert witnesses. Some state nurses associations are developing resource banks of nurse expert witnesses. Nurses may need to submit a letter of intent describing their qualifications as a nurse expert, resume, and letters of reference. Some state nurses associations provide continuing education regarding legal issues and being an expert witness to ensure a pool of adequately prepared expert witnesses.

Attorneys often want to meet experts before selecting them. They also need resumes and letters of reference. Attorneys often contact experts by telephone and provide brief case summaries. Then the nurse must decide which cases to accept. The case must match the expert's area of expertise. Experts should review only records that are within their specialty. The expert compares the facts of the case with standards of care and offers a professional opinion. The expert should understand clearly whether the attorney wants the expert to defend the nurse or dispute the nurse's credibility. The cases selected should not involve matters concerning places where the expert has worked or people with whom the expert has worked because the issue of bias could be raised. Fees negotiated should include time required to review the records, write report, and provide testimony (Holburn, Bond, Solon, & Burn, 2000; Pozgar, 2004).

CHAPTER SUMMARY

The Institute of Medicine report *To Error Is Human* indicated there is considerable mortality related to medical errors; *Crossing the Quality Chasm* concluded that merely making incremental improvements would not solve the problems, and it presented a comprehensive strategy and action plan for future health care; and *Keeping Patients Safe* recommended adopting evidence-based management and leadership practices, maximization of the capability of the workforce, and design of work and workspace to reduce error. *Keeping Patients Safe* also recommended creating and sustaining a culture of safety through governing boards that focus on safety, leadership, and evidence-based management structures and processes, effective nursing transformational leadership, adequate staffing, organizational support for ongoing learning and decision support, mechanisms that promote interdisciplinary collaboration, work design that promotes safety, and an organizational culture that continuously strengthens patient safety. Related to that, continuous quality improvement, evidence-based practice, program evaluation, and the differences between research and evaluation are related issues.

Nurses need to know regulations, legal issues, and risk management because nurses are legally responsible and accountable for assessing, diagnosing, planning, implementing, and evaluating nursing care. Nurses need to understand the regulations and legal issues, adhere to legal guidelines, policies, and procedures, and participate in risk management to reduce the organization's legal risk. The doctrine of respondeat superior establishes that the employer is responsible for the employee's actions, while the state boards of nursing develop nurse practice acts to regulate the practice of nursing.

CRITICAL THINKING ACTIVITY

Reflective Journal: Make observations in a clinical setting, or reflect on past experiences. Describe the continuous quality improvement program in a health care facility. What tools and processes are used for continuous quality improvement? What procedures are used to monitor for risk management? Who is responsible for the program? Have there been lawsuits against the agency?

CASE STUDY

You are the evening charge nurse caring for 20 critically ill patients with the help of one licensed practical nurse (LPN) and two aides. There are many medications and treatments to give. You do not think it is possible for you and the LPN to do all the medications and treatments and do not believe the aides are qualified to do most of the work that needs to be done. What are you going to do?

ONLINE RESOURCES

evolve Additional critical thinking activities, worksheets, and case studies are available online at http://evolve.elsevier.com/Marriner/guide8e.

REFERENCES

Allen DE, Bockenhauer B, Egan C, et al: Relating outcomes to excellent nursing practice, *JONA* 36(3):140-147, 2006.

American Bar Association: *Complete and easy guide to health care law*, New York, 2001, Three Rivers Press.

American Nurses Association: *Nursing care report card for acute care*, Washington, DC, 1995, The Association.

American Nurses Association: *Nursing quality indicators: Definitions and implications*, Washington, DC, 1996a, The Association.

American Nurses Association: *Nursing quality indicators: Guide for implementation*, Washington, DC, 1996b, The Association.

American Nurses Association: *Standards of clinical nursing practice*, ed 2, Washington, DC, 1998, The Association.

American Nurses Association: *Work release during a disaster—guidelines for employers*, Washington DC, 2002, The Association.

Autrey P, Moss J: High-reliability teams and situation awareness: Implementing a hospital emergency incident command system, *JONA* 36(2):67-72, 2006.

Bauer-Wu S, Epshtein A, Ponte R: Promoting excellence in nursing research and scholarship in the clinical setting, *JONA* 36(5):224-227, 2006.

Berwick DM: Sounding board: Continuous quality improvement as the deal in health care, *N Eng. J Med* 320(1):53-56, 1989.

Bradley D, Moore H: Preventing workplace violence from negligent hiring healthcare, *JONA* 34(3):157-161, 2004.

Burke TA, McKee JR, Wilson HC, et al: A comparison of time-and-motion and self-reporting methods of work measurement, *JONA* 30(3):118-125, 2000.

Burns N, Grove SK: *The practice of nursing research: Conduct, critique, & utilization*, ed 5, Philadelphia, 2005, WB Saunders.

Campbell DT, Stanley JC: *Experimental and quasi-experimental designs for research*, Chicago, 2005, Houghton Mifflin Company.

Carpenter D & Hoppszallern S: Still booming, *Hospitals & Health Networks* March, pp. 44–48, 2007.

Centers for Medicare and Medicaid Services: *Overview of OASIS*, 2007 (website): www.cms.hhs.gov/oasis. Accessed August 27, 2007.

Cherry B, Jacob SR: *Contemporary nursing: Issues, trends, & management*, St. Louis, 2002, Mosby.

Cofer JI, Greeley HP: *Continuous quality improvement for health information management*, Marblehead, MA, 1998, Opus Communications.

Cooper RW: Legal and ethical issues. In Huber DL, editor: *Leadership and nursing care management*, ed 3, Philadelphia, 2006, Saunders/Elsevier.

Craig JV, Smyth RL: *The evidence-based practice manual for nurses*, St. Louis, 2002, Churchill Livingstone.

Crosby PB: *Let's talk quality*, New York, 1989, McGraw-Hill.

Crosby PB: *Completeness: Quality for the 21st century*, New York, 1992a, Dutton.

Crosby PB: *Quality is free: The art of making quality certain*, New York, 1992b, Mentor Books.

Crosby PB: *Quality without tears: The art of hassle-free management*, New York, 1995, McGraw-Hill.

Darling v. Charleston Community Memorial Hospital, 33 Ill.2d 326, 211 N.E.2d 253, 14 A.L.R.3d 860 (IL, 1965).

Deming WE: *Quality, productivity, and competitive position*, Cambridge, MA, 1982, Massachusetts Institute of Technology Press.

Donabedian A: Criteria and standards for quality assessment and monitoring, *Qual Rev Bull* 3:99-108, 1986.

Engelke MK, Marshburn DM: Collaborative strategies to enhance research and evidence-based practice, *JONA* 36(3):131-135, 2006.

Ervin N: Does patient satisfaction contribute to nursing care quality?, *JONA* 36(3):126-130, 2006.

Fleming v. Correctional Healthcare Solutions, Inc, 751 A2d 1035 (NJ, 2000).

Folse VN: Managing quality and risk. In Yoder-Wise PS, editor: *Leading and managing in nursing*, ed 4, St. Louis, 2007, Elsevier.

Force MVO, Deering L, Hubble J, et al: Effective strategies to increase reporting of medication errors in hospitals, *JONA* 36(1):24-41, 2006.

Fortune v. National Cash Register Company, 272 Mass 96, 264 NE2d 1251 (1977).

Gates D, Fitzwater E, Succop P: Reducing assaults against nursing home caregivers, *Nursing Research* 54(2):119-127, March/April 2005.

Grohar-Murray ME, DiCroce HR: *Leadership and management in nursing*, Stamford, CT, 2003, Appleton & Lange.

Gross v. Allen, 22 Cal App 4th 354 (1994).

Guido GW: Legal and ethical issues. In Yoder-Wise P, editor: *Leading and managing in nursing*, St. Louis, 2007, Mosby.

Harris MJ: Medicare quality initiative, *Policy, Politics & Nursing Practice* 4(4):263-265, 2003.

Heinen M, Coyle G, Hamilton A: Dare to shift cultural behaviors, *Nsg Man* 35(9):14, 2004.

Holburn CJ, Bond C, Solon M, Burn S: *Health care professionals as witnesses in the court*, Cambridge, UK, 2000, Greenwich Medical Media.

Huber DL: Measuring and managing outcomes. In Huber DL, editor: *Leadership and nursing care management*, ed 3, Philadelphia, 2006, Elsevier.

Institute of Medicine: *Quality first: Better health care for all Americans*, Washington, DC, 1998, National Academy Press.

Institute of Medicine: *To error is human: Building a safer health system*, Washington, DC, 1999, National Academy Press.

Institute of Medicine: *Crossing the quality chasm: A new health system for the 21st century*, Washington, DC, 2001a, National Academy Press.

Institute of Medicine: *Envisioning the national health care quality report*, Washington, DC, 2001b, National Academy Press.

Institute of Medicine: *Leadership by example: Coordinating government roles in improving health care quality*, Washington, DC, 2002, National Academy Press.

Institute of Medicine: *Health professions education: A bridge to quality*, Washington, DC, 2003a, National Academy Press.

Institute of Medicine: *Patient safety: Achieving a new standard for care*, Washington, DC, 2003b, National Academy Press.

Institute of Medicine: *Priority areas for national action: Transforming health care quality*, Washington, DC, 2003c, National Academy Press.

Institute of Medicine: *Who will keep the public healthy? Educating public health professionals for the 21st century*, Washington, DC, 2003d, National Academy Press.

Institute of Medicine: *Keeping patients safe: Transforming the work environment of nurses*, Washington, DC, 2004, National Academy Press.

Joanna Briggs Institute: Strategies to reduce medication errors with reference to older adults, *Australian Nursing Journal* 14(4):26-29, 2006.

Joint Commission on Accreditation of Healthcare Organizations: *Sentinel event alert*, Issue 6—Lessons learned: Wrong site surgery, 1998a.

Joint Commission on Accreditation of Healthcare Organizations: *Sentinel event alert*, Issue 7—Inpatient suicides: Recommendations for prevention, 1998b.

Joint Commission on Accreditation of Healthcare Organizations: *BOJ's guide to 1999 standards and scoring,* Oakbrook Terrace, 1999, JCAHO.

Joint Commission on Accreditation of Healthcare Organizations: *Sentinel event alert*, Issue 12—Operative and post-operative complications: lessons learned for the future, 2000a.

Joint Commission on Accreditation of Healthcare Organizations: *Sentinel event alert*, Issue 14—Fatal falls: Lessons for the future, 2000b.

Joint Commission on Accreditation of Healthcare Organizations: *Sentinel event alert*, Issue 26—Delays in treatment, 2002.

Judge v. Rockford Memorial Hospital, 150 NE 2d 202 (Ill App Ct, 1958).

Juran JM: Product quality: A prescription for the West. I. Training and improvement programs, *Man Rev* 70: 8-14, 1981.

Juran JM: *Juran on planning for quality*, New York, 1988, Free Press.

Juran JM: *Juran on leadership for quality: An executive handbook*, New York, 1989, Free Press.

Juran JM: *Juran on quality by design: The new steps for planning quality into goods and services*, New York, 1992, Free Press.

Juran JM, Goyna FM, Jr Bingham RS, Jr editors: *Quality control handbook*, New York, 1988, McGraw-Hill.

Karkos B, Peters K: A magnet community hospital: Fewer barriers to nursing research, *JONA* 36 (7–8):277-283, 2006.

Kavianian JR, Wentz CA: *Occupational and environmental safety engineering and management*, New York, 1997, John Wiley & Sons.

Kelly LP, Bassendowski SL: Evidence-based nursing in clinical practice: Implications for nurse educators, *J of Continuing Education in Nursing* 37(6):240-255, 2006.

Killion SW, Dempski KM: *Legal and ethical issues*, Thorofare, NJ, 2000, Slack.

Koch MW, Fairly TM: *Integrated quality management: The key to improving nursing care quality*, St Louis, 1993, Mosby.

Kruger N, Hurley A, Gustafson M: Framing patient safety initiatives: Working model and case example, *JONA*: 200-204, 2006.

Lorah M: personal correspondence, February 2007.

Marquis BL, Huston CJ: *Leadership roles and management functions in nursing: Theory and application*, ed 5, Philadelphia, 2006, Lippincott.

McDavid JC, Hawthorn LRL: *Program evaluation and performance measurement: An introduction to practice*, London, 2006, Sage Publications.

McLaughlin CP, Kaluzny AD: *Continuous quality improvement in health care*, Sudbury, MA, 2004, Jones & Bartlett Publishers.

Milstead JA, Furlong E: *Handbook of nursing leadership: Creative skills for a culture of safety*, Boston, 2006, Jones and Bartlett Publishers.

Monson M: Disclosing adverse events: You said it, now write it, *Nsg Man* 37(8):16-17, 2006.

Moody R: Creating and sustaining safety cultures in acute care health contexts: Evaluation of relationships among nurse-sensitive variables that may make a difference, *JONA* 36(5):228, 2006.

National League for Nursing: *National League for Nursing 1998 annual report*, New York, 1998, The League.

Newhouse RP: Selecting measures for safety and quality improvement initiatives, *JONA* 36(3):109-113, 2006.

Ogle K: Preventing wrong-site surgery: How the American Academy of Surgeons wants to eliminate this surgical nightmare, *Today's Surgical Nurse,* September/October:28-31, 1998.

O'Keefe ME: *Nursing practice and the law: Avoiding malpractice and other legal risks*, Philadelphia, 2001, FA Davis.

Olson v. Molland, 232 NW 625 (Minn, 1930).

Pape TM: Searching for the final answer: Factors contributing to medication administration errors, *J Contin Educ Nurs* 32(4):152-160, 2001.

Pelletier LR, Albright LA: Quality improvement and health care safety. In Huber DL, editor: *Leadership and nursing care management*, ed 3, Philadelphia, 2006, Saunders/Elsevier.

Polit DF, Beck CT, Hunger BP: *Essentials of nursing research: Methods, appraisals, and utilization*, Philadelphia, 2005, Lippincott.

Pozgar GD: *Legal aspects of health care administration*, ed 9, Sudbury, MD, 2004, Jones & Bartlett Publishers.

Rabert A, Sebastian M: The future is now: Implementation of a tele-intensivist program, *JONA* 36(1):49-54, 2006.

Rossi PH, Lipsey M, Freeman H: *Evaluation: A systematic approach*, London, 2004, Sage Publications.

Roulston v. Tendercare (Michigan), Inc, 608 NW 2d 525 (Mich App), 2000.

Roussel L, Swansburg RC, Swansburg RJ: *Management and leadership for nurse administrators*, ed 4, Sudbury, MA, 2006, Jones and Bartlett Publishers.

Saba VK, McCormick KA: *Essentials of computers for nurses: Information for the new millennium*, ed 4, New York, 2005, McGraw-Hill/Medical.

Simonson v. Meader Distribution Co., 413 N.W.2d 146, 148. (Minn.Ct.App.1987).

Spielberger CD: *State-Trait Anger Expression Inventory-2 (STAXI-2)*, Odessa, FL, 1999, Psychological Assessment Resource Inc.

Sullivan EJ, Decker PJ: *Effective leadership and management in nursing*, ed 6, Upper Saddle River, NJ, 2005, Prentice Hall.

Swansburg RC, Swansburg RJ: *Introductory management and leadership for nurses: An interactive text*, ed 3, Boston, 2002, Jones and Bartlett.

Tarasoff v. Regents of the University of California, 17 Cal 3d 425, 444 (1976).

Taylor v. Memorial Health Systems, Inc, 770 So2d 752 (Fla App, 2000).

Tourangeau A: Determinants of 30-day mortality for hospitalized medical and surgical patients, *JONA* 36(5):228-229, 2006.

Trombley v. Southwestern Vermont Medical Center, 738 A2d 103 (VT, 1999).

Tucker SM, Canobbio MM, Paquette EV, et al : *Patient care standards: Collaborative planning & nursing interventions*, St. Louis, 2000, Mosby.

UTMB v. Hohman, 6 SW 3d 767 (Tex App, 1999).

Walton M: *Deming management at work,* New York, 1990, Putnam's Sons.

Watkins v. Unemployment Compensation Board of Review, 689 A2d 1019 (Pa Commonwealth, 1997).

Weidman v. Ketcham, 15, NW 2d 426 (NY, 1938).

Weir C, Hoffman J, Nebeker J, Hurdle J: Nurse's role in tracking adverse drug events: The impact of provider order entry, *Nur Adm Q* 29(1):39-44, 2005.

Wertenberger S, Wilson J: The development of a patient safety program across the continuum of care, *Nur Adm Q* 29(4):303-307, 2005.

White House Domestic Policy Council: *Health security: The president's report to the American people*, Washington, DC, 1993, The Council.

Yount L: *Patients' rights in the age of managed care,* New York, 2001, Facts On File.

Zuzelo P, McGoldrick TB, Seminara P, Karbach H: Shared governance and EBP: A logical partnership? *Nsg Man* 37(6):45-50, 2006.

Index

Page numbers followed by *f, t* and *b* indicate figures, tables, and boxes respectively